Practical Standard Prescriber

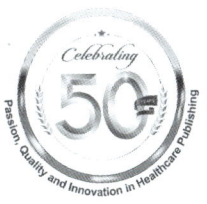

Practical Standard Prescriber

Author

ABM Abdullah MRCP (UK) FRCP (Edin)
UGC Professor
Ex-Dean
Faculty of Medicine
Ex-Chairman and Professor
Department of Medicine
Bangabandhu Sheikh Mujib Medical University
Dhaka, Bangladesh

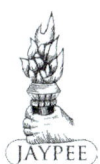

JAYPEE BROTHERS MEDICAL PUBLISHERS
The Health Sciences Publisher
New Delhi | London

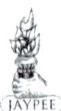 **Jaypee Brothers Medical Publishers (P) Ltd**

Headquarters

Jaypee Brothers Medical Publishers (P) Ltd
4838/24, Ansari Road, Daryaganj
New Delhi 110 002, India
Phone: +91-11-43574357
Fax: +91-11-43574314
Email: jaypee@jaypeebrothers.com

Overseas Offices

J.P. Medical Ltd
83 Victoria Street, London
SW1H 0HW (UK)
Phone: +44 20 3170 8910
Fax: +44 (0)20 3008 6180
Email: info@jpmedpub.com

Website: www.jaypeebrothers.com
Website: www.jaypeedigital.com

© 2020, Jaypee Brothers Medical Publishers

The views and opinions expressed in this book are solely those of the original contributor(s)/author(s) and do not necessarily represent those of editor(s) of the book.

All rights reserved. No part of this publication may be reproduced, stored or transmitted in any form or by any means, electronic, mechanical, photocopying, recording or otherwise, without the prior permission in writing of the publishers.

All brand names and product names used in this book are trade names, service marks, trademarks or registered trademarks of their respective owners. The publisher is not associated with any product or vendor mentioned in this book.

Medical knowledge and practice change constantly. This book is designed to provide accurate, authoritative information about the subject matter in question. However, readers are advised to check the most current information available on procedures included and check information from the manufacturer of each product to be administered, to verify the recommended dose, formula, method and duration of administration, adverse effects and contraindications. It is the responsibility of the practitioner to take all appropriate safety precautions. Neither the publisher nor the author(s)/editor(s) assume any liability for any injury and/or damage to persons or property arising from or related to use of material in this book.

This book is sold on the understanding that the publisher is not engaged in providing professional medical services. If such advice or services are required, the services of a competent medical professional should be sought.

Every effort has been made where necessary to contact holders of copyright to obtain permission to reproduce copyright material. If any have been inadvertently overlooked, the publisher will be pleased to make the necessary arrangements at the first opportunity. The **CD/DVD-ROM** (if any) provided in the sealed envelope with this book is complimentary and free of cost. **Not meant for sale.**

Inquiries for bulk sales may be solicited at: jaypee@jaypeebrothers.com

Practical Standard Prescriber / ABM Abdullah

First Edition: **2020**

ISBN: 978-93-89188-45-5

Printed in India

Dedicated to

*My wife **Mrs Mahmuda Begum***
*My son **Dr Sadi Abdullah***
*My daughter **Dr Sadia Sabah***

Preface

By the good grace of Almighty, I have succeeded to bring out the first edition of *"Practical Standard Prescriber"*.

A sound knowledge of medical science, optimum clinical skills, good interpersonal communication and adequate time management are all needed to be a good doctor.

The art of diagnosing any disease is by history taking, physical examination and good communication with the patient must be practiced. On the other hand, management or giving treatment is the ultimate goal for a doctor. Hence, writing a good prescription or giving organized management is the reflection of a physician's knowledge and skills.

From my experience as a teacher and an examiner in medicine, I feel that it is important to acquire knowledge from the textbooks. However, most of the textbooks are voluminous which are difficult to consume for a new junior doctor or even for a general practitioner. With this in mind, I have written this book in a concise and simplified way so that it can be palatable and practiced practically in day-to-day life.

For a general practitioner, apart from common diseases of internal medicine, I have added some additional chapters of Eye, ENT, Gynecology and Obstetrics in a very brief manner. These chapters have been reviewed by the respective experts in these subjects. I hope this book will provide an algorithmic approach to diagnose and will be helpful to give proper management.

I would like to invite constructive criticism from valued readers of this book, so that any error or omission may be corrected in future edition.

ABM Abdullah MRCP (UK) FRCP (Edin)
UGC Professor
Ex-Dean, Faculty of Medicine
Ex-Chairman and Professor, Department of Medicine
Bangabandhu Sheikh Mujib Medical University
Dhaka, Bangladesh

Acknowledgments

I would like to take the opportunity to extend my sincere gratitude to Professor Kanak Kanti Barua, Vice Chancellor, Bangabandhu Sheikh Mujib Medical University, for his encouragement and valuable suggestions in preparing this book.

I am also highly grateful to Dr Mustasin Haider Sami and Dr Abhishek Bhadra for computer composing of the entire book. They have also gone through the whole manuscript and made necessary corrections and modifications. I can, without any hesitation, mention that they have worked as the co-authors.

I must acknowledge the contributions of my colleagues, doctors and students who were kind enough to help me in writing such a book of its kind. They are always a source of my inspiration and encouragement.

- Professor Sunil Kumar Biswas MCPS (Medicine) MD (Internal Medicine)
- Professor Tahmida Hassan DDV MD
- Dr Tazin Afrose Shah FCPS
- Dr Ahmed-Al-Muntasir-Niloy MD internist (USA)
- Dr Omar Serajul Hasan MD internist (USA)
- Dr Tanjim Sultana MD internist (USA)
- Dr Sadi Abdullah MBBS DTCD MRCP (UK)
- Dr Sadia Sabah MBBS MD (Resident)
- Dr Imtiaz Ahmed MBBS MRCP (UK)
- Dr Md. Shakhawat Hossain Rokan
- Dr Manjurul Alam MRCP (UK)
- Dr Mohammad Abul Kalam Azad FCPS MD (Rheumatology)
- Dr Md. Razibul Alam MBBS MD (Gastroenterology)
- Dr Samprity Islam MBBS MD (Pulmonology)
- Dr Parvin Akhter MBBS MD
- Dr Nazma Azim Daizy MBBS
- Dr Sadia Shamsad MBBS
- Dr Nuzhat Nadia MBBS
- Dr Nazia Hasin MBBS
- Dr Israt Rubaiya MBBS
- Dr Sumayia Sultana MBBS
- Dr Nazmun Nahar MBBS
- Dr Dolon Sarkar MBBS

My special thanks to Shri Jitender P Vij (Group Chairman), Dr Ekta (Senior Development Editor), Mr Sabysachi Hazra (Commissioning Editor), Mr Sanjay Chakraborty (Branch Manager, Kolkata) and all the staff of Jaypee Brothers Medical Publishers (P) Ltd. for their untiring endeavor and hard work, which made it possible for "painless delivery" of this book. They have also notably enhanced the physical quality of the book making it beautiful and attractive.

I must be grateful to my students who are always my source of inspiration.

Last, but not the least, I would like to express my gratitude to my wife, whose untiring support and sacrifice has made it possible to bring out such a nice book. I am also grateful to my daughter Dr Sadia Sabah and my son Dr Sadi Abdullah for their encouragement and inspiration in preparing such a book.

Chapter Reviewer

Following individual chapters are thoroughly reviewed and checked by the eminent specialists:

Chapter 20: Diseases of the Eye

Mehjabin Haque MS Fellowship in Glaucoma
Assistant Professor
Department of Ophthalmology
Bangabandhu Sheikh Mujib Medical University
Dhaka, Bangladesh

Chapter 21: Diseases of the Ear, Nose and Throat

Pran Gopal Dutta MCPS ACORL (Odessa) PhD (Kiev)
MSc in Audiology (UK) FCPS FRCS (Glasgow)
Professor
Department of Ear, Nose and Throat
Ex-Vice Chancellor
Bangabandhu Sheikh Mujib Medical University
Dhaka, Bangladesh

Chapter 22: Gynecology and Chapter 23: Obstetrics

Joya Sree Roy MCPS MS
Professor
Department of Gynecology and Obstetrics
Green Life Medical College
Ex-Professor
Department of Gynecology and Obstetrics
Dhaka Medical College
Dhaka, Bangladesh

Contents

1. Cardiovascular System — 1
2. Respiratory Diseases — 39
3. Gastrointestinal Diseases — 64
4. Hematology — 90
5. Hepatology — 117
6. Endocrinology — 135
7. Infectious Disease and Tropical Medicine — 164
8. Nephrology — 196
9. Rheumatology — 221
10. Dermatology — 236
11. Sexually Transmitted Diseases — 252
12. Neurology — 257
13. Poisoning — 298
14. Psychiatric Diseases — 306
15. Vitamins — 318
16. Electrolyte and Acid-base Imbalance — 325
17. Pediatrics — 330
18. Genetics — 341
19. Miscellaneous — 345
20. Diseases of the Eye — 375
21. Diseases of the Ear, Nose and Throat — 386
22. Gynecology — 401
23. Obstetrics — 417

Bibliography — 429
Index — 431

CHAPTER 1

Cardiovascular System

MITRAL STENOSIS

Cause: Chronic rheumatic heart disease is the most common cause. It is rarely congenital.

Symptoms: Breathlessness, usually on exertion, palpitation and cough, may be hemoptysis, and weakness.

Signs: Pulse—low volume and jugular venous pressure (JVP)—normal (but raised in pulmonary hypertension).

In precordium:
- *Inspection*: Visible cardiac impulse in mitral area
- *Palpation*: Tapping apex beat. Diastolic apical thrill
- *Auscultation*:
  - First heart sound—loud in all areas, more in mitral area. Second heart sound—normal in all the areas
  - Mid-diastolic murmur (MDM) in mitral area, which is low-pitched, localized, rough, rumbling (LLRR), and best heard with the bell of stethoscope, in left lateral position with breathing hold after expiration, with presystolic accentuation
  - Opening snap, just medial to the mitral area.

Investigations:
- *X-ray of chest posteroanterior(P/A) view*: It shows straightening of left border of heart and double border on right side
- Electrocardiogram (ECG) and color Doppler echocardiogram. Cardiac catheter in some cases.

Complications:
- Atrial fibrillation (AF)
- Pulmonary edema, pulmonary hypertension causing congestive cardiac failure (CCF), embolism and infarction
- Left atrial thrombus with systemic embolism
- Ortner's syndrome (enlarged left atrium gives pressure on left recurrent laryngeal nerve, causing hoarseness of voice). Dysphagia due to enlarged left atrium.

Treatment:
- *Medical*: Restriction of activity
  - Low-dose diuretic (thiazide or frusemide)
  - Anticoagulant (e.g. warfarin) to reduce the risk of embolism
  - If AF—digoxin, beta-blocker and rate-limiting calcium antagonist (e.g. verapamil and diltiazem)
  - If CCF—diuretics and digoxin.
- *Surgical*: Valvuloplasty, valvotomy and valve replacement.

MYXOMA OF HEART

It is the common primary tumor of heart, usually benign, attached by a pedicle to atrial septum. It occurs in 3rd–6th decade and is seen more in females.

Sites of origin: Left atrium (75%).

Clinical features: Three groups of manifestations—
1. Obstructive features like mitral stenosis (MS), signs vary with posture. It may be syncope or vertigo
2. Embolic features either systemic or pulmonary embolism
3. *Constitutional features*: Fever, malaise, weakness, loss of weight, myalgia, arthralgia, clubbing, skin rash and Raynaud's phenomenon.

Investigations:
- Complete blood count (CBC) [Leukocytosis, polycythemia and high erythrocyte sedimentation rate (ESR)]
- Chest X-ray (may be similar to MS)
- 2D or transesophageal echocardiogram
- Computed tomography (CT) scan or magnetic resonance imaging (MRI) may be done.

Treatment: Surgical excision. Recurrence may occur.

MITRAL REGURGITATION

Causes:
- Chronic rheumatic heart disease
- Mitral valve prolapse (MVP)
- Papillary muscle dysfunction
- Infective endocarditis
- Trauma or mitral valvotomy
- Connective tissue diseases [rheumatoid arthritis (RA), systemic lupus erythematosus (SLE), Marfan syndrome and Ehlers–Danlos syndrome]
- *Others*: Ankylosing spondylitis, cardiomyopathy, and secondary to LV dilatation.

Symptoms: Breathlessness on exertion, palpitation, cough and weakness.

Signs: In precordium—
- *Inspection*: Visible cardiac impulse in mitral area
- *Palpation*: Apex beat is shifted, diffused and thrusting in character. Systolic thrill in mitral area
- *Auscultation*: First heart sound—soft in mitral area and normal in other areas; second heart sound—normal in all the areas, and pansystolic murmur in mitral area and radiates to left axilla.

Investigations: X-ray of chest P/A view, ECG and color Doppler echocardiogram. Cardiac catheterization is done in some cases.

Complications: Acute left ventricular failure (LVF), infective endocarditis, embolism, arrhythmia (AF and ectopics) and CCF.

Treatment:
- *In mild to moderate case*:
   o Diuretic (frusemide or thiazide). Vasodilator—angiotensin-converting enzyme (ACE) inhibitor (captopril, ramipril and lisinopril)
   o If fast AF—digoxin. Anticoagulant—if AF or history of pulmonary embolism
   o Prophylactic penicillin to prevent endocarditis. Follow up every 6 months by echocardiogram.
- In severe MR—replacement of valve.

MITRAL VALVE PROLAPSE

It is also called as Barlow's syndrome or floppy mitral valve. It can cause MR, may be congenital or due to degenerative myxomatous change. It is common in thin and young women, and may be familial.

Symptoms: Atypical chest pain in left submammary region, stabbing in quality, and confused with anginal pain. May be palpitation, dyspnea and fatigue.

Signs: Mid-systolic click is followed by late systolic murmur (cardinal sign). Later, signs of MR appear.

Investigation: Echocardiogram.

Treatment: If asymptomatic—reassurance and periodic echocardiography. If chest pain and palpitation–beta-blockers (propranolol, atenolol and metoprolol). Prophylactic penicillin is given to prevent infective endocarditis. If MR develops, treatment as in MR.

TRICUSPID REGURGITATION

Causes:
- *Functional*: Secondary to pulmonary hypertension, cor pulmonale and right heart failure (common cause)
- Chronic rheumatic heart disease
- Infective endocarditis (commonly involved in drug addicts)
- *Others*: Congenital heart disease (e.g. Ebstein's anomaly), carcinoid syndrome, right ventricular papillary muscle infarction, and trauma or steering wheel injury in chest.

Symptoms: May be asymptomatic. Symptoms of primary disease.

Signs: Pulse—normal, JVP—raised and giant "v" wave, oscillating up to ear lobule.

Precordium:
- *Palpation*: Left parasternal lift and epigastric pulsation [due to RVH (right ventricular hypertrophy)]
- *Auscultation*:
   o First heart sound—soft in tricuspid area and normal in other areas. Second heart sound—normal in all areas

- Pansystolic murmur in left lower parasternal area with no radiation and loud with inspiration.
- *Others*: Liver may be enlarged, tender and pulsatile.

Investigations: Chest X-ray, ECG and color Doppler echocardiogram.

Complications: Right-sided heart failure and infective endocarditis.

Treatment: Treatment of primary cause. In severe organic tricuspid regurgitation (TR), valve replacement is done.

EBSTEIN'S ANOMALY

It is a congenital heart disease associated with downward displacement of tricuspid valve into the right ventricle. Hence, right atrium is large and right ventricle is small. Characteristically, multiple clicks occur due to asynchronous closure of tricuspid valve. Atrial septal defect (ASD) is commonly associated with this anomaly.

PULMONARY STENOSIS

Causes: Congenital (common). It is associated with carcinoid syndrome, Noonan syndrome and Fallot's tetralogy. May occur, if rubella in pregnancy. Three types—(1) valvular, (2) subvalvular, and (3) supravalvular.

Symptoms: May be asymptomatic. May be fatigue, weakness and effort syncope.

Signs: In precordium—
- *Palpation*: Left parasternal lift and epigastric pulsation (due to RVH). Systolic thrill in pulmonary area
- *Auscultation*:
  - First heart sound—normal in all areas
  - Second heart sound—P2 is soft in pulmonary area, and A2 is normal (wide splitting of second sound may be present).
- Ejection systolic murmur in pulmonary area radiates to neck
  - Fourth heart sound may be present (due to right atrial contraction).

Investigations: ECG, chest X-ray and color Doppler echocardiogram.

Complications: Right heart failure and pulmonary embolism.

Treatment: In mild case, compatible with normal life. In severe symptomatic case, balloon valvuloplasty is done. Infective endocarditis is unusual in pulmonary stenosis (PS) and prophylactic antibiotic is unnecessary.

PULMONARY REGURGITATION

Causes:
- Dilatation of pulmonary valve secondary to pulmonary hypertension
- Secondary to MS
- Rarely rheumatic fever (RF) and carcinoid syndrome.

Symptoms: May be asymptomatic or symptoms of primary disease. Features of right heart failure.

Signs: Left parasternal lift and P2 may be soft. Early diastolic murmur in 3rd or 4th left intercostal space.

Investigations: Chest X-ray, ECG and echocardiogram.

Treatment: Treatment of underlying cause. In severe regurgitation, valve replacement is done.

AORTIC STENOSIS

Causes:
- Chronic rheumatic heart disease
- Congenital bicuspid aortic valve (common in male)
- *Others*: Calcification in old age and congenital (in early age).

Symptoms:
- Breathlessness, mainly on exertion, palpitation and anginal chest pain
- Syncope (transient loss of consciousness) during effort
- Sudden death [probably due to ventricular fibrillation (VF)].

Signs: Pulse—low volume, slow rising, blood pressure (BP)—low systolic, normal diastolic and narrow pulse pressure.

In precordium:
- *Inspection*: Visible cardiac impulse in mitral area
- *Palpation*: Palpable apex beat and heaving. Systolic thrill in aortic area
- *Auscultation*:
  - First heart sound—normal in all areas
  - Second heart sound—A2 is soft in all the areas, and P2 is normal. May be reversed splitting of second heart sound
  - Ejection systolic murmur in aortic area radiates to the neck.

Investigations: X-ray of chest, ECG and color Doppler echocardiogram. Cardiac catheterization is done in some cases.

Complications: Left ventricular failure, infective endocarditis (in 10%), sudden death due to VF, complete heart block (CHB) (in calcification of aortic valve), and systemic embolism.

Treatment: If aortic stenosis (AS) is asymptomatic, follow-up is done with periodic echocardiogram. Avoid strenuous activity or exercise.
- If symptomatic or syncopal attack or asymptomatic with severe AS—valve replacement
- If patient is unfit for surgery—percutaneous valvuloplasty
- In children, elderly or pregnancy—valvotomy.

AORTIC REGURGITATION

Causes:
- Chronic rheumatic heart disease
- Infective endocarditis
- Syphilitic aortitis
- Bicuspid aortic valve
- *Others*: Dissecting aneurysm of ascending aorta, Marfan's syndrome, seronegative arthritis (ankylosing spondylitis), RA, cystic medial necrosis and congenital.

Symptoms: It may be asymptomatic. Some of the other symptoms may be palpitation, breathlessness on exertion, cough and anginal pain.

Signs: Pulse—high volume, collapsing and dancing carotid pulse in neck (Corrigan's sign). BP—high systolic, low diastolic and wide pulse pressure.

Precordium:
- *Inspection*: Visible cardiac impulse
- *Palpation*: Apex beat is shifted, thrusting. Diastolic thrill may be present in left parasternal area
- *Auscultation*:
  - First heart sound—normal in all the areas. Second heart sound—A2 is absent, and P2 is normal
  - Early diastolic murmur in left lower parasternal area with patient bending forward and breathing hold after expiration. Ejection systolic murmur may be present in aortic area due to increased flow.

Formula of 3 to diagnose aortic regurgitation (AR):
- *3 pulse*: Collapsing (water hammer), dancing carotid and capillary pulsation
- *3 BP*: Rise of systolic, fall of diastolic and wide pulse pressure
- *3 murmur*: Early diastolic murmur, Austin Flint murmur and ejection systolic murmur.

Investigations: X-ray of chest, ECG and color Doppler echocardiogram. Cardiac catheterization is done in some cases.

Complications: Acute LVF, infective endocarditis and arrhythmia.

Treatment: In mild asymptomatic case, follow-up.
- In asymptomatic, moderate-to-severe AR with normal left ventricular (LV) function, conservative treatment. Systolic BP should be controlled with vasodilator drugs (nifedipine or ACE inhibitors)
- In severe case—valve replacement.

HEART FAILURE

It is the failure of heart to maintain adequate cardiac output to meet the demand of tissue or can do so only at the expense of an elevated filling pressure. Three types—(1) left-sided, (2) right-sided, and (3) biventricular failure.

Acute left ventricular failure: It is the failure of left ventricle to propel blood in systemic circulation. As a result, there is accumulation of blood in pulmonary circulation, causing pulmonary edema.

Causes of LVF (or pulmonary edema):
- Systemic hypertension
- Acute myocardial infarction (MI)
- Aortic valvular disease (stenosis and regurgitation)
- Mitral regurgitation (MR)
- *Others*: Cardiomyopathy, coarctation of aorta, and rapid or excess infusion of fluid or blood or plasma.

Symptoms: Breathlessness, may be orthopnea. Cough with frothy sputum, palpitation, restlessness, sweating and oliguria.

Signs: Patient looks dyspneic with propped up position, and cyanosis. Pulse—tachycardia, may be pulsus alternans. BP—low but may be high, if the patient is hypertensive.

In precordium:
- *Apex beat*: It may be shifted, thrusting or heaving in character
- *On auscultation*: Gallop rhythm (tachycardia with third or fourth heart sound). In lungs—bilateral basal crepitations

- Signs of primary cause may be present.

Investigations: Chest X-ray shows pulmonary edema (perihilar bat wing appearance), ECG and echocardiogram.

Treatment of acute LVF (pulmonary edema):
- Bed rest. Propped up position. High flow O_2 inhalation
- *Diuretic*: Injection frusemide IV, 80–120 mg. It may be repeated
- Morphine [if no contraindications such as bronchial asthma, chronic obstructive Pulmonary disease (COPD), emphysema and chronic bronchitis]: 10–20 mg intravenous (IV) slowly with antiemetic metoclopramide or cyclizine
- *ACE inhibitors*: Ramipril, captopril and enalapril
- If there is no response, inotropic agents like dopamine and dobutamine are given
- Treatment of primary cause. Anti-arrhythmic drug is given, if arrhythmia occurs.

CONGESTIVE CARDIAC FAILURE

It means right heart failure. There is inability of right ventricle to propel blood resulting in backflow of blood to systemic veins, causing engorged vein, enlarged liver and dependent edema.

Causes:
- Secondary to left-sided heart failure (common cause)
- Mitral stenosis with pulmonary hypertension
- Chronic cor pulmonale due to any cause
- Pulmonary hypertension
- *Others*: PS or regurgitation, TR, shunt anomaly [ASD, ventricular septal defect (VSD)], reversal of shunt (Eisenmenger syndrome), cardiomyopathy, and right ventricular MI.

Symptoms:
- Breathlessness on exertion, cough with mucoid sputum, and palpitation
- Pain in right upper abdomen (due to hepatomegaly) and swelling of legs
- *Others*: Weakness, weight loss, anorexia, nausea, vomiting, oliguria and nocturia.

Signs: Pulse (low volume), BP (low) and JVP (engorged and pulsatile). Dependent pitting edema in legs.

In precordium:
- *Inspection*: Visible cardiac impulse
- *Palpation*: Apex beat may be shifted. Thrill—absent or present according cause
- *Auscultation*: Heart sounds and murmur according to the vulvular lesion.

Abdomen: Liver is enlarged and tender.

Three cardinal signs of CCF: (1) engorged and pulsatile neck veins, (2) enlarged and tender liver, and (3) dependent pitting edema.

Investigations: X-ray of chest, ECG, and echocardiogram. Others—CBC, ESR, urea, creatinine and electrolytes.

Treatment:
- Complete rest. Restriction of fluid and salt
- *Diuretics*: Frusemide and spironolactone

- Vasodilator [ACE inhibitor or angiotensin II receptor blockers (ARB)]
- Beta-blocker (bisoprolol 1.25 mg daily, gradually increases the dose over 12 weeks up to 10 mg daily)
- Digoxin (helpful in CCF with AF)
- Treatment of arrhythmia (e.g. amiodarone) and treatment of underlying cause
- Heart transplantation—if all above measures fail.

Causes of biventricular failure: Dilated cardiomyopathy, myocarditis, extensive MI, right heart failure secondary to left heart failure (MR, AS or AR), hyperdynamic circulation (in severe anemia, thyrotoxicosis, arteriovenous shunt and beriberi), myxedema and multiple vulvular diseases.

HYPERTENSION

It means persistent rise of arterial BP above the arbitrarily normal range. If systolic BP is >140 mm Hg and diastolic BP is >90 mm Hg, the patient is diagnosed as hypertensive.

Causes:
- Primary or essential hypertension (95%)—cause unknown
- *Secondary (5%)*:
  - *Renal (common)*: Chronic glomerulonephritis, chronic pyelonephritis, diabetic nephropathy, adult polycystic kidney disease and renal artery stenosis
  - *Endocrine*: Cushing's syndrome, Conn's syndrome (primary aldosteronism), pheochromocytoma, congenital adrenal hyperplasia, hyperparathyroidism, primary hypothyroidism, hyperthyroidism, and acromegaly
  - *Drugs*: Alcohol, oral contraceptive pill, steroid and erythropoietin
  - *Others*: Preeclampsia and eclampsia (toxemia of pregnancy), pregnancy-induced hypertension, coarctation of aorta, and cerebral tumor.

Clinical features: It may be asymptomatic and is detected in routine examination. Symptoms are headache, dizziness, giddiness, insomnia and blurring of vision. Features of complication such as heart failure, cerebrovascular disease (CVD), and renal failure.

Complications of hypertension:
- *Cardiovascular*: Ischemic heart disease (IHD), acute LVF, and dissecting aneurysm
- *Renal*: Renal failure
- *Ocular*: Retinopathy
- *Neurological*: CVD (intracerebral or subarachnoid hemorrhage), and hypertensive encephalopathy.

Note: Following points are important—
- A single reading is not sufficient. At least three readings in different times should be taken to label as hypertensive
- BP should be measured at least 5 minutes after the patient has taken rest comfortably in sitting or supine position
- BP should be measured at least 30 minutes after smoking or coffee ingestion.

White coat hypertension: When BP is recorded in the doctor's chamber, there may be transient rise in BP in a normal individual. This is called white coat hypertension.

Grades of hypertension:

Grade	Systolic	Diastolic
Grade 1 (mild)	140–159 mm Hg and/or	90–99 mm Hg
Grade 2 (moderate)	160–179 mm Hg and/or	100–109 mm Hg
Grade 3 (severe)	≥180 mm Hg and/or	≥110 mm Hg

Hypertensive encephalopathy: It is characterized by very high BP with neurological abnormalities such as severe headache, loss of consciousness, convulsion, paresthesia, transient disturbance of speech or vision, and retinopathy.

Malignant hypertension: It is characterized by severe hypertension with diastolic BP >130 mm Hg, associated with grade III or IV retinopathy (retinal hemorrhage or exudates and papilledema) and renal failure or encephalopathy. If untreated, death occurs within months.

Treatment: Complete rest. Slow and controlled reduction of BP by oral antihypertensive over 24–48 hours is ideal (rapid reduction is avoided as it reduces tissue perfusion, can cause cerebral damage, and may even precipitate coronary or renal insufficiency). Sometimes IV or intramuscular (IM) labetalol, IV glyceryl trinitrate, and IM hydralazine may be used.

Refractory hypertension: When there is no response to antihypertensive drugs, it is called refractory hypertension. Causes are irregular and inadequate drug therapy (common cause) or undiagnosed cause (renal artery stenosis or pheochromocytoma).

Resistant hypertension: It means failure to control BP with full dose of appropriate three drugs including a diuretic.

Following things should be seen:
- Improper BP measurement
- Volume overload due to excess sodium intake, renal disease or inadequate diuretic therapy
- Inadequate dose and improper combination of drugs or noncompliance
- Patient may take nonsteroidal anti-inflammatory drugs (NSAIDs), steroid, oral contraceptive pills, cyclosporine and erythropoietin
- Other secondary causes of hypertension and associated obesity, and excess alcohol intake.

Investigations in hypertension: History, physical examination and laboratory investigation should be done.

Laboratory investigations:
- *Routine*: Urine examination [routine/microbial (R/M)], blood urea, creatinine, serum electrolytes, blood sugar, lipid profile. X-ray of chest P/A view, ECG and echocardiogram
- *Other investigations according to suspicion of cause*:
    - If renal cause: Ultrasonography (USG) of kidney, intravenous urogram (IVU), computed tomography (CT) scan, and isotope renogram
    - Cushing's syndrome, pheochromocytoma, Conn's syndrome, and coarctation of aorta—investigate accordingly.

Treatment of hypertension:
- *General measures (nondrug treatment):*
  - Salt restriction, smoking should be stopped, weight reduction if obese, dietary modification (low fat, increase fruits and vegetables), avoid anxiety and tension, and restriction of tea, coffee and alcohol
  - Regular exercise (at least 30 minutes daily)
  - Control of diabetes mellitus (DM) and other modifiable risk factors.
- *Drug treatment:*
  - Diuretic: Thiazide
  - ACE inhibitors: Enalapril, lisinopril and ramipril
  - ARB: Losartan, valsartan and irbesartan
  - Calcium channel blockers: Amlodipine, cilnidipine, nifedipine, diltiazem and verapamil
  - Beta-blockers: Atenolol, metoprolol, and bisoprolol
  - Combined alpha and beta-blocker: Labetalol and carvedilol
  - Alpha-blocker: Prazosin
  - *Others*: Methyldopa (used in pregnancy)
  - Management of primary cause, if any.

How to start drug in treatment of hypertension: Single drug is started (diuretic or beta-blocker or calcium channel blocker or ACE inhibitor). If no response, combination therapy.

Contraindications of beta-blocker:
- *Respiratory*: Bronchial asthma, COPD, emphysema and chronic bronchitis
- *Cardiovascular system (CVS)*: Bradycardia, partial or CHB, CCF, peripheral vascular disease (Raynaud's phenomenon)
- *Endocrine*: Pheochromocytoma (beta-blocker alone is avoided), DM receiving insulin (masks the features of hypoglycemia).

Treatment of hypertension in specific conditions

Hypertension in bronchial asthma: Avoid β-blockers. May be used—diuretics, calcium channel blocker, ARB, and ACE inhibitor (it may cause cough).

Hypertension in chronic kidney disease (Target BP is <130/80 mm Hg):
- Angiotensin-converting enzyme inhibitors and ARB may delay progression of kidney disease (if creatinine is >2.5 mmol/L, these should be avoided)
- Calcium channel blockers may be used
- Loop diuretic (frusemide).

Hypertension in pregnancy:
- Methyldopa or labetalol
- Calcium channel blocker (nifedipine) may be used. Beta-blocker may be used (avoid in first trimester)
- Angiotensin-converting enzyme inhibitor is contraindicated. Diuretic is also avoided
- Severe hypertension or eclampsia may be treated with intravenous hydralazine.

Hypertension in diabetes mellitus:
- Angiotensin-converting enzyme inhibitor, ARB, and calcium channel blocker may be used
- Avoid thiazide (it aggravates diabetes). Avoid β-blocker in patient who is on insulin (it masks symptoms of hypoglycemia).

Hypertension in peripheral vascular disease:
- Calcium channel blocker, alpha-blocker and ACE inhibitor
- Avoid beta-blocker.

Hypertension in dyslipidemia:
- Alpha-blocker, ACE inhibitor, ARB, and calcium channel blocker
- Avoid beta-blocker and diuretic (which worsen lipid profile).

Hypertension in psoriasis: Calcium channel blocker may be used. Avoid β-blocker and ACE inhibitor (which aggravates).

Hypertension in angina: Beta-blocker, calcium channel blocker and nitrate.

RHEUMATIC FEVER

It is a multisystem disorder that occurs as a sequela to pharyngitis by group A beta-hemolytic streptococcus. It is common in children and young adults, 5–15 years of age.

Diagnostic criteria of RF: Diagnosed revised by Jones criteria. After *Streptococcus pharyngitis*, usually a latent period of 1–3 weeks.
- *Major criteria (5 criterions)*:
    - Shifting or migrating polyarthritis involving big joints (knee, elbow, ankle and wrist)
    - Carditis
    - Rheumatic chorea
    - Erythema marginatum
    - Subcutaneous nodule.
- *Minor criteria*: Fever, arthralgia, previous history of RF, high ESR or C-reactive protein (CRP), leukocytosis, and first- or second-degree AV block in ECG
- *Supportive evidence of previous streptococcal infection*—such as recent streptococcal sore throat, scarlet fever, high antistreptolysin O (ASO) (>200) or other *streptococcal* antibody titer (anti-DNAse or antihyaluronidase) or positive throat swab culture.

Diagnosis is made by two or more major criteria, or one major and two or more minor criteria *plus* supportive evidence of streptococcal infection.

Signs of carditis: RF can cause carditis involving all the layers of heart (endocardium, myocardium and pericardium), called pancarditis.
- *Signs of endocarditis*: Soft heart sounds, pansystolic murmur (due to MR), mild diastolic murmur (Carey Coombs murmur), and early diastolic murmur (due to AR)
- *Signs of myocarditis*: Tachycardia, soft heart sounds, S3 gallop, cardiomegaly and heart failure
- *Signs of pericarditis*: Pericardial rub and pericardial effusion may develop.

Investigations:
- CBC and ESR (high ESR and leukocytosis)
- CRP: High ASO titer—high (in adult >200, in children >300)
- Throat swab culture (to find *Streptococcus* beta-hemolyticus)
- Chest X-ray, ECG and echocardiography.

Complications:
- Congestive cardiac failure, arrhythmia, pericarditis and pericardial effusion

- Later, rheumatic heart disease causing vulvular stenosis and regurgitation.

Treatment of acute RF:
- Complete bed rest
- Oral phenoxymethyl penicillin—250 mg 6 hourly for 10 days or single injection benzathine penicillin 1.2 million units, deep IM in buttock. Erythromycin may be given, if allergic to penicillin
- Analgesic (for pain). Aspirin 60 mg/kg/day in divided doses. Higher dose may be required
- *Other treatment*: If carditis or severe arthritis, prednisolone 1–2 mg/kg daily. If chorea, diazepam for mild case or haloperidol in severe case.
- Treatment of complications like cardiac failure, valvular lesion, heart block, arrhythmia, etc., if needed.

Prophylactic of RF: To prevent recurrence, oral phenoxymethyl penicillin 250 mg 12 hourly or injection benzathine penicillin, 1.2 million units deep IM in buttock every 4 weeks should be given. In penicillin-sensitive cases, erythromycin (250 mg 12 hourly) may be used. It should be continued up to 21 years of age or 5 years after the last attack (recurrence after 5 years is rare), whichever comes last.

Antibiotic prophylaxis should be given for dental or surgical procedure.

Note: Following points are important—
- Skin infection with *Streptococci* is not associated with RF
- *Streptococcal* sore throat may not be present in some cases
- More than 50% patients of RF with carditis will develop chronic valvular disease after 10–20 years. All the cardiac valves may be involved, but commonly mitral valve is affected (90%). Also aortic valve may be involved. Involvement of tricuspid and pulmonary valves is rare (5%)
- In chronic rheumatic heart disease, may not be history of RF in 50–60% cases
- Arthritis in RF recovers completely without any residual change (RF licks the joints, kills the heart).

CONGENITAL HEART DISEASES

It may be cyanotic and acyanotic.

Cyanotic: Tetralogy of Fallot (TOF), transposition of great vessels, truncus arteriosus, pulmonary atresia, tricuspid atresia and Ebstein's anomaly.

Acyanotic: Left to right shunt [ASD, VSD and patent ductus arteriosus (PDA)], obstructive lesion (coarctation of aorta, AS and PS), and abnormal position of heart (dextrocardia).

VENTRICULAR SEPTAL DEFECT

Causes: Commonly congenital. Also acquired due to rupture of interventricular septum after acute MI, rarely trauma.

Three types according to size:
- *Small*: It is asymptomatic, closes spontaneously
- *Moderate*: Patient presents with fatigue and dyspnea
- *Large*: Murmur is soft.

Site of VSD: Common in perimembranous part of intraventricular septum (in 90% cases).

Symptoms: May be asymptomatic. Symptoms are breathlessness, palpitation, fatigue and weakness.

Signs: In precordium—
- *Inspection*: Visible cardiac impulse in left parasternal area
- *Palpation*: Systolic thrill in left parasternal area in 4th or 5th intercostal space
- *Auscultation*: Pansystolic murmur in left parasternal area in 4th or 5th intercostal space.

Complications: Infective endocarditis (common in small VSD), pulmonary hypertension with reversal of shunt (Eisenmenger syndrome), and heart failure.

Investigations: ECG, X-ray of chest, color Doppler echocardiography, cardiac catheterization. CMR (cardiac magnetic resonance angiography) may be helpful.

Treatment:
- *Small VSD*: No surgery. Prophylactic penicillin for subacute bacterial endocarditis (SBE)
- *Moderate to large VSD*: Surgical correction
- *When Eisenmenger syndrome develops*: Surgery is contraindicated, as it aggravates right-sided heart failure. Following treatments are given—
  - Diuretic and digoxin in some cases. Venesection, if polycythemia
  - Heart lung transplantation may be done.

ATRIAL SEPTAL DEFECT

It is common in female. It is of two types:
1. *Ostium primum (15%)*: Due to atrioventricular (AV) defect in septum
2. *Ostium secundum (75%)*: Defect at fossa ovalis in atrial mid septum.

Symptoms: May be asymptomatic. Symptoms may be breathlessness on exertion, palpitation and weakness.

Signs: In precordium—
- *On auscultation*:
- First heart sound is normal. Wide and fixed splitting of second heart sound
- Ejection systolic murmur in left 2nd and 3rd intercostal space. High-pitched MDM in tricuspid area.

Note: When there is reversal of shunt, features of Eisenmenger syndrome will be found.

Investigations: X-ray of chest, ECG and color Doppler echocardiogram. Cardiac catheterization or CMR may be done.

Complications: Pulmonary hypertension with reversal of shunt (Eisenmenger syndrome), AF (common), embolism (pulmonary and systemic) and brain abscess.

Treatment:
- No surgery in small ASD. Surgical closure in moderate to large ASD
- Angiographic closure is possible with transcatheter clamshell device
- *In Eisenmenger syndrome*: surgical closer is contraindicated (see in Eisenmenger syndrome).

PATENT DUCTUS ARTERIOSUS

Common in female, M:F = 1:3. Probable causes are maternal rubella in first trimester, birth at high altitude, prematurity.

Symptoms: May be asymptomatic. May be breathlessness on exertion, palpitation, weakness, anorexia.

Signs: Pulse—may be high volume, BP—wide pulse pressure, JVP—normal.

In precordium:
- *Palpation*: Apex beat is thrusting or heaving. Systolic thrill in pulmonary area
- *Auscultation*: Continuous murmur in left 2nd and 3rd intercostal space, called machinery murmur like "train in a tunnel".

Complications: Pulmonary hypertension with reversal of shunt (Eisenmenger syndrome), CCF, infective endocarditis, and AF. Duct may rupture or calcify.

Investigations: ECG, X-ray of chest and color Doppler echocardiogram. Cardiac catheterization, MRI or CMR may be done.

Treatment:
- Small PDA can be closed during cardiac catheterization by using implantable occlusive device
- *Large PDA*: surgical closure
- Prophylactic penicillin for infective endocarditis
- If Eisenmenger syndrome develops, surgery is contraindicated (see Eisenmenger syndrome).

EISENMENGER SYNDROME

Pulmonary hypertension with reversal of shunt is called Eisenmenger syndrome. Causes are ventricular septal defect (VSD), ASF, and patent ductus arteriosus (PDA). Persistently raised pulmonary flow (due to left to right shunt) causes high pulmonary resistance, pulmonary hypertension, and high pressure in right ventricle with reversal of shunt (from right to left side).

Symptoms: Dyspnea, fatigue, syncope, angina, hemoptysis and features of CCF.

Signs:
- Central cyanosis. In PDA, differential cyanosis occurs (cyanosis in toes, not in the hands)
- Clubbing. In PDA, differential clubbing occurs (clubbing in toes, not in the hands)
- Pulse: Low volume. Prominent "a" wave in JVP
- *Other signs of pulmonary hypertension*: Palpable P2, left parasternal lift, and epigastric pulsation
- Tricuspid regurgitation (TR) may occur. Original murmur of VSD, ASD or PDA decrease in intensity, may disappear.

Treatment:
- Diuretic. Digoxin may be given in some cases. Venesection may be required in polycythemia

- Heart lung transplantation may be done
- Surgery is contraindicated in Eisenmenger syndrome, as it aggravates right-sided heart failure.

TETRALOGY OF FALLOT

It is a cyanotic congenital heart disease consisting of four components:
1. Pulmonary stenosis (right ventricular outflow tract obstruction)
2. Overriding and dextroposition of aorta (aortic origin two-thirds from left ventricle and one-third from right ventricle)
3. Right ventricular hypertrophy
4. VSD.

Symptoms:
- Breathlessness, weakness, cough, chest pain and palpitation
- Bluish discoloration of lips and fingers during exertion
- Young child usually presents with cyanotic spell (Fallot's spell) during exertion, feeding or crying. The child becomes apneic and unconscious. Squatting relieves cyanosis
- Growth retardation. Syncope, seizure, cerebrovascular events or even sudden death.

Signs:
- Short stature and cyanosis (both central and peripheral). Generalized clubbing involving fingers and toes
- Pulse—low volume, BP—low, JVP—prominent "a" wave (due to RVH).

Precordium:
- *Inspection*: Visible cardiac impulse in apical and epigastric region
- *Palpation*: Left parasternal lift and epigastric pulsation (due to RVH), systolic thrill in pulmonary area
- *Auscultation*: First heart sound is normal in all areas, second heart sound is soft (or absent) in pulmonary area, and A2 is normal. Ejection systolic murmur in pulmonary area, radiates to neck.

Investigations: CBC and ESR (may be polycythemia, ESR may be low). Chest X-ray (boot-shaped heart), ECG. 2D and color Doppler echoardiogram. Cardiac catheterization may be done.

Complications: Infective endocarditis (common), paradoxical emboli, cerebral abscess (10% cases), polycythemia (due to hypoxemia, may cause CVD and MI), and coagulation abnormality.

Acyanotic Fallot: When TOF is associated with infundibular PS. Outflow obstruction is mild, no cyanosis.

Treatment: Total surgical correction should be done before 5 years of age.
- If pulmonary artery is hypoplastic or anatomy is unfavorable, temporarily palliative surgery called Blalock–Taussig shunt is done. Corrective surgery is done later
- Prophylactic penicillin to prevent infective endocarditis.

Blalock–Taussig shunt: It is the anastomosis between left subclavian artery with left pulmonary artery. It improves pulmonary blood flow and pulmonary artery development, and may help definitive surgery later on.

COARCTATION OF AORTA

It is the narrowing of aorta.

Causes: Congenital. Rarely, acquired in trauma, Takayasu disease. It is of two types:
1. *Postductal (adult type)*: Below the origin of left subclavian artery, where ductus arteriosus joins the aorta
2. *Preductal (infantile type, 2%)*: Above the origin of left subclavian artery.

Symptoms: More common in male. May be asymptomatic. Symptoms are headache, nose bleeding and claudication of lower limbs and cold legs (due to poor blood flow in lower limbs).

Signs: BP—High in upper limb, low in lower limb. Pulse—Normal in upper limb, feeble in lower limb with radiofemoral delay.

Precordium:
- *Inspection*: Visible cardiac impulse. Visible dilated tortuous artery around the scapula, anterior axilla and over the left sternal border (due to collateral vessels)
- *Palpation*: Heaving apex beat and thrill over the collateral vessels
- *Auscultation*: Both first and second heart sounds are normal. Systolic murmur is audible near sternum, better heard in 4th intercostal space posteriorly (site of coarctation).

Investigations:
- X-ray of chest P/A view—shows heart is enlarged, rib notching, and figure of '3' sign (constriction at coarctation, prestenotic and poststenotic dilatation)
- ECG [LV hypertrophy (LVH)] and echocardiogram. CT scan and CMR may be done.

Complications:
- Hypertension and its complication [LVF and cerebrovascular accident (CVA)]
- Infective endocarditis
- Rupture at the coarctation site
- Dissecting aneurysm and aneurysm of aorta
- Subarachnoid hemorrhage (rupture of Berry aneurysm or circle of Willis).

Treatment: Surgery as early as possible, before 5 years of age.

ISCHEMIC HEART DISEASE

It is due to reduced coronary blood flow to myocardium, when there is imbalance between supply of oxygen and myocardial demand. IHD includes angina pectoris and myocardial infarction.

Causes of IHD: Coronary blood flow may be reduced due to atherosclerosis (most common), thrombosis, spasm, embolus, coronary ostial stenosis and coronary arteritis.

Common presentations of IHD: Angina pectoris, acute MI, arrhythmia, heart failure and sudden death.

Risk factors for coronary artery disease: Following factors are responsible for atherosclerosis–

Nonmodifiable:
- *Age*: Common in elderly
- *Sex*: More in male. After menopause in female, incidence is same
- *Family history*: More common, if there is family history of IHD
- *Genetic factors*: A number of genetic factors have been linked with coronary artery disease.

Modifiable:
- *Smoking*: IHD is more in smokers
- *Alcohol*: Moderate alcohol consumption is associated with less risk but high intake increases the risk
- *Diet*: High fats are associated with IHD. Diet low in fresh fruits, vegetables and polyunsaturated fatty acids are associated with increased risk
- *Obesity*: Overweight has an increased risk
- *Exercise*: More in sedentary workers
- *Others*: Hypertension, DM, hyperlipidemia, psychosocial factors (stress, depression, and anxiety).

ANGINA PECTORIS

It is defined as paroxysmal precordial pain of short duration due to transient myocardial ischemia.

Symptoms: Main symptom is pain, which has the following characters—
- *Site*: Central, retrosternal chest
- *Character*: Stabbing or squeezing or constricting
- *Radiation*: Lower jaw, neck and inner side of left arm up to the finger
- Precipitated by exertion, eating or emotion (3 E)
- Relieved by rest and nitroglycerine
- *Duration*: 5-10 minutes (less than half hour).

Signs: Usually no definitive physical sign.

Investigations:
- ECG is often normal. During attack—ST depression, T inversion
- Chest X-ray, echocardiography, exercise tolerance test (ETT) and coronary arteriography
- *Other stress testing*: Myocardial perfusion scan, stress echocardiography and transthoracic echocardiography
- *For risk factor*: Fasting lipid profile and blood sugar.

Treatment:

During acute attack: Sublingual glyceryl trinitrate (GTN) as aerosol or tablet under the tongue. It will relieve attack of angina in 2-3 minutes. If no response, it can be repeated. But if still no response, myocardial infarction should be excluded.

Prevention of further attack:
- *Antiplatelet therapy*: Low-dose (75–150 mg) aspirin and clopidogrel (75 mg daily)
- *Antianginal drugs*:
    - To prevent angina pain: Oral nitrates such as isosorbide dinitrate (10–20 mg, 8 hourly), isosorbide mononitrate (20–60 mg, once or twice a day) can be given by mouth
    - *Other drugs*: Beta-blockers (atenolol, metoprolol, and bisoprolol). Calcium antagonists (nifedipine, nicardipine, verapamil and

diltiazem) and potassium channel activators (nicorandil) may be used
  - If recurrent or persistent pain: Coronary angiogram should be done. If coronary artery blockage, then stenting or percutaneous transluminal coronary angioplasty (PTCA) or coronary artery bypass surgery (CABG) may be required.
- Risk factors should be controlled
  - Lifestyle modification. No smoking, and avoid alcohol. Avoid anxiety, tension and depression
  - Reduction of weight if obese. Regular exercise, at least 30 minutes daily
  - Control of hypertension and DM. Lipid-lowering drugs—atorvastatin and rosuvastatin.

Treatment of unstable angina:
- Hospitalization. Complete bed rest, oxygen and sedation, if needed
- Aspirin or clopidogrel or combined. Nitroglycerine, beta-blocker and calcium channel blocker
- *Heparin*: Low-molecular-weight (LMW) heparin [enoxaparin subcutaneous (SC)] for 5–7 days
- If pain persists, nitroglycerine infusion
- If all fail, urgent coronary angiography and revascularization, if necessary.

MYOCARDIAL INFARCTION

It is defined as myocardial necrosis, which occurs as result of critical imbalance between coronary blood flow and myocardial demand due to occlusion of coronary artery by thrombus.

Types:
- Q wave (Transmural) or ST-elevated MI
- Non-Q wave or non-ST-elevated (NSTEMI) or subendocardial MI.

Symptoms:
- Central chest pain which is severe, stabbing or squeezing or constricting, radiates to lower jaw, neck and inner side of left arm up to finger, and not relieved by rest or nitroglycerine, persist for >30 minutes
- Sweating and fear of impending death. Nausea and vomiting (more in inferior MI) and breathlessness
- Collapse or cardiogenic shock.

Signs:
- The patient is restless with pallor, sweating and tachycardia (bradycardia in inferior MI)
- Hypotension, oliguria and cold peripheries
- Signs of complications such as cardiogenic shock, acute LVF, arrhythmia, mitral regurgitation and pericarditis.

Investigations:
- *ECG*: It shows ST elevation (with upward convexity), pathological Q wave, and T inversion
- *Enzymatic changes in acute MI*:
  - Troponin I: rise in 2–4 hours, may persist up to 7 days
  - Creatine kinase-muscle/brain (CK-MB): rise in 4–6 hours, peak in 12 hours, returns to normal within 48–72 hours

- Serum glutamic oxaloacetic transaminase (SGOT): increases after 12 hours, peak in 24 hours, returns to normal in 3-4 days
- LDH: rises after 12 hours, peak in 3-4 days, and normal after 7-10 days.
- *Others*: Chest x-ray and echocardiography may be done.

Complications of MI: May be early and late.
- *Early complications*:
  - Arrhythmia: Ventricular ectopics (more common), VF, ventricular tachycardia, sinus bradycardia (common in inferior MI), sinus tachycardia, AF and heart block
  - Cardiogenic shock
  - Cardiac failure (LVF and biventricular failure)
  - Acute pericarditis (common in 2nd or 3rd day)
  - Thromboembolism (systemic and pulmonary)
  - Rupture of papillary muscle or chordae tendineae resulting in MR, rupture of interventricular septum causing VSD, rupture of ventricular wall.
- *Late complications*: Ventricular aneurysm (10%), post-myocardial infarction syndrome (Dressler's syndrome), frozen shoulder and postinfarction angina.

Treatment of acute myocardial infarction:
- Admission in coronary care unit (CCU) and complete bed rest. High flow O_2 inhalation (60%) 2-4 L/min by nasal cannula
- *To relieve pain*: Injection morphine (5-10 mg) or dimorphine (2.5-5 mg) *plus* antiemetic (cyclizine or metoclopramide) IV. May be repeated, if necessary
- Chewable aspirin 300 mg and clopidogrel 300 mg
- Primary percutaneous coronary intervention (PCI), if available. Should be performed as early as possible
- *Or thrombolytic therapy*: Streptokinase, if no contraindication
- *Other therapy*: β-blocker (if no contraindication), IV bolus atenolol 5-10 mg or metoprolol 5-15 mg slowly over 5 minutes. Oral atenolol 25-50 mg BD, or bisoprolol 5 mg daily or metoprolol 25-50 mg BD or TDS may be given
- Sublingual nitroglycerin—0.3-1 mg
- *Anticoagulants*: Heparin 5,000 IU, IV, bolus, and then 0.25 U/kg/hour. Or low-molecular-weight heparin (S/C enoxaparin 1 mg/kg body weight 12 hourly)
- Angiotensin-converting enzyme inhibitor.

Follow-up after acute MI:
- Patient should be reviewed after 6-8 weeks.
- Risk factors should be reviewed and modified accordingly:
  - Lifestyle modification (avoid stress and heavy work). Regular exercise. Weight control, if obese
  - Smoking should be stopped. Avoid fatty and oily food
  - Control of hypertension and DM
  - Antiplatelet (aspirin or clopidogrel) should be continued indefinitely
  - ACE inhibitor should be continued indefinitely in patient with persistent LV dysfunction (EF <40%)
  - Beta-blocker and lipid-lowering agents
  - Rehabilitation.

VENTRICULAR ANEURYSM

If in ECG, ST remains elevated after few months of acute MI, the diagnosis is ventricular aneurysm. X-ray of chest shows enlarged heart, bulge or rounded protrusion from LV wall, and calcification may occur at the wall of aneurysm. Confirmed by echocardiogram.

ACUTE PERICARDITIS

It is the acute inflammation of pericardium.

Causes:
- Viral (coxsackie B virus and echovirus)—common cause
- Acute RF
- After acute MI (in 2nd or 3rd day)
- Bacterial (*Staphaylococcus aureus* and *Hemophilus influenza*), tuberculous and fungal (histoplasmosis, and coccidioidomycosis).
- *Others*: Acute renal failure, trauma, radiation, drugs (doxorubicin and cyclophosphamide), and collagen disease (SLE and scleroderma)

Symptoms: Chest pain, which is retrosternal, sharp or stabbing in nature, aggravated by movement, lying down and deep breathing, exercise and swallowing. Pain may be relieved by sitting or bending forward. Other symptoms are according to cause [e.g. low grade evening rise of temperature, night sweat and weight loss in tuberculosis (TB)].

Signs: Pericardial rub.

Investigations:
- *ECG*: ST elevated with upward concavity (chair shaped or saddle shaped)
- Chest X-ray P/A view and echocardiography. CT and cardiac MRI may be done in some cases
- *Others*: According to suspicion of cause.

Treatment:
- If pain—NSAID (indomethacin or ibuprofen). In severe or recurrent pain, steroid is given
- *If no response to steroid*: azathioprine or colchicine may be added
- If recurrence with no response to medical treatment—pericardiotomy may be done
- Treatment of primary cause—antibiotic, if bacterial infection. Anti-Koch's, if tuberculosis is suspected.

PERICARDIAL EFFUSION

Accumulation of fluid in the space between parietal and visceral pericardium.

Causes:
- After acute pericarditis (bacterial and viral), and tuberculosis (the most common)
- Collagen diseases (SLE and RA)
- *Others*: Myxedema, lymphoma, secondary metastasis, renal failure and dialysis, after radiotherapy.

Symptoms: Heaviness in chest, breathlessness and palpitation. Symptoms of primary cause.

Signs:
- Pulse—low volume, tachycardia, there may be pulsus paradoxus (indicating cardiac tamponade)
- JVP—raised, Kussmaul's sign positive (rise of JVP during inspiration)
- Blood pressure—low systolic, normal diastolic and narrow pulse pressure
- Liver is enlarged and tender.

In precordium:
- Area of cardiac dullness is increased (on percussion)
- Apex beat is difficult to palpate
- Heart sounds are muffled or distant
- Bronchial sound at the left inferior angle of scapula (Ewart sign).

Investigations:
- Chest X-ray (heart is globular and lung fields are oligemic), CBC, ECG, and echocardiogram (shows echo-free zone)
- Paracentesis—to see color, analysis of pericardial fluid [Gram staining, cytology, biochemistry, AFB, culture/sensitivity (C/S), and ADA]
- MRI—very helpful
- Other investigations according to the suspicion of causes.

Confirmation of diagnosis: By echocardiogram (shows the echo free zone). Paracentesis is definitive.

Treatment: According to cause—
- If tuberculosis, antituberculosis drug *plus* prednisolone
- If bacterial cause is suspected—broad-spectrum antibiotic
- Other treatment of primary cause (e.g. hypothyroidism, SLE, RA and lymphoma)
- Paracentesis, if cardiac tamponade develops.

CARDIAC TAMPONADE

It is a state of compression of heart in rapidly developing pericardial effusion. It interferes with diastolic filling of heart and the patient develops features of shock.

Causes:
- Trauma or cardiac surgery (causing hemopericardium)
- Malignancy (repeated effusion may occur)
- Myocardial rupture
- Dissecting aortic aneurysm
- Any cause of pericardial effusion can cause.

Symptoms: Heaviness and compression in chest, dyspnea and features of shock.

Signs: See above in pericardial effusion.

Treatment: Immediate pericardiocentesis and treatment of primary cause.

CHRONIC CONSTRICTIVE PERICARDITIS

It is a disease characterized by progressive thickening, fibrosis and calcification of pericardium.

Causes:
- *Infection*: TB, coxsackie B virus and histoplasmosis
- Hemopericardium (due to trauma and myocardial rupture after infarction or dissecting aneurysm)
- Collagen disease (RA)
- *Others*: Cardiac operation, mediastinal irradiation and idiopathic, rarely after acute purulent pericarditis.

Symptoms: Cough, breathlessness on exertion, may be orthopnea and paroxysmal nocturnal dyspnea. Weakness, dizziness, giddiness, anorexia, nausea and vomiting. Abdominal swelling and later ankle swelling.

Signs:
- Tachycardia and low-volume pulse. Pulsus paradoxus may be present
- JVP—raised, fall of Y descent (Friedreich's sign). Kussmaul's sign is positive (raised JVP on inspiration)
- Pericardial knock (a third heart sound due to rapid ventricular filling)
- Enlarged tender liver and ascites
- Peripheral edema later on.

Complications: Atrial fibrillation (in 30% cases), ascites and myocardial fibrosis.

Investigations:
- Chest X-ray (pericardial calcification in 50% cases) and ECG
- Echocardiogram, CT scan or CMR. Cardiac catheterization is done in some cases
- Other investigations according to suspicion of cause [Mantoux test (MT), RA and antinuclear antibodies (ANA)].

Treatment: Complete resection of pericardium. Treatment of primary cause should be done.

MYOCARDITIS

It is the inflammation of the myocardium of heart.

Causes:
- *Infection*: Viral (coxsackie A and B and influenza A and B), bacterial (*Streptococcus*, *Pneumococcus*, and Lyme disease), protozoal (Chagas disease), and fungal (*Candida* and *Actinomyces*)
- Rheumatic fever
- Diphtheritic myocarditis
- *Others*: Drugs and toxins (doxorubicin and lithium), radiation and autoimmune (SLE and RA).

Symptoms: Palpitation, breathlessness and chest pain. Features of cardiac failure or primary disease, if any.

Signs:
- Pulse—low volume and tachycardia
- Apex beat may be displaced downward and outward due to cardiomegaly
- First and second heart sounds may be soft. Third or fourth heart sound may be present
- Features of heart failure and arrhythmia may be present.

Investigations:
- Chest X-ray, ECG, echocardiography and MRI
- Endomyocardial biopsy may be needed for confirmation.

Treatment: Complete bed rest and low-salt diet. Diuretics and ACE inhibitors may be helpful. Treatment of arrhythmia. Treatment of primary cause, if any.

ENDOCARDITIS

It is the infection of endocardium, mainly the lining of chamber or heart valve or in congenital anomaly, usually occurs at the site of preexisting heart disease or septal defect. Infection with virulent organism may cause acute endocarditis in normal heart (e.g. by *Staphylococcus aureus*).

Acute Endocarditis

It is usually caused by highly virulent and invasive organism (*S. aureus*, *Streptococcus* and *Pneumococcus*). It can affect damaged as well as normal heart. Vegetations are usually very large and valve destruction is more than in subacute endocarditis.

Symptoms: Fever, usually very high with chill and rigor. Headache, bodyache, malaise, weakness, chest pain and breathlessness.

Signs: Patient looks toxic with very high temperature. Prominent and changing heart murmur. Stigmata of subacute or chronic endocarditis are usually absent.

Treatment: Vancomycin (1 g twice daily IV) and gentamicin (1 mg/kg twice daily IV).

Subacute Bacterial Endocarditis

It is usually caused by organisms of low virulence, affecting rheumatic or congenitally abnormal valves.

Predisposing factors or causes of SBE:
- Rheumatic valve lesion (e.g. AR and MR)
- Congenital heart disease (VSD, PDA, bicuspid aortic valve, coarctation of aorta and TOF)
- Prosthetic valve
- Dental extraction
- Instrumentation (IV cannula, central venous (CV) line, and cardiac catheterization)
- Cardiac surgery
- IV drug abuse (right-sided endocarditis is more common, especially tricuspid valve).

Organisms causing infective endocarditis:
- *Subacute bacterial endocarditis*:
  - *Streptococcus viridans*: Most common (35–50%)
  - *Enterococcus faecalis* and *Enterococcus faecium*
  - *Streptococcus bovis* (associated with large bowel carcinoma), *Streptococcus milleri* and other *Streptococci*
  - *Staphylococcus aureus* or epidermidis
  - HACEK organisms (*Haemophilus*, *Actinobacillus*, *Cardiobacterium hominis*, *Eikenella* and *Kingella*).
- *Acute bacterial endocarditis*: *S. aureus* (common). Others—*Pseudomonas*, *Candida*, *Streptococcus pneumoniae*, and *Neisseria gonorrhoeae*
- *Postoperative endocarditis*: *Staphylococcus albus*, *Candida*, *Aspergillus* and all other organisms causing subacute and acute endocarditis.

Symptoms of SBE:
- Fever, usually low grade and continuous, is persistent and does not respond to usual antibiotics
- Chest pain and palpitation, difficulty in breathing. Anorexia, weight loss, malaise, weakness, night sweat and arthralgia
- Symptoms of embolism according to involvement like brain (CVD), kidney (renal infarction), and lung (pulmonary infarction).

Signs:

General examination:
- *Appearance*: Ill-looking, emaciated and toxic, and anemia
- *In hands*:
  - Clubbing involving all fingers and toes
  - Osler's node (small painful violaceous raised nodule, present on the tip of the fingers)
  - Janeway lesion (large painless erythematous macules on the palm and sole)
  - Infarction at the tip of fingers or toes, petechiae on the dorsum or other parts
  - Splinter hemorrage (subungual)
  - Infarction due to embolism.
- Pulse—tachycardia, BP—may be low
- Precordium
- Signs of previous heart disease (AR, MR, ASD, VSD and PDA)
  - Murmur—appearance of new murmur or changing character of previous murmur.
- *Abdomen*: Splenomegaly may be present
- *Fundoscopy*: Roth's spot (white-centered retinal hemorrhage).

Investigations:
- CBC, ESR (high) and CRP (high)
- *Blood C/S (both aerobic and anaerobic)*: Three samples from different sites at 1 hour apart
  1. Echocardiography (preferably transesophageal echocardiography) to see vegetation, valvular lesion or congenital anomaly
  2. Urine examination (R/M) (hematuria and proteinuria may be present). Serum urea and creatinine
  3. Chest X-ray (shows cardiomegaly) and ECG.

Complications of SBE:
- Heart failure (LVF is a common cause of death), valve destruction, regurgitation and obstruction
- Aortic root abscess and systemic embolism
- Right-sided endocarditis involves the pulmonary valve and may cause septic pulmonary emboli, occasionally infarction and lung abscess.

Causes of noninfective endocarditis:
- Libman–Sacks (nonbacterial verrucous endocarditis in SLE)
- Marantic endocarditis (nonbacterial thrombotic or verrucous endocarditis found in malignancy, such as bronchial carcinoma).

Treatment: Antibiotic is given according to C/S, should be started after sending blood for C/S.

- *For Viridans streptococci*: Benzyl penicillin 1.2 g IV 4 hourly and gentamycin 1 mg/kg IV 8 hourly for 4 weeks or ceftriaxone 2 g once daily IV or vancomycin 15 mg/kg IV 12 hourly for 4 weeks
- *In penicillin allergy or methicillin resistant Staphylococcus aureus (MRSA)*: Triple therapy with vancomycin, gentamycin with oral rifampicin. Or another regimen—Vancomycin 1 g 12 hourly IV with ceftriaxone 2 g every 24 hours
- *In prosthetic valve endocarditis*: IV penicillin 6 weeks and IV gentamicin 2 weeks
- *For HACEK organisms*: Ceftriaxone 2 g IV once daily for 4 weeks. If prosthetic valve is involved, then treatment should be given for 6 weeks.
- *Q fever endocarditis*: Prolonged treatment with doxycycline and rifampicin or ciprofloxacin.

Prevention during dental procedure: Antibiotic is given in high risk cases, such as prosthetic heart valve, previous infective endocarditis, and congenital heart disease.

Drugs used for prophylaxis:
- Amoxicillin 2 g 1 hour before procedure
- *If penicillin allergy*: Clindamycin 600 mg or cephalexin 2 g or azithromycin or clarithromycin 500 mg 1 hour before procedure.

CARDIOMYOPATHY

Cardiomyopathies are a group of diseases involving the heart muscle and not due to congenital, valvular, hypertension and coronary arterial or pericardial abnormalities.

Three types: (1) Hypertrophic, (2) dilated (ischemic), and (3) restrictive cardiomyopathy.

Hypertrophic cardiomyopathy (HCM): It is a disease of heart muscle characterized by hypertrophy of cardiac muscle with misalignment of cardiac fibers. Hypertrophy may be generalized or localized to the interventricular septum (asymmetrical septal hypertrophy) or other regions (apical hypertrophic cardiomyopathy).

Types are:
- Asymmetrical septal hypertrophy (70%)
- Basal septal hypertrophy (15–20%)
- Concentric (8–10%)
- Apical or lateral wall (<2%).

Symptoms: May be asymptomatic. May be angina or breathlessness or presyncope or syncope on exertion, palpitation and sudden death.

Signs: Pulse—Carotid pulse is jerky. BP—low systolic, normal diastolic and narrow pulse pressure.

Precordium:
- *Palpation*: Apex beat—heaving (may be double apical impulse). Systolic thrill may be palpable at apex
- *Auscultation*: Ejection systolic murmur at left lower sternal border. Pansystolic murmur at the apex due to mitral regurgitation.

Investigations: Chest X-ray, ECG, echocardiogram (diagnostic), cardiac MR, and genetic analysis.

Treatment:
- *In nonobstructive case*: Beta-blocker and rate-limiting calcium channel blocker (verapamil and diltiazem). Amiodarone may be helpful in arrhythmia
- *In left ventricular outflow obstruction*: Dual chamber pacing may be needed. Partial surgical resection (myectomy) may be needed
- *Other treatment*: Implantable cardioverter-defibrillator (ICD) (if clinical risk factors for sudden death). Cardiac transplantation may be needed in congestive heart failure (CHF) not responding to treatment. Infective endocarditis prophylaxis may be needed.

Advice to be given in HCM:
- Vigorous exercise and dehydration should be avoided
- Genetic counseling, as in 50% cases, may be inherited as autosomal dominant
- First-degree family members should be screened by echocardiogram.

Drugs to be avoided in HCM: Digoxin, vasodilators, diuretics, nitrates, dihydropyridine calcium channel blockers, and alcohol (may cause vasodilatation).

Dilated cardiomyopathy (DCM): It is characterized by dilatation and impaired contraction of left and sometimes right ventricle causing progressive left-sided and later right-sided heart failure. Functional mitral or TR may occur.

Causes:
- Alcohol
- 25% cases are inherited as autosomal dominant trait
- Autoimmune reaction to viral myocarditis
- Ischemic heart disease
- Nutritional—thiamine (Vitamin B1) deficiency
- *Others*: Muscular dystrophies (Duchenne or Becker thyrotoxicosis), pregnancy, infiltrative disease (hemochromatosis and sarcoidosis), and idiopathic in many cases.

Symptoms: Breathlessness on exertion. Features of heart failure (palpitation, swelling of legs and fatigue), sporadic chest pain and sudden death.

Signs: Signs of cardiac failure (left or right or biventricular) and arrhythmia.

Investigations: ECG, chest X-ray and echocardiography.

Treatment: Mainly of heart failure.
- Rest, salt and fluid restriction, and avoid exercise
- *Medical therapy*: β-blockers, ACE inhibitors or angiotensin receptor blocker, diuretics and nitrates. Anti-arrhythmic drugs, if arrhythmia (amiodarone)
- In some patients—implantation of ICD
- Treatment of primary cause, if any
- Cardiac transplantation may be indicated.

Restrictive cardiomyopathy (RCM): Rare, ventricular filling is impaired, as ventricles are "stiff". This leads to high atrial pressures with atrial hypertrophy, dilatation and later AF.

Diagnosis: Color Doppler echocardiography, CT or MRI, and endomyocardial biopsy.

Treatment: Symptomatic but prognosis is usually poor and transplantation may be indicated.

Postpartum cardiomyopathy: If any patient develops cardiac failure in last trimester of pregnancy or within 6 months after delivery in absence of previous heart disease, it is called postpartum or peripartum cardiomyopathy. It is a type of dilated cardiomyopathy. Cause is unknown. Immune and viral causes are postulated. Other factors are advanced age, multiple pregnancy, multiparity, and hypertension in pregnancy. Commonly occurs immediately after or in the month before delivery (peripartum).

Symptoms: Common in multipara, age above 30 years. Respiratory distress, orthopnea and heart failure. Cough with frothy sputum due to pulmonary edema.

Signs: Signs of heart failure. AF or other arrhythmia may occur.

Diagnostic criteria (four criteria):
1. Presentation in last month of pregnancy or within 6 months of delivery
2. Absence of an obvious cause for heart failure
3. Previously normal cardiac status
4. Echocardiographic evidence of systolic LV dysfunction.

Treatment: Symptomatic for heart failure (diuretics, ACE inhibitor, and digoxin). Beta-blocker may be helpful in some cases. Inotropic agent may be given.

ARRHYTHMIA

It is defined as the disorder of rate, rhythm and conduction of cardiac impulse.

Types:
- *Impulse arising from sinoatrial (SA) node*: Sinus arrhythmia, sinus tachycardia, sinus bradycardia, and sick sinus syndrome
- *Impulse arising from atria*: AF, atrial flutter, atrial tachycardia and atrial ectopics
- *Impulse arising from AV junction or nodal*: Nodal or junctional rhythm, nodal tachycardia, and nodal ectopics
- *Impulse arising from ventricles*: Ventricular tachycardia, VF and ventricular ectopics
- *Heart block*: SA block, AV block, and bundle branch block [left bundle branch block (LBBB) and right bundle branch block (RBBB)].

Sinus arrhythmia: It is an arrhythmia in which heart rate increases in inspiration and decreases in expiration. It is a benign condition, common in children and young adults, sometimes in healthy old person. ECG findings—PP or RR interval (Short in inspiration and long in expiration).

Sinus tachycardia: When heart rate is more than 100/min in sinus rhythm.
Causes:
- *Physiological*: Anxiety, emotion, exercise, pain and pregnancy
- *Pathological*: Anemia, fever, thyrotoxicosis, shock (except vasovagal attack, in which bradycardia is present), heart failure, bleeding, hypovolemia, chronic constrictive pericarditis, acute anterior MI, and drugs (salbutamol, propantheline, and thyroxine).

Symptoms: Palpitation and features of primary disease if any.

Treatment: If symptomatic—beta-blockers (propranolol and atenolol) or calcium channel blocker (verapamil). Treatment of primary cause if any.

Sinus bradycardia: When heart rate is less than 60/min in sinus rhythm.

Causes:
- *Physiological (due to increased vagal tone)*: Athlete and sleep. Occasionally, healthy elderly
- *Pathological*: Hypothyroidism, hypothermia, raised intracranial pressure, drugs (digoxin, β-blockers and verapamil), acute inferior MI, obstructive jaundice, and hypokalemia.

Causes of bradycardia:
- Sinus bradycardia due to any cause
- Second-degree heart block (Mobitz type II) and CHB
- Nodal rhythm, idioventricular rhythm and drugs (β-blocker, digoxin).

Treatment: Treatment of primary cause.

SICK SINUS SYNDROME

It is the dysfunction of SA node characterized by sinus bradycardia, sinus arrest or junctional rhythm which may lead to dizziness or syncope, followed by episodes of paroxysmal tachycardia, so called tachy-brady syndrome. It is due to fibrosis, degenerative changes or ischemia of SA node. Probable causes are elderly, IHD, drug (digoxin), cardiomyopathy, rheumatic heart disease and idiopathic.

Symptoms: May be asymptomatic. May be dizziness, syncope and palpitation.

Signs: Pulse (bradycardia or tachycardia or drop beat). Features of primary disease.

Investigations: ECG and Holter monitoring (single ECG may sometimes be normal).

Treatment: If asymptomatic—no specific therapy. Follow-up. If symptomatic—permanent dual chamber pacemaker. Anti-arrhythmic drug may be required.

Supraventricular tachycardia (SVT): It is a type of tachycardia that occurs due to reentry or rapidly firing ectopic focus in atria or AV node.

Causes:
- *Physiological*: Anxiety, tension, tea, coffee and alcohol
- *Pathological*: Thyrotoxicosis, IHD, Wolff–Parkinson–White (WPW) syndrome and digitalis toxicity.

Symptoms: Palpitation, dizziness, syncope, breathlessness, and chest pain. Polyuria after the attack.

Complications: Short diastolic filling time, so less stroke volume and precipitate heart failure.

Treatment:
- Rest. Carotid sinus massage or Valsalva maneuver. It acts by increasing the vagal tone
- *If no response*:
    - IV adenosine, 3 mg over 2 seconds. If no response in 1–2 minute, then 6 mg IV. If still no response in 1–2 minutes, then 12 mg (maximum dose)

- Or IV verapamil 10 mg slowly over 5–10 minutes (verapamil should be avoided if QRS >0.12 second or history of WPW syndrome or if the patient is on β-blocker).
- *Other drugs*: β-blocker or digoxin may be used
- *If patient is hemodynamically unstable (hypotension and pulmonary edema)*: Direct current (DC) shock
- *If attack is frequent*: Prophylactic oral β-blocker, verapamil or digoxin may be given
- *In WPW syndrome*: Transvenous radiofrequency catheter ablation is the treatment of choice
- In some cases—antitachycardia pacing is done (overdrive atrial pacing).

WPW SYNDROME

It is a syndrome in which there is an accessory pathway that bypasses AV node and connects the atrium and ventricle (by bundles of Kent).

It is of two types:
1. *Type A*: Accessory pathway on left side (in ECG, tall R in V1 and V2)
2. *Type B*: Accessory pathway on right side (in ECG, deep Q in V1 and V2).

Clinical features: May be asymptomatic. May present with palpitation, paroxysmal attack of atrial or SVT, and AF. Syncope and sudden death (due to AF). Rarely, features of ventricular tachycardia and VF.

Investigations: ECG shows short PR interval (<0.12 second) and wide QRS. Delta wave in the upstroke of QRS (slurred QRS). Q wave may be present in lead II, III, and a VF (confused with inferior MI). Electrophysiological study may be done.

Treatment: If asymptomatic—no treatment is required. If symptomatic, transvenous radiofrequency catheter ablation of accessory pathway is the specific treatment. If not available, prophylactic anti-arrhythmic drug should be given (β-blocker and amiodarone). Surgical resection of accessory pathway may be done.

Drugs to be avoided in WPW syndrome: Digoxin, and IV verapamil. These shorten refractory period of accessory pathway.

ATRIAL FIBRILLATION

It is an arrhythmia where atria beat rapidly, chaotically, and ineffectively, while the ventricles respond at irregular intervals, producing the characteristic irregularly irregular pulse.

Clinically, five types:
1. First detected—not diagnosed previously, irrespective of duration or severity of symptoms
2. *Paroxysmal*: Self-limiting and stops spontaneously within 7 days
3. Persistent—continuous >7 days
4. Long-standing persistent—continuous >1 year
5. Permanent—continuous, with a joint decision between the patient and the physician to cease further attempts to regain sinus rhythm.

According to heart rate, two types:
1. *Fast AF*: Heart rate >100 beats/min
2. *Slow AF*: Heart rate <100 beats/min.

Causes:
- Chronic rheumatic heart disease with valvular lesions, commonly MS
- Coronary artery disease (commonly, acute myocardial infarction)
- Thyrotoxicosis
- Hypertension
- Lone AF (idiopathic in 10%)
- *Others*: ASD, chronic constrictive pericarditis, acute pericarditis, cardiomyopathy, myocarditis, sick sinus syndrome, coronary bypass surgery, pneumonia, thoracic surgery, electrolyte imbalance (hypokalemia and hyponatremia), alcohol, and pulmonary embolism.

Complications: Systemic and pulmonary embolism (systemic from left atrium and pulmonary from right atrium) and heart failure.

Symptoms: Palpitation, breathlessness and weakness.

Signs:
- *Pulse*: Irregularly irregular (irregular in rhythm and volume)
- Examination of heart (heart rate to see pulsus deficit, mitral valvular or other cardiac disease)
- Thyroid status (warm sweaty hands, tremor, tachycardia, exophthalmos and thyroid gland size)
- Check BP in hypertensive case.

Investigations:
- ECG shows absent P wave (replaced by fibrillary "*f*" wave) with irregularly irregular (R-R interval is irregular)
- Chest X-ray and echocardiography. Thyroid function test, if thyrotoxicosis is suspected.

Treatment:

Aims of treatment: Control of heart rate, restoration of sinus rhythm, prevention of recurrence, and treatment of primary cause.
- To control rate—digoxin, β-blocker or calcium channel blocker (verapamil or diltiazem) may be given
- *If no response, cardioversion (medical or DC shock) should be done as follows*:
  - Intravenous anti-arrhythmic drug such as flecainide, propafenone, vernakalant or amiodarone. Oral flecainide or propafenone may be given
  - If no response—DC shock should be given.
- *Long-term treatment (according to types)*:
  - Paroxysmal AF:
    - If asymptomatic: No treatment. Treatment of primary cause, regular follow-up
    - If symptomatic: β-blocker. If no response, flecainide or propafenone may be given. Amiodarone is effective in prevention. Low-dose aspirin to prevent thromboembolism
    - If bradycardia (SA disease): Permanent overdrive atrial pacing
    - In intractable cases: Radiofrequency ablation may be done, if no structural heart disease.
  - Persistent AF:
    - To control heart rate—β-blocker, digoxin or calcium channel blocker (verapamil, diltiazem). Combination of digoxin and atenolol may be used

- To control rhythm: DC cardioversion. May be repeated, if relapse
- β-blocker or amiodarone may be used to prevent recurrence
- If no response—transvenous radiofrequency ablation may be done.

Lone AF: It means AF without any cause. Usually life span is normal.

ATRIAL FLUTTER

It is characterized by rapid atrial rate associated with 2:1, 3:1, 4:1 or more AV block.

Causes: These causes are like atrial fibrillation (AF). AF and flutter may be present together, it is called flutter-fibrillation.

Symptoms: Palpitation, breathlessness, fatigue, weakness, light headedness, dizziness and even syncope.

ECG findings: Saw-tooth appearance of P wave (normal P is replaced by flutter or F wave). RR is regular (may be irregular, when there is variable block).

Treatment: To control heart rate, digoxin, β-blocker or verapamil. β-blocker or amiodarone can be used to prevent recurrence. If no response, DC cardioversion or atrial overdrive pacing may be done. In persistent or troublesome symptoms, radiofrequency catheter ablation.

Ectopics: Ectopic beat or extrasystole is a premature beat which arises from other than SA node and comes earlier than normal beat. It arises from abnormal focus such as atria, AV node or ventricle.

Types: Atrial, nodal, and ventricular.

Atrial ectopics: May occur in normal people. Other causes are, excess tea, coffee and smoking. Any organic heart disease (myocarditis and cardiomyopathy), electrolyte imbalance, and COPD.

ECG findings: P (small or inverted), PR interval (short) and PP interval (irregular).

Ventricular ectopics: It may be unifocal, multifocal, bigeminy, trigeminy, and quadrigeminy.

Causes:
- Normally in young adults, also in anxiety, excess caffeine, and alcohol
- Myocarditis and cardiomyopathy
- Valvular heart disease and MVP
- *Others*: Hypertensive heart disease, hypokalemia, digoxin toxicity and hypoxemia.

Treatment: In absence of any heart disease and asymptomatic case, no treatment is necessary. β-blocker may be used. If organic heart disease, treatment of primary cause. Anti-arrhythmic drug does not improve, may even worsen the prognosis.

Ventricular tachycardia (VT): It is defined as three or more consecutive ectopic beats and heart rate usually 140–220 beats/min with regular rhythm. It may be sustained or nonsustained.

Causes:
- Acute MI
- Myocarditis, cardiomyopathy

- Chronic IHD (especially with poor LV function)
- *Others*: Ventricular aneurysm, MVP, hypokalemia, hypomagnesemia, and idiopathic.

Symptoms: Palpitation, dyspnea, dizziness and giddiness.

Treatment:
- *If patient is hemodynamically unstable (such as hypotension, systolic BP <90 mm Hg or heart failure)*: DC shock. If hemodynamically stable, IV amiodarone bolus followed by IV infusion. If fails, DC shock should be done
- *To prevent recurrence*: β-blocker and oral amiodarone may be used. Correction of hypokalemia, hypomagnesemia, hypoxemia and acidosis should be done
- *If all fail*: Implantable cardioverter-defibrillator or radiofrequency ablation of focus.

Ventricular fibrillation: It is characterized by rapid, irregular, ineffective, and uncoordinated ventricular activation with no mechanical effect. There is chaotic electrical disturbance of ventricles, with impulse occurring irregularly at 300–500/min. Cardiac output falls to zero. It is the most common cause of sudden death. It may occur as a primary arrhythmia or as a complication in acute MI.

Causes: Acute MI, and electrolyte imbalance (hypokalemia and hypomagnesemia). Others—Electrocution, drowning, and drug overdose (digitalis, adrenaline and isoprenaline).

Signs: Patient is unconscious. Pulse is absent and BP is not recordable. Respiration is absent. Pupils are dilated and less or no reaction to light. Heart sounds are absent.

Treatment:
- Immediate defibrillation—200 Joules. If no response, another shock with 200 Joules. If still no response, another shock with 360 Joules. If three shocks unsuccessful—adrenaline IV, followed by cardiopulmonary resuscitation
- If defibrillator is not available—cardiopulmonary resuscitation should be given
- The patient who survives from VF in absence of any cause is at high risk of sudden death. It is treated with ICD.

HEART BLOCK

It is defined as defect in either initiation or conduction of cardiac impulse.

Sites: SA node, AV node, bundle of His and branches of bundle of His (left and right).

Types:
- SA block
- *Atrioventricular block. It is of three types*:
  - First-degree AV block
  - Second-degree AV block. Two types: (i) Mobitz type I (Wenckebach's phenomenon) and (ii) Mobitz type II
  - Complete heart block or third-degree heart block.
- *Bundle branch block*: Right bundle branch block and left bundle branch block.

Hemiblock: It means when there is block involving one of the fascicles of left bundle branch.

There are two types:
1. When left axis deviation, it is called left anterior hemiblock
2. When right axis deviation, it is called left posterior hemiblock.

Note: There may be two or three blocks. In such case, it is called bifascicular or trifascicular block.

Sinoatrial block: Failure to initiate an impulse from SA node.

Causes: Degenerative changes in elderly, IHD (involving SA node), drugs (digoxin), and increased vagal tone.

Symptoms: May be asymptomatic. May be dizziness and giddiness.

Signs: Drop beat and no heart sound at the time of drop beat.

Investigations: ECG and Holter monitoring may show the block.

Treatment: No treatment, if asymptomatic. Withdrawal of offensive drug, if any. If syncopal attack or sick sinus syndrome, permanent pacemaker should be given.

First-degree AV Block: It is the prolongation of PR >0.22 second

Causes: Normally in athlete (due to increased vagal tone), drugs (digitalis toxicity), acute MI (common in inferior MI), acute rheumatic carditis, in elderly (atherosclerosis), and hyperkalemia.

Symptoms: Usually asymptomatic. ECG shows prolonged PR interval, >0.22 second.

Treatment: No specific treatment is necessary.

Second-degree AV Block: Three types: (1) Mobitz type I (Wenckebach phenomenon), (2) Mobitz type II, and (3) 2:1 or 3:1 heart block.

Mobitz type I (Wenckebach phenomenon): Progressive prolongation of PR interval followed by drop beat.

Site of block: Higher area of AV node (proximal to bundle of His).

Causes: Physiological—in athlete, during rest, sleep (due to increased vagal tone), digoxin toxicity and acute MI (commonly inferior).

Symptoms: Usually asymptomatic, may be features of primary disease.

Sign: Pulse is irregular (drop beat occurs).

ECG findings: Progressive lengthening of PR interval followed by absent QRS complex.

Treatment: No treatment is necessary. Primary cause should be treated.

Mobitz type II: Site of lesion is in His-Purkinje system.

Cause: Acute anterior MI.

ECG: Some P waves are not followed by QRS, PR and PP interval is constant, and wide QRS.

(In 2:1 AV block, alternate P wave is conducted. It may be 3:1, 4:1). This type of AV block is rare and more severe. It is generally a sign of severe conduction system disease.

Treatment:
- *If due to inferior MI*: If asymptomatic, close monitoring and follow-up. If symptomatic, injection atropine 0.6 mg IV. If fails, temporary pacemaker. Majority will resolve in 7–10 days

- *If due to anterior MI*: Temporary pacing followed by permanent pacemaker.

COMPLETE HEART BLOCK

No impulse from atria transmitted to the ventricles. So ventricles generate their own rhythm.

Causes:
- *Acute CHB*: Acute MI (commonly inferior)
- *Chronic CHB*:
  - Progressive fibrosis of distal His-Purkinje system (Lev's disease) in elderly
  - Progressive fibrosis of proximal His-Purkinje system (Lenegre's disease) in younger
- *Other causes*: Cardiomyopathy, myocarditis, drugs (digoxin, β-blocker, amiodarone), cardiac surgery (aortic valve replacement, VSD repair), radiofrequency AV node ablation, infiltrative disease (sarcoidosis, amyloidosis, and hemochromatosis), infection (infective endocarditis, Chagas disease, Lyme disease), collagen disease (SLE and RA), congenital CHB [common in child of mother with SLE due to transplacental transfer of anti-Ro antibody/anti-Sjögren's-syndrome-related antigen A (SSA)].

Symptoms: Weakness, dizziness, giddiness, syncope (Stokes Adams attack), and breathlessness on exertion.

Signs:
- *Pulse*: Bradycardia, 20–40 beats/min (<40 beats/min), high volume, does not increase by exercise or injection atropine
- *BP*: High systolic, normal diastolic, and high pulse pressure
- *Neck vein*: Cannon waves (large "a" wave) may be present
- *Heart sounds*: Variable intensity of first heart sound
- *Murmur*: Systolic flow murmur.

ECG criteria: Atrial rate more, ventricular rate <40. PP interval is constant. No relationship between P wave and QRS complex (PR looks variable).

Treatment: If the patient is symptomatic, permanent pacemaker should be given. In congenital CHB, pulse rate is high, and no pacemaker is necessary.

Stokes–Adam attack: Syncope or blackout in patient with CHB due to ventricular asystole.

Symptoms and signs:
- Syncope or blackout with or without preceding dizziness. During attack, the patient is unconscious, looks pale and may have convulsion. If asystole persists, there may be cyanosis, absent pulse, fixed and dilated pupil, and incontinence of urine. Plantar is extensor
- Usually consciousness recovers rapidly followed by flushing.

Treatment: Permanent pacemaker.

RIGHT BUNDLE BRANCH BLOCK

ECG criteria: RSR in V1 and V2 (M pattern). QRS (wide, >0.12 second).

Causes:
- Normal variant (common)
- Coronary artery disease (acute myocardial infarction)

- Atrial septal defect
- *Others*: Right ventricular hypertrophy, chronic cor pulmonale, pulmonary embolism, cardiomyopathy, and conduction system fibrosis.

Fascicular block (hemiblock): Two types—
1. Right bundle branch block with left anterior hemiblock (block in anterior fascicle). ECG shows RBBB with left axis deviation
2. Right bundle branch block with left posterior hemiblock (block in posterior fascicle). ECG shows RBBB with right axis deviation.

LEFT BUNDLE BRANCH BLOCK

Causes: Severe coronary artery disease, acute MI, cardiomyopathy, myocarditis, aortic valve disease (stenosis or regurgitation), LV hypertrophy, and hypertension.

Symptoms: Features of primary disease.

Signs: On auscultation, there is reverse splitting of second heart sound.

Treatment: Treatment of primary cause. In acute MI, if new LBBB occurs and temporary pacemaker is indicated.

TAKAYASU'S DISEASE

It is a chronic, inflammatory, and granulomatous panarteritis of unknown cause involving the elastic arteries commonly aorta and its major branches such as carotid, ulnar, brachial, radial, and axillary. Occasionally, it may involve pulmonary artery, rarely abdominal aorta, and renal artery resulting in obstruction. It is also called pulseless disease or aortic arch syndrome.

Types: There are four types—
- *Type 1*: Involves aortic arch and its major branches
- *Type 2*: Involves descending aorta and abdominal aorta
- *Type 3*: Involves both type 1 and type 2. This may be complicated by aortic regurgitation
- *Type 4*: Involves the pulmonary arteries.

Clinical features: Common in young female, 25–30 years (F:M ratio is 8:1), more in Asians.
- In acute stage—may present with fever, malaise, weight loss, arthralgia, myalgia and high ESR
- In chronic case—dizziness, giddiness, headache, blurring of vision, syncope and claudication of upper limb. There may be features of aortic regurgitation, renal artery stenosis or anginal pain, and hypertension.

Signs: All pulses of upper limbs are absent, but present in lower limbs. BP is undetectable in upper limb and normal or high in lower limb. Bruit may be present over the carotid, also renal bruit. Fundoscopy (shows wreath-like anastomosis around the optic disk).

Investigations:
- Complete blood count (high ESR and normocytic normochromic anemia), and CRP (high)
- Chest X-ray shows cardiomegaly and widening of aorta
- MRI—helpful to detect inflammatory thickening of the affected vessel walls

- CT angiography—helpful to detect stenosis, occlusion and condition of arteries
- Aortography of aortic arch and its branches (shows narrowing, coarctation and aneurysmal dilatation)
- Serum immunoglobulin—high.

Treatment:
- Prednisolone 40–60 mg daily or 1–2 mg/kg. If difficult to taper, or in refractory case, methotrexate 25 mg/week may be given with prednisolone. Or methotrexate, mycophenolate mofetil or azathioprine may be added with prednisolone
- Cyclophosphamide may be used in resistant case
- Anti-TNF agents such as etanercept and infliximab may be given in relapse
- Reconstructive vascular surgery in selected case
- Angioplasty, stenting or bypass surgery may be done, if vascular complication occurs
- Treatment of hypertension.

Complications: Heart failure, stroke, seizure, organ failure, retinopathy and renovascular hypertension.

PACEMAKER

It is an artificial device used to electrically stimulate the heart. It is composed of two parts—battery powered generator and wire electrode (attached to the heart chamber to be stimulated, atrium or ventricle or both).

Pacemaker may be single chamber or dual chamber. Two types—Temporary and permanent.

Indications of temporary pacemaker:
- Acute inferior MI with AV block or severe bradycardia with hemodynamic change
- Acute extensive anterior MI with second- or third-degree AV block or new bifascicular block
- Atrioventricular reentry tachycardia and ventricular tachycardia can be terminated by overdrive pacing.

Indications of permanent pacemaker: Commonly CHB with syncope or Stokes Adams syndrome and sick sinus syndrome.

ECG findings (atrial pacing): There is a spike followed by P wave.

ECG findings (ventricular pacing): There is a spike followed by wide QRS (looks like LBBB).

Complications of pacemaker:
- *Early*: Pneumothorax, infection, lead displacement, cardiac tamponade and pocket hematoma
- *Late*: Infection, erosion of generator or lead, chronic pain at implant site, lead fracture, malfunction, perforation of ventricular wall, ventricular arrhythmia [premature ventricular contraction (PVC)], electromagnetic interference, pacemaker failure, pacemaker-mediated tachycardia (by dual chamber pacing), and pacemaker syndrome (by single-chamber pacing).

PULMONARY HYPERTENSION

Mean pulmonary arterial pressure >25 mm Hg at rest and >30 mm Hg during exercise.

Types:
- Primary or idiopathic pulmonary hypertension—no underlying cause. May have genetic predisposition
- Secondary pulmonary hypertension—more common than idiopathic pulmonary hypertension.

Causes:
- *Respiratory*: COPD, emphysema, chronic bronchitis, diffuse parenchymal lung disease (DPLD), and pulmonary thromboembolism
- *Cardiac*: Left-sided heart failure, MS and reversal of shunt (ASD, VSD and PDA)
- *Connective tissue disorders*: Scleroderma and SLE
- Sleep apnea syndrome and other sleep disorders
- *Drugs*: Cocaine.

Symptoms: Asymptomatic. May be shortness of breath (orthopnea or paroxysmal nocturnal dyspnea), chest pain, palpitations, cough, and hemoptysis (rarely). Fatigue, ankle swelling, dizziness and syncope.

Signs:
- Epigastric pulsation (indicates RVH)
- Palpable P2, prominent "a" wave in JVP, and left parasternal heave (indicates RVH)
- Loud P2 on auscultation, and early diastolic murmur [Graham Steel murmur due to pulmonary regurgitation (PR)].

Complications: Right-sided heart failure and cor pulmonale, and arrhythmia.

Investigations:
- CBC and ESR
- Chest X-ray P/A view (shows enlargement of pulmonary arteries) and CT scan of chest
- ECG [shows RVH and right atrial hypertrophy (RAH)], and Doppler echocardiography
- Pulmonary function test and ventilation-perfusion (V/Q) scan
- Open lung biopsy and genetic tests
- Other investigations according to suspicion of cause.

Treatment: Reduction of weight, avoid heavy exercise and smoking must be stopped. Oxygen inhalation.
- Diuretics, digoxin, and vasodilator drugs (ACE inhibitors, sildenafil and tadalafil)
- *Other drugs*: Endothelin receptor antagonists (bosentan and ambrisentan), calcium channel blockers (amlodipine and nifedipine), and anticoagulants (warfarin)
- *Surgery*: Atrial septostomy, heart-lung transplantation in selected cases, and pulmonary thromboendarterectomy.

CARDIAC ARREST

It is defined as sudden loss of cardiac function, when the heart abruptly stops beating.

Causes:
- Ventricular fibrillation (most common cause)
- Ventricular tachycardia (pulseless)
- Asystole
- Electromechanical dissociation
- *Others*: Myocardial rupture, cardiac tamponade, respiratory arrest (loss of breathing function), massive pulmonary embolism, tension pneumothorax, electrocution and drowning.

Clinical features: Sudden collapse and loss of consciousness. No pulse, no BP, and no breathing. Permanent brain damage and death can occur unless the flow of blood to the brain is restored within 5 minutes.

Treatment:
- *A*: Airway restoration
- *B*: Breathing should be ensured (mouth to mouth breathing)
- *C*: Circulation [cardiopulmonary resuscitation (CPR) should be started, 15 compression—2 breaths]
- Precordial thump
- *Defibrillation*: In ventricular fibrillation
- *Other supportive therapy*: Injection adrenaline and transvenous pacemaker.

MARFAN'S SYNDROME

It is a connective tissue disorder, inherited as autosomal dominant. Male and female are equally affected. It is characterized by triad of eye, skeletal, and cardiac abnormalities.

- *Eye*: Blue sclera, subluxation or dislocation of lens (ectopia lentis), iridodonesis (tremor of iris), heterochromia iris (various color of iris), myopia, retinal detachment and glaucoma
- *Skeletal*: Tall, lean and thin, arachnodactyly, hyperextensibility of joints, high arch palate, kyphosis, scoliosis or both, and pes planus. Pectus excavatum or carinatum or asymmetry of chest. Arm span > height. Lower segment > upper segment
- *CVS*: AR (due to aortic root dilatation and secondary to cystic medial necrosis involving aorta), MR (with MVP).

Complications: Dissecting aneurysm, infective endocarditis and heart failure.

Investigations: X-ray of chest, ECG, echocardiogram, and CT or CMR (to see aortic dilatation).

Treatment:
- *Medical treatment*:
  - β-blocker: It reduces aortic dilatation and prevents the risk of aortic rupture or dissecting aneurysm. Atenolol is more preferable
  - ACE receptor blocker: It prevents aortic root dilatation
  - Prophylaxis for infective endocarditis.
- *Surgery*: Replacement of ascending aorta and aortic valve if progressive dilatation of aorta (>5 cm)
- *Advice to patient*: Avoid strenuous exercise to prevent aortic dissection. Genetic counselling and orthopedic measures. Regular checkup and echocardiography should be done annually.

CHAPTER 2

Respiratory Diseases

BRONCHIAL ASTHMA

It is a chronic airway inflammatory disorder characterized by hyperresponsiveness of airways to various stimuli presenting with breathlessness, cough, chest tightness and wheeze. It is reversible.

Causes:
- *Genetic factors*: Asthma and atopy are common in family members
- *Allergens*: Indoor (such as house dust, mite, pet allergens, dander and fungal spores), outdoor (grass and flower pollens) and food allergens (egg, crab and fish)
- *Irritants*: Tobacco smoke, wood smoke, strong odors, perfume, sprays, cosmetics, paints and vehicle smoke
- *Upper respiratory tract infection*: Respiratory syncytial virus (RSV) or bacterial infection (*Haemophilus influenzae*)
- Occupational asthma
- *Others*: Exercise, psychological factors (anxiety and stress), drugs [nonsteroidal anti-inflammatory drugs (NSAIDs) and β-blockers] and changes in weather or temperature
- *Conditions associated with asthma*: Atopic dermatitis, allergic rhinitis and allergic conjunctivitis.

Symptoms:
- Recurrent dyspnea, cough with mucoid sputum and wheeze. May be spontaneous or precipitated by exercise, cold weather, exposure to allergens or pollens and infection
- Diurnal variation, symptoms more in early morning and during sleep at night called "nocturnal asthma"
- Cough may be the only symptom, called "cough variant asthma".

Signs: Breath sound is vesicular with prolonged expiration. Multiple rhonchi in both inspiration and expiration, present all over the lungs.

Investigations:
- *X-ray of chest*: Normal in early

- *Lung function tests*:
  - Spirometry: Forced expiratory volume in 1 second (FEV1) and forced vital capacity (FVC) (obstructive airway disease)
  - FEV1 >15% increase after bronchodilator (reversibility test)
  - Peak expiratory flow rate (PEFR): Patient should record after rising in morning and before retiring in evening. Diurnal variation >20% (low value in the morning, called "morning dipping").
- *Others*: Complete blood count (CBC) (high eosinophil), sputum for eosinophil (high), serum immunoglobulin E (IgE) (high in atopic patient), skin prick test to identify allergic factors and methacholine provocation test.

Types of bronchial asthma:

There are four groups:
- *Intermittent or episodic asthma*: Between attacks, the patient is symptom free
- *Persistent or chronic asthma*: Frequent asthmatic attacks
- Acute exacerbation
- *Special variants*: Five types—(1) cough variant asthma, (2) exercise-induced asthma, (3) occupational asthma, (4) drug-induced asthma, and (5) seasonal asthma

Management of bronchial asthma:
- *General measures*: Avoid smoking, allergens (house dust, mite, pets and pollens) and drugs which aggravate asthma
- *Drug therapy*: Bronchodilator therapy and preventive drug therapy.

Drugs used in bronchial asthma:
- β_2 *adrenoceptor agonist*: Short-acting (salbutamol and terbutaline) and long-acting (salmeterol and formoterol). Given as inhalation, nebulized solution or dry powder
- *Anticholinergic drug*: Ipratropium bromide or oxitropium bromide (as inhaler or nebulizer, may be combined with salbutamol)
- *Methyl xanthines*: Theophylline, aminophylline and doxofylline
- *Corticosteroid*: Inhaled beclomethasone dipropionate, budesonide, fluticasone propionate or mometasone furoate. Combined corticosteroid and long-acting β_2 agonist (budesonide plus formoterol or fluticasone and salmeterol). Oral prednisolone and intravenous (IV) hydrocortisone
- *Chromones*: Sodium cromoglycate, nedocromil sodium or ketotifen in mild asthma
- *Leukotriene receptor antagonist*: Oral montelukast and zafirlukast
- *Anti-IgE*: Omalizumab is effective in allergic asthma.

Acute Severe Asthma

It is defined as severe acute persistent attack of asthma without any remission, not controlled by conventional bronchodilator. Previously, it was called "status asthmaticus".

Signs:
- Inability to complete a sentence in one breath
- Respiratory rate ≥25/min
- Pulse rate ≥110/min (pulsus paradoxus may be present)
- PEFR <50% of predicted normal (<200 L/min).

Respiratory Diseases

Treatment:
- *High flow O_2*: 40–60%
- Nebulized salbutamol or terbutaline, repeated every 20–30 minutes or if necessary. Nebulized ipratropium bromide may be added
- Injection hydrocortisone 200 mg IV 6 hourly. When improves, oral prednisolone 60 mg daily for 2 weeks, then taper
- If no response, magnesium sulfate IV 1.2–2 g over 20 minutes
- In some cases, injection aminophylline 5 mg/kg loading dose over 20 minutes, then continuous infusion at 1 mg/kg/h
- If no response, the patient should be shifted to intensive care unit (ICU) for assisted ventilation.

Cough Variant Asthma

It is a type of asthma in which cough is the only symptom, mostly at night. Cough may be increased with exercise, exposure to dust, strong fragrances or cold air.

Treatment:
- Allergic rhinitis should be treated, if present
- Gastroesophageal reflux disease should be treated with proton pump inhibitor (omeprazole) and prokinetic agent (domperidone)
- Environmental factors like cold, dust and fume should be avoided
- Nedocromil sodium is effective.

Exercise-induced Asthma

It occurs during exercise.

Treatment: Before exercise, salbutamol, sodium cromoglycate or nedocromil sodium should be used. Inhaled corticosteroid twice daily for 8–12 weeks reduces severity.

Occupational Asthma

It means asthma occurs due to inhaled occupation related agents at the work place. Main feature is symptoms that worsen on work days and improve on holidays. Found in chemical workers, farmers, grain handlers, cigarette manufacturers, press and printing workers, laboratory workers, poultry breeders, and wood and bakery workers.

Treatment: Avoidance of further exposure using mask at work. If no response, management of asthma should be given.

Drug-induced asthma

After use of certain drugs, asthmatic attack may occur, such as aspirin, β-blocker and NSAID. These drugs should be avoided.

Management of asthma with other diseases:
- *Asthma with diabetes mellitus*: Any drugs are used. Steroid can be used if needed, regular sugar monitoring should be done. In severe acute asthma, insulin therapy may be necessary. Metformin should be avoided in uncontrolled asthma and contraindicated in acute severe asthma
- *Asthma in pregnancy*:
  - During pregnancy: All inhalers are safe and effective. $β_2$ agonist (both short and long-acting), inhaled steroid, theophylline, oral

prednisolone and sodium cromoglycate are safe. If the patient was getting leukotriene receptor blockers (e.g. montelukast and zafirlukast), it can be continued
- During labor: Treatment as usual should be continued. If patient is on prednisolone, it should be changed to IV hydrocortisone, 100 mg 6–8 hourly. Breastfeeding should be continued.
- *Asthma with hypertension*: β-blocker should be avoided. Calcium channel blocker or angiotensin-receptor blocker (losartan and valsartan) may be used. Angiotensin-converting enzyme (ACE) inhibitor is avoided as it may induce cough.

BRONCHIECTASIS

It is the abnormal, permanent dilatation of one or more bronchi with destruction of bronchial wall proximal to the terminal bronchiole. Three types are—Saccular or cystic (more severe form), cylindrical and fusiform. The most common site of bronchiectasis is left lower lobe and lingula.

Causes:
- *Congenital or hereditary*: Cystic fibrosis, Kartagener syndrome (triad of bronchiectasis, dextrocardia and sinusitis or frontal sinus agenesis), primary ciliary dyskinesia, hypogammaglobulinemia, yellow nail syndrome and Young's syndrome
- *Acquired*: In children, pneumonia (complicating measles and whooping cough), primary tuberculosis (TB) and foreign body. In adults, bronchial neoplasm, pulmonary TB and recurrent aspiration.

Symptoms: Recurrent cough with profuse expectoration of sputum, more marked in morning after waking from sleep and hemoptysis.

Signs: Generalized clubbing in fingers and toes. In chest, multiple coarse crepitations in affected side, altered by cough.

Dry Bronchiectasis (Bronchiectasis Sicca)

It is a type of bronchiectasis in which dry cough is associated with intermittent episodes of hemoptysis.

Investigations: Chest X-ray (CXR) posteroanterior (PA) view (shows ring with or without fluid level) and high-resolution computed tomography (HRCT) scan (definitive).

Treatment:
- Postural drainage, keeping the affected part remaining up and percussion over it, done for 5–10 minutes, once or twice daily. Chest physiotherapy
- Antibiotic, if infection
- Bronchodilator drugs. Nebulized salbutamol may be used. Inhaled or oral steroid can decrease the rate of progression
- Surgery (lobectomy). Done in unilateral, localized to single lobe.

Indications of surgery: Unilateral, localized to single lobe, severe and recurrent hemoptysis.

Complications: Secondary infection, lung abscess, pleural effusion, empyema or pneumothorax, pulmonary hypertension, cor pulmonale, respiratory failure, amyloidosis, brain abscess and aspergilloma.

BRONCHIAL CARCINOMA

Types of bronchial carcinoma:
Two types are:
1. *Small cell carcinoma*: 20%
2. *Nonsmall cell carcinoma*: Squamous cell carcinoma (35%), adenocarcinoma (30%) and large cell carcinoma (15%).

Causes or risk factors:
- Cigarette smoking; even passive smoking can cause
- Exposure to asbestos, silica, beryllium, cadmium, chromium, arsenic, radiation, petroleum products and oils, and coal tar
- Adenocarcinoma may develop in nonsmokers and in old scar.

Symptoms: Usually in elderly patients with history of smoking.
- *Due to lung lesion*: Cough. changing pattern of regular cough is highly suspicious. Hemoptysis, breathlessness and chest pain
- *Due to local spread in mediastinum*: Hoarseness of voice, bovine cough (due to recurrent laryngeal nerve palsy), dysphagia (due to esophageal involvement), puffiness with plethoric face [due to superior vena cava (SVC) obstruction] and Horner's syndrome (due to involvement of cervical sympathetic chain). If pericardium is invaded, there may be pericardial effusion. Stridor, if lower trachea, carina, and main bronchi are compressed by tumor
- Features of distant metastasis (in liver, brain and bone)
- Nonmetastatic extrapulmonary manifestations
- *General features of malignancy*: Anorexia, weight loss, malaise and fatigue.

Nonmetastatic extrapulmonary manifestations (paraneoplastic syndrome):
- *Endocrine (10%, more in small cell carcinoma)*: Syndrome of inappropriate antidiuretic hormone, adrenocorticotropic hormone secretion causing Cushing's syndrome, carcinoid syndrome, hypercalcemia and gynecomastia. Rarely, hypoglycemia and thyrotoxicosis
- *Neurological*: Peripheral neuropathy (usually sensory-motor), cerebellar and cortical degeneration, myelopathy and retinal blindness
- *Musculoskeletal*: Polymyositis or dermatomyositis, myasthenic myopathic syndrome (Eaton–Lambert syndrome), and clubbing and hypertrophic osteoarthropathy
- *Hematological*: Migrating thrombophlebitis, disseminated intravascular coagulation, thrombotic thrombocytopenic purpura, normocytic normochromic anemia, occasionally hemolytic and eosinophilia
- *Heart*: Marantic endocarditis (nonbacterial, thrombotic or verrucous endocarditis)
- *Skin*: Acanthosis nigricans, dermatomyositis and herpes zoster
- *Renal*: Nephrotic syndrome due to membranous glomerulonephritis (rare)
- *Metabolic*: Loss of weight, lassitude and anorexia.

Investigations:
- X-ray of chest PA view and computed tomography (CT) scan of chest
- Sputum for malignant cells

- CT-guided fine needle aspiration cytology (FNAC) and FNAC (or biopsy) of lymph nodes (if present)
- Fiber optic bronchoscopy and biopsy
- Positron emission tomography scan
- *To see metastasis*: Ultrasonography (USG) of whole abdomen, X-ray of skull and isotope bone scan.

Treatment: Staging should be done before therapy.
- *Nonsmall cell carcinoma*: Surgery, if the tumor is localized to a lobe or segment. If not possible, radiotherapy or chemotherapy or combination should be given. In squamous carcinoma, radiotherapy. Chemotherapy is less helpful in nonsmall cell type
- *Small cell carcinoma*: Metastasis occurs early. Surgery is less helpful. Chemotherapy is given. Radiotherapy may be added. Chemotherapy—CDV (cyclophosphamide, doxorubicin and vincristine) or CE (cisplatin plus etoposide), every 3 weeks for 3–6 cycles
- *Other treatments*: Usually palliative. Laser therapy, endobronchial therapy, radiofrequency thermal ablation and pleural drainage or pleurodesis (in pleural effusion).

PNEUMONIA (CONSOLIDATION)

It is defined as inflammation of the lung parenchyma characterized by accumulation of secretion and inflammatory cells in alveoli.

Types of pneumonia (consolidation):
- *Anatomically two types*:
  - Lobar: Commonly involves one or more lobe
  - Lobular (bronchopneumonia): Characterized by patchy alveolar opacity with bronchial and bronchiolar inflammation, commonly involves both lower lobes.
- *Clinically four types*:
  - Community-acquired pneumonia (CAP)
  - Nosocomial (hospital acquired)
  - Pneumonia in immunocompromised
  - Suppurative and aspiration pneumonia.

Causes of community-acquired pneumonia:
- *Typical organism*: *Streptococcus pneumoniae* (50%), *Klebsiella pneumoniae, H. influenzae* and *Staphylococcus aureus*
- *Atypical organism*: *Mycoplasma pneumoniae, Legionella pneumophila, Chlamydia psittaci* and *Coxiella burnetii*
- *Others*: Viral (*influenza, parainfluenza, measles, respiratory syncytial virus in infancy, varicella and cytomegalovirus*) and *Actinomyces israelii*.

Symptoms: Fever, may be high with chill and rigor. Cough, initially dry. Later on, expectoration (during resolution). Rusty sputum (due to *S. pneumoniae*). May be dyspnea, hemoptysis and pleuritic chest pain.

Signs (on affected site):
- *Inspection*: Restricted movement
- *Palpation*: Vocal fremitus is increased
- *Percussion*: Dullness (woody)
- *Auscultation*: Breath sound is bronchial. Vocal resonance is increased with whispering pectoriloquy. Pleural rub (due to pleurisy) and crepitations (during resolution).

Complications of pneumonia:
- *Pulmonary*: Lung abscess, pleurisy, pleural effusion, empyema thoracis, pneumothorax by *S. aureus* and acute respiratory distress syndrome (ARDS)
- *Cardiovascular*: Pericarditis, myocarditis, endocarditis, arrhythmia and peripheral circulatory failure
- *Neurological*: Meningism and meningoencephalitis
- *Musculoskeletal*: Septic arthritis
- *Gastrointestinal tract*: Meteorism (gaseous distension of stomach, intestine or abdomen).

Causes of slow or delayed resolution of pneumonia: Delayed resolution means when the physical signs persist for >2 weeks and radiological features persist for >4 weeks after antibiotic therapy.

Causes: Incorrect diagnosis, improper antibiotic or insufficient dose, fungal, tubercular or atypical pneumonia, bronchial obstruction (bronchial carcinoma, adenoma and foreign body), empyema or atelectasis, and immunocompromised patient [human immunodeficiency virus (HIV), diabetes mellitus (DM), lymphoma, leukemia and multiple myeloma].

Causes of recurrent pneumonia (three or more separate attack):
- Bronchial obstruction (bronchial carcinoma, adenoma and foreign body) and bronchiectasis
- Aspiration (achalasia cardia and pharyngeal pouch)
- Immunocompromised patient (HIV, DM, lymphoma, leukemia and multiple myeloma).

Investigations:
- Complete blood count and erythrocyte sedimentation rate (ESR)
- *X-ray of chest*: Homogeneous opacity with air bronchogram
- *Sputum*: Gram staining and culture and sensitivity (C/S) (aerobic and anaerobic)
- Blood C/S (positive in pneumococcal pneumonia)
- Arterial blood gas analysis
- *Others (according to etiology)*: Mycoplasma antibody [agglutination and complement fixation test (CFT)], Coombs test and C/S in special media. Antibody against virus, chlamydia, and legionella. Urinary legionella pneumophila antigen. C-reactive protein (high).

Treatment of pneumonia: Sputum should be sent for C/S before starting antibiotic.
- *General treatment*: Rest, O_2 therapy, adequate hydration and chest physiotherapy
- Antibiotic (empirically with suspicion of cause) as follows.

Community-acquired pneumonia:
- *Mild CAP*:
  - Amoxicillin 500 mg 8 hourly orally or erythromycin 500 mg 6 hourly or clarithromycin 500 mg 12 hourly or azithromycin 500 mg daily
  - If *S. aureus* is suspected: Clarithromycin 500 mg 12 hourly orally or IV, plus flucloxacillin 1–2 g 6 hourly IV
  - If *K. pneumoniae* is suspected: Ciprofloxacin 200 mg IV 12 hourly plus gentamycin 60–80 mg IV 8 hourly or gentamycin plus ceftazidime 1 g IV 8 hourly
    Duration of treatment: 7–10 days (up to 14 days)

- If *mycoplasma, legionella* or atypical organism is suspected: Clarithromycin 500 mg 12 hourly orally or erythromycin 500 mg 6 hourly orally or doxycycline may be used
- Duration of treatment: 2–3 weeks.
- *Severe CAP*: Clarithromycin 500 mg twice daily IV or erythromycin 500 mg 6 hourly IV plus co-amoxiclav or cefuroxime or ceftriaxone.

Nosocomial pneumonia: New episode of pneumonia occurring at least 2 days after admission in the hospital is called nosocomial pneumonia. If occurs within 4–5 days of admission (early onset), organisms are similar to CAP. If occurs later (late onset), organisms, *Escherichia coli*, *K. pneumoniae* and *Pseudomonas aeruginosa*, are common. Others—*S. aureus* including methicillin resistant *S. aureus* (MRSA). Anaerobic organisms.

Predisposing factors: Elderly patient, bedbound, unconscious, postoperative case, malignancy, DM, use of steroid, cytotoxic drugs, antibiotics, prolonged anesthesia, intubation, tracheostomy, IV cannula, achalasia of cardia, vomiting and bulbar or vocal cord palsy.

Treatment:
Empirically, antibiotic should be started which cover Gram-negative organisms:
- *In early onset*: If no antibiotic was given, co-amoxiclav or cefuroxime may be given. If antibiotic was given, piperacillin/tazobactam or cefotaxime should be added
- *In late onset*: Antibiotic must cover Gram-negative organisms, *S. aureus* (including MRSA) and anaerobes:
  - Cefotaxime with gentamicin or aztreonam with flucloxacillin
  - If MRSA: IV vancomycin or oral doxycycline, rifampicin or linezolid
  - If pseudomonas: IV ciprofloxacin or ceftazidime or doripenem, carbapenem (meropenem)
  - Chest physiotherapy and oxygen, fluid and nutritional support.

Bronchopneumonia: It is defined as widespread diffused patchy alveolar opacity associated with bronchial and bronchiolar inflammation, often affecting both lower lobes. In children, it occurs as a complication of measles or whooping cough and in elderly, complication following bronchitis or influenza.

Atypical pneumonia: When pneumonia is caused by mycoplasma, legionella, coxiella or chlamydia, constitutional symptoms are more than respiratory symptoms.

Features are gradual onset, dry cough, and low-grade fever. Constitutional symptoms like headache, myalgia, fatigue, nausea and vomiting. Less physical finding in the chest.

Investigations: White blood cell (normal), CXR (involves lower lobe, may be bilateral patchy consolidation) and cold agglutinin (positive in 50%). Rising antibody titer for *M. pneumoniae*.

Extrapulmonary complications of *M. pneumoniae*:
- Maculopapular skin rash, erythema multiforme and Stevens-Johnson syndrome
- Myocarditis and pericarditis
- Hemolytic anemia (Coombs test may be positive) and thrombocytopenia

- Meningoencephalitis, Guillain-Barré syndrome (GBS) and other neurological abnormalities
- Myalgia and arthralgia
- Hepatitis and gastrointestinal symptoms like vomiting and diarrhea.

Treatment: Clarithromycin 500 mg twice daily orally or IV or erythromycin 500 mg 6 hourly orally or IV for 7–10 days. Or, doxycycline 100 mg twice daily. Or, Rifampicin 600 mg 12 hourly orally for 7–10 days.

CHRONIC BRONCHITIS

It is defined as "presence of cough, productive of sputum, not attributable to other causes, on most of the days, for three consecutive months, at least for two successive years".

Causes: Smoking, exposure to dust, fume, foggy environment (may be occupational), dampness, sudden change in temperature and infection (*H. influenzae, S. pneumoniae and Moraxella catarrhalis*).

Symptoms: Cough with mucoid or mucopurulent sputum, chest tightness and breathlessness on exertion. In advanced stage, features of pulmonary hypertension and cor pulmonale.

Signs: The patient looks blue bloater (cyanosed and edematous). Breath sound is vesicular with prolonged expiration, plenty of rhonchi in both lung fields.

Complications: Emphysema, pulmonary hypertension, cor pulmonale and respiratory failure.

Investigations:
- Complete blood count, CXR PA view, electrocardiography (ECG), blood gas analysis
- *Lung function tests*: FEV1 and FVC (reduced). Ratio of FEV1—FVC (reduced) and PEFR (reduced)
- CT scan of chest in some cases.

Treatment: Smoking must be stopped, avoid air pollution (dust and fume). Control of infection with appropriate antibiotic.
- *Bronchodilator*: Inhaled β agonist— salbutamol and terbutaline. Inhaled ipratropium, tiotropium and oxitropium. Long-acting β agonist— salmeterol and formoterol. Oral theophylline may be used
- *Inhaled corticosteroid*: Beclomethasone or budesonide or fluticasone
- In severe case, oral prednisolone 30 mg for 2 weeks, followed by maintenance dose
- Mucolytic agents like bromhexine or N-acetylcysteine may be given
- *Other measures*: Chest physiotherapy, exercise and weight reduction, if obese, long-term domiciliary oxygen and pulmonary rehabilitation. Annual influenza vaccine, 5-yearly pneumococcal vaccine and *H. influenzae* vaccine may be given.

Treatment of acute exacerbations:
- Nebulized bronchodilator (salbutamol, terbutaline and ipratropium bromide)
- Oxygen inhalation (24%, 1–3 L/min)
- Intravenous hydrocortisone. When improved, oral prednisolone
- Antibiotic to control infection.

ACUTE BRONCHITIS

Symptoms: Dry or productive cough, fever may be present, if secondary infection.

Signs: Breath sound is vesicular with prolonged expiration, multiple rhonchi in both lungs.

Treatment: Smoking must be stopped; hot drinks such as tea and coffee; steam or tincture benzoin co-inhalation to relieve cough. Anti-histamine may be used. Antibiotic may be used, if secondary infection. Oral aminophylline, theophylline and ketotifen may be used.

ACUTE RESPIRATORY DISTRESS SYNDROME

It is defined as severe diffuse acute inflammatory process in lungs associated with hypoxemia, in which there is damage of both capillary endothelium and alveolar epithelium causing noncardiogenic pulmonary edema. There is increased capillary permeability, accumulation of protein rich cellular fluid within alveoli, alveolar collapse and reduced lung compliance which results in hypoxemia due to ventilation-perfusion mismatch and increased pulmonary shunt.

Causes: Aspiration of gastric contents, pneumonia, blast injury, inhalational injury (smoke or corrosive gases), fat embolism, amniotic fluid embolism, near-drowning, septicemia, multiple trauma, acute pancreatitis, cardiopulmonary bypass, severe burns, major transfusion reaction, anaphylaxis and obstetric crisis (eclampsia and pre-eclampsia).

Symptoms: Dyspnea, cough and tachypnea.

Signs: Cyanosis, bilateral extensive crepitations in both lungs.

Investigations: Arterial blood gas analysis shows hypoxemia and hypocapnia. CXR shows diffused bilateral fluffy opacities (mostly peripheral).

Treatment: Patient should be treated in ICU.
- High flow oxygen via mask or endotracheal tube
- Treatment of underlying cause
- Broad spectrum antibiotic, if sepsis
- Mechanical ventilation is usually necessary
- *Steroid*: Methylprednisolone 500 mg to 1 g in 5% DA 200 cc IV for 3–5 days.

EMPHYSEMA

It is the permanent distension of alveoli with destruction of their walls distal to the terminal bronchioles.

Causes: Smoking, cold, dust (centrilobular) and α_1-antitrypsin deficiency.

Symptoms: Common in elderly smokers. Breathlessness on exertion and minimum cough with lip pursing.

Signs:
- *Inspections*:
  - The patient is dyspneic with lip pursing
  - Barrel-shaped chest with indrawing of lower intercostal space during inspiration
  - Horizontal ribs with wide intercostal spaces
  - Wide subcostal angle. Prominent sternomastoid and scalene muscles

- Suprasternal and supraclavicular excavation during inspiration, tracheal tug.
- *Palpation*: Reduced cricosternal distance (length of trachea above suprasternal notch). Apex beat cannot be palpated. Vocal fremitus is reduced on both sides
- *Percussion*: Increased resonance in both lung fields, upper border of liver dullness (lower down) and cardiac dullness (obliterated)
- *Auscultation*: Breath sound (reduced vesicular with prolonged expiration). No added sound.

Investigations:
- X-ray of chest PA view
- *Lung function tests*: FEV1 and FVC are reduced. Ratio of FEV1—FVC is reduced. PEFR—reduced. Lung volume with increased TLC and RV
- *Arterial blood gas analysis*: Low PCO_2, low PO_2 and impaired gas transfer of CO
- *Other investigations*: CBC, ESR and HRCT of chest. In young patient, serum α_1 antitrypsin may be done. ECG, Echocardiography.

Treatment:
- Smoking must be stopped
- *For breathlessness*: Inhaled salbutamol or ipratropium or tiotropium or oxitropium. If no response, inhaled beclomethasone. In severe case, oral prednisolone 30 mg for 2 weeks, followed by maintenance dose
- Antibiotic, if secondary infection
- *Others*: In chronic cough—mucolytic therapy. Domiciliary O_2 may be given. Vaccination, annual influenza vaccine, 5-yearly pneumococcal vaccine, and *H. influenzae* vaccine may be given.

PLEURAL EFFUSION

It means accumulation of excessive amount of fluid in pleural cavity.
- *Four common causes are*: TB, parapneumonic, bronchial carcinoma and pulmonary infarction
- *Other causes are*: Lymphoma, systemic lupus erythematosus (SLE), liver abscess bursting in pleural cavity, rheumatoid arthritis, congestive cardiac failure, nephrotic syndrome and Meigs syndrome (triad of ovarian fibroma, ascites and right-sided pleural effusion).

Causes of bilateral effusion:
- All causes of transudative effusion [congestive cardiac failure (CCF), nephrotic syndrome, cirrhosis of liver and hypoproteinemia]
- *Others*: Collagen diseases (rheumatoid arthritis and SLE), lymphoma, bilateral extensive pulmonary TB.

Causes of recurrent pleural effusion: Bronchial carcinoma, lymphoma, collagen diseases (rheumatoid arthritis and SLE), all causes of transudate.

Types of pleural effusion:
According to color:
- Serous (hydrothorax)
- Straw
- Purulent (empyema or pyothorax)
- Milky or chylous (chylothorax)
- Pleural effusion may be exudative or transudative.

Causes of exudative effusion (pleural fluid protein >3 g%): TB, parapneumonic, bronchial carcinoma, pulmonary infarction, lymphoma and collagen diseases (rheumatoid arthritis and SLE).

Causes of transudative effusion (pleural fluid protein <3 g%): CCF, nephrotic syndrome, cirrhosis of liver and hypoproteinemia.

Symptoms: May by asymptomatic. Cough, chest pain, breathlessness and heaviness in the chest.

Signs (in chest):
- *Inspection*: Restricted movement in affected side
- *Palpation*: Trachea and apex beat (shifted to the opposite side). Vocal fremitus (reduced or absent in affected side). Chest expansion is reduced
- *Percussion*: Stony dull in affected side
- *Auscultation*: Breath sound (diminished or absent), vocal resonance (diminished or absent).

Investigations:
- Chest X-ray PA view (if small effusion, lateral decubitus view)
- Complete blood count and ESR (high ESR in TB, leukocytosis in pneumonia)
- Mantoux test (MT)
- Aspiration of fluid for analysis:
    - Physical appearance (straw-colored, serous, hemorrhagic and chylous)
    - Gram staining, cytology (routine), exfoliative cytology (malignant cells) and C/S
    - Biochemistry (protein and sugar) and adenosine deaminase (ADA) (high in TB)
    - Acid-fast bacillus (AFB) and mycobacterial C/S.
- Others (of pleural fluid), according to suspicion of causes:
    - Cholesterol, lactate dehydrogenase (LDH) and rheumatoid factor (in RA)
    - Amylase (high in acute pancreatitis, esophageal rupture and malignancy)
    - Triglyceride (in chylothorax).
- Pleural biopsy (positive in 80% cases in TB, 40–60% cases in bronchial carcinoma)
- *If palpable lymph node*: FNAC or biopsy (for lymphoma and metastasis)
- *Other investigations according to suspicion of causes*: Antinuclear antibody, anti-dsDNA (SLE), liver function test (chronic liver disease), urine for protein and serum total protein (nephrotic syndrome), and CT scan in some cases.

Treatment:
- *If TB*: Anti-TB therapy plus prednisolone 20–30 mg daily for 4–6 weeks
- *If parapneumonic*: Aspiration of fluid. Antibiotics should be given
- *If malignancy*: Treatment accordingly. If recurrent effusion, pleurodesis is necessary.

EMPYEMA

It means presence of pus in the pleural space. Clinically, it looks like pleural effusion.

Causes: Bacterial pneumonia, lung abscess (bursting in pleural cavity), bronchiectasis, TB, secondary infection after aspiration of pleural fluid, rupture of subphrenic or liver abscess and infected hemothorax.

Symptoms:
- High fever, sometimes hectic, may be associated with chill, rigor and sweating
- Malaise and weight loss. Pleuritic chest pain, breathlessness and cough
- Copious purulent sputum if empyema ruptures into a bronchus (bronchopleural fistula).

Signs: Patient is toxic, emaciated, tachypneic, tachycardia and clubbing. In chest, signs of pleural effusion (as above).

Investigations: CXR PA view. CBC, ESR (high ESR in TB, leukocytosis in pneumonia) and MT. Aspiration of fluid and analysis (as in pleural fluid).

Treatment:
- *Nontuberculous*:
  - Drainage of pus with wide bore intercostal tube using water seal drainage
  - Antibiotics for 2-6 weeks. IV co-amoxyclav or cefuroxime plus metronidazole. May be given according to C/S
  - Surgical intervention if pus is thick or loculated.
- *Tuberculous empyema*: Antitubercular drug. Wide bore needle aspiration or intercostal tube drainage. Sometimes surgical ablation of pleura.

LUNG ABSCESS

It is the localized area of suppuration within the lung parenchyma that leads to parenchymal destruction, manifested radiologically as cavity with air fluid level.

Causes:
- Aspiration of nasopharyngeal or oropharyngeal contents such as in vomiting, anesthesia, tooth extraction, tonsillectomy, unconscious patient, alcoholism and achalasia of cardia
- Specific infections (*S. pneumoniae* type 3, *S. aureus*, *K. pneumoniae*, and fungal). In HIV, *Pneumocystis jirovecii* and *Cryptococcus neoformans*
- Bronchial obstruction by carcinoma, adenoma and foreign body
- Infection in pulmonary infarction
- Spread from liver abscess and subphrenic abscess (due to transdiaphragmatic spread)
- Hematogenous from other infection as septic emboli (pelvic abscess, salpingitis, right-sided endocarditis and IV drug abuse).

Symptoms:
- Cough with profuse foul-smelling sputum, may be fetid (due to anaerobic infection)
- Hemoptysis and chest pain (pleuritic)
- High fever, chill and rigor with profuse sweating. Malaise, weakness and weight loss.

Signs: Depends on site. If deep-seated within the lung parenchyma, there may not be any physical findings. If it is near the surface, findings are:
- Features of consolidation, usually
- Rarely, features of cavitation

- Sometimes, combined features of consolidation and cavitation, if large abscess.

Investigations:
- Complete blood count (leukocytosis) and blood sugar
- X-ray of chest (cavity with air fluid level)
- Sputum for Gram staining, C/S (aerobic and anaerobic), AFB, fungus and malignant cells
- Bronchoscopy (to exclude mass and foreign body), CT or MRI (in some cases).

Treatment: Sputum is sent for C/S and broad spectrum antibiotic should be started.
- Clindamycin 600 mg IV 8 hourly or coamoxiclav orally 8 hourly or amoxicillin 500 mg 8 hourly. Add metronidazole (500 mg orally or IV 8-12 hourly)
- Or, cefuroxime 1 g IV 6 hourly plus metronidazole 500 mg IV 8 hourly
- In MRSA, vancomycin 15 mg/kg IV 12 hourly or linezolid 600 mg IV 12 hourly
- If improves, continue the therapy. If no response, antibiotic given according to be C/S finding
- Treatment continued for 4–6 weeks
- If no response to medical therapy, percutaneous aspiration (USG or CT guided). Sometimes, lobectomy may be done (if no clinical response, increasing size of abscess, massive hemorrhage and hemoptysis)
- General measures for fever, weakness and dehydration. Postural drainage and chest physiotherapy.

SUPERIOR VENACAVAL OBSTRUCTION

Causes:
- Bronchial carcinoma (common, in 75%)
- Lymphoma (in early age, also in the elderly)
- *Other causes*: Retrosternal thyroid, thymoma, mediastinal fibrosis, metastasis to the mediastinum, giant aortic aneurysm, carcinoma of esophagus, rarely thrombosis, invasion by malignancy and chronic constrictive pericarditis.

Symptoms:
- Breathlessness, cough, hoarseness of voice, stridor and dysphagia
- Flushing, red, puffy and edematous face
- Headache (early morning), which becomes severe with coughing. May be syncope, dizziness or blackout, stupor and seizure (due to increased intracranial pressure).

Signs:
- *Face*: Edematous or puffy, red, plethoric and cyanosed
- *Eyes*: Periorbital edema, red eyes, congested conjunctiva (blood shot eyes) and chemosis (conjunctival edema)
- *Neck*: Swollen, neck veins are engorged and nonpulsatile
- Visible tortuous veins in chest wall and abdomen, flow is downward
- Upper limb may be edematous with prominent engorged veins.

Investigations: CXR, CT or MRI of chest. Sputum for malignant cells. If palpable lymph node—FNAC or biopsy.

Treatment:
According to cause:
- *If bronchial carcinoma*: Radiotherapy in nonsmall cell carcinoma and chemotherapy for small cell carcinoma
- *If lymphoma*: Treatment should be given accordingly (usually chemotherapy)
- *To relieve edema*: IV furosemide, head should be raised. Dexamethasone may be used
- *To relieve severe obstruction*: Balloon angioplasty and expandable metallic stent may be used (placed in SVC) as palliative measure.

PNEUMOTHORAX

It means presence of air in pleural cavity.

Causes:
- *Spontaneous*:
  - Primary: Without underlying lung disease. May be due to rupture of apical subpleural bleb, rupture of subpleural emphysematous bullae or pulmonary end of pleural adhesion
  - Secondary: Due to pre-existing lung disease, such as chronic obstructive pulmonary disease (COPD) and TB, lung abscess, acute severe asthma, bronchial carcinoma and pulmonary infarction.
- *Traumatic*: During aspiration of pleural fluid, thoracic surgery, lung or pleural biopsy and chest wall injury.

Three types (anatomical):
- *Closed*: Communication between lung and pleural space is sealed off. Trapped air is slowly reabsorbed, lung re-expands in 2–4 weeks
- *Open*: Communication between lung and pleural space persists (bronchopleural fistula). Infection is common. Hydropneumothorax and empyema develop
- *Valvular*: Communication between pleura and lung, which acts as one-way valve. Air enters into the pleural space during inspiration, but does not come out during expiration.

Symptoms: Sudden unilateral pleuritic chest pain and breathlessness.

Signs (in chest):
In affected side:
- *Inspection*: Restricted movement of chest
- *Palpation*: Trachea and apex beat shifted to opposite side. Vocal fremitus reduced in affected side. Chest expansion reduced in affected side
- *Percussion*: Hyper-resonance
- *Auscultation*: Breath sound diminished or absent, vocal resonance diminished or absent.

Investigations: CXR PA view. Sometimes, CT scan of chest.

Treatment:
- *In primary pneumothorax*: If small, spontaneous resolution occurs. Follow up at 2 weeks interval (repeat CXR). Avoid strenuous exercise. If moderate to large with breathlessness, percutaneous needle aspiration (2–5 liter)
- *In secondary pneumothorax*: All patients should be hospitalized for observation

- If small (<1 cm) or isolated apical pneumothorax in asymptomatic patient, observation
- If age <50 years, asymptomatic or small pneumothorax, simple aspiration. If successful, 24 hours observation, then discharge. If unsuccessful, intercostal drain tube
- If age >50 years, symptomatic or large pneumothorax, intercostal drain tube should be inserted.
- *Open pneumothorax*: Surgery
- Tension pneumothorax (see below).

Advice to the patient: Must stop smoking. Avoid air travel for 6 weeks after normal CXR. Diving should be permanently avoided.

Tension pneumothorax

It is a valvular type of pneumothorax, where there is communication between lung and pleural cavity with one-way valve, which allows air to enter during inspiration and prevents to leave during expiration. It results in compression of lung, shifting of mediastinum to opposite side, compression of heart and opposite lung also.

Features: Severe and progressively increasing dyspnea, features of shock (hypotension, central cyanosis and tachycardia), severe chest pain, tachypnea and pulsus paradoxus. Raised jugular venous pressure (JVP), engorged neck vein due to compression of heart, death may occur within minutes.

Treatment: High flow oxygen inhalation.
- Immediate insertion of wide bore needle in 2nd intercostal space in mid-clavicular line
- Intrathoracic tube is inserted in 4th, 5th or 6th intercostal space in midaxillary line, tip should be in apical direction, connected to underwater seal or one-way Heimlich valve
- Patient should be kept propped up. Morphine 5–10 mg subcutaneously
- If bubbling ceases, repeat CXR. If lung re-expands, tube may be removed
- If no response or continued bubbling for 5–7 days, surgical treatment may be necessary.

SARCOIDOSIS

It is a multisystem granulomatous disease of unknown cause, characterized by noncaseating granuloma in different organs. Cause is unknown. Histologically, noncaseating granuloma.

Symptoms: Common in young, in 3rd or 4th decade, more in female. May be asymptomatic.
- *Constitutional symptoms*: Fever, arthralgia and polyarthritis
- *Pulmonary symptom*: Cough and breathlessness on exertion
- *Other features*: According to the involvement of organ.

Signs:

Depending on involvement of organs:
- *In skin*: Erythema nodosum, lupus pernio, maculopapular rash, plaque, subcutaneous nodules and hypo- or hyperpigmentation
- Generalized lymphadenopathy, bilateral parotid enlargement and hepatosplenomegaly

- *Ocular*: Episcleritis, scleritis, uveitis, keratoconjunctivitis sicca and lacrimal gland enlargement
- Hypercalcemia (in 10% cases) and bone cysts (in the digits)
- *Central nervous system (CNS)*: Rare (2%), called neurosarcoid. Cranial nerve palsy, meningism, seizure, psychosis and diabetes insipidus
- *Cardiac*: Arrhythmias, conduction defects, cardiomyopathy and congestive cardiac failure.

Note: Presence of fever, arthritis or arthralgia, erythema nodosum with bilateral hilar lymphadenopathy (BHL) in CXR is highly suggestive of sarcoidosis.

Investigations:
- Complete blood count and ESR (lymphopenia and high ESR). MT (usually negative)
- X-ray of chest, X-ray of hands or feet and X-ray of kidney
- High-resolution computed tomography of chest
- Serum calcium and γ-globulin (usually high)
- Lung and liver function tests
- Bronchoscopy (shows cobble-stone appearance of mucosa)
- Bronchoalveolar lavage (shows increased CD4:CD8 ratio)
- Lung biopsy-transbronchial or percutaneous or open biopsy (shows noncaseating granuloma)
- *Fine needle aspiration cytology or biopsy from*: Lymph node, skin nodule, liver and lacrimal gland
- *Others*: ACE in blood and ^{67}Gallium scanning of lung.

Treatment:
- *Acute with erythema nodosum*: Bed rest and NSAID. Spontaneous resolution may occur
- *If no improvement in 6 months*: Prednisolone, 20–40 mg for 6 weeks, then alternate day 15 mg for 6–12 months
- *Other treatment*: Avoid strong sunlight. Topical steroid for uveitis, inhaled corticosteroid if breathlessness. Chloroquine, hydroxychloroquine and thalidomide—useful in cutaneous sarcoid
    - In severe disease with no response to steroid: Methotrexate 10–20 mg weekly or azathioprine 50–100 mg daily or TNF-α blocker (infliximab and etanercept)
    - Single lung transplantation may be done in selected case.

CHRONIC OBSTRUCTIVE PULMONARY DISEASE

It is a preventable and treatable disease characterized by persistent airflow limitation, usually progressive, associated with an enhanced chronic inflammatory response in the airways and the lung to noxious particles or gases. Multiple factors are responsible, such as:
- Exposure to active or passive smoking, air pollution, exposure to dust, fumes, chemicals (coal miners and cadmium workers). Urban dweller, low socioeconomic status and low birth weight. Recurrent lung infection and persistent adenovirus in lung tissue
- *Host factors*: α_1 antitrypsin deficiency and airway hyperreactivity.

Symptoms: Usually above 40 years, male, smoker. Chronic cough with sputum and breathlessness.

Signs (in chest):
- *Inspection*: Patient is dyspneic. Barrel-shaped chest, indrawing of lower intercostal space on inspiration. Suprasternal and supraclavicular space excavation with prominent accessory muscles of respiration
- *Palpation*: Tracheal tug is present (descent of trachea during inspiration). Cricosternal distance is reduced (normally three fingers or more). Chest expansion is reduced and chest movement is vertical. Vocal fremitus is reduced on both sides
- *Percussion*: Increased resonance in both lung fields. Obliteration of liver and cardiac dullness
- *Auscultation*: Breath sound is diminished, vesicular with prolonged expiration. Rhonchi may be present. Vocal resonance is normal.

Investigations:
- *CBC*: May be polycythemia
- Chest X-ray PA view. HRCT of chest may be done
- Lung function test
- *Arterial blood gas analysis*: Normal at rest, pO_2 (reduced), pCO_2 (normal or high) and pH (acidosis).

Treatment: Smoking must be stopped. Avoidance of dust, fume and smoke. Reduction of obesity.
- *Drug therapy*:
    - Short-acting inhaled bronchodilator: Salbutamol, terbutaline or ipratropium
    - Long-acting bronchodilator: Salmeterol and formoterol
    - Inhaled steroid (fluticasone)
    - Mucolytic (N-acetylcysteine), antibiotic (if infection) and diuretic (if edema).
- Oxygen, if needed. Long-term oxygen, if chronic respiratory failure
- Pneumococcal and influenza vaccination
- *Surgery*: Bullectomy, lung volume reduction surgery and lung transplantation.

Management acute exacerbation of COPD (type II respiratory failure):
- Continuous low flow oxygen via venturi mask
- Nebulized salbutamol with ipratropium
- Oral prednisolone 30 mg daily for 10 days
- Antibiotic, if infection. Diuretic, if edema
- *Chest physiotherapy*: Secretions should be removed by suction
- If above treatment fail, bilevel positive airway pressure (BiPAP) or continuous positive airway pressure (CPAP).

DIFFUSE PARENCHYMAL LUNG DISEASE (DPLD)

Diffuse parenchymal lung disease (DPLD) is a heterogenous group of diseases characterized by diffuse lung injury and inflammation that can progress to lung fibrosis. Previously, it was called interstitial lung disease (ILD). Its types are:
- Granulomatous DPLD (e.g. sarcoidosis)
- Granulomatous DPLD with vasculitis (e.g. Wegener granulomatosis, Churg–Strauss syndrome and microscopic vasculitis)

- *Idiopathic interstitial pneumonia (IIP)*:
  - Idiopathic pulmonary fibrosis (IPF) (90%)
  - Idiopathic interstitial pneumonia other than IPF (10%).
- Pulmonary autoimmune rheumatic diseases (e.g. rheumatoid arthritis and SLE)
- Drugs (busulfan, bleomycin, methotrexate, nitrofurantoin and amiodarone)
- *Other types*: Histiocytosis X, Goodpasture syndrome, and idiopathic pulmonary hemosiderosis.

Symptoms: Patient is usually elderly above 50 years. Cough with progressive breathlessness.

Signs: Patient is dyspneic, hyperventilating with cyanosis and finger clubbing. Chest expansion is reduced. Breath sound is vesicular with prolonged expiration. Bilateral basal end-inspiratory fine crepitations, unaltered by coughing.

Investigations:
- Complete blood count with ESR
- X-ray of chest. HRCT of chest
- Lung function tests
- Bronchoscopy
- For confirmation, lung biopsy. Others (according to suspicion of cause).

Treatment: Smoking must be stopped, avoid air pollution (dust and fume).
- Control of infection by antibiotic
- *Bronchodilator*: Salbutamol, terbutaline, ipratropium, tiotropium and oxitropium
- *Long-acting β agonist*: Salmeterol and formoterol. Oral theophylline (in some cases)
- Prednisolone 0.5 mg/kg with azathioprine 2–3 mg/kg for 2 months
- *Antifibrotic therapy*: Pirfenidone and N-acetylcysteine
- Single lung transplantation in young patient at advanced stage. Survival is 1 year in 60% cases.

HYPERSENSITIVITY PNEUMONITIS (EXTRINSIC ALLERGIC ALVEOLITIS)

It results from inhalation of organic antigens which gives rise to widespread diffuse inflammatory reaction in alveoli and bronchioles. The most common causes are farmer's lung and bird fancier's lung. Repeated episodes of pneumonitis progress to pulmonary fibrosis.

Symptoms: History of work in farm, breathlessness, dry cough, weight loss, fever and night sweat.

Investigations:
- Chest X-ray and HRCT of chest
- Lung function test
- Complete blood count
- *Others*: Antibodies in the serum. Bronchoalveolar lavage.

Treatment: Avoid allergen. Prednisolone 30–40 mg daily for 1–2 weeks, then taper over next 2–4 weeks.

RESPIRATORY FAILURE

It is defined as when pulmonary gas exchange fails to maintain normal arterial oxygen and carbon dioxide levels. There are two types:
1. Type I: Hypoxemia (PaO_2 <60 mm Hg) with normal or low $PaCO_2$
2. Type II: Hypoxemia and hypercapnia ($PaCO_2$ >50 mm Hg).

Causes of type I respiratory failure: Acute bronchial asthma, pulmonary edema, pneumonia, pneumothorax, pulmonary embolism (PE), ARDS and emphysema.

Treatment: Oxygen inhalation in high concentration (40–60% via venturi mask), treatment of underlying cause. Mechanical ventilation may be needed.

Causes of type II respiratory failure: COPD, severe bronchial asthma, obstructive sleep apnea syndrome and foreign body causing upper airway obstruction. Extrapulmonary causes—drugs causing CNS depression (narcotics and sedatives), respiratory muscle paralysis (GBS, myasthenia gravis and poliomyelitis), and kyphoscoliosis.

Clinical features: Features of primary cause, features of CO_2 retention. There may be headache, drowsiness, confusion, even coma. Signs are warm periphery, bounding pulse, flapping tremor, muscles twitching and papilledema.

Investigations: Chest X-ray, ECG, arterial blood gas analysis, and pulse oxymetry. Other investigations according to cause.

Treatment: Oxygen in low concentration (24–28%). Maintenance of airway, suction and chest physiotherapy. Mechanical ventilation may be required, if condition deteriorates. Treatment of cause.

TUBERCULOSIS

Three types of mycobacteria: *Mycobacterium tuberculosis* (causes TB in human), *Mycobacterium bovis* (endemic in cattle and rarely infects human), and atypical mycobacteria.
- *Types*: Primary, postprimary or secondary and miliary.
- *Sites*: Lung, lymph node, spine (Pott disease), kidney, intestine (ileocecal), fallopian tube, meninges and pericardium.

Primary Tuberculosis

First infection of lung is called primary pulmonary TB. It is due to inhalation of bacillus. Primary lesion in lung is called "Ghon focus", common in subpleural at lower part of upper lobe or upper part of lower lobe. From primary site, bacilli are carried to hilar lymph nodes. The primary lesion with the hilar lymphadenopathy is called "Ghon complex".

Symptoms: Mostly asymptomatic, may have low-grade fever, malaise, weakness and loss of weight.

Signs: Usually no physical sign. Erythema nodosum may be present.

Fate of primary pulmonary tuberculosis:
- Majority heals completely (80–90%). May calcify
- Some remain dormant, reactivate later in immunosuppressed condition, e.g. lymphoma, leukemia, chemotherapy and HIV infection

- Some may be active, progress from the beginning
- In few cases, bacilli may enter into the bloodstream, cause miliary TB and also spread to the other organs.

Postprimary TB

After primary infection, which is completely cured, if again TB, it is called postprimary TB. Usually involves the lung, commonly apex. Cavitation may occur.

Features of pulmonary TB: Cough, dry or expectorant, hemoptysis. Patient may present with pyrexia of unknown origin (PUO), pleural effusion and pneumothorax. General features are low-grade fever (evening rise), weight loss, night sweating, weakness and loss of appetite.

Investigations:
- Complete blood count, ESR (usually high), CXR, and tuberculin test (MT)
- Sputum for AFB staining, mycobacterial C/S, polymerase chain reaction (PCR), and Gene Xpert
- In child, sputum collected from gastric lavage or laryngeal swab (to see AFB).

Treatment:
- *First 2 months (intensive phase)*: Combination of rifampicin, isonicotinylhydrazide (INH), ethambutol and pyrazinamide
- *Next 4 months (continuation phase)*: Rifampicin and INH
- Pyridoxine 10–20 mg to prevent peripheral neuropathy.

First- and second-line antitubercular drugs:
- *First-line drugs*: Rifampicin, INH, ethambutol and pyrazinamide (streptomycin and thioacetazone are less used)
- *Second-line drugs*: Ethionamide, prothionamide, kanamycin, amikacin, ciprofloxacin, ofloxacin, clarithromycin, azithromycin, amoxiclav and cycloserine. These drugs are used only when first-line drugs fail or in multidrug-resistant TB (MDR-TB).

Common side effects of antitubercular drugs:
- *Rifampicin*: Hepatitis and skin rash
- *Isonicotinylhydrazide*: Peripheral neuropathy
- *Ethambutol*: Optic neuritis
- *Pyrazinamide*: Hepatitis and gout.

MT (tuberculin test) with its interpretation—MT is done by using 10 tuberculin unit (0.1 mL of 1:1,000 strength purified protein derivative). Injection is given intradermally in forearm, reading is taken after 72 hours. It is positive, when induration (not erythema) is 10 mm or above. Only positive MT does not indicate TB.

Positive MT may occur in the following cases—BCG (Bacillus Calmette–Guérin) vaccination, Previous sufferer of TB or exposure to TB bacillus, present infection (should be correlated with clinical features).

Negative MT may occur in (even patient may have TB)
- Immunocompromised patient (lymphoma, leukemia and malignancy), HIV infection and immunosuppressive drugs (cytotoxic drug and steroid)
- *Others*: Malnutrition, elderly, newborn, some cases of severe TB (negative in 25%) and sarcoidosis.

Treatment of TB in pregnancy:
- Isonicotinylhydrazide, rifampicin, ethambutol and pyrazinamide are given as usual doses. These drugs do not cause harm to the fetus. Breastfeeding should be continued
- Injection streptomycin should never be given in any stage of pregnancy, because it causes damage of 8th cranial nerve of the fetus.

MDR-TB: When tubercular bacilli are resistant to both INH and rifampicin.

Diagnosis of MDR-TB: To diagnose MDR-TB, high degree of suspicion is the key point.
- *Clinically, suggestive features are*: Persistent symptoms for 2 months or more (fever, cough and hemoptysis), history of contact with MDR-TB patient and worsening of symptoms with therapy
- *Laboratory criteria for diagnosis*: With treatment, sputum for AFB is positive after 5 months, culture is positive after 3 months, and C/S show resistance.

Treatment of MDR-TB: Treatment is expensive, difficult and lengthy, because of lack of available drugs, costs and side effects. Combination of drugs may be given—ethambutol, ethionamide, ofloxacin or ciprofloxacin, pyrazinamide and streptomycin.
- *Initial phase*: At least 6 months or till the culture is negative
- *Continuation phase (sterilizing)*: At least 18 months after culture becomes negative. Total duration may be 24 months, which may increase up to 36 months.

Miliary TB: It is the acute dissemination of pulmonary TB, characterized radiologically by multiple small nodules in the lungs. It is due to rupture of tuberculous focus in bloodstream. It occurs in primary TB, not in postprimary TB.

Symptoms: Fever, malaise, weight loss, night sweat, cough, usually dry, headache, drowsiness, confusion, only PUO.

Signs: May not be any sign. May be hepatosplenomegaly in 25% cases. Lung examination may be normal, there may be few crepitations. Fundoscopy shows choroid tubercle.

Complications: Tuberculous meningitis and Addisonian crisis.

Investigations:
- *Chest X-ray*: Shows multiple military shadow in both lung fields
- CBC and ESR (usually high)
- Sputum for AFB staining, and mycobacterial C/S, PCR and MT
- *Other test*: Fiberoptic bronchoscopy and bronchial washing for AFB
- Sometimes bone marrow study.

Miliary mottling: It means multiple, small shadows, usually 1–2 mm, involving all zones of both lung fields.

Tuberculous meningitis is diagnosed by:
- History of TB
- *On examination*: Neck rigidity and Kernig's sign
- Fundoscopy shows choroid tubercle (in 5–10% cases)
- Lumbar puncture and cerebrospinal fluid (CSF) study (shows high pressure, high lymphocyte; biochemistry shows high protein and low sugar, high ADA).

PULMONARY THROMBOEMBOLISM

It is the occlusion of main pulmonary artery or its branches by embolus arising from thrombus in right heart or systemic veins. Causes are DVT from legs and pelvis. Thrombus in right heart (in atrial fibrillation).

Types of pulmonary thromboembolism:
- Acute massive PE, embolus occlude the main pulmonary artery
- *Small PE*: embolus occludes the small branches of pulmonary artery causing pulmonary infarction.

Risk factors for thromboembolism:
- *Surgery*: Abdominal or pelvic surgery, hip or knee surgery, postoperative cases.
- *Obstetrical*: Pregnancy and puerperium
- *Cardiac*: Atrial fibrillation
- *Malignancy*: Carcinoma of pancreas, ovary and stomach
- *Hypercoagulable diseases*: Antiphospholipid syndrome, polycythemia rubra vera and nephrotic syndrome
- *Miscellaneous*: Prolonged immobility, trauma, oral contraceptive pill, fracture and varicose veins.

Acute Massive PE

Occlusion of major proximal artery causes reduced cardiac output and acute right heart failure.

Symptoms: Severe central chest pain, crushing in nature, severe dyspnea, faintness or syncope, and features of shock or sudden death.

Signs: Tachycardia, tachypnea, cyanosis, raised JVP, loud P2, wide splitting of 2nd heart sound, right ventricular gallop, and features of shock.

Small or Medium Sized PE

Occlusion of segmental pulmonary or small pulmonary artery causes infarction of lung tissue.

Features: Pleuritic chest pain, restricted breathing, low-grade fever and hemoptysis. Tachycardia, pleural rub, raised hemidiaphragm, crepitations (localized) and effusion (often bloodstained).

Investigations:
- Chest X-ray PA view
- CT pulmonary angiography (CTPA)
- *Plasma D-dimer*: If low or undetectable, it excludes PE
- Ventilation and perfusion scan (VQ scan)
- USG of leg veins
- Blood gas analysis shows low PaO_2 and low $PaCO_2$
- Electrocardiography ($S_1Q_3T_3$ pattern) and echocardiogram
- *If pulmonary infarction*: Neutrophil leukocytosis, high ESR and high LDH
- *Spiral CT angiography*: It is sensitive and specific for medium size embolism
- MRI (if CT is contraindicated).

Treatment:
- High flow oxygen (60–100%). Relief of pain by morphine or pethidine

- *Anticoagulant*: Injection heparin 10,000 units IV bolus, followed by continuous infusion 1,000–2,000 units/hour. Or low molecular heparin (enoxaparin and dalteparin) given subcutaneously
- *Oral anticoagulant (warfarin)*: Started after 48 hours of heparin therapy. Heparin is usually stopped after 5 days. Warfarin is continued for 6 weeks to 6 months. In recurrent PE, it may be required to continue for lifelong
- Alternately, rivaroxaban (an oral factor Xa inhibitor) may be used. Dose is 15 mg 12 hourly for 21 days, then 20 mg for 6 months. Dose is reduced in renal failure
- *Fibrinolytic therapy*: Streptokinase (2,50,000 units by IV infusion over 30 min followed by streptokinase 1,00,000 units IV hourly for up to 12–72 h). Or alteplase (60 mg IV over 15 min). Heparin should be given subsequently
- *In massive PE with severe hemodynamic compromise*: Surgical embolectomy is necessary
- In recurrent PE, insertion of a filter in inferior vena cava above the level of renal veins may be done.

PNEUMOCONIOSIS (OCCUPATIONAL LUNG DISEASE)

It is defined as fibrosis of lung due to inhalation of mineral dust. Common diseases are Coal worker's pneumoconiosis due to coal dust, silicosis due to silica, asbestosis due to asbestos, siderosis due to iron oxidem, byssinosis due to cotton dust, stannosis due to tin oxide, and berylliosis due to beryllium.

Symptoms are common in all pneumoconiosis such as breathlessness, cough, with or without sputum, later pulmonary hypertension, and cor pulmonale.

Coal Worker's Pneumoconiosis

It is due to prolonged inhalation of coal dust. There are two types:
- *Simple coal worker's pneumoconiosis*: Small radiographic nodules in an otherwise asymptomatic individual. Does not impair lung function and not progress once exposure ceases
- *Progressive massive fibrosis*: Formation of fibrotic masses mainly in upper lobes, may cavitate.

Clinical features: Cough, sputum which may be black, and breathlessness. Fibrosis leads to respiratory failure and right ventricular failure. Rheumatoid arthritis associated with coal worker's pneumoconiosis is called Caplan's syndrome.

Treatment: No satisfactory treatment. Exposure should be avoided.

Asbestosis

It is defined as disease of lung caused by asbestos dust. Asbestosis-related lung disease occurs in ship workers. Also, mining and milling of mineral.
- *In the pleura*: Benign pleural plaques or calcification, pleural effusion, and mesothelioma (blue asbestos is the common cause)
- *In the lung*: ILD (progressive pulmonary fibrosis), carcinoma and Honeycomb lung. Others—carcinoma of larynx and mesothelioma of peritoneum.

Three types—Chrysotile (white asbestos, 90%), crocidolite (blue asbestos), and amosite (brown asbestos).

Pleural Mesothelioma

It is the primary malignant tumor of pleura due to prolonged exposure to asbestos, mainly blue. Latent period between exposure and development of mesothelioma is 20–40 years. Features are chest pain (pleuritic), features of pleural effusion (bloodstained), and breathlessness.

Investigations: CXR, CT scan or MRI, FNAC and biopsy.

Treatment: No satisfactory treatment. Does not respond to chemotherapy. Radiotherapy may be given.

SLEEP APNEA

It is defined as intermittent cessation of airflow in nose and mouth during sleep. Apnea means cessation of airflow through nose for at least 10 seconds. There are two types: obstructive and central.

Obstructive Sleep Apnea (OSA)

During sleep, apnea occurs due to obstruction of upper airway. Common in obese and middle-aged male.

Risk factors: Obesity, craniofacial abnormalities, upper airway soft tissue abnormalities, nasal obstruction, smokers, alcoholism, associated with certain medical illnesses, such as heart failure, cerebrovascular diseases (CVD), hypothyroidism and acromegaly.

Diagnosis: Overnight polysomnography.

Clinical features: Nocturnal symptoms are loud snoring, cessation of breathing, insomnia with frequent awakening with choking, vivid dreams and restlessness. Daytime symptoms are sleepiness, morning headache, lack of concentration, fatigue, cognitive deficit and changes in mood.

Treatment: If obese, weight reduction. Avoidance of alcohol and sedatives. Correction of cause (nasal polyp, deviated nasal septum, enlarged tonsil, hypothyroidism and acromegaly). Specific therapy—CPAP and oral appliances. In some cases, surgery (uvulopalatopharyngoplasty).

Central Sleep Apnea

It is a disorder in which apnea occurs during sleep without obstruction of airway. Common in elderly, male with comorbid conditions.

Causes: CNS diseases (CVD and CNS suppressing drugs), neuromuscular diseases, acromegaly, renal failure, kyphoscoliosis, high altitude, and cardiovascular diseases.

Clinical features: Disrupted sleep, excessive daytime sleep, poor sleep quality, insomnia, inattention, poor concentration, fatigue, decreased libido and impotence. Feature of primary disease.

Treatment: O_2 during sleep, CPAP. Treatment of primary cause.

CHAPTER 3

Gastrointestinal Diseases

MOUTH ULCER

Causes of Mouth Ulcer
- Aphthous ulcer
- Trauma
- *Local infection*: Viral (herpes simplex), candidiasis, Vincent's angina, and syphilis (chance in primary and snail tract ulcer in secondary syphilis)
- *Gastrointestinal tract (GIT) disease*: Crohn's disease, ulcerative colitis, celiac disease
- *Rheumatological disease*: Systemic lupus erythematosus (SLE), Behçet's syndrome and Reiter's syndrome
- *Drugs*: Hypersensitivity (Stevens-Johnson syndrome) and cytotoxic drugs
- *Dermatological*: Pemphigus vulgaris, pemphigoid and lichen planus
- *Neoplastic*: Carcinoma, leukemia and Kaposi's sarcoma.

Aphthous Ulcer

It is characterized by superficial, painful, and usually recurrent ulcer in any part of mouth. Single or multiple round or oval ulcers with inflammatory halo. It may be associated with inflammatory bowel disease and emotional stress.

Treatment: Avoid trauma, tobacco, spicy and hot food. Maintenance of oral hygiene.
- Chlorhexidine 0.2% mouthwash. Tetracycline mouthwash
- Topical triamcinolone 0.1%, applied 2–3 times daily
- In severe and recurrent case, oral prednisolone may be given for a short period
- Sometimes dapsone, colchicine, thalidomide, and azathioprine may be used
- Pain may be relieved by using local anesthetic mouthwash and anesthetic lozenge.

Candidiasis (Oral Thrush)

It is characterized by multiple white patches over the surface of tongue with some denuded area on the margin, caused by *Candida albicans*.

Creamy white curd-like patches in mouth and tongue. Factors associated with oral candidiasis are poor oral hygiene, diabetes mellitus (DM), immunosuppressive disease [lymphoma, leukemia, malignancy and human immunodeficiency virus (HIV)], prolonged use of antibiotic, steroid and immunosuppressive drug, and steroid inhaler use.

Treatment:
- Topical antifungal (nystatin, econazole and miconazole). Systemic antifungal (fluconazole or clotrimazole)
- Maintenance of oral hygiene, antiseptic mouthwash. Treatment of underlying disease.

DISEASES OF ESOPHAGUS

Dysphagia

It means difficulty in swallowing. Causes are:
- *Oropharyngeal disease*: Acute tonsillitis, peritonsillar abscess, pharyngeal web, carcinoma of pharynx, Plummer–Vinson syndrome, pharyngeal diverticulum, stomatitis and aphthous ulcer
- *Esophageal causes*:
  - Cause in the lumen: Foreign body
  - Cause in the wall: Achalasia cardia, carcinoma of esophagus, stricture, and esophagitis (due to candidiasis and peptic esophagitis), and diffuse esophageal spasm, scleroderma and Chagas disease
  - Pressure from outside: Retrosternal goiter, mediastinal mass, enlarged left atrium due to mitral stenosis and giant aortic aneurysm.
- *Neurogenic causes*: Bulbar or pseudobulbar palsy and myasthenia gravis.

Odynophagia

It means pain during swallowing. Causes are:
- Esophagitis due to herpes simplex infection, candidiasis, esophageal ulceration or perforation due to corrosive poisoning, radiation and reflux esophagitis
- *Drugs*: Doxycycline, aspirin, nonsteroidal anti-inflammatory drug (NSAID), ferrous sulfate and bisphosphonate.

Globus Hystericus

It means feeling of a lump in throat without any organic cause, found in conversion disorder (HCR).

Hematemesis

It means vomiting of blood. Causes are:
- Chronic duodenal ulcer and chronic gastric ulcer
- Gastric erosion due to NSAID, steroid, and carcinoma of stomach
- Rupture of esophageal varices and Mallory–Weiss syndrome
- *Bleeding disorder*: Hemophilia and immune thrombocytopenic purpura (ITP)
- *Others*: Dengue hemorrhagic fever, hereditary hemorrhagic telangiectasia, prolonged use of antiplatelet (aspirin and clopidogrel) and anticoagulant (warfarin).

Hematochezia

It means passage of fresh blood per rectum. It indicates bleeding from lower GIT (usually large gut).

Causes:
- Hemorrhoid, anal fissure, and carcinoma of rectum
- Bacillary dysentery
- *Others*: Diverticular disease, angiodysplasia of colon, inflammatory bowel disease (commonly ulcerative colitis) and ischemic colitis.

Melena

It means passage of black tarry stool per rectum, indicates bleeding from upper GIT. Causes are as in hematemesis.

Gastroesophageal Reflux Disease

It means regurgitation of gastroduodenal contents into esophagus. In some patients of gastroesophageal reflux disease (GERD), there is reduced lower esophageal sphincter tone, allowing reflux when intra-abdominal pressure rises.

Symptoms: Heartburn, pain and regurgitation. Symptoms aggravated by bending, straining or lying down. Nocturnal regurgitation with cough and dyspnea. Atypical chest pain which confuses with anginal pain.

Investigations: Barium swallow X-ray of esophagus in Trendelenburg position (shows hiatus hernia) and endoscopy.

Treatment:
- *General*:
  - Weight reduction, if obese. Avoid tight belts, corsets, diet which aggravates symptoms, smoking and alcohol
  - Patient is advised not to lie down immediately after food, also should avoid drinking water while eating (should be taken sometimes after eating food)
  - Straining during defecation, lifting heavy object should be avoided
  - Head end of bed should be raised, especially for those who have nocturnal symptoms.
- *Drug treatment*: Antacid gives symptomatic relief. Proton-pump inhibitor (PPI) (omeprazole and lansoprazole) or H2 receptor blocker (ranitidine and famotidine). Domperidone may be given. If medical treatment fails, laparoscopic anti-reflux surgery may be considered. Large hiatus hernia may require surgery.

Barrett's Esophagus

It is the metaplasia of normal squamous epithelium to columnar epithelium of lower esophagus. It is more in male above 50 years. Usually, secondary to reflux esophagitis. Smoking may be a cause (but not alcohol). Hiatus hernia is common.

Complication: Malignant change, usually adenocarcinoma.

Investigations: Endoscopy and biopsy. If dysplastic change is found, endoscopy and biopsy should be done every 6 months.

Treatment: Regular follow-up. If dysplastic change, surgical intervention may be necessary.

Hiatus Hernia

It is the herniation of part of the stomach into chest through the esophageal hiatus of diaphragm.

Three types—sliding or esophagogastric, rolling or paraesophageal. Rarely, a mixed type.

Clinical features: It may be asymptomatic. It may be heartburn, regurgitation of food and retrosternal chest pain. Dysphagia, if esophageal stricture develops.

Investigations: Barium swallow X-ray of esophagus in Trendelenburg position and endoscopy.

Treatment: As in GERD. Surgery, if symptoms persist despite adequate medical therapy (fundoplication).

Achalasia Cardia

Achalasia of esophagus or cardia is a motility disorder, characterized by failure of relaxation of lower esophageal sphincter due to absence or reduction of ganglion cells of Auerbach's plexus. As a result, food is collected in esophagus resulting in progressive dilation.

Causes: Causes are unknown. There is failure of nonadrenergic noncholinergic (NANC) innervations related to abnormal nitric oxide synthesis in lower esophageal sphincter. Degeneration of ganglion cells in sphincter and body of esophagus occurs.

Symptoms: Dysphagia both for solid and liquid and regurgitation of food. Retrosternal chest pain (due to esophageal spasm) may be severe. Repeated respiratory infection and aspiration pneumonia. Cough and dyspnea due to pressure of dilated esophagus on trachea and bronchi. Loss of weight.

Investigations:
- *Barium swallow X-ray of esophagus*: Shows smooth tapering of lower end with dilatation above, with loss of peristalsis
- Endoscopy and biopsy
- *Esophageal manometry*: Gold standard (for diagnosis).

Complications:
- *Respiratory*: Recurrent aspiration pneumonia, bronchiectasis, and collapse of lung
- Carcinoma of esophagus (squamous type in 5–10%)
- Malnutrition (due to dysphagia).

Treatment:
- Endoscopic dilatation by pneumatic bougie
- *If repeated dilatation fails*: Surgery, open or laparoscopic (Heller's cardiomyotomy) or endoscopic myomectomy
- *Medical treatment*: Long-acting nitrate, calcium channel blocker (nifedipine) may be used. Injection botulinum toxin in lower esophageal sphincter may be given.

Carcinoma of Esophagus

Types: Mainly two types—squamous cell carcinoma (involves upper and middle parts) and adenocarcinoma (involves lower third).

Sites: Upper part (15%), middle part (45%) and lower part (40%).

Causes: Causes are unknown. Predisposing factors are smoking, chewing of betel nuts or tobacco, alcoholism, achalasia of esophagus, Plummer–Vinson syndrome, Barrett's esophagus, tylosis (familial hyperkeratosis of palm and sole and dysphagia), and celiac disease.

Symptoms: Dysphagia initially for solid, later for both solid and liquid diets. It is progressive and painless. Retrosternal discomfort or chest pain at the site of obstruction. Anorexia, regurgitation and weight loss. Features of metastases (lymph node, lung, liver, brain and bone) and tracheoesophageal fistula (cough, dyspnea and pneumonia).

Signs: Patient is cachexic. Anemia and signs of metastasis (lymphadenopathy and hepatomegaly).

Investigations:
- Barium swallow of esophagus (shows irregular filling defect, shouldering, and narrowing like rat-tail appearance)
- Endoscopy and biopsy
- *Others (to see metastasis)*: Chest X-ray (CXR), ultrasonography (USG) of whole abdomen, computed tomography (CT) scan or magnetic resonance imaging (MRI) of chest and abdomen, endoscopic USG, complete blood count (CBC) and erythrocyte sedimentation rate (ESR).

Treatment:
- *Upper and middle parts*: High-voltage radiotherapy
- *Lower part*: Surgery (esophagogastrectomy)
- Chemotherapy (using 5-fluorouracil and cisplatin may be tried)
- *Palliative therapy*: Endoscopic laser therapy, repeated dilatation of stricture, endoscopic insertion of stent in esophagus, endoscopic gastrostomy and tube feeding, and palliative radiotherapy.

ACUTE GASTRITIS

It means inflammation associated with mucosal injury of stomach. It is often erosive and hemorrhagic.

Causes: Mostly due to pain killers like aspirin, indomethacin, diclofenac or other NSAID. Also due to corticosteroid and alcohol.

Symptoms: Anorexia, nausea, vomiting, epigastric fullness or pain. Hematemesis and melena.

Sign: Epigastric tenderness.

Investigation: Endoscopy.

Treatment:
- Antacid, PPI (omeprazole, lansoprazole and esomeprazole) and H2 receptor blockers (ranitidine and famotidine)
- Prokinetic drug (domperidone). Sucralfate 1 g 8 hourly in NSAID-induced erosions
- Soft or liquid diet.

CHRONIC GASTRITIS

Mostly associated with *Helicobacter pylori* infection.

Symptoms: Asymptomatic. May be anorexia, nausea, vomiting, epigastric fullness or pain, hematemesis and melena.

Sign: Epigastric tenderness.

Investigation: Endoscopy and biopsy.

Treatment: As in acute gastritis. Anti-helicobacter therapy may be given.

PEPTIC ULCER DISEASE

It is the break of superficial epithelial cells either in the stomach or duodenum.

Sites: First part of duodenum, lesser curvature of stomach, lower end of esophagus, in gastrojejunostomy stoma. Rarely, in Meckel's diverticulum.

Causes:
- *H. pylori* infection
- *Drugs*: Aspirin or other NSAIDs, steroid and bisphosphonate
- Smoking and alcohol
- *Others*: Acid hypersecretory disorder (Zollinger–Ellison syndrome), hyperparathyroidism, Crohn's disease, genetic, blood group "O", and other associated diseases [chronic obstructive pulmonary disease (COPD), cirrhosis of liver, chronic kidney disease (CKD)].

Diagnosis of *H. pylori* infection:
- *Noninvasive tests*:
  - Serology: Anti *H. pylori* antibody [immunoglobulin G (IgG)], 90% sensitive and 83% specific
  - ^{13}C urea breath test: 90% sensitive and 96% specific. False negative result may occur if the patient is taking PPI or antibiotic
  - Fecal *H. pylori* antigen test: 97.6% sensitive and 96% specific. It is useful in diagnosis and monitoring the efficacy of eradication. The patient should stop taking PPI for 1 week before the test, but can continue H2 blocker.
- *Invasive tests (antral biopsy by endoscopy)*:
  - Rapid urease tests, e.g. Campylobacter-like organism (CLO), PyloriTek (its specificity is 95% and sensitivity is 85%). Sample is taken by biopsy from antrum of stomach
  - Histology (Giemsa stain of gastric biopsy): *H. pylori* can be detected from gastric mucosa
  - Microbiological culture (biopsy material in a special media): It is slow and less sensitive.

Treatment of *H. pylori* infection:
- *First-line therapy (given for 7 days)*: Omeprazole (20–40 mg) or lansoprazole (30 mg) or pantoprazole (40 mg) or rabeprazole (20 mg) 12 hourly plus clarithromycin 500 mg 12 hourly plus amoxicillin 1 g 12 hourly or metronidazole 400 mg 12 hourly
- *Second-line therapy*: Given if failure of first-line therapy or in areas of clarithromycin resistance, given for 14 days—PPI 20–40 mg 12 hourly plus bismuth citrate 120 mg 6 hourly plus metronidazole 400 mg 8 hourly plus tetracycline 500 mg 6 hourly.

DUODENAL ULCER

Symptoms: Pain in epigastrium, burning in nature, more in empty stomach (hunger pain), also late hours of night. Pain is relieved by taking food, antacid or after vomiting. Heartburn, dyspepsia, and sometimes vomiting. Pain comes and goes every 2–3 months (called periodicity).

Sign: Tenderness at epigastric region.

Investigations: Endoscopy (definitive). Barium meal X-ray of stomach and duodenum (shows ulcer crater or deformity of bulb).

Complications: Bleeding (hematemesis and melena), perforation, gastric outlet obstruction (pyloric stenosis).

Treatment:
- *H. pylori* eradication (see above)
- *General measures*: Avoid smoking, aspirin, and NSAID (moderate alcohol is not harmful). No special dietary advice
- *Other drugs*: Antacid, H2 antagonist, PPI, and sucralfate
- Maintenance treatment may be needed in some cases
- *Surgical treatment*: Less needed nowadays. Gastrojejunostomy with vagotomy is usually done. Sometimes partial gastrectomy may be done. Indications are—Emergency (perforation or hemorrhage) and elective (complications such as pyloric stenosis and recurrent ulcer following gastric surgery).

Management of peptic ulcer bleeding: The patient should be assessed and managed simultaneously:
- Intravenous (IV) access and resuscitation by IV normal saline (crystalloid) or colloid solution
- *Initial clinical assessment*:
  - To check: Pulse, blood pressure (BP), urine output, features of shock (pallor, cold nose, cold clammy extremities, systolic BP <100 mm Hg, and pulse >100/min). Central venous pressure (CVP) is monitored in severe bleeding
  - Other systems: Cardiorespiratory, cerebrovascular or renal diseases should be assessed
  - Evidence of liver disease should be sought.
- *Blood tests*: Blood grouping and cross matching, CBC, urea and electrolytes, liver function tests and prothrombin time
- Blood transfusion should be given if hemoglobin is less than 10 g/dL or the patient is in shock. CVP is monitored and fluid replacement should be adjusted accordingly
- *Oxygen*: If the patient is in shock
- Intravenous PPI therapy (omeprazole 80 mg followed by infusion 8 mg/h for 72 h). Followed by oral therapy according to improvement
- Endoscopy of upper GIT should be performed after resuscitation. If persistent bleeding, patient may be treated with heater probe, injection of dilute adrenaline or by metallic clips to stop bleeding
- Pulse, BP, and urine output should be monitored hourly
- *Surgical management*: Urgent surgery is indicated when endoscopic management fails to stop bleeding or rebleeding occurs once in an elderly or frail patient, or twice in younger fit patient
- If patient is suffering from chronic peptic ulcer, eradication therapy for *H. pylori* should be started. PPI should be continued for 4 weeks to ensure healing.

GASTRIC ULCER

Symptoms: Epigastric distress, pain which is relieved by vomiting or antacid. Dyspepsia or early satiety. Even after small amount of eating, patient feels fullness of abdomen. There may be pain after eating.

Sign: Epigastric tenderness.

Investigations: Endoscopy and barium meal X-ray of stomach (if the patient cannot tolerate endoscopy).

Treatment: Same as duodenal ulcer.

NONULCER DYSPEPSIA

It is defined as chronic dyspepsia characterized by pain or upper abdominal discomfort without any organic cause. Cause is unknown, probably due to spectrum of mucosal motility and psychiatric disorder. Patient is usually young <40 years, women are twice more affected.

Symptoms: Upper abdominal pain or discomfort, early satiety, fullness, bloating, and nausea after meal. Symptoms are more in the morning. There is no weight loss. Patient looks anxious. Symptoms may be disproportionate to clinical well-being. Abdomen may be inappropriately tender.

Investigation: Diagnosis is from history. No investigation is needed in young patient. For older patients or with alarming symptoms, endoscopy to exclude other disease. In young female, pregnancy should be excluded. Other investigations such as USG of whole abdomen (to exclude hepatobiliary or pancreatic disease), liver function test, CBC, stool for occult blood test (OBT), colonoscopy, and CT abdomen when appropriate.

Treatment: Explanation, reassurance, and lifestyle change. Restriction of fat, coffee and alcohol. Smoking must be stopped.

- *Drugs*: Antacid, metoclopramide, domperidone (if nausea, vomiting or bloating is prominent), H2 blocker or PPI may be given. Amitriptyline may be helpful
- Sometimes *H. pylori* eradication regimen may be given but the role is controversial
- Psychotherapy should be given.

ZOLLINGER–ELLISON SYNDROME (GASTRINOMA)

It is a syndrome characterized by severe peptic ulceration due to excess secretion of gastrin from a nonbeta cell tumor of pancreas arising from G-cells that stimulate gastric acid hypersecretion. It is also called gastrinoma.

Symptoms: Epigastric pain due to multiple and severe ulcers in stomach, duodenum, jejunum and esophagus. Nausea, vomiting, chronic diarrhea and weight loss. Ulcer does not respond to standard therapy or recurrence of ulcer after standard surgery. Bleeding and perforation are common.

Complications: Gastrointestinal hemorrhage, perforation, gastric outlet obstruction or stricture and metastasis (commonly in liver).

Investigations:
- Upper GI endoscopy (shows multiple ulcers)
- Barium meal X-ray (shows coarse gastric mucosa)

- High basal gastric acid secretion, no or little increase after pentagastrin
- Serum gastrin is high
- Computed tomography scan and selective arteriography of pancreas.

Treatment: High dose PPI (omeprazole 60–80 mg daily) and octreotide (subcutaneously, reduces gastrin secretion). Surgical resection, if tumor is single. Occasionally, total gastrectomy. If wide metastasis or incurable gastrinoma, debulking surgery and chemotherapy are indicated.

PYLORIC STENOSIS (GASTRIC OUTLET OBSTRUCTION)

Causes: Chronic duodenal ulcer (common cause) and carcinoma of pylorus. Others (rare)—congenital hypertrophic pyloric stenosis.

Symptoms:
- History of duodenal ulcer for long time but loss of pain and periodicity
- Anorexia, nausea, and vomiting (which is recurrent, projectile, large in volume, contains previous day's food, but no blood or bile. History of self-induced vomiting, which relieves abdominal discomfort)
- Food habit (patient eats breakfast, little lunch, and little or nothing at dinner), constipation and weight loss.

Signs: Patient looks emaciated with signs of dehydration. Abdomen is distended with visible peristalsis. Succussion splash (present 4 h or more after the last meal or drink).

Investigations:
- Complete blood count with ESR. Serum electrolytes—low sodium, low potassium and high bicarbonate (metabolic alkalosis). Blood urea and serum creatinine
- Endoscopy of upper GIT with biopsy (if needed). Barium meal X-ray of stomach and duodenum.

Treatment:
- *Resuscitation of the patient*: Correction of dehydration and electrolyte imbalance (by normal saline 3–4 L and potassium)
- Nasogastric aspiration may be given
- *Surgery*: Partial gastrectomy or gastrojejunostomy with vagotomy followed by PPI to prevent stomal ulcer.

CARCINOMA OF STOMACH

Sites: Antrum (50%), greater curvature (20–30%), and cardia of stomach (20%).

Causes:
Causes are unknown. Predisposing factors are:
- *Diet*: Preservatives (nitrites and nitrates converted to N-nitroso compounds, which are carcinogenic), diet rich in salted, smoked or pickled food, diet lacking fresh fruits, vegetables, vitamin C and A may be a contributing factor. Diet with high vegetables, fruits, and low salt protects from carcinoma of stomach
- *Others*: Smoking, alcohol, gastric surgery (partial gastrectomy), *H. pylori* infection, pernicious anemia, familial adenomatous polyposis, Ménétrier's disease, blood group A, and first degree relatives. Rarely, familial.

Clinical features:
- Any patient above 40 years of age presenting with "3A" (anemia, anorexia and asthenia)
- Vomiting (if tumor in pyloric end) and dysphagia (if tumor at the cardiac end)
- Epigastric pain or discomfort, not relieved by antacid, food or vomiting. Mass in the epigastrium
- Hematemesis and melena or features of anemia (unexplained)
- *Features of metastasis*: Hepatomegaly, ascites due to peritoneal metastasis, Virchow's gland (enlarged left supraclavicular lymph node—Troisier's sign), hard nodule around umbilicus (Sister Mary Joseph's nodule), ovarian involvement (Krukenberg tumor) and prerectal pouch (a shelf-like mass, Blumer's shelf)
- Paraneoplastic syndrome (acanthosis nigricans, dermatomyositis and thrombophlebitis migrans).

Investigations:
- Complete blood count and ESR
- Endoscopy and biopsy. Barium meal double contrast—shows filling defect and irregular ulcer
- Ultrasonography of whole abdomen (to see any metastasis). CT scan may be needed
- Stool for occult blood test
- *To monitor recurrence*: Carcinoembryonic antigen (CEA).

Treatment:
- Surgery is the only curative treatment in early stage
- *Perioperative chemotherapy*: Extracellular fluid (ECF) (epirubicin, cisplatin and fluorouracil) has improved 5-year survival in operable gastric and lower esophageal adenocarcinoma
- *Chemotherapy*: Not much helpful. FAM (5-fluorouracil, adriamycin and mitomycin C) may be given
- *Palliative*: Radiotherapy (very little role). Endoscopic laser ablation of tumor tissue. Endoscopic dilatation or insertion of stent may be used for relief of dysphagia or vomiting.

Early gastric cancer: When carcinoma is confined to mucosa or submucosa regardless of lymph node involvement, it is called early gastric cancer. It is associated with 5-year survival in 90%. Many may survive 5 years even without treatment. It may be cured by endoscopic mucosal resection or endoscopic submucosal dissection.

ACUTE PANCREATITIS

It is the acute inflammation of pancreas in which activated pancreatic enzymes leak into the substance of pancreas causing autodigestion of the gland.

Causes:
- *Common (90%)*: Gallstones, alcohol, idiopathic and post endoscopic retrograde cholangiopancreatography (ERCP)
- *Rare*: Postsurgical (abdominal and cardiopulmonary bypass), trauma, drugs (azathioprine, thiazide diuretics and sodium valproate), metabolic (hypercalcemia and hypertriglyceridemia), sphincter of Oddi dysfunction, infection (mumps and coxsackie B virus) and hereditary.

Symptoms:
- Abdominal pain mainly in upper abdomen which is severe, agonizing, radiating to the back, and reduced by bending forward (called Mohammedan's prayer position)
- Nausea, vomiting, fainting attack and sweating
- In severe case, hypovolemic shock.

Signs:
- Patient looks exhausted and distressed. Features of shock (cold clammy skin, tachycardia and low BP)
- Tenderness in the upper abdomen
- Bluish-red or green-brown discoloration of flanks (Grey Turner's sign) or bluish discoloration around periumbilical region (Cullen's sign) are features of severe pancreatitis with hemorrhage
- Mass due to pseudocyst may be found.

Investigations:
- Serum amylase and lipase (high)
- Ultrasonography or CT scan of abdomen, plain X-ray abdomen
- Blood sugar (high), serum calcium (low), serum electrolytes, CBC and CXR
- Blood gas analysis.

Complications:
- *Pancreatic*: Pseudocyst, abscess and necrosis
- *Systemic*: Shock, multiorgan dysfunction and systemic inflammatory response syndrome (SIRS)
- *Respiratory*: Acute respiratory distress syndrome (ARDS) and pleural effusion
- *Kidney*: Acute renal failure
- *Gastrointestinal tract*: Bleeding from gastric or duodenal erosion and paralytic ileus
- *Hepatobiliary*: Jaundice and common bile duct obstruction
- *Metabolic*: Hypoglycemia or hyperglycemia, hypocalcemia and hypoalbuminemia
- *Hematologic*: Disseminated intravascular coagulation (DIC).

Treatment:
- Nil per os (NPO) i.e., nothing from mouth and nasogastric suction. O_2 inhalation
- Intravenous fluid and correction of electrolytes. Control of blood sugar
- Relief of pain by tramadol or other opiates (meperidine or fentanyl). Or, injection pethidine 100 mg intramuscularly (IM) or morphine 15 mg IM with atropine in severe case
- *Broad-spectrum antibiotic*: Imipenem and cefuroxime with metronidazole
- Low-molecular weight heparin for deep vein thrombosis (DVT) prophylaxis
- Treatment of primary cause and complications, if any
- Early enteral nutrition in the first 72 hours through a nasojejunal tube
- In patients with gallstone pancreatitis, ERCP may be done to remove stone in common bile duct and sphincterotomy for those who have a high suspicion of cholestasis
- Cholecystectomy should be performed after recovery in all patients with gallstone pancreatitis.

CHRONIC PANCREATITIS

It is a chronic inflammatory disease of pancreas characterized by fibrosis, permanent and progressive morphologic or functional damage of pancreas.

Causes: Alcohol, tropical or idiopathic, chronic calcific pancreatitis (possibly due to malnutrition or cassava consumption). Others—hereditary, autoimmune, cystic fibrosis, recurrent acute pancreatitis and obstructive (stenosis of ampulla of Vater and pancreas divisum).

Symptoms: Recurrent or chronic persistent epigastric pain, recurrent attack of pancreatitis, diarrhea, steatorrhea, weight loss and DM.

Complications: Pseudocyst, pancreatic ascites, pleural effusion, obstructive jaundice, portal or splenic vein thrombosis and pancreatic cancer.

Investigations:
- Serum amylase and lipase (high during acute attack)
- X-ray (may show calcification), USG, and CT scan of abdomen
- Magnetic resonance cholangiopancreatography (MRCP). Endoscopic ultrasound. Blood sugar to see DM.

Treatment:
- Alcohol must be stopped
- Pain relief by tramadol. Sometimes in chronic pain, amitriptyline or pregabalin may be used
- *Endoscopic therapy*: Dilatation or stenting of pancreatic duct strictures and removal of calculi
- *Surgical*: Partial pancreatic resection and pancreaticojejunostomy may be necessary
- *For steatorrhea*: Oral pancreatic enzyme, H2 receptor antagonist or PPI.

CARCINOMA OF PANCREAS

Usually, adenocarcinoma (90%). Causes are unknown and factors are—age above 70 years, common in male, chronic pancreatitis, alcohol, smoking, environmental factors, and genetic (hereditary pancreatitis, multiple endocrine neoplasia and hereditary nonpolyposis colon cancer). Sites are 60% in head, 25% in body and 15% in tail.

Symptoms:
- *Painless obstructive jaundice with palpable gallbladder*: In carcinoma of head of pancreas
- *Carcinoma involving the body and tail*: Pain in epigastrium, which is deep-seated, dull aching, radiates to the back, more on lying flat, feels better with bending forward
- Weight loss, anorexia and nausea. Mass in upper abdomen (in 20% cases)
- *Others*: DM, acute pancreatitis and marantic endocarditis.

Signs: Emaciation, jaundice (if carcinoma of head), mass in epigastrium, hepatomegaly and lymphadenopathy.

Investigations:
- Ultrasonography of abdomen. Contrast enhanced CT scan. Endoscopic USG, MRCP
- Ultrasonography-guided fine needle aspiration cytology (FNAC)
- *Other tests*: Liver function tests, blood sugar and CA 19-9.

Treatment:
- *In early stage*: Whipple's operation (pancreas, duodenum, draining lymph node, and part of mesentery are removed)
- *Other treatment (usually palliative)*:
  - For pain: Analgesic and injection of alcohol in celiac plexus (USG or endoscopic USG-guided)
  - Endoscopic insertion of stent to relieve intractable itching
  - *Chemotherapy*: 5FU, adriamycin, and cisplatin or 5FU plus gemcitabine may be given
  - Radiotherapy is not much helpful.

ACUTE APPENDICITIS

It is the acute inflammation of appendix. Cause are obstruction of the lumen of appendix by faecolith, inflammation, worm, and infection by *Escherichia coli,* enterococci, *Proteus* and anaerobes.

Symptoms: Abdominal pain, colicky, initially in periumbilical region. After few hours, pain is shifted to the right iliac fossa. Vomiting once or twice (due to reflex pylorospasm). Low-grade fever.

Signs:
- Tenderness at McBurney's point (it is the point in the medial two-third and lateral one-third of a line joining right anterior superior iliac spine and umbilicus). Rebound tenderness
- *Rovsing's sign*: Pressure over left iliac fossa produces pain over right iliac fossa
- *If not treated in time*: Appendicular lump may develop.

Investigations: Diagnosis is clinical.
- *Complete blood count*: Polymorphonuclear leukocytosis
- Ultrasonography of abdomen
- CECT (contrast-enhanced CT scan) may be done if diagnosis is doubtful.

Treatment: Appendicectomy should be done after resuscitation of the patient—NPO, IV fluids, nasogastric suction, and antibiotic (IV broad-spectrum antibiotic with metronidazole).

Treatment of appendicular lump: Usually conservative. Surgery is done later on.
- NPO and nasogastric suction by Ryle's tube
- *Intravenous fluid*: 5% DNS and broad-spectrum antibiotic plus metronidazole
- *After 3–4 days*: When abdomen is soft, tenderness is less and stool has passed, then Ryle's tube is removed and oral liquid is given followed by soft diet
- Appendicectomy should be done after 6–8 weeks.

Note: No purgative and no exploratory laparotomy.

INTESTINAL OBSTRUCTION

It is the failure of onward propulsion of the contents of intestine.

Causes:
- *Cause in the lumen*: Impacted fecal matter and ascariasis

- *Cause in the wall*: Carcinoma of colon, stricture [due to tuberculosis (TB), Crohn's disease] and adhesions
- *Cause outside the wall*: Hernia, band, adhesion, volvulus and intussusception.

The most common causes according to age:
- *Neonate*: Imperforate anus
- *Children*: Ascariasis and intussusception
- *Younger age*: Hernia
- *Elderly*: Malignancy (carcinoma of colon and rectum).

Symptoms: There are four typical symptoms—abdominal pain, vomiting, abdominal distension and absolute constipation (no flatus and no feces).

Signs: Visible peristalsis and distended abdomen. On auscultation, excess borborygmi. When paralytic ileus develops, no bowel sound.

Investigations:
- Plain X-ray of abdomen in erect posture (shows multiple air-fluid level)
- Complete blood count, ESR and serum electrolytes
- Ultrasonography of whole abdomen and CT scan.

Treatment: NPO and nasogastric suction by Ryle's tube. IV fluid (5% DNS) and correction of electrolytes. Broad-spectrum antibiotic with metronidazole. Surgery may be necessary.

INFLAMMATORY BOWEL DISEASE

It includes Crohn's disease and ulcerative colitis.

Crohn's Disease

It is a chronic inflammatory bowel disease of unknown cause, characterized by localized areas of nonspecific granulomatous inflammation of bowel. Common in female, M:F = 1:1.2, more in young (mean age is 26 years). Any part of GIT from mouth to anus may be affected, but commonly involves terminal ileum (hence, it was previously called regional ileitis). Lesion is transmural (all layers are involved). Causes are unknown. Probable factors are:
- Genetic and familial
- *Diet*: High sugar and fat, but low residue diet
- *Others*: Smoking, probable association with mycobacteria and measles virus (not proved), and abnormal immunological response.

Symptoms:
- Frequent diarrhea, colicky abdominal pain, weight loss, subacute or acute intestinal obstruction
- *General features*: Malaise, lethargy, low-grade fever, anorexia, nausea and vomiting
- Patient may present like acute appendicitis. May be recurrent aphthous ulcer of mouth, mass in right iliac fossa, and anal fissures or perianal abscess. If colitis, may present with bloody diarrhea
- Extraintestinal manifestations.

Extraintestinal features:
- *Eyes*: Conjunctivitis, episcleritis, uveitis or iritis
- *Mouth*: Aphthous ulcer and thickened lip

- *Skin*: Erythema nodosum, pyoderma gangrenosum, and fistula in abdominal wall
- *Bones and joints*: Acute peripheral arthritis, ankylosing spondylitis or sacroiliitis and clubbing
- *Perianal region*: Perianal fistula, skin tag and abscess
- *Liver or hepatobiliary*: Fatty liver, pericholangitis, sclerosing cholangitis (common in ulcerative colitis), autoimmune hepatitis, cirrhosis of liver, granuloma, liver abscess or portal pyemia, gallstone and cholangiocarcinoma
- *Kidney*: Nephrolithiasis (oxalate stone), hydronephrosis and pyelonephritis
- *Others*: Amyloidosis and venous thrombosis.

Investigations:
- Complete blood count (anemia, normocytic, may be megaloblastic due to vitamin B12 deficiency), ESR and C-reactive protein (CRP) (both high). Total protein and albumin to globulin (A/G) ratio (low albumin).
- Liver function tests (may be abnormal)
- Stool for routine examination and culture/sensitivity
- Ultrasonography of whole abdomen
- Barium follow through or small bowel enema (shows narrowing of affected segment, called "*string sign*" which is pathognomonic of Crohn's disease). Barium enema may be done
- Colonoscopy (in colonic Crohn's disease) with biopsy
- Enteroscopy. Capsule endoscopy (in assessing small bowel disease)
- Computed tomography scan or MRI of abdomen.

Complications: Intestinal obstruction, enteric fistula, perianal disease (fissure, skin tag, fistula, perianal abscess and hemorrhoid), carcinoma (rare, may occur if Crohn's disease involves colon), toxic dilatation of colon (common in ulcerative colitis) and malabsorption syndrome.

Treatment: Induction of remission in active disease and maintenance of remission.

Induction of remission:
- *General measures*:
  - Diet: High protein, low fat and milk free. If needed, enteral or parenteral feeding
  - For anemia: Iron, vitamin B12, folic acid and zinc. Erythropoietin may be given
  - Symptomatic treatment for diarrhea (loperamide, codeine phosphate or co-phenotrope). In long-standing diarrhea, cholestyramine may be helpful.
- *Drugs*:
  - Prednisolone, 40–60 mg/day
  - Combination of prednisolone and azathioprine or 6-mercaptopurine (6-MP) may be used
  - For perianal disease: Metronidazole plus ciprofloxacin (for 14 days). 6-MP or azathioprine may be used in chronic case. Infliximab and adalimumab are effective in healing fistula and perianal disease
  - Oral and per-rectal aminosalicylate plus per-rectal steroid should be given.

- In severe colitis or in patient who fails to maximum oral therapy—patient should be hospitalized and treated as follows:
  - Intravenous fluid and nutritional support
  - Intravenous methylprednisolone or hydrocortisone 100 mg 6 hourly
  - Topical and oral aminosalicylates
  - If the patient does not respond to steroid therapy—IV cyclosporine or infliximab may be given. Otherwise urgent surgery should be done.

Maintenance of remission:
- Smoking must be stopped
- Aminosalicylate may be given, but has minimal efficacy
- Thiopurine (azathioprine or 6-MP) is given in patient who relapses more than once a year
- *If fails*: Weekly methotrexate should be given
- *In aggressive disease*: Combination of immunosuppressive and anti-tumor necrosis factor (TNF) therapy should be given.

Surgical treatment: Surgery should be avoided if possible and minimum resection should be done, as the disease is multicentric and recurrence is common. Indications of surgery are:
- Failure of medical therapy, intractable disease or fulminant disease
- Complications like toxic megacolon, obstruction, perforation, massive hemorrhage, refractory fistula and abscess, etc.
- Extraintestinal complications like severe arthritis or pyoderma gangrenosum, not responding to medical treatment
- Failure to grow in children despite medical treatment
- Suspicion of malignancy or severe dysplasia.

Ulcerative Colitis

It is a type of inflammatory bowel disease characterized by ulceration of mucosa of colon (not the deeper layers of bowel wall). There is crypt distortion, cryptitis, crypt abscess, loss of goblet cells and pseudopolyp formation.

Sites of involvement: Large gut, rectum is invariably involved in 95% cases.

Types of ulcerative colitis:
According to the site of involvement:
- Proctitis (when the disease is limited to rectum)
- Distal colitis (when sigmoid and descending colons are involved)
- Pancolitis or total colitis (when whole colon is involved).

Symptoms: Frequent bloody diarrhea with passage of mucous and tenesmus. In severe case—anorexia, weight loss, abdominal pain, patient is toxic with fever and tachycardia. Extraintestinal features like Crohn's disease.

Investigations: Same as Crohn's disease.
- *Barium enema*: In early stage, mucosal irregularity, pseudopolyp, and stricture may be seen. In chronic case, there is shortening and narrowing of the bowel with loss of haustrations
- *Sigmoidoscopy*: Uniform continuous involvement of the mucosa, loss of mucosal vascularity, diffuse erythema, multiple ulcers, blood, mucous or pus, and pseudopolyp.

Complications:
- *Intestinal*: Perforation of colon, toxic megacolon, severe hemorrhage, and malignant change
- *Extraintestinal*: Similar to that for Crohn's disease.

Treatment: Objective of treatment is to control of active disease and maintenance of remission.

Control of active disease:
- *Active proctitis or extensive proctocolitis*: Oral aminosalicylate (mesalazine) plus mesalazine enema or suppository. Rectal steroid (10% hydrocortisone foam or prednisolone 20 mg enema or foam) may be used. If no response or moderate to severe case, oral prednisolone 40 mg daily
- In severe ulcerative colitis, the patient should be hospitalized
- Intravenous methylprednisolone 60 mg or hydrocortisone 100 mg 6 hourly *plus* oral and topical aminosalicylate
    - Intravenous antibiotic, if necessary
    - General measures: IV fluid, blood transfusion, and nutrition
    - If no response: IV cyclosporine or infliximab may be given
    - In colonic dilatation >6 cm, or if clinical condition deteriorates or who do not respond after 7–10 days with conservative therapy, urgent surgery (colectomy) may be needed
    - After recovery: Oral prednisolone should be given. Once remission, it should be tapered 5–10 mg weekly.

Maintenance of remission:
- *After recovery*: Oral aminosalicylate either mesalazine or balsalazide is given to prevent relapse
- In chronic cases with frequent relapse or who require steroid in high dose, azathioprine (1.5–2 mg/kg) may be given. Cyclosporine may also help.

Note: Prednisolone is used only in active disease, no role in preventing relapse. 5-aminosalicylates are mesalazine or olsalazine or balsalazide.

TOXIC MEGACOLON

It is characterized by huge dilatation of colon with severe colitis associated with fever, tachycardia, shock and cessation of diarrhea, and commonly involve transverse colon. Usually, occurs in first attack of ulcerative colitis. Patient is toxic and abdomen is distended. In plain X-ray, if transverse colon is >6 cm, colonic perforation with peritonitis may occur. Cause is—ulcerative colitis (common cause). Rarely, Crohn's disease. Other causes are ischemic colitis and pseudomembranous colitis. Plain X-ray abdomen should be taken daily. Barium enema is contraindicated and CT scan may be done.

Treatment:
- NPO, nutritional support, IV fluid, and correction of electrolytes. Blood transfusion, if Hb <10 g%
- Hydrocortisone 100–200 mg 6 hourly IV or methylprednisolone
- Antibiotic, if infection
- *Surgery*: If no response within 5–7 days, or if the condition deteriorates.

CARCINOMA OF COLON (COLORECTAL CANCER)

Sites: Rectosigmoid (the most common), rectum, cecum, ascending, transverse and descending colon.

Gastrointestinal Diseases

Types:
- *Macroscopically*: Polypoid and fungating, annular and constricting
- *Microscopically*: Adenocarcinoma.

Causes:
Causes are unknown. Predisposing factors are:
- *Dietary factors*: Excess consumption of red meat, saturated animal fat, less dietary fibers, less intake of vegetables and fruits (high vegetables and fruits may be preventive for carcinoma), and excess and prolonged sugar consumption
- *Nondietary factors*:
  - Increasing age: Family history of colon cancer
  - Genetic factors: Benign adenomatous polyp or familial adenomatous polyposis. Hereditary nonpolyposis colon cancer
  - Long standing extensive ulcerative colitis or Crohn's colitis
  - Others: History of breast cancer, ureterosigmoidostomy, acromegaly, pelvic radiotherapy, alcohol (weak association), smoking (relative risk 1.5–3.0), obesity and sedentary lifestyle, cholecystectomy and type 2 diabetes mellitus (T2DM) (hyperinsulinemia).

Factors which Decrease Risk of Colorectal Carcinoma
- *Diet*: Increase fiber, fruits, vegetables, garlic and milk
- Exercise
- *Drugs*: Aspirin or other NSAID, calcium, folic acid, omega-3 fatty acid, and combined estrogen and progesterone hormone replacement therapy.

Symptoms:
Depend on the site (may be asymptomatic):
- *If on the left side*: Bleeding per rectum, alteration of bowel habit, and mass in left iliac fossa
- *If on the right side*: Alteration of bowel habit, intestinal obstruction, and mass in right iliac fossa.

Signs: Depend on site—mass in left iliac fossa or right iliac fossa, hepatomegaly, if metastasis. Others—anemia, lymphadenopathy, etc.

Investigations:
- Ultrasonography of whole abdomen. Sigmoidoscopy or colonoscopy and biopsy (gold standard)
- Computed tomography colonography. CT scan of whole abdomen
- Endoanal ultrasound or pelvic MRI
- Positron emission tomography (PET) scan is useful for detecting occult metastases
- Barium enema (double contrast)
- *Others*: CBC, stool for occult blood, CEA (to see recurrence), and X-ray of chest
- Fine needle aspiration cytology (CT-guided or USG-guided)
- Sometimes, laparotomy may be needed.

Treatment:
- *Curative*: Surgical resection of tumor with pericolic lymph nodes. Adjuvant postoperative chemotherapy (with five fluorouracil and folinic acid)

- *Palliative*: Chemotherapy with 5FU may improve survival. If this fails, second-line drug such as irinotecan may be given. Endoscopic laser therapy or insertion of an expandable metal stent can be used to relieve obstruction.

Screening in Carcinoma of Colon
- Any person >50 years of age, stool for OBT
- Colonoscopy (gold standard). Flexible sigmoidoscopy is an alternative to colonoscopy
- Computed tomography colonoscopy may be used in screening program.

ILEOCECAL TUBERCULOSIS

It is caused by reactivation of primary disease by *Mycobacterium tuberculosis*. May be secondary to pulmonary TB (by swallowing of sputum).

Symptoms:
- History of pulmonary TB may be present. Abdominal pain (usually in right iliac fossa, occasionally generalized), and colicky in nature. Features of intestinal obstruction (acute or subacute)
- Tuberculous peritonitis or ascites. Diarrhea or malabsorption syndrome. Mass in right iliac fossa
- *General features of TB*: Low-grade fever with evening rise, night sweat, malaise and weight loss.

Investigations:
- Complete blood count with ESR, CXR (shows TB in 50%), and Mantoux test
- Ultrasonography of whole abdomen and colonoscopy. CT scan of abdomen
- Barium follow through with spot film in ileocecal region
- Laparoscopy to see tubercle in peritoneum and biopsy.

Complications of Ileocecal Tuberculosis

Intestinal obstruction, fistula (enteroenteric or enterocutaneous), malabsorption and perforation (rare).

Treatment: Standard anti-TB chemotherapy (using four drugs)
- Treatment to be continued for at least 1 year
- Occasionally, surgery (if intestinal obstruction or fistula).

TUBERCULOUS PERITONITIS

Infection of the peritoneum due to *M. tuberculosis*. It may be secondary to pulmonary TB. May occur from direct spread of tubercular bacilli from ruptured abdominal lymph nodes or hematogenous seeding secondary to intestinal TB.

Symptoms: Fever, weight loss, night sweat, diffuse abdominal pain, and unexplained ascites.

Signs: Abdomen is distended due to ascites. Doughy feeling.

Investigations:
- Complete blood count with ESR. X-ray of chest (shows TB in 50%)
- Mantoux test (MT)

- Ultrasonography and CT scan of abdomen
- Ascitic fluid analysis [cytology, biochemistry, adenosine deaminase (ADA), acid-fast bacillus (AFB), and polymerase chain reaction (PCR)]
- Laparoscopy: Shows tubercle which is taken for biopsy.

Finding in ascitic fluid: Straw-colored, exudative (high protein and low glucose), high lymphocyte, and high ADA. AFB and PCR may be positive.

Treatment: Anti-Koch's therapy, continued for 1 year. Steroid may be added.

IRRITABLE BOWEL SYNDROME

Irritable bowel syndrome (IBS) is characterized by recurrent abdominal pain associated with abnormal defecations in the absence of any structural abnormality of the gut. Common in female. Coexisting conditions such as nonulcer dyspepsia, chronic fatigue syndrome, fibromyalgia and dysmenorrhea may be present. Causes are unknown, some factors may trigger:
- *Affective disorder*: Anxiety and depression. Psychological factors (e.g. stress and trauma)
- Gastrointestinal infection
- Antibiotic therapy
- Sexual, physical and verbal abuse
- Eating disorder
- *Dietary factors*: Lactose and fructose containing diet may be responsible
- May be triggered by some organisms like salmonella, campylobacter, etc.

Irritable Bowel Syndrome

Irritable bowel syndrome with diarrhea, IBS with constipation, and mixed (alternating constipation and diarrhea).

Symptoms:
- Abdominal pain, bloating, alternating diarrhea, and constipation. Pain is relieved after defecation
- Diarrhea is usually painless, sometimes in the morning, and usually not at night
- Stools are usually pellet or ribbon-like, mixed with mucus
- Feeling of incomplete evacuation of bowel, dyspepsia, flatulence, heart burn or pain in the upper abdomen
- Sometimes, frequency of micturition and urgency may be present.

Signs: No abnormality, may be tenderness in the left iliac fossa and palpable sigmoid colon.

Investigations: No specific investigation. Some tests are done to exclude any organic disease—
- Stool to see ova, cyst, parasite and occult blood
- Ultrasonography of whole abdomen
- Sigmoidoscopy or colonoscopy
- Barium enema
- Computed tomography scan of abdomen
- Thyroid function tests, if necessary.

Treatment:
- *General measures*:
  - Reassurance and explanation. Psychotherapy, behavior therapy, and hypnotherapy may be needed. Avoid stress and depression. Regular meals and adequate sleep is essential
  - Avoid fried foods, milk and milk products, alcohol, tea and coffee.
- *If pain and distension or bloating*:
  - Dietary modification, spasmolytic (mebeverine, alverine or peppermint oil or hyoscine)
  - Probiotic. Rifaximin may be given
  - Amitriptyline or imipramine may be added at night.
- *If diarrhea is predominant*: Dietary modification (gluten free, milk or milk product free), loperamide or codeine or cholestyramine may be given, spasmolytic (mebeverine, alverine or peppermint oil or hyoscine)
- *If constipation is predominant*: High fiber diet, ispaghula husk, and lactulose may be given. 5-HT receptor agonist (prucalopride or linaclotide) may be given. If symptoms persist, duloxetine or paroxetine may be tried.

VOMITING

Causes of Vomiting
- *Physiological*: Pregnancy
- *Gastrointestinal tract disorders*: Gastroenteritis, pyloric stenosis, peptic ulcer disease (PUD), carcinoma of stomach, acute cholecystitis, acute appendicitis, acute pancreatitis, and intestinal obstruction
- *Hepatic*: Acute hepatitis
- *Renal*: Acute kidney injury (AKI) and chronic kidney disease (CKD)
- *Central nervous system (CNS)*: Raised intracranial pressure, migraine, meningitis, encephalitis and vestibular neuronitis
- *Endocrine disorders*: Diabetic ketoacidosis, lactic acidosis, and Addisonian crisis
- *Drugs*: Morphine, digoxin, cytotoxic drugs, NSAID and alcohol
- *Others*: Psychogenic vomiting, hysterical conversion reaction, and anorexia nervosa.

Investigations: According to suspicion of cause.

Treatment: Antiemetic (e.g. prochlorperazine, ondansetron, metoclopramide and domperidone) may be given. Psychotherapy in psychogenic vomiting. Treatment of primary cause.

CONSTIPATION

It means passage of hard stool or bowel movement less than three times a week. Patient may complain of straining, sensation of incomplete evacuation of stool or anorectal blockage. Causes are:
- *General*: Lack of fiber diet and fluid intake, pregnancy and immobility
- *Gastrointestinal tract causes*: IBS, intestinal obstruction, diverticular disease, carcinoma of colon, Hirschsprung's disease, and anorectal diseases (Crohn's disease, anal fissures and hemorrhoid)

- *Neurological causes*: Multiple sclerosis, cerebrovascular disease (CVD), Parkinsonism, and spinal cord disease
- *Endocrine and metabolic*: Hypothyroidism, DM, hyperparathyroidism and hypercalcemia
- *Drugs*: Opiates, anticholinergics, calcium, iron, verapamil and aluminum-containing antacids
- *Psychological*: Depression, anxiety and anorexia nervosa.

Symptoms: Infrequent bowel movement, abdominal pain, fullness, nausea and vomiting. Features of underlying disease.

Investigations: Should be done according to suspicion of cause.

Treatment: Diet—high fiber such as bran, raw fruits, vegetables, plenty of fluids and ispaghula husk.
- Laxatives in some cases
- Glycerine suppository or sometimes enema
- Treatment of primary cause.

DIARRHEA

It means frequent passage of loose stool more than 200 g daily or passage of frequent stool three times per day. There are two types:
1. *Acute diarrhea*: Persists less than 2 weeks
2. *Chronic diarrhea*: Persists more than 4 weeks.

Acute Diarrhea

Causes:
- *Infection*:
  - Bacterial: Enterotoxigenic *E. coli, Vibrio cholerae, Shigella, Salmonella, Campylobacter, Bacillus cereus, Staphylococcus aureus,* and *Clostridium difficile*
  - Viruses: *Rota virus, Norwalk virus,* and *Corona virus*
  - Parasitic: *Entamoeba histolytica, Giardia lamblia,* and *Cryptosporidium parvum.*
- *Drugs*: Antibiotics, laxatives, domperidone, antacid, digitalis, colchicine and chemotherapeutic agents.

Symptoms: Passage of loose stool, abdominal discomfort or pain, vomiting and fever, if infective cause. Increased thirst, decreased urination, fatigue and altered consciousness.

Signs: Signs of dehydration (dry tongue, loss of skin turgor, tachycardia and low BP). Localized or diffuse abdominal tenderness.

Complications: Hypovolemia and shock, renal failure, electrolyte imbalance (hypokalemia, hypernatremia and metabolic acidosis).

Investigations:
- Complete blood count
- Stool for R/M/E and C/S
- Serum electrolytes. Blood urea and serum creatinine
- In chronic case: Investigation according to suspicion of cause.

Treatment: Fluid and electrolyte replacement—oral rehydration solution (ORS) and IV cholera saline. Antibiotic therapy (if bacterial infection is suspected). Treatment of cause.

Chronic Diarrhea

Diarrhea more than weeks or months, usually >4 weeks, may be persistent or intermittent. Causes are:
- *Gastrointestinal tract causes*: IBS, inflammatory bowel disease, infectious (giardiasis, amoebiasis and intestinal TB), radiation colitis, colon cancer, diverticulitis, ischemic colitis, malabsorption syndrome, chronic pancreatitis, Celiac disease, tropical sprue, intestinal lymphoma, gastrinoma, and VIPoma
- *Extraintestinal causes*: Hyperthyroidism, Addisonian crisis, DM (due to autonomic neuropathy), drugs (laxative, statin, metformin and anticancer drug), factitious diarrhea (due to purgative abuse), and Zollinger–Ellison syndrome.

Investigations: According to suspicious of cause.

Treatment: Symptomatic and supportive. Treatment of cause.

Causes of Bloody Diarrhea

Bacillary dysentery, ulcerative colitis, carcinoma of large gut, pseudo-membranous colitis, mesenteric vasculitis, angiodysplasia of colon, ischemic colitis, and radiation enteritis.

MALABSORPTION SYNDROME

It is a group of disorders associated with disturbance of digestion and defective mucosal absorption of essential constituents of food like nutrients, electrolytes, minerals and vitamins. It is usually associated with chronic diarrhea and features of malnutrition.

Causes: According to the organ involved—
- *Stomach*: Gastrectomy (partial or total), carcinoma of stomach, Ménétrier's disease, and bariatric surgery
- *Intestine*:
    - Celiac disease, tropical sprue, and Whipple's disease
    - Intestinal TB and carcinoid syndrome
    - Intestinal resection: Ileal resection or massive intestinal resection (short bowel syndrome)
    - Inflammatory bowel disease
    - Bacterial overgrowth and parasites (giardiasis and *Diphyllobothrium latum*)
    - Others: Radiation enteritis, fistulae, diverticular disease, strictures, amyloidosis and lymphoma.
- *Pancreatic causes*: Fibrocystic disease of the pancreas, chronic pancreatitis, and carcinoma of pancreas
- *Liver disease*: Obstructive jaundice and primary biliary cirrhosis
- *Systemic causes*: Hyperthyroidism, Addison's disease, DM and systemic sclerosis
- *Due to enzyme deficiencies*:
    - Lactase deficiency causing lactose intolerance
    - Intestinal disaccharidase deficiency
    - Intestinal enteropeptidase deficiency
    - Sucrose intolerance.

Gastrointestinal Diseases

- *Drugs*: Cholestyramine, neomycin, orlistat, colchicine and cytotoxic drugs
- *Miscellaneous*: HIV, intestinal lymphoma, and abetalipoproteinemia.

Clinical features:
- Diarrhea or steatorrhea (frothy, bulky, pale, offensive and floats on the toilet), abdominal discomfort, bloating, undigested food in stool, and mucus and blood in stool
- Other features are due to defective absorption of specific nutrients
- *Protein malabsorption*: Muscle wasting, edema, weight loss and leukonychia
- *Fat malabsorption*: Weight loss and bulky pale frothy stool
- *Carbohydrate malabsorption*: Bloating, abdominal distension, borborygmi and flatus
- Growth retardation
- *Iron and folic acid*: Anemia, glossitis and koilonychia
- *Vitamin B1 and B2*: Angular stomatitis, cheilosis and glossitis
- *Vitamin B12*: Anemia, smooth shiny tongue, peripheral neuropathy, and subacute combined degeneration of spinal cord
- *Vitamin K*: Bleeding tendency (bruise and ecchymosis)
- *Vitamin A*: Night blindness, xerosis, xerophthalmia and toad skin
- *Vitamin D and calcium*: Rickets or osteomalacia, bone and muscle pain, and tetany
- *Zinc*: Acrodermatitis enteropathica, poor wound healing, and tingling
- *Magnesium*: Weakness, tetany and paresthesia
- *Potassium*: Muscular weakness, abdominal distension, and arrhythmia
- *Sodium*: Weakness, hypotension and muscle cramp.

Investigations:
- *Routine investigations*:
  - Complete blood count, ESR, peripheral blood film (PBF), and blood sugar
  - Stool: Microscopy to see, ova, cyst and larva. Also stool for C/S
  - Liver function tests. Total protein and Albumin:Globulin (A/G) Ratio (A:G) ratio
  - Serum iron, folic acid, B12, calcium, magnesium and electrolytes
  - Ultrasonography of whole abdomen. Plain X-ray and CT scan of abdomen
  - Barium meal and follow through
  - Endoscopy.
- *Specific*: According to suspicion of cause.

Treatment: According to the cause.
- Replacement nutrients, electrolytes and fluids
- Pancreatic enzyme in pancreatic insufficiency
- *Dietary modification*: Gluten-free diet in celiac disease and lactose avoidance in lactose intolerance
- Antibiotic therapy in bowel infection
- Cholestyramine in bile acid malabsorption
- Treatment of specific disease like Crohn's disease and ulcerative colitis.

CELIAC DISEASE

It is a gluten-sensitive enteropathy characterized by mucosal destruction mainly of jejunum due to hypersensitivity to gliadin fraction of gluten protein. There is atrophy of villi, crypt hypertrophy, infiltration of plasma cells, and lymphocytes in lamina propria.

Symptoms:
- Diarrhea or steatorrhea. Anorexia, nausea, weight loss, abdominal pain, bloating, flatulence and distension. May be associated with itchy vascular rash due to dermatitis herpetiformis
- *Features of intestinal malabsorption*: Anemia, muscle cramps, bone pain, osteomalacia, bleeding manifestation, and ankle edema. Failure to thrive (in children).

Investigations:
- Stool routine microbial examination. Complete blood count shows dimorphic anemia (both macrocytic and microcytic), due to deficiency of iron, folic acid, and rarely B12. PBF shows Howell–Jolly body and target cells
- Ultrasonography of whole abdomen (to exclude other disease)
- *Antibody*: Serum antiendomysial antibody, tissue transglutaminase antibody (anti-tTG). Antireticulin antibody (very sensitive, but less specific), and anti-gliadin antibody (less sensitive)
- Endoscopic jejunal biopsy shows subtotal villous atrophy and crypts hyperplasia
- Low serum albumin, calcium, iron or folate level.

Complications: Hyposplenism, gastric or small bowel T-cell lymphoma, esophageal squamous cell and small bowel carcinoma, ulcerative jejunoileitis. Dermatitis herpetiformis may be associated with celiac disease.

Treatment: Avoid gluten-free diet (wheat, rye, barley and oat). Iron, folic acid, calcium and magnesium should be given. If lactose intolerance, milk and milk products should be avoided.

TROPICAL SPRUE

It is a chronic, progressive malabsorption in a patient residing in and from the tropical region, characterized by inflammation and flattening of villi of small intestine. Cause is unknown. Probably due to bacterial, viral, amoebial or parasitic infection. Small bowel bacterial overgrowth with *E. coli*, *Enterobacter*, and *Klebsiella* is frequently seen.

Clinical features: Like celiac disease. Relapse and remission may occur.

Investigations:
- *Complete blood count*: Like celiac disease. Stool for R/M/E
- Endoscopy with small bowel biopsy shows inflammation of the lining and flattening of villi of small intestine. Jejunal biopsy reveals presence of inflammatory cells (mostly lymphocytes)
- Low serum albumin, calcium, iron or folate level. Low vitamin A, B12, E, D and K level.

Treatment:
- Tetracycline 250 mg four times daily for 28 days, may be required more (up to 6 months)
- Folic acid 5 mg daily

- Correction of fluid and electrolytes. Other deficiencies should be corrected, e.g. iron, vitamin B12, etc.

DIVERTICULAR DISEASES

Diverticula are the sac-like outpouching of colonic mucosa and submucosa through weaknesses of muscle layers in the colon wall. Presence of diverticula is called diverticulosis and inflammation of the diverticula is called diverticulitis. Diverticula are common in elderly, occurs in 50% over 50 years.

Diverticulosis

It is characterized by presence of diverticula in the colon. These are associated with hypertrophy of circular muscle layer. Sites are any part of colon, common in sigmoid colon.

Risk factors: Diet—low fiber diets, refined diet, and relative deficiency of fibers is thought to be responsible for diverticula. Also, positive family history.

Mechanism: High intracolonic pressure that occurs due to low fiber diet causes herniation of mucosa through areas of weakness in colonic muscular wall where blood vessels penetrate the muscle.

Symptoms: Asymptomatic in 95% cases.
- *In symptomatic case*: Pain or discomfort in left iliac fossa, bloating, constipation or diarrhea
- *During severe episode*: There may be diarrhea, bleeding per rectum, and fever.

Signs: Tenderness in the left iliac fossa.

Complications: Rectal bleeding, perforation, pericolic abscess, fistula formation (into bladder, small bowel, and vagina), and diverticulitis.

Investigations:
- Sigmoidoscopy or colonoscopy
- Ultrasonography of abdomen to exclude other disease
- Computed tomography scan of abdomen
- Barium enema (avoided in acute attack).

Treatment:
- *If asymptomatic*: High fiber diet and plenty of fluids are sufficient
- *In acute attack*: Metronidazole 400 mg 8 hourly plus antibiotic (ciprofloxacin or ampicillin) for 7 days.

Diverticulitis

It means when diverticula are inflamed. It occurs when fecal matter obstructs the neck of diverticulum causing stagnation, allowing bacteria to multiply and produce inflammation.

Symptoms: Fever, pain in left iliac fossa, vomiting and alternation of bowel habits (constipation or diarrhea).

Signs: Tenderness and rigidity in left iliac fossa, colonic mass may be felt.

Complications: Abscess formation, obstruction, bowel perforation, fistula into the adjacent organ, and generalized peritonitis.

Investigations: As in diverticulosis.

Treatment:
- NPO, IV fluids, and IV broad-spectrum antibiotic with metronidazole
- Surgery is recommended (resection of involved segment), once acute inflammation resolves.

CHAPTER 4

Hematology

ANEMIA

It is a clinical condition characterized by reduced hemoglobin concentration according to the age and sex of the individual.

Classification:
- Etiological (based on cause)
- Morphological [based on morphology of red blood cell (RBC)].

Etiological:
- *Hemorrhagic anemia (due to blood loss)*:
    - Acute: Trauma, postpartum bleeding, hematemesis, melena and epistaxis
    - Chronic: Hookworm, hemorrhoid, excessive menstrual loss, and bleeding peptic ulcer.
- *Deficiency anemia*:
    - Iron deficiency anemia
    - Vitamin B12 and folic acid deficiency (megaloblastic anemia).
- *Dyshemopoietic anemia (less production of RBC)*:
    - Aplastic anemia (bone marrow failure, may be primary or secondary)
    - Anemia of chronic disorder: Systemic lupus erythematosus (SLE), rheumatoid arthritis (RA), sideroblastic anemia, chronic kidney disease (CKD), hypothyroidism and malignancy.
- *Hemolytic anemia (due to breakdown of RBC)*:
    - Genetic: Red cell membrane defect (e.g. hereditary spherocytosis, elliptocytosis and stomatocytosis), hemoglobin abnormality (thalassemia, and sickle cell anemia), and enzyme defects [glucose-6-phosphate dehydrogenase (G6PD) deficiency and pyruvate kinase deficiency]
    - Acquired: Autoimmune, toxic, mechanical and infectious causes.

Morphological [depending on mean corpuscular volume (MCV) and mean corpuscular hemoglobin concentration (MCHC)]:
- Normocytic normochromic anemia (normal MCV and MCHC)
- Microcytic hypochromic anemia (low MCV <76 fL, low MCHC <30 g/dL)
- Macrocytic anemia (high MCV >96 fL)

- Dimorphic anemia (combination of two cell lines—macrocytes and microcytes).

Causes of normocytic normochromic anemia: Hemorrhagic and hemolytic anemia, aplastic anemia, anemia of chronic disorder, malignancy, endocrine disease, and sideroblastic anemia.

Causes of microcytic hypochromic anemia: Iron deficiency, thalassemia, sideroblastic and anemia of chronic disorder.

Causes of macrocytic anemia:
- *Macrocytosis with megaloblastic marrow*: Vitamin B12 or folic acid deficiency
- *Macrocytosis with normoblastic marrow*: Chronic liver disease (CLD), chronic alcoholism, hypothyroidism, hemorrhage, hemolysis, sideroblastic anemia, pure red cell aplasia, and azathioprine.

DIMORPHIC ANEMIA

When both microcytes and macrocytes are found in peripheral blood film (PBF), this is called dimorphic anemia.

Causes: Combined iron, B12 or folate deficiency, and sideroblastic anemia, during treatment of anemia.

Signs that may point to a specific cause of anemia:
- *Hemolytic anemia*: Triad of anemia, jaundice and splenomegaly
- *Iron deficiency anemia*: Angular stomatitis, cheilitis, glossitis and koilonychia
- *Glossitis*: Iron deficiency anemia, vitamin B12 deficiency, and folate deficiency
- *Vitamin B12 deficiency (megaloblastic anemia)*: Neurological changes (dementia, optic atrophy, and features of subacute combined degeneration of spinal cord) and lemon yellow tint.

Investigations of anemia: Detailed history, physical examination, and relevant laboratory investigations are done.

History:
- Dietary history and malabsorption
- History of bleeding (hemorrhoid, epistaxis, hematemesis, melena and menorrhagia in female)
- *In female*: Multiple pregnancies, repeated abortion, and menorrhagia
- *Drug history*: Nonsteroidal anti-inflammatory drugs (NSAIDs) drugs causing bone marrow suppression (e.g. cytotoxic drugs), and drugs causing hemolysis (e.g. sulfasalazine and methyldopa)
- *History of surgery*: Gastrectomy or partial gastrectomy and ileal surgery (causes deficiency of vitamin B12)
- Family history (in hereditary hemolytic anemia)
- History of chronic disease (e.g. SLE, RA, CKD and CLD).

Clinical examination: See above.

Laboratory investigations:
- Complete blood count (CBC), erythrocyte sedimentation rate (ESR), platelet, and PBF (to see normocytic, microcytic, macrocytic or dimorphic)
- Reticulocyte count—high in hemolytic anemia
- MCV and MCHC

- Bone marrow examination—to detect megaloblastic anemia, aplastic anemia, bone marrow infiltration (secondary deposit), and ring sideroblasts (in sideroblastic anemia)
- Other investigations according to suspicion of cause.

Investigations of microcytic hypochromic anemia (low MCV and low MCHC):
- *For iron deficiency anemia*: Serum iron, total iron-binding capacity (TIBC), and serum ferritin
- *For hereditary hemolytic anemia*: Hemoglobin electrophoresis and skeletal survey
- *For sideroblastic anemia*: According to history, bone marrow examination (to see ring sideroblasts)
- *For anemia of chronic disease*: Test should be done according to the cause.

Investigations for macrocytic anemia (high MCV): Serum B12 and folic acid assay. Bone marrow study, if needed.

SIDEROBLASTIC ANEMIA

It is defined as a group of anemia characterized by refractory anemia, variable number of hypochromic cells in the peripheral blood, excess iron, and ring sideroblast.

Types:
- Hereditary
- *Acquired, which may be primary and secondary*:
  - Primary sideroblastic anemia (refractory anemia with ring sideroblast)
  - Secondary sideroblastic anemia may be due to—(1) Drugs and chemicals [isonicotinylhydrazide (INH), alcohol and lead], (2) Hematological disease [myelofibrosis, polycythemia rubra vera (PRV), myeloma, Hodgkin's lymphoma, hemolytic anemia, and leukemia], (3) Inflammatory disease (RA, and SLE), and (4) Others (carcinoma, myxedema and malabsorption).

Treatment: Treatment of primary cause, e.g. withdrawal of drug and stop alcohol. Some cases may respond to pyridoxine and folic acid. Correction of anemia is done by blood transfusion.

IRON DEFICIENCY ANEMIA

Anemia secondary is due to deficiency of iron.

Causes:
- *Bleeding due to any cause*: Gastrointestinal tract (GIT) (hemorrhoid, colorectal carcinoma, carcinoma of stomach, diverticulitis and angiodysplasia of colon), and menorrhagia in female
- Hookworm (also schistosomiasis)
- Less intake of food
- Malabsorption
- More demand (e.g. pregnancy).

Symptoms: Weakness, vertigo, dizziness, lightheadedness, tingling, numbness, anorexia, weight loss, palpitation, breathlessness on exertion, and pica (eating of unusual material, e.g. earth).

Signs: The patient is pale and anemic. Koilonychia, glossitis and angular stomatitis.

Investigations:
- *Test to confirm iron deficiency anemia*:
  - Complete blood count with PBF (microcytic hypochromic blood picture)
  - Serum iron, TIBC and ferritin (low iron, low ferritin, and increased TIBC).
- *Test to find out causes*:
  - Stool for ova or cyst of hookworm and occult blood test
  - Upper gastrointestinal (GI) endoscopy (to see esophageal varices, peptic ulcer, and carcinoma stomach)
  - Proctoscopy (hemorrhoid), sigmoidoscopy or colonoscopy (neoplasm, polyp, diverticulum, ulcer and angiodysplasia of colon)
  - Ultrasonography (USG) of abdomen (any mass and fibroid uterus in female).

Treatment:
- Severe anemia should be corrected by blood transfusion
- *Iron therapy*: Oral ferrous sulfate, ferrous gluconate or ferrous fumarate, for 3–6 months after hemoglobin is normal to replenish the iron store. If the patient is unable to take iron orally, it can be given intravenous (IV)
- Treatment of cause (e.g. menorrhagia and hemorrhoid).

MEGALOBLASTIC ANEMIA

It is a type of anemia which is due to deficiency of vitamin B12, folic acid or both, characterized by macrocyte in peripheral blood and megaloblast in bone marrow.

Causes of megaloblastic anemia due to vitamin B12 deficiency:
- *Diet*: Strict vegetarians
- *Stomach pathology*: Total or partial gastrectomy, carcinoma of stomach, and pernicious anemia
- *Small bowel pathology*:
  - Ileal disease: Crohn's disease and ileal resection
  - Pancreatic exocrine insufficiency: Vitamin B12 deficiency occurs in 30% patients
  - Motility disorders: It can cause bacterial overgrowth and vitamin B12 deficiency
  - Fish tapeworm (Diphyllobothrium latum).

Pernicious Anemia

It is an autoimmune disease in which there is atrophy of gastric mucosa with loss of parietal cells causing intrinsic factor deficiency. So, vitamin B12 is not absorbed due to deficiency of intrinsic factor. There are anti-intrinsic factor antibodies and also anti-parietal cell antibodies in serum.

Symptoms of megaloblastic anemia: Weakness, malaise, weight loss, breathlessness and sore mouth. Paresthesia, poor memory, depression, hallucinations, and visual disturbance.

Signs:
- Angular cheilitis. Tongue—smooth and shiny with atrophy of papillae
- Skin pigmentation, lemon yellow tint, and vitiligo

- *Neurological*:
  - Peripheral neuropathy
  - Spinal cord (subacute combined degeneration): Loss of vibration and position sense (posterior column lesion), and upper motor neuron signs (corticospinal tract lesion)
  - Cerebral: Dementia
  - Optic atrophy.

Investigations:
- *CBC*: Low hemoglobin (Hb)% may indicate pancytopenia. PBF shows macrocytes and hypersegmented neutrophils
- Serum vitamin B12 (low)
- Parietal cell and intrinsic factor antibodies for pernicious anemia
- *Bone marrow aspiration*: Shows increase cellularity and megaloblasts
- *Others*: Low reticulocyte count and high lactic acid dehydrogenase (LDH).

Treatment: Blood transfusion in severe anemia. Injection hydroxycobalamin 1,000 µg intramuscular (IM) daily six dose, for 2 or 3 days apart. Then 1,000 µg every 3 months (lifelong for pernicious anemia).

Causes of megaloblastic anemia due to folic acid deficiency:
- Less intake of vegetables
- *Malabsorption*: Due to any cause (e.g. celiac disease and tropical sprue)
- *Increased demand*: Pregnancy and hemolysis
- *Drugs*: Methotrexate and phenytoin.

Investigation: Serum folate level (low) and red cell folate level (low).

Treatment: Tablet folic acid 5 mg is given daily for 3 weeks and then it is given 5 mg weekly. Prophylactic folic acid should be given in pregnancy and also in hemolytic anemia.

Note: Folic acid alone should not be given if there is vitamin B12 deficiency, otherwise it may aggravate neurological lesion. In such cases, both should be given.

HEMOLYTIC ANEMIA

Anemia occurs due to destruction or breakdown of RBC.

There are two types:
- *Inherited*:
  - Red cell membrane abnormality: Hereditary spherocytosis and elliptocytosis
  - Red cell enzyme deficiency: G6PD deficiency and pyruvate kinase deficiency
  - Hemoglobinopathy: Thalassemia, sickle cell disease, and other hemoglobinopathies.
- *Acquired*:
  - Autoimmune:
    - Warm antibodies (primary or idiopathic and secondary in SLE, RA, chronic lymphatic leukemia (CLL), and lymphoma, drugs such as methyldopa and quinidine)
    - Cold antibodies (primary or idiopathic, secondary in Mycoplasma pneumoniae, and lymphoma).

Hematology

- Nonimmune:
    - Mechanical (microangiopathic hemolytic anemia and prosthetic valve)
    - Infection (falciparum malaria)
    - *Chemicals*: Dapsone, sulfasalazine and maloprim
    - *Acquired membrane abnormality*: Paroxysmal nocturnal hemoglobinuria (PNH).

Evidence of Hemolysis

- *Clinical*: Triad of anemia, jaundice and splenomegaly (in hereditary hemolytic anemia)
- *In the blood*:
    - High serum bilirubin
    - High urinary urobilinogen
    - Low haptoglobin
    - High LDH
    - High reticulocytes
    - Erythroid hyperplasia in bone marrow.

THALASSEMIA

It is an inherited disorder characterized by impaired hemoglobin production due to partial or complete failure to synthesize specific type of globin chain.

There are two types:
1. *Beta-Thalassemia*: Less production of β chain, causing less production of HbA. It is of two types—
    i. β-Thalassemia major: HbA is less and HbF is high
    ii. β-Thalassemia minor: HbA2 is high.
2. *Alpha-Thalassemia*: Inadequate production of α chain, so less HbA, HbF and HbA2, as all of them contain α chain.

Beta-thalassemia Major

It is characterized by reduced or absent synthesis of β chain of globin. Family history may be present.

Symptoms: Weakness, palpitation and dizziness. Yellow coloration of eyes, high colored urine. Feeling of a mass in the left upper abdomen (due to splenomegaly).

Note: If the patient develops severe abdominal pain, likely cause is cholelithiasis. There may also be splenic infarction and acute pancreatitis.

Signs: Triad of hemolytic anemia (anemia, jaundice and splenomegaly). Frontal and parietal bossing, and mongoloid facies with prominent malar bones. Short stature and retardation of growth.

Investigations:
- CBC and PBF (shows microcytic hypochromic blood picture), and reticulocyte count (high)
- Hemoglobin electrophoresis
- *Others*: X-ray of skull and hand, and other skeletal survey, and serum bilirubin (high). Serum iron profile—ferritin (high), iron and TIBC.

Treatment:
- *Correction of anemia*: Blood transfusion to keep Hb% above 10 g/dL, every 4 months (because life span of RBC is 4 months)

- Folic acid 5 mg daily, to be continued
- Iron-containing drugs and diet are avoided (iron can only be given if deficiency)
- Repeated blood transfusion may cause hemosiderosis, which can be prevented by chelating agent. (see below)
- Injection erythropoietin
- Hydroxyurea 1–2 g daily may be helpful
- *Specific therapy*: Allogeneic bone marrow transplantation. Also, gene therapy
- Splenectomy may be needed in some cases
- Genetic counselling should be offered.

Complications of Repeated Blood Transfusion
- Hemosiderosis (usually when more than 30–50 L of blood is transfused)
- Infections such as hepatitis B, C and D, and human immunodeficiency virus (HIV).

Prevention of Hemosiderosis

It can be prevented by using chelating agent desferrioxamine (1.5–2 g with each unit of blood), usually given subcutaneously in the anterior abdominal wall with infusion pump for 12 hours. It may also be given with infusion drip (normal saline or aqua). Oral chelating agents such as deferiprone and deferasirox. Vitamin C 200 mg daily orally also helps in iron excretion.

Thalassemia Minor

Usually asymptomatic or mild anemia.

Investigations: CBC shows microcytic hypochromic blood picture. Hemoglobin electrophoresis shows high A2.

Differential diagnoses: It confuses with iron deficiency anemia. However, anemia is more marked in iron deficiency and relatively less in thalassemia minor. Also, in iron deficiency, there is low iron, low ferritin, and high TIBC.

Alpha-Thalassemia

It is characterized by reduced or absent alpha globin chain synthesis. Normally, adults have four alpha globin chain genes.
- When 1 alpha gene is absent—patient is hematologically normal (silent carrier)
- When 2 alpha genes are absent—called alpha thalassemia trait. The patient is clinically normal, life expectancy is normal
- When 3 alpha genes are absent—the patient has HbH disease. There is chronic hemolytic anemia with variable severity. Examination shows severe anemia with splenomegaly
- If all 4 alpha globin chains are absent—affected fetus is stillborn due to hydrops fetalis.

AUTOIMMUNE HEMOLYTIC ANEMIA

It is group of hemolytic anemia that occurs due to red cell autoantibodies causing increased red cell destruction. Antibodies may be IgG or IgM. Antibodies are of two types depending on temperature at which the antibody reacts with red cells.

- Warm antibodies bind at 37°C, common (80% cases). Antibody is IgG
- Cold antibodies bind at 4°C but can bind up to 37°C in some cases. Antibody is IgM. Less common (20% cases).

Warm Autoimmune Hemolytic Anemia

Occurs at all ages, common in middle age, more in females.

Causes:
- Primary or idiopathic (50% cases)
- *Secondary*: Infection (*M. pneumoniae*, infectious mononucleosis, and cytomegalovirus), collagen diseases (SLE and RA), drugs (methyldopa and quinidine), neoplastic (CLL, and lymphoma), and others (carcinoma and sarcoidosis).

Clinical features: May be asymptomatic or features of primary cause or features of hemolytic anemia (anemia, jaundice and splenomegaly).

Investigations: CBC with PBF shows macrocytes and spherocytes. Direct Coombs or antiglobulin test is positive. Serum IgG is high.

Treatment: Underlying cause should be treated, offending drugs must be stopped. Prednisolone 1 mg/kg orally. When Hb and reticulocyte count are normal, dose can be reduced slowly over 10 weeks. Blood transfusion is done in case of severe anemia. If there is no response to prednisolone, splenectomy should be considered. If splenectomy is not possible, azathioprine or cyclophosphamide may be given. Anti-CD20 monoclonal antibody, rituximab is helpful in some cases.

Cold Agglutinin Disease

It is an autoimmune hemolytic anemia which is due to cold antibodies. It is of two types—(1) Cold hemagglutinin disease (CHAD), and (2) paroxysmal cold hemoglobinuria (PCH).

Chronic cold agglutinin disease occurs in elderly and may be associated with an underlying low-grade B-cell lymphoma. It causes low-grade intravascular hemolysis with cold, painful, blue fingers, toes and ears or nose (called acrocyanosis).

Causes:
- Idiopathic in most cases
- *Secondary*: Lymphoma, CLL, SLE and Waldenström's macroglobulinemia. Also in *M. pneumoniae* and infectious mononucleosis.

Investigation: The CBC with PBF shows cold agglutination at low temperature. Direct Coombs test is positive with complements. Serum IgM is high.

Treatment: Treatment of underlying causes. If idiopathic—patients must keep extremities warm, especially in winter. Some respond to steroid; blood transfusion may be needed in severe anemia. Folic acid should be given.

SICKLE CELL ANEMIA

It is a hereditary disorder, inherited as autosomal recessive trait, in which the red cells contain an abnormal hemoglobin called HbS.

There are two types:
1. Homozygotes produce abnormal β-chains that make hemoglobin S (called AS). This causes clinical syndrome of sickle cell disease

2. Heterozygotes produce normal and abnormal β-chains that make normal HbA and HbS. This causes sickle cell trait, which is clinically asymptomatic.

When hemoglobin S is deoxygenated and red cell membrane is distorted, then it produces sickle-shaped cells.

Clinical features: Usually present in childhood before 2 years.
- Features of hemolytic anemia, frequent infection, leg ulcers, gall stone, and dactylitis (due to microinfarction of medulla of carpal and metatarsal bones)
- Splenomegaly is present, but repeated infarction of spleen causes atrophy (autosplenectomy) at the age of 8 years. So spleen is no longer palpable
- *May present with following crises called sickle cell crises*:
  - Vaso-occlusive crisis: Plugging of small vessels in bone produces acute severe bone pain. Mesenteric infarction causes acute abdominal pain. Papillary necrosis may occur in kidney. Cerebral infarction is due to involvement of brain
  - Sickle chest syndrome: Bone marrow infarction results in fat emboli to lungs, which causes further infarction, leading to ventilatory failure
  - Sequestration crisis: There is splenic pooling of red cells and hypovolemia, leading to circulatory collapse and death. Liver sequestration can also occur
  - Aplastic crisis: Red cell aplasia causes very low hemoglobin.

Investigations:
- Complete blood count with PBF shows sickle cells, target cells, and features of hyposplenism
- Reticulocyte count—high
- Sickle solubility test
- Hemoglobin electrophoresis shows high HbS, absence of HbA, and 2–20% HbF.

Treatment:
- Phenoxymethylpenicillin is given to protect pneumococcal infection
- Folic acid. Blood transfusion, if severe anemia. Hydroxyurea may be helpful
- Vaccination against *Pneumococcus*, *Meningococcus*, *Haemophilus influenzae* B, hepatitis B, and influenza
- Allogeneic stem cell transplantation from human leukocyte antigen (HLA)-matched siblings may be curative.

MICROANGIOPATHIC HEMOLYTIC ANEMIA

It is a type of mechanical hemolytic anemia in which anemia is associated with fragmented RBC (schistocyte and helmet cell). Red cell fragmentation is due to contact between red cells and abnormal intima of partially thrombosed, narrowed or necrotic vessels.

Causes:
- Disseminated intravascular coagulation (DIC)
- Thrombotic thrombocytopenic purpura (TTP)
- Hemolytic uremic syndrome (HUS)
- Disseminated malignancy
- Vasculitis

- Metallic cardiac valve prosthesis
- Malignant hypertension.

Investigations: CBC with PBF (shows anemia with fragmented RBC). Others—bilirubin and high reticulocyte count.

Treatment: Treatment of primary cause.

PAROXYSMAL NOCTURNAL HEMOGLOBINURIA

It is an acquired clonal abnormality of red cells, which are destroyed by activated complement resulting in intravascular hemolysis. Platelet and granulocyte are involved, causing thrombocytopenia and leukopenia.

Clinical features: Commonly, urine, voided at night and in morning on waking from sleep, is dark colored. Hemolysis may be precipitated by infection, surgery or iron therapy.

Complications:
- Venous thrombosis involves mesenteric, portal (Budd–Chiari syndrome) or cerebral veins, and calf muscles
- Aplastic anemia may precede PNH in 25% cases, acute myeloid leukemia (AML) may occur
- *Others*: Infection, iron deficiency, and pigment gallstone.

Investigations:
- Complete blood count shows anemia, leukopenia and thrombocytopenia
- Ham acid serum test may be positive
- Flow cytometric analysis of red cells with CD55 and CD59 has replaced Ham test
- Bone marrow may be hypoplastic or aplastic.

Treatment:
- Supportive (blood transfusion, and iron), and prednisolone (in some cases)
- *In marrow failure*: Antithymocyte globulin and cyclosporin or bone marrow transplantation
- Recombinant humanized monoclonal antibody (eculizumab) may be helpful
- *Antiplatelet may be used*: Aspirin and clopidogrel
- Gene therapy.

Prognosis: Survival is 10–15 years.

HEMOLYTIC UREMIC SYNDROME

It is characterized by rapid onset of microangiopathic hemolytic anemia, thrombocytopenia, and acute renal failure (triad) due to thrombosis in small arteries and arteriole.

Causes: Verotoxin producing organisms, such as enterohemorrhagic *Escherichia coli* 0157:H7, also *E. coli* 0104:H4. HUS may be diarrheal (D+HUS) or non-diarrheal HUS (D-HUS or atypical HUS).

Clinical features: Common in children, <3 years. It usually follows gastroenteritis.
- Fever, vomiting and diarrhea, often bloody, called diarrhea associated HUS (D+HUS)

- Intravascular hemolysis is followed by oliguria or anuria
- Purpura, anemia, bleeding, drowsiness and hypertension may occur.

Investigations:
- *Complete blood count*: Anemia and marked thrombocytopenia. PBF shows features of microangiopathic hemolytic anemia (schistocyte) and spherocyte
- *Creatinine*: Very high
- *Other features of intravascular hemolysis*: High bilirubin, high LDH, reduced haptoglobin, and increased reticulocyte count
- Confused with DIC, but coagulation tests are normal in HUS.

Treatment: In diarrheal HUS, treatment is mainly supportive—
- Correction of water and electrolyte balance, and maintenance of nutrition
- Control of hypertension
- FFP transfusion and dialysis may be needed
- Heparin or antiplatelet drug may be helpful
- Plasmapheresis is not helpful.

In atypical HUS:
- Supportive, as above
- Plasmapheresis or plasma transfusion
- *Monoclonal antibody (anti-CD5 antibody)*: Eculizumab may be effective.

Prognosis: About 5% die in acute episode, 5% develop CKD, and 30% develop persistent proteinuria.

THROMBOTIC THROMBOCYTOPENIC PURPURA

Thrombotic thrombocytopenic purpura (TTP) is a disorder of unknown etiology characterized by fever, microangiopathic hemolytic anemia, thrombocytopenia, neurological signs, and renal failure.

Clinical features: Common in young female. Fever and purpuric spot due to thrombocytopenia, fluctuating neurological features, microangiopathic hemolytic anemia, and renal failure.

It confuses with HUS, but neurological features are absent in HUS. These two conditions are probably the part of same disorder.

Diagnosis: Diagnostic *pentad* in TTP—
1. Fever
2. Neurological features: Headache, seizure and coma
3. Thrombocytopenia
4. Microangiopathic hemolytic anemia
5. Renal failure.

Investigations:
- *Complete blood count and PBF*: Thrombocytopenia and fragmented RBC (schistocyte). Reticulocytes (high)
- *Bleeding time*: Prolonged
- *Bilirubin and LDH*: High. Also haptoglobin is reduced
- *Coagulation screen*: Activated partial thromboplastin time (APTT), D-dimer, fibrin degradation product (FDP), and prothrombin time (PT) are all normal. Usually no DIC.

Treatment:
- Plasma exchange. Fresh frozen plasma or cryoprecipitate infusion
- Pulse intravenous (IV) methylprednisolone may be given
- Rituximab is also very helpful
- Platelet transfusion is contraindicated, as it may aggravate the disease.

Prognosis: Mortality 90% in untreated and 10–30% in treated cases.

APLASTIC ANEMIA

It is a disorder due to bone marrow failure leading to pancytopenia. Diagnosis is done by bone marrow aspiration and biopsy.

Causes: It may be primary and acquired or secondary.
- *Primary*: Cause unknown
- *Acquired or secondary*:
  - Drugs: Cytotoxic drugs, antibiotics (chloramphenicol and sulfonamide), antithyroid drugs (carbimazole), carbamazepine, and penicillamine
  - Secondary deposits in bone marrow
  - Radiotherapy
  - Chemicals: Benzene, lindane and dichlorodiphenyltrichloroethane (DDT)
  - Infection: Viral hepatitis, Epstein-Barr virus (EBV) infection, HIV and parvovirus infection
  - Others: Lymphoma, multiple myeloma, and PNH.

Symptoms (Primary):
- *Features of anemia*: Weakness, palpitation, dizziness and vertigo
- *Bleeding manifestations*: Gum bleeding, nasal bleeding, multiple bleeding spots such as bruise, and ecchymosis in different parts of the body
- *Infection*: Sore throat, other infections, and septicemia.

Signs:
- Anemia. Bleeding spots (e.g. purpura, ecchymosis and bruise)
- No lymphadenopathy, hepatomegaly and splenomegaly or bony tenderness (which may be present in secondary deposit or secondary causes of aplastic anemia).

Note: In secondary aplastic anemia, features of primary are the predominant features.

Investigations:
- *Complete blood count*: Shows pancytopenia (anemia, leukopenia and thrombocytopenia)
- *Bone marrow (aspiration and trephine biopsy)*: Dry tap or acellular or hypocellular marrow.

Treatment:
- Removal of causative agent, if any
- *Supportive therapy*: Blood transfusion and control of infection
- *Allogeneic bone marrow transplantation (with HLA-matched siblings)*: If the patient is below 30 years with severe idiopathic aplastic anemia
- *In older patient or if HLA-matched donor is not available*: Immunosuppressive therapy with cyclosporine and antithymocyte globulin should be given. Tacrolimus may be used

- *Other treatment (if bone marrow transplantation is not possible)*:
    - Androgen (e.g. oxymetholone) is useful, prednisolone in some cases
    - If associated with thymoma in adult pure red cell aplasia, thymectomy may be done.

POLYCYTHEMIA

It is defined as increase in RBC, hemoglobin and hematocrit.

There are two types:
1. *Relative (pseudopolycythemia)*: Due to reduced plasma volume (e.g. dehydration and diuretic)
2. *True polycythemia*: Red cell mass is increased. True polycythemia may be—
    - Primary: Polycythemia rubra vera
    - Secondary: Causes are physiological (high altitude), cyanotic heart disease such as tetralogy of fallot (TOF), chronic obstructive pulmonary disease (COPD), emphysema, chronic bronchitis, and smoking. Inappropriate and excess erythropoietin secretion (renal cyst, renal cell carcinoma, cerebellar hemangioblastoma, hepatoma and uterine fibroids).

MYELOPROLIFERATIVE DISORDER

It is a group of disorder characterized by clonal proliferation of bone marrow stem cells which causes uncontrolled proliferation of erythroid, myeloid and megakaryocytic series.

It includes four diseases:
1. Polycythemia rubra vera
2. Essential thrombocythemia
3. Myelofibrosis
4. Chronic myeloid leukemia (CML).

All myeloproliferative disorders may lead to acute leukemia.

Myelofibrosis

It is a myeloproliferative disorder characterized by bone marrow fibrosis, extramedullary hematopoiesis, and leukoerythroblastic blood picture. There is clonal proliferation of stem cells.

Clinical features: Common above 50 years. History of polycythemia rubra vera in 25% cases and 50% have *JAK-2* mutation, seen in polycythemia rubra vera.

Features:
- *May be asymptomatic*: Mass in the left hypochondrium or hepatosplenomegaly
- *General features*: Malaise, weakness, weight loss, night sweat, repeated infection, and bleeding
- There may be peptic ulcer, pruritus after hot bath, and gout.

Investigations:
- *CBC and PBF*: Leukoerythroblastic blood picture (immature nucleated RBC and premature cells of white blood cell (WBC) series, myelocytes and myeloblasts). Teardrop RBCs (teardrop poikilocytes). Platelets (very high

and later decreased). Anemia (usually macrocytic, pancytopenia may occur)
- *Bone marrow*: May be dry tap. Trephine biopsy should be done (which shows increased megakaryocyte, increased reticulin, and fibrous tissue)
- *Others*:
  - Leukocyte alkaline phosphatase (LAP) score—increased
  - Uric acid is high and folic acid is low
  - Genetic test may show *JAK-2* mutation.

Treatment:
- Correction of anemia by blood transfusion and folic acid
- Hydroxyurea (it reduces WBC and splenomegaly)
- *If huge spleen*: Radiotherapy and splenectomy (if pressure symptoms or hypersplenism)
- Bone marrow transplantation (if the patient is young)
- Ruxolitinib (inhibitor of JAK-1 and JAK-2) may be used in some patients.

Prognosis: Median survival is 4 years (ranges from 1 year to 20 years).

Polycythemia Rubra Vera

It is a stem cell disorder in which there is excess proliferation of erythroid, myeloid, and megakaryocyte progenitor cells. It is characterized by increased hemoglobin, RBC, hematocrit, WBC and platelet. Bone marrow is hypercellular with increased megakaryocyte.

Symptoms: Polycythemia rubra vera is common in males, after 40 years. Features of hyperviscosity syndrome (headache, dizziness, blackout and blurring of vision), thrombosis [cardiovascular disease (CVD) and peripheral vascular disease], hypertension, angina and intermittent claudication. Pruritus after hot bath or with warm body. Peptic ulcer is common, in which bleeding may occur.

Signs: Face is plethoric, deep dusky, cyanosed, redness of conjunctiva, and engorged retinal vessels on fundoscopy. Splenomegaly (70%) and hepatomegaly (50%).

Complications: May transform to myelofibrosis (15%), AML and refractory state with anemia. Thromboembolism (cerebral and coronary). Hypertension, gout and peptic ulcer.

Investigations:
- *CBC and platelet*: High hemoglobin, RBC, WBC, platelet and high hematocrit
- Red cell mass (increased)
- Erythropoietin is low or absent (high in secondary polycythemia)
- Bone marrow shows erythroid hyperplasia and increased megakaryocyte
- *Others*: High LAP score, high vitamin B12 and serum uric acid (high).

Note: Plethoric appearance, splenomegaly, high RBC, WBC and platelets are highly suggestive of PRV.

Treatment:
- Venesection (400–500 mL of blood, every 5–7 days) until hematocrit is <45% and platelet <400 × 10^9/L
- Radioactive phosphorus for elderly (5 mCi of 32P IV)
- *Other drugs*: Hydroxyurea, and interferon may be given
- Aspirin reduces risk of thrombosis.

Median survival is 10 years, some 20 years.

Myelodysplastic Syndrome

It is a group of acquired bone marrow disorders due to defect in stem cells, characterized by increasing marrow failure with quantitative and qualitative abnormality of all three cell lines. There are anemia, neutropenia or leukopenia and thrombocytopenia, usually with hypercellular or normocellular marrow.

Clinical features: Common in elderly, transform to AML in 30% cases. May be asymptomatic. May present with anemia, recurrent infection or bleeding manifestations.

Investigations:
- *CBC*: It shows thrombocytopenia and leukopenia, hypogranular and hyposegmented neutrophil (Pelger cells) or hypersegmented neutrophil. MCV is high (macrocytic) or normal
- *Bone marrow*: Hypercellular with dysplastic change despite pancytopenia. Megaloblastic changes, ring sideroblast, dyserythropoiesis, granulocyte precursor, and megakaryocyte show abnormal morphology
- *Chromosome analysis*: Abnormality in chromosome 5 or 7.

Treatment:
- *If blast <5%*: Supportive therapy with platelet, and red cell transfusion. Erythropoietin and granulocyte-colony stimulating factor (G-CSF) may be given
- *If blast >5%*: Supportive therapy. Chemotherapy (low-dose hydroxyurea or etoposide). Lenalidomide (a thalidomide analog) may be effective in early stage of myelodysplastic syndrome (MDS) with chromosome 5q deletion. Allogeneic stem cell transplantation in young <55 years. Azacytidine may be given, which is helpful especially if patient is not eligible for transplantation.

LEUKEMIA

It is a malignant disorder of hematopoietic stem cell characterized by increased number of primitive WBC in marrow and peripheral blood.

Types:
- *Acute*: Characterized by presence of primitive blast cell in marrow and blood. There are two types:
  i. Acute lymphoblastic leukemia (ALL): Common in children, 80% improves with chemotherapy. Central nervous system (CNS) involvement is common
  ii. Acute myeloid leukemia: Common in adult, CNS involvement is rare and cure rate is less.
- *Chronic*: Characterized by presence of excess mature cells in marrow and blood. There are two types:
  i. Chronic lymphocytic leukemia
  ii. Chronic myeloid leukemia.
- *Other types*:
  - Subleukemic: When WBC count is normal but blast cells are seen in the blood
  - Aleukemic: When WBC count is normal or subnormal but no blast cell is present in the blood. Diagnosis is done by bone marrow.

Acute Leukemia

Symptoms: Features of anemia (weakness, dizziness and giddiness). Fever, malaise and infection of mouth and throat. Bleeding—nasal, gum, persistent bleeding after operation. Pain in the bones and joints (common in childhood).

Signs: Anemia, hepatosplenomegaly and generalized lymphadenopathy in ALL. Bruise, ecchymosis and petechiae. Bony tenderness.

Investigations: CBC and PBF—WBC is high, Hb and platelet are low. PBF shows blast cell (In ALL, mostly lymphoblast and in AML, myeloblast). Bone marrow—hypercellular with leukemic blast cell.

Treatment:
- *General measures*: Correction of anemia, control of infection by antibiotics, control of bleeding, and psychological support
- *Specific*: By chemotherapy (induction of remission, consolidation and maintenance)
- Bone marrow transplantation (either allogeneic or autologous may be done).

Chronic Myeloid Leukemia

It is a myeloproliferative stem cell disorder, characterized by proliferation of all hematopoietic cells, predominantly granulocyte series. Philadelphia chromosome is present in 95% cases, and is common in 40–60 years, peak age is 55 years.

Symptoms: May be asymptomatic. Weakness, tiredness, lethargy, anorexia, weight loss, fever and night sweat. Repeated infection, bleeding and priapism (painful erection of penis). Patient may complain of mass, discomfort and heaviness or pain in left upper abdomen (due to splenomegaly).

Signs: Splenomegaly may be huge. Hepatomegaly (in 50%), bony tenderness, and lymphadenopathy occur in blast crisis.

Investigations:
- *CBC*: WBC (very high. 50,000–500,000/mm^3). Differential count—high myelocyte, promyelocyte and metamyelocyte. Myeloblast <10%, increase in neutrophil, also basophil and eosinophil. Platelets are increased
- *Bone marrow study*: Hypercellular marrow with increased myeloid precursors
- Cytogenetic analysis for Philadelphia chromosome, also RNA analysis to see the presence of *BCR-ABL* gene product
- *Other tests*: The LAP score (low), serum uric acid (high), serum vitamin B12 (high), and serum LDH (high).

Clinical phases or types of CML: Three phases—
1. Chronic phase
2. Accelerated phase
3. Blast crisis.

Blast crisis in CML: It means the disease is transformed to acute leukemia. It may be myeloid (70%) or lymphatic (30%). It is difficult to treat. Blast crisis in CML can be suspected, if there is rapid deterioration of patient, increasing splenomegaly, and if blood picture shows increase in blast cells with increasing basophil.

Treatment of CML: Depends on phase of disease—
- *Treatment of chronic phase*:
    - Imatinib: 400 mg daily. 600–800 mg may be given, can be continued indefinitely
    - If there is no response to imatinib, in that case dasatinib or nilotinib or allogeneic bone marrow transplantation should be considered
    - Hydroxyurea or α-interferon is also useful
    - Bone marrow transplantation from HLA-matched sibling donor (usually below 40 years and in early chronic phase).
- *Treatment of accelerated phase and blast crisis*:
    - Treatment is difficult; imatinib is indicated if the patient has not received it
    - Hydroxyurea can be effective or low-dose cytarabine can be given.

Chronic Lymphatic Leukemia

It is a neoplastic disorder, usually involving B lymphocytes (95%) and rarely T lymphocytes (5%). More in elderly male, 65–70 years.

Symptoms: Asymptomatic in many cases, diagnosed incidentally during routine examination. There may be malaise, weakness, fatigue, weight loss, night sweating, and recurrent infections.

Signs: Generalized lymphadenopathy and hepatosplenomegaly.

Stages of CLL: Three stages—
1. *Stage A (60%)*: Survival >10 years
    - No anemia
    - No thrombocytopenia
    - Less than 3 areas of lymph nodes involvement.
2. *Stage B (30%)*: Survival 7 years
    - No anemia
    - No thrombocytopenia
    - Three or more areas of lymph nodes involvement.
3. *Stage C (10%)*: Survival 2 years.
    - Anemia
    - With or without thrombocytopenia
    - Regardless of area of lymph nodes involvement.

Investigations:
- *CBC*: Hb% (low), WBC (very high, 50–200 × 10^9/mm^3). Differential count shows increased lymphocytes (95%), mostly small lymphocyte. Platelet is normal, low or slightly increased
- Bone marrow shows increased lymphocytes
- *Others*:
    - Reticulocyte (high in autoimmune hemolytic anemia)
    - Coombs test (positive in autoimmune hemolytic anemia)
    - Uric acid (high)
    - Immunophenotyping of B cell antigen (CD19 and CD23) and T cell antigen (CD5).

Treatment: Early indolent case requires no treatment. Otherwise, treatment depends on stage—
- *Stage A*: No treatment, unless progression occurs. The patient survives for long time (reassurance and follow-up). Life expectancy is normal in older patient

- *Stage B*: No treatment, if the patient is asymptomatic
- *Stage C*: Usually treatment is necessary.

Modes of treatment:
- *Symptomatic*:
  - For anemia and thrombocytopenia: Prednisolone and blood transfusion
  - Infection: Antibiotic and immunoglobulin (gamma globulin 0.4 g/kg/month)
  - Local radiotherapy for lymph node (LN) causing discomfort or local obstruction and symptomatic splenomegaly.
- *Specific*:
  - Chlorambucil 5 mg daily, dose is adjusted according to blood count
  - Fludarabine alone or with cyclophosphamide or mitoxantrone (with or without steroid) is very helpful. Usually rituximab *plus* fludarabine with or without cyclophosphamide is the treatment of choice
  - Alemtuzumab may be used in patient that progresses after fludarabine
  - Allogeneic stem cell transplantation may be curative, but only used in those patients whose disease cannot be controlled by standard therapies.

LEUKEMOID REACTION

It means PBF resembles leukemia but there is no leukemia. It is of two types—myeloid and lymphoid.

1. *Myeloid*: PBF resembles myeloid leukemia.

Causes: Remember **LIMA**—
- **L**eukoerythroblastic blood picture due to any cause
- **I**nfection: Pneumonia, meningitis and disseminated tuberculosis
- **M**alignancy
- **A**cute hemolysis.

2. *Lymphoid*: PBF resembles lymphocytic leukemia.

Causes:
- *Viral infection*: Infectious mononucleosis, cytomegalovirus, measles and chickenpox
- Whooping cough
- Tuberculosis
- Malignancy.

Leukoerythroblastic blood picture: It means presence of immature myeloid and nucleated RBC in peripheral blood due to involvement of bone marrow by abnormal tissue.

Causes:
- Secondary deposit of bone marrow
- Myelofibrosis
- Thalassemia major, especially after splenectomy
- Active hemolytic anemia
- Rarely, multiple myeloma and lymphoma.

PURPURA

It is the spontaneous bleeding or extravasation of blood from capillary in skin and mucous membrane that does not blanch on pressure with progressive color change.

Causes of purpura: Thrombocytopenic, vascular and coagulation defect.

Thrombocytopenic purpura
- Primary or idiopathic thrombocytopenic purpura (ITP)
- *Secondary*: Aplastic anemia (due to any cause), leukemia, secondary deposit in bone marrow, drugs, radiotherapy, SLE and DIC.

Vascular purpura
- *Congenital*: Hereditary hemorrhagic telangiectasia and Ehlers–Danlos syndrome
- *Acquired*: Senile (in elderly), Henoch–Schönlein purpura, drug-induced (NSAID, steroid, sulfonamide and penicillin), infections [subacute bacterial endocarditis (SBE), meningococcal infection, septicemia, dengue and hemorrhagic fever], scurvy, metabolic disorder (CKD and Cushing's syndrome), collagen disease (RA and SLE), multiple myeloma, and amyloidosis (periorbital).

Coagulation defect
Hemophilia, Christmas disease, and anticoagulant therapy.

Investigations in purpura:
- CBC, ESR, platelet and PBF
- If pancytopenia or thrombocytopenia: Bone marrow study (dry tap in aplastic anemia and increased megakaryocyte in ITP)
- *Other investigations (according to suspicion of causes)*: Coagulation screen [bleeding time (BT), clotting time (CT), PT, APTT and FDP], test for hemophilia and Christmas disease. Blood culture (if septicemia), antinuclear antibody (ANA), anti-dsDNA (for SLE), and antiphospholipid antibody.

IDIOPATHIC THROMBOCYTOPENIC PURPURA

It is a type of thrombocytopenic purpura due to autoantibody against platelet (IgG type), which causes premature removal of platelet.

Types: Acute (common in children) and chronic (common in adult women).

Symptoms:
- *In child*: Common age is 2–6 years, usually acute presentation, previous history of viral infection followed by bleeding or purpura, easy bruising, etc.
- *In adult*: Common in adult female, 20–40 years, usually insidious onset without preceding viral infection. There are purpura, easy bruising, epistaxis or menorrhagia. May be relapse and remission.

Signs: Apart from bleeding points or purpura, no other physical findings.

Note: Following points are important—
- If platelet count is <20,000/mm^3, then spontaneous bleeding occurs
- If platelet count is >50,000/mm^3, there may not be any bleeding.

Investigations:
- Complete blood count shows thrombocytopenia
- *Bone marrow*: increased immature megakaryocytes
- Bleeding time is prolonged, but clotting time is normal
- Antiplatelet antibody is present in 60–70% cases
- Anti-cardiolipin antibody is positive in 30% cases.

Treatment:

In children, self-limiting, does not require treatment in most cases. If no improvement:
- Prednisolone (2 mg/kg), if platelet is <10,000/mm^3 and bruising, epistaxis or other bleeding
- If still persistent bleeding, IV immunoglobulin should be given
- In some cases, platelet transfusion may be required if persistent bleeding (epistaxis, GIT bleeding, retinal hemorrhage, and intracranial bleeding).

In Adult, persistent thrombocytopenia is common. Most patients with platelet count >30,000/mm^3 are stable and do not require treatment. Even with low platelet, treatment is not necessary unless there is spontaneous bruise or bleeding.

- *First-line therapy*:
  ○ Prednisolone 1 mg/kg, given for 4–6 weeks, then taper. Relapse is common when steroid is reduced or stopped. If relapse occurs, steroid should be started again
  ○ IV immunoglobulin may be given if severe hemostatic failure or slow response to steroid alone or surgery is required. Steroid may be added with immunoglobulin.
- *Second line therapy*: If there is frequent relapse or requirement of high dose of steroid, then splenectomy should be done
- *Third line therapy*: If failure after splenectomy, corticosteroid and IV immunoglobulin—danazol, dapsone, azathioprine, vincristine, vinblastine, cyclosporin, mycophenolate mofetil or monoclonal antibody like rituximab, and recombinant thrombopoietin may be given.

Note: Platelet transfusion is not usually necessary. However, it is used only if there is persistent or potentially life-threatening bleeding or where emergency splenectomy is done.

Henoch-Schönlein Purpura

It is a small vessel vasculitis characterized by purpura or skin rash, joint pain (in big joints), abdominal pain, and glomerulonephritis. It occurs 1–3 weeks after upper respiratory infection (usually viral). Other factors are foods, drugs or vaccination.

Symptoms: More common in boys, 5–15 years of age, but may occur at any age.
- *Skin lesion*: Purpura, common in legs and buttock. Resolves in 2–4 weeks, fresh crops may appear
- *Polyarthralgia*: Commonly involves knee and ankle, may be fleeting type
- *Abdominal pain*: Colicky in nature, associated with nausea, vomiting and bloody diarrhea
- *Renal disease*: May be hematuria, proteinuria, nephrotic syndrome, and rarely renal failure.

Investigations:
- *CBC and platelet*: Normal (nonthrombocytopenic purpura)
- Urine (proteinuria and hematuria)
- Serum IgA is high in 50% cases
- Skin biopsy from normal and involved skin (shows leukocytoclastic vasculitis)

- *Kidney biopsy*: Shows focal and segmental proliferative glomerulonephritis with IgA deposition.

Treatment of Henoch-Schönlein purpura:
- Usually self-limiting and spontaneous cure in most cases
- Prednisolone, if GIT and joint symptoms. Abdominal pain may be improved in 24 hours after steroid therapy
- *In renal involvement*: Pulse IV methylprednisolone and cytotoxic drugs should be given
- *Recurrence may occur*: Dapsone is helpful, if cutaneous recurrence.

HEMOPHILIA

It is an X-linked inherited disorder due to deficiency of factor VIII or antihemophilic factor, characterized by prolonged bleeding. Male is the sufferer and female is the carrier. Normal factor VIII level is 50–150 IU/dL.

According to severity, it is of three types:
1. *Mild*: Factor VIII is 10–50% (>5 but <40 IU/dL). Bleeding occurs after injury or surgery
2. *Moderate*: Factor VIII is 2–10% (1–5 IU/dL). There is severe bleeding after injury or surgery, also spontaneous bleeding sometimes
3. *Severe*: Factor VIII is <2% (<1 IU/dL). There is frequent spontaneous bleeding, also bleeding into the joints and muscles.

Pedigree of hemophilia
- *If father is affected*:
  - All daughters are carriers
  - All sons are normal.
- *If mother is carrier*:
  - 50% daughters are carriers
  - 50% sons are sufferers.

When a female can be a sufferer in hemophilia:
- If a carrier female is married to an affected male, the female baby may be a sufferer
- Turner's syndrome (because there is XO, if the only X is affected)
- According to lyonization theory, there is randomized inactivation of one X chromosome in fetus. Female may be affected, if normal X chromosome is inactivated.

Symptoms: Depends on whether factor VIII deficiency is mild, moderate or severe. Prolonged and persistent bleeding after trauma or injury and tooth extraction. Spontaneous bleeding may occur in severe case. Bleeding into the large joints and muscles (psoas and calf muscle) is also common.

Complications:
- *Due to repeated hemorrhage*: Arthropathy due to repeated bleeding in joint (e.g. knee and elbow). Death may occur due to intracerebral hemorrhage
- *Due to therapy*: Infections (hepatitis A, B, C and D, and HIV), and factor VIII antibody (20–30%).

Treatment:
- Bleeding episodes are treated with intravenous infusion of factor VIII concentrate, usually 2–3 times daily

Hematology

- If factor VIII is not available, cryoprecipitate, fresh frozen plasma or fresh blood can be given
- *Synthetic vasopressin (desmopressin)*: Intravenous, subcutaneous or intranasal, increases factor VIII
- Genetic counselling.

Christmas disease (Hemophilia B)

It is a coagulation disorder due to deficiency of factor IX. Features are like hemophilia. Severe bleeding may occur, if severe deficiency of factor IX. In such cases, treatment with factor IX concentrate should be given.

LYMPHOMA

It is defined as neoplastic disorder of lymphoid tissues. It is of two types: (1) Hodgkin's disease (HD); and (2) non-Hodgkin's lymphoma (NHL).

Hodgkin's Disease

It is a type of lymphoma characterized by painless and progressive enlargement of lymph nodes associated with Reed–Sternberg giant cell (hallmark of disease). It usually occurs in adolescence and young adults (20–35 years of age), also after 45 years (50–70 years, two peaks of incidence).

Symptoms:
- May be asymptomatic. May present with lumps in the neck, axilla and inguinal region.
- *Systemic features*:
  - Fever may be low grade, sometimes Pel–Ebstein type (recurrent bouts of pyrexia followed by apyrexial period)
  - Night sweat, cough, weight loss, anorexia, malaise, weakness, pruritus (10%), and shortness of breath (due to mediastinal lymphadenopathy)
  - Pain at the site of disease after drinking alcohol
  - Superior vena cava (SVC) obstruction occurs due to pressure by mediastinal lymph nodes.

Signs: Generalized lymphadenopathy involving cervical, axillary and inguinal regions. Lymph nodes are soft, rubbery and discrete. Hepatosplenomegaly with abdominal para-aortic lymphadenopathy.

Investigations:
- *CBC*: Anemia, lymphopenia, high eosinophil, and high ESR. Blood count may be normal.
- Chest X-ray (shows bilateral hilar lymphadenopathy and widening of mediastinal shadow)
- Fine-needle aspiration cytology (FNAC) or preferably biopsy of lymph node
- USG of whole abdomen
- Computed tomography (CT) scan of chest and abdomen including pelvis
- *Others*:
  - Bone marrow study
  - Renal function tests (serum creatinine) and liver function tests [serum glutamic pyruvic transaminase (SGPT)]
  - Serum uric acid and serum LDH.

Staging of HD: For staging, chest X-ray, bone marrow, USG of whole abdomen, and CT scan (whole abdomen and chest).

Stages of HD: Ann Arbor staging.

Four stages:
1. *Stage I*: Involvement of a single LN region (I) or extralymphatic site (IE)
2. *Stage II*: Involvement of two or more LN regions (II) or an extralymphatic site and LN regions on the same side of diaphragm (IIE)
3. *Stage III*: Involvement of LN regions on both sides of diaphragm with (IIIE) or without (III) localized extralymphatic involvement or involvement of spleen (IIIS) or both (IIISE)
4. *Stage IV*: Diffuse involvement of one or more extralymphatic tissue with or without LN involvement (bone marrow, liver and lung).

Depending on systemic features, each stage is divided into two:
1. *"A" symptoms*: No systemic features
2. *"B" symptoms, with systemic features*: Fever >38°C, drenching sweats, unexplained loss of body weight >10% within the previous 6 months.

Treatment:
- *Chemotherapy and adjunctive radiotherapy*: ABVD (adriamycin or doxorubicin, bleomycin, vinblastine and dacarbazine) regimen is widely used
- Patient with early stage HD (IA, IIA and no bulk) is treated with 2–4 cycles of ABVD followed by radiotherapy to the involved lymph nodes
- Patient with advanced disease is usually treated with chemotherapy alone. Usually 6–8 cycles of ABVD is given
- *Patients resistant to chemotherapy*: Autologous bone marrow transplantation
- *Other chemotherapeutic regimen that were previously used are as follows*:
  - MOPP: Mechlorethamine, oncovin (vincristine), procarbazine and prednisolone
  - COPP: Cyclophosphamide, oncovin (vincristine), procarbazine and prednisolone.

Non-Hodgkin's Lymphoma

It is characterized by malignant proliferation of lymphoid cells, majority are B cells (70%) and few T cells (30%).

Types or grading:
- *Low grade shows the following characteristics*:
  - Asymptomatic for many years. Low cell proliferation rate
  - Slow indolent course. Remitting and relapsing course
  - Good response to minimal therapy
  - Most nodular lymphoma is of low grade
  - Incurable, but the patient survives for long time
  - Small cell disease (mature lymphocyte) is associated with low-grade lymphoma
  - No treatment is required, if the disease is not advanced and asymptomatic
  - Median survival up to 10 years
  - Transformation to high grade is associated with poor prognosis, occurs in 3% per annum
  - Bone marrow involvement is more common (50–60%).

- *High grade shows the following characteristics*:
  - Cell divisions occur quickly. Early symptoms are common. Fatal, if untreated
  - Responds better to treatment and patient may achieve a long-term remission if treated properly
  - About 80% respond to initial therapy and 35% are disease-free for 5 years
  - Large cell disease (immature lymphoid cells) is of high grade
  - Most diffuse lymphomas are of high grade
  - Bone marrow involvement is less common (10%).

Stages of NHL are similar to HD, but NHL is more likely to be stage III or IV at presentation.

Symptoms: It can occur at any age, but common in 65–70 years.
- Generalized lymphadenopathy
- "B" symptoms: Fever, night sweats and weight loss may be present
- Extranodal presentations are more common than Hodgkin's disease. It may involve gastrointestinal tract (stomach), lung, thyroid, skin, testes and CNS.

Signs: Discrete, painless, firm, lymph nodal enlargement, and hepatosplenomegaly.

Investigations: Similar to HL, *plus* the following—
- Routine bone marrow aspiration and trephine
- Immunotyping of surface antigen-CD20 should be done.

Treatment:

Low-grade NHL: It is not curable. So, if asymptomatic, no therapy. Follow-up should be done.

Indications of treatment:
- Marked systemic symptoms
- Bone marrow failure
- *Features of compression*: SVC obstruction, spinal cord, gut obstruction, and ascites
- Large lymphadenopathy causing discomfort or disfigurement.

Treatment options:
- Radiotherapy, for stage I
- *Chemotherapy*: Oral chlorambucil may be used. More aggressive combination therapy may be tried in younger age
- *Monoclonal antibody therapy*: Rituximab (anti-CD20 antibody) is effective in 60% cases. Synergistic effects are seen with standard chemotherapy [rituximab, cyclophosphamide, vincristine sulfate, and prednisone (R-CVP)]
- Autologous stem cell transplantation can also be given (if failure to chemotherapy).

High-grade NHL:
- Chemotherapy (R-CHOP—rituximab, cyclophosphamide, hydroxydaunorubicin, vincristine and prednisolone), 4–6 cycles every 3 weeks
- *Radiotherapy*: For stage I without bulky disease. Also indicated for residual localized site of bulk disease after chemotherapy, for spinal cord and other compression syndrome
- Autologous stem cell transplantation for relapse chemosensitive disease.

MULTIPLE MYELOMA

It is characterized by malignant proliferation of plasma cells of bone marrow, associated with excessive production of paraprotein. Plasma cells produce monoclonal paraprotein, which may be associated with the excretion of light chain in urine, called Bence–Jones protein, either kappa or lambda.

Types: IgG (55%), IgA (21%), light chains (22%), and others (D, E and nonsecretory, 2%).

Symptoms: Common in elderly, above 60 years, more in male, M:F = 2:1. May be asymptomatic, diagnosis is suspected on routine blood test.

Usual presentations:
- Bone pain, commonly backache, generalized body ache, rheumatic-like pain. Spontaneous fracture and collapse of vertebrae (with shortening of stature)
- Unexplained anemia. Recurrent infection (respiratory and urinary tract). Bleeding manifestations. Renal failure. Features of hyperviscosity syndrome (dizziness, giddiness, headache, vertigo, blurring of vision, stupor, confusion and coma).

Investigations:
- CBC, ESR and PBF (high ESR, and marked rouleaux formation)
- Bone marrow (to see atypical plasma cells)
- Plasma protein electrophoresis or immunoelectrophoresis (myeloma band)
- Urine for Bence–Jones protein. Serum total protein (high), and albumin (low)
- X-ray Skull and other bones
- Serum calcium (high), C-reactive protein (CRP) (high), LDH (high), and uric acid (normal or high)
- Renal function (urea, creatinine and electrolytes)
- Serum alkaline phosphatase (normal, and it may be high, if fracture occurs)
- Serum β2-microglobulin (high).

Treatment: In asymptomatic case with no evidence of organ damage (e.g. kidney, bone marrow or bone), no treatment is necessary. Only follow-up is done. Treatment is given in symptomatic patient.

- *Supportive therapy*: Correction of anemia (blood transfusion and erythropoietin) and control of infection with antibiotics and vaccination (pneumococcal and yearly influenza vaccine). Control of renal failure and allopurinol to prevent urate nephropathy. Plasmapheresis is done for hyperviscosity. Analgesic and bisphosphonate (zolendronate) for bone pain
- *Specific therapy*:
  - *In older patient*: Melphalan with prednisolone *plus* thalidomide (MPT)
  - *In young patient*: Cyclophosphamide, thalidomide and dexamethasone (CTD) or bortezomib, thalidomide and dexamethasone (BTD)
  - Then autologous hematopoietic stem cell transplantation (HSCT) improves quality of life and prolongs survival

- Lenalidomide may be used for maintenance in patients who have achieved maximal response
- *Radiotherapy*: For localized bone pain or pathological fractures or spinal cord compression
- Carfilzomib (second-generation proteasome inhibitor) and daratumumab (anti-CD38 antibody) may be used in relapse or refractory disease. Responding patients may benefit from a second autologous HSCT.

Note: Therapy should be continued until a plateau phase is attained (patient is clinically improved and Hb%, paraprotein and β2-microglobulin are stable for 3 months).

DISSEMINATED INTRAVASCULAR COAGULATION

It is a hemorrhagic disorder in which diffuse intravascular clotting causes a hemostatic defect resulting from utilization of coagulation factor and platelet in clotting process, also called consumption coagulopathy.

Causes:
- *Obstetrical*: Abruptio placentae, amniotic fluid embolism, and abortion
- Surgery, especially heart and lung
- Hemolytic transfusion reaction and septicemia (due to Gram-negative and meningococcus)
- *Others*: Pulmonary embolism, falciparum malaria, malignant disease, liver disease, trauma, burn, snake bite and heat stroke.

Chronic DIC may occur in acute leukemia (usually promyelocytic), intrauterine device, septicemia and disseminated malignancy.

Investigations:
- *CBC*: Thrombocytopenia
- *Prothrombin time and APTT*: Prolonged
- *Fibrinogen*: low
- *D-dimer and FDP*: High.

Treatment: Treatment of underlying cause. Broad-spectrum antibiotic, if septicemia. Fresh frozen plasma and platelet transfusion.

BLOOD TRANSFUSION

It is usually needed in severe anemia, after severe bleeding. It is also required in DIC and hereditary hemolytic anemia.

Complications:
- *Allergic reaction*: Itching, urticaria and anaphylaxis
- *Febrile reaction or pyrogenic reaction*: Rise of temperature, chill and rigor
- *Circulatory overload*: leading to pulmonary edema or acute left ventricular failure
- *Infections*: Hepatitis B and C, HIV, cytomegalovirus (CMV), and EBV
- *Transmission of disease*: Malaria, kala-azar, toxoplasma and Brucella
- Hemolytic transfusion reaction is mostly due to incompatibility
- Repeated transmission may cause hemosiderosis
- Thrombophlebitis
- Air embolism.

Treatment during reaction:
- Transfusion should be stopped
- Grouping and cross matching must be checked
- Injection hydrocortisone 100 mg IV or dexamethasone IV
- *Antihistamine*: Chlorpheniramine IV
- When there is reaction, the bag of blood should be stored in refrigerator. After management of reaction, if the grouping and cross matching is normal, same blood may be transfused again.

CHAPTER 5

Hepatology

JAUNDICE

It is the yellow discoloration of skin and mucous membrane due to excess bilirubin in the blood. Clinically, jaundice is seen when serum bilirubin is >3 mg/dL. There are three types:
1. Prehepatic (unconjugated hyperbilirubinemia)
2. Hepatocellular (both conjugated and unconjugated hyperbilirubinemia)
3. Posthepatic or obstructive (conjugated hyperbilirubinemia).

Causes of prehepatic (unconjugated hyperbilirubinemia):
- *Excess production of bilirubin [due to breakdown of red blood cell (RBC)]*: Hemolytic anemia due to any cause
- *Reduced hepatic uptake of bilirubin or impaired conjugation*: Gilbert's syndrome, Crigler–Najjar syndrome Type 1 and 2, drugs (sulfonamides, penicillin and rifampicin), and physiological jaundice of newborn.

Causes of hepatocellular (conjugated hyperbilirubinemia):
- *Hepatitis*: Viral infections [Hepatitis-A, B, C, D, E, Epstein-Barr virus (EBV), cytomegalovirus (CMV), yellow fever and dengue). Nonviral infections (leptospirosis and Q fever)
- *Drugs*: Anti-TB (tuberculosis) [rifampicin, pyrazinamide and isonicotinylhydrazide (INH)], phenothiazines (chlorpromazine and haloperidol), cyclosporine and alcohol
- *Metabolic*: Wilson's disease and hemochromatosis
- Autoimmune
- *Inherited disorders*: Dubin-Johnson syndrome and Rotor syndrome.

Causes of posthepatic or obstructive (conjugated hyperbilirubinemia):
- *Extrahepatic*: Choledocholithiasis, carcinoma of head of pancreas, cholangiocarcinoma, periampullary carcinoma, extrahepatic biliary atresia, roundworm in common bile duct (CBD), and biliary stricture (due to trauma and sclerosing cholangitis)
- *Intrahepatic*: Primary biliary cirrhosis (PBC), primary sclerosing cholangitis and viral hepatitis (causes transient intrahepatic cholestasis).

History to be taken in jaundice patient:
- History of contact with jaundiced patient or sexual exposure

- Family history of jaundice, consanguinity of marriage among parents, and associated pallor (indicates hereditary hemolytic anemia)
- Anorexia, nausea and vomiting (indicate viral hepatitis)
- Color of stool (yellowish, pale and dark) and itching (indicates obstructive jaundice)
- History of injection, infusion or blood transfusion, intravenous (IV) drug abuse, tattooing or surgery [hepatitis B virus (HBV) or hepatitis C virus (HCV)]
- History of alcohol or any drugs
- History of high fever and urinary complain (indicates leptospirosis)
- Recurrent jaundice associated with neurological abnormality (indicates Wilson's disease)
- Abdominal pain and fluctuating jaundice (indicates bile duct stricture or stone)
- History of traveling abroad (hepatitis B).

Features of prehepatic jaundice:
- Usually in hereditary hemolytic anemia. There is triad of anemia, jaundice and splenomegaly. Other features are frontal and parietal bossing and mongoloid facies
- *Other causes of hemolytic anemia*: Malaria and autoimmune hemolytic anemia.

Features of hepatocellular jaundice:
- Anorexia, nausea, vomiting and weakness
- Stool is yellow in early stage, but dark or clay-colored in later stage due to intrahepatic cholestasis
- *Liver*: Enlarged and tender.

Features of obstructive jaundice:
- Pale, dark or clay-colored stool, itching of whole body, abdominal pain and mass in the epigastrium
- Other features depend upon cause (xanthelasma or xanthoma in PBC)
- Bleeding tendency (due to deficiency of vitamin K, resulting in deficiency in vitamin K-dependent clotting factors—factor II, VII, IX and X)
- Bone pain (due to osteomalacia).

Investigations of jaundice:
- *Liver function tests (LFTs)*: Serum bilirubin, serum glutamate-pyruvate transaminase (SGPT), serum glutamic-oxaloacetic transaminase (SGOT), alkaline phosphatase and prothrombin time (PT)
- Ultrasonography (USG) of hepatobiliary system (HBS). Sometimes computed tomography (CT) scan
- *Viral markers*: For A [anti-hepatitis A virus (HAV) immunoglobulin M (IgM)], for E [anti-hepatitis E virus (HEV) IgM], for B (HBsAg, HBeAg, anti HBc), for C (anti-HCV)
- Other investigation according to suspicion of cause.

ALCOHOLIC LIVER DISEASE

One unit of alcohol contains 8 g ethanol. Effects of alcohol are worse in women. Alcohol intake 21 units/week in male and 14 units/week in female is considered to be safe.

Definition: Alcoholic liver disease (ALD) means hepatic manifestations due to excess alcohol consumption, depends on duration and amount of alcohol intake. Alcohol can produce fatty liver, alcoholic hepatitis and alcoholic cirrhosis.

Clinical features: Depend on type of hepatic involvement
- *General*: Loss of appetite, fatigue, weight loss, nausea, vomiting and upper abdominal pain
- *Alcoholic fatty liver disease*: May be asymptomatic. There is high SGPT and SGOT on routine investigation. Prognosis is good after 3 months of alcohol abstinence
- *Acute alcoholic hepatitis*: Features like acute viral hepatitis
- *In chronic hepatitis or chronic liver disease (CLD) or cirrhosis*: Stigmata of CLD (bilateral parotid enlargement, Dupuytren's contracture and spider angioma).

Investigations:
- Complete blood count (shows macrocytosis)
- Liver function tests [aspartate aminotransferase (AST) > alanine aminotransferase (ALT)] and gamma glutamyltransferase (GT) (high)
- Ultrasonography or CT of HBS
- Liver biopsy.

Treatment:
- Alcohol should be stopped. Nutritional supplementation—Vitamin B1, folic acid and protein
- Corticosteroid is helpful acute alcoholic hepatitis
- Pentoxifylline may be given in severe acute alcoholic hepatitis
- *If cirrhosis*: Manage accordingly. Liver transplantation may be done, and patient must stop alcohol.

NONALCOHOLIC FATTY LIVER DISEASE

It means liver disease in the absence of excessive alcohol consumption. Usually asymptomatic, but liver is enlarged due to lipid deposition within hepatocytes, usually associated with obesity, insulin resistance, dyslipidemia and type 2 diabetes mellitus (DM). Patients are at high risk of developing cardiovascular disease. There are two types:
1. *Nonalcoholic fatty liver (NAFL)*: Hepatic steatosis without evidence of inflammation
2. *Nonalcoholic steatohepatitis (NASH)*: Hepatic steatosis is associated with hepatic inflammation. May lead to progressive liver fibrosis, cirrhosis and liver cancer, also cardiovascular risk.

Investigations: LFT, USG or CT scan of HBS, and liver biopsy (confirmatory). Other investigations to exclude other cause of liver disease.

Treatment:
- Reduction of weight and orlistat for obesity. Exercise is effective in reducing weight and insulin resistance
- Control of DM and hypertension. Metformin for insulin resistance associated with nonalcoholic fatty liver disease (NAFLD)
- Atorvastatin for dyslipidemia. Omega-3 fatty acids may also be used.

ACUTE VIRAL HEPATITIS

Hepatitis caused by the virus.

Causes:
- *Hepatotropic viruses*: A, B, C, D and E virus
- *Non-hepatotropic viruses*: EBV, CMV, yellow fever and dengue virus.

Symptoms: Anorexia, nausea, vomiting, fever, malaise and weakness. Yellow coloration of skin and sclera, and high colored urine. Pain in the right upper abdomen, pale stools may develop later (due to intrahepatic cholestasis).

Signs: Jaundice (mild-to-moderate) and tender hepatomegaly.

Note: Hepatitis E infection is only serious during pregnancy.

Investigations:
- Complete blood count (may be leukopenia with relative lymphocytosis)
- *Liver function test*: Serum bilirubin (high), SGPT (high), SGOT (high, more in drug-induced hepatitis), and alkaline phosphatase (slightly high). In cholestatic hepatitis, alkaline phosphatase is high and PT (prolonged in severe hepatitis)
- *Viral markers*:
  - Virus A (anti-HAV IgM, indicates acute infection)
  - Virus B (HBsAg, HBeAg and anti-HBc)
  - Virus E (anti-HEV and IgM indicates acute infection)
  - Virus C (anti-HCV).
- Ultrasonography or CT scan of HBS
- *Others*: Blood sugar and urine routine examination (R/E).

Complications:
- Acute fulminating hepatic failure (by B and sometimes with E in pregnancy, rare by HAV)
- Relapsing hepatitis
- Cholestatic hepatitis mostly by HAV, may persist for 7–20 weeks
- Posthepatitis syndrome is seen in anxious patient
- Chronic liver disease (due to B and C virus), which may cause cirrhosis and hepatoma
- *Others*: Aplastic anemia (usually reversible), rarely Coomb's positive hemolytic anemia, polyarteritis nodosa, Henoch–Schönlein purpura and glomerulonephritis.

Management: Symptomatic and supportive, no specific dietary modifications are needed. Alcohol and hepatotoxic drugs should be avoided during acute illness.

OBSTRUCTIVE JAUNDICE

Obstruction usually occurs in CBD. Causes may be in the lumen, in the wall, and outside the wall.
- *Causes in the lumen*: Stone in CBD (choledocholithiasis) and worms (roundworm)
- *Causes in the wall*: Sclerosing cholangitis, cholangiocarcinoma, periampullary carcinoma and stricture (due to surgery and trauma)
- *Causes outside the wall*: Carcinoma head of pancreas, lymphoma, and enlarged lymph node in porta hepatis.

Intrahepatic causes of cholestatic (obstructive) jaundice:
- Primary biliary cirrhosis
- Primary sclerosing cholangitis
- Viral hepatitis
- Drugs and alcohol
- *Others*: Autoimmune hepatitis, cystic fibrosis, postoperative, benign recurrent intrahepatic cholestasis and pregnancy.

Clinical features:
- Deep jaundice, dark yellow skin, deep yellow or mustard oil-like urine, pale or clay-colored stool
- Generalized itching with scratch mark. Weight loss and steatorrhea
- *Deep-seated abdominal pain*: Due to stone in the CBD (choledocholithiasis), choledochal cyst, and sometimes due to carcinoma of head of pancreas
- In prolonged case, osteomalacia due to vitamin D deficiency, bleeding disorder due to vitamin K deficiency, and night blindness due to vitamin A deficiency
- Palpable gallbladder and mass due to carcinoma of head of pancreas.

Investigations:
- *Liver function tests*: Serum bilirubin, SGPT (slightly high), alkaline phosphatase (very high), γ-GT (very high), PT (prolong), serum total protein, and A:G ratio (altered)
- Ultrasonography of HBS and pancreas. CT scan or magnetic resonance imaging (MRI) of upper abdomen, magnetic resonance cholangiopancreatography (MRCP) or endoscopic retrograde cholangiopancreatography (ERCP).

Treatment:
- Rest and maintenance of nutrition. If patient cannot take orally, IV fluid
- Injection vitamin K IV 10 mg to prevent bleeding. For itching, cholestyramine
- Treatment of primary cause.

LIVER ABSCESS

There are two types of liver abscess—Pyogenic and amoebic.

Pyogenic Liver Abscess

Causes:
- Ascending cholangitis in biliary obstruction
- *Hematogenous*: Portal pyemia from intra-abdominal sepsis, suppurative appendicitis and perforation. Septicemia or bacteremia (along the hepatic artery)
- Direct extension from peripheral abscess
- Trauma (penetrating injury) and infection of liver tumor or cyst.

Organisms: *Escherichia coli, Streptococcus milleri, Streptococcus faecalis* or other *Streptococcus* species, *Staphylococcus aureus*, anaerobic organisms or bacteroids.

Symptoms:
- Fever, may be high with chill and rigor, malaise, anorexia and weight loss. Only pyrexia of unknown origin (PUO) may be present

- Pain in right upper abdomen, may radiate to right shoulder, and pleuritic right lower chest pain
- Jaundice is usually mild, may be severe in multiple abscesses causing biliary obstruction.

Investigations:
- *Complete blood count*: Neutrophilic leukocytosis
- Ultrasonography of abdomen. Sometimes CT scan or MRI of upper abdomen may be done
- *Liver function test*: Alkaline phosphatase (high), SGPT (normal, may be slightly high), and serum albumin (low)
- Chest X-ray shows raised right dome of diaphragm and small right-sided pleural effusion
- *Blood for culture/sensitivity (C/S)*: Positive in 30% cases.

Treatment: Amoxicillin plus gentamicin plus metronidazole. *Or*, cefoperazone (1–2 g IV 12 hourly) with metronidazole (500 mg 8 hourly) for 2–3 weeks, sometimes up to 6 weeks. If large abscess or not responding to antibiotic therapy, ultrasonography-guided aspiration.

Amoebic Liver Abscess

It is caused by *Entamoeba histolytica* carried from the bowel to liver through portal circulation. It is common in right lobe and usually single. Pus is chocolate or anchovy sauce-colored.

Symptoms: History of diarrhea (may be absent in 50% cases), fever (low grade), malaise, pain in the right upper abdomen, anorexia, nausea and weight loss.

Signs: Liver is enlarged and tender, local edema in right lower chest with fullness in intercostal space, and right lower chest is tender (punched tenderness).

Investigations:
- Complete blood count (shows leukocytosis) and LFT
- Ultrasonography of abdomen. CT scan or MRI of the upper abdomen may be done
- Serum albumin (low)
- Chest X-ray shows raised right dome of diaphragm and small right-sided pleural effusion
- *Stool RME*: To see cyst of *E. histolytica*
- *Others*: Immunofluorescent antibody test (positive in 95%), indirect hemagglutination test (positive in 95%), complement fixation test, enzyme-linked immunosorbent assay (ELISA), lectin antigen (positive in serum, liver pus or saliva but not in stool), polymerase chain reaction (PCR) from liver pus (100% sensitive), and sigmoidoscopy in some cases (shows flask-shaped ulcer).

Complication: Abscess may rupture into pleural cavity, pericardial sac or peritoneal cavity, and hepatobronchial fistula.

Treatment:
- Metronidazole 800 mg 8 hourly for 10 days or secnidazole 2 g daily for 5 days or tinidazole or ornidazole 2 g daily for 3 days, or nitazoxanide 500 mg 12 hourly for 3 days
- *After treatment*: Diloxanide furoate 500 mg 8 hourly for 10 days or paromomycin in intestinal infection to eradicate luminal cyst

- *If large abscess or not responding to therapy*: USG-guided aspiration should be done.

Other treatment: Mixed infections are common. So, antibiotic plus antiamoebic drugs should be given. Abscess may rupture into pleural cavity, pericardial sac or peritoneal cavity. In such cases, immediate aspiration or surgical drainage is needed.

Differences between pyogenic and amoebic liver abscess

Points	Pyogenic	Amoebic
Organism	*E. coli* and others	*E. histolytica*
History	Cholangitis and septicemia	Amoebiasis
Fever	High with chill and rigor	Mild-to-moderate, no chill and rigor
Neutrophil leukocytosis	Common	Less
Ultrasonography	Multiple lesion	Usually single
Aspiration	Frank pus	Chocolate and anchovy sauce
Prognosis	More fatal (mortality 16%)	Less fatal (<1%)

PRIMARY BILIARY CIRRHOSIS

It is a chronic, progressive and cholestatic liver disease, characterized by granulomatous destruction of interlobular bile ducts, inflammatory damage with fibrosis spreading from portal tract to liver parenchyma and eventual cirrhosis. Probably an autoimmune disease with genetic predisposition.

Symptoms: It is common in middle-aged females, 40–60 years. It may be asymptomatic and may be isolated hepatomegaly and high alkaline phosphatase on routine examination.

- Pruritus may be the early feature, may precede jaundice by many months or years
- Jaundice with pruritus, abdominal pain or discomfort, and malabsorption (steatorrhea)
- Malaise, weakness, loss of weight and hyperpigmentation
- *Others*: Hepatic osteodystrophy (characterized by bony pain or fracture due to osteoporosis or osteomalacia from malabsorption).

Signs:
- Ill-looking, emaciated and hyperpigmented. Multiple scratch marks (due to pruritus)
- Moderate jaundice. Xanthelasma around both eyes. Spider angioma may be present
- Generalized clubbing, leukonychia and palmer erythema
- Liver is enlarged and spleen may be palpable.

Investigations:
- *Liver function test*: Alkaline phosphatase is very high. SGPT is slightly high. γ-GT is also high. Serum total protein and albumin is reduced
- Ultrasonography (shows hepatomegaly with cirrhotic change, splenomegaly and ascites)

- *Anti-mitochondrial antibody (AMA)*: Positive in 95% cases. Other antibodies such as antismooth muscle antibody and antinuclear antibody may be present
- Serum IgM may be very high
- Liver biopsy
- Magnetic resonance cholangiopancreatography or ERCP (to rule out extrahepatic biliary obstruction)
- *Others*: Serum cholesterol and triglyceride (high).

Treatment:
- Ursodeoxycholic acid 10–15 mg/kg
- *For pruritus*: Cholestyramine 4–16 g/day orally with orange juice
- Vitamins A, D, E, K and calcium supplement, alfacalcidol (1 mg/day orally)
- *If osteoporosis*: Bisphosphonate (risedronate may be used)
- Liver transplantation is considered in liver failure
- Steroid should be avoided. Azathioprine, penicillamine and cyclosporine have no role.

ASCITES

It is the pathological accumulation of free fluid in peritoneal cavity. Usually, 2 liters fluid is necessary to detect clinically (1 liter in thin person).

Causes:
- *Liver diseases*: Cirrhosis of liver with portal hypertension, hepatoma with secondary in peritoneum, and Budd–Chiari syndrome
- *Abdominal causes*: Intra-abdominal malignancy (carcinoma of kidney, stomach, colon and ovary) with peritoneal metastasis
- *Peritoneal causes*: Peritonitis (tuberculous or pyogenic), secondaries in the peritoneum
- *Cardiovascular*: Chronic constrictive pericarditis (early ascites) and congestive cardiac failure (CCF) (ascites in advanced stage)
- Hypoproteinemia due to nephrotic syndrome, malnutrition and malabsorption
- *Others*: Collagen disease [systemic lupus erythematosus (SLE) and polyarteritis nodosa], lymphoma, leukemia, Meigs syndrome (ovarian fibroma, ascites and right-sided pleural effusion), acute pancreatitis and myxedema.

Common causes: Cirrhosis of liver with portal hypertension (in 80% cases), intra-abdominal malignancy with peritoneal metastasis, and CCF.

Investigations:
- Ultrasonography of abdomen
- *If CLD*: LFT should be done
- Complete blood count (high ESR in TB and leukocytosis in pyogenic infection)
- Chest X-ray (may be TB, cardiomegaly or chronic constrictive pericarditis)
- *Ascitic fluid aspiration for the following tests*:
  - Naked eye examination (straw-colored, blood-stained, and serous or chylous)
  - Gram staining and C/S (in pyogenic infection)

- Cytology [neutrophil >250 or white blood cell (WBC) >500 in spontaneous bacterial peritonitis (SBP), and high lymphocyte in TB peritonitis]
- Biochemistry for protein and sugar (high protein in exudative and low protein in transudative). Simultaneous serum albumin to see serum ascitic albumin gradient
- In tuberculous peritonitis: Fluid for acid-fast bacillus (AFB), adenosine deaminase (ADA), mycobacterial C/S and PCR
- Malignant cells.
- *Other tests (according to suspicion of cause)*:
  - For tuberculous peritonitis: MT
  - Urine for proteinuria and serum total protein (nephrotic syndrome)
  - Ascitic fluid amylase in acute pancreatitis (>1,000 is highly suggestive)
  - Computed tomography scan or MRI (if any mass suspected)
  - Laparoscopy and biopsy in some cases.

Ascitic fluid color indicates the following:
- *Serous*: Cirrhosis of liver
- *Straw*: Tuberculosis
- *Purulent or hazy*: Pyogenic
- *Bloodstained*: Malignancy
- *Chylous*: Lymphatic obstruction.

Treatment:
- Bed rest. Sodium and water restriction
- Weight, abdominal girth, and urinary output should be seen daily. Weight loss should be 0.5–1 kg/day
- *Diuretic*: Spironolactone 100–400 mg/day. If no response, frusemide (20–40 mg daily) or bumetanide (1 mg daily) is added. If no response, with spironolactone 400 mg plus frusemide 160 mg daily, it is considered as refractory ascites
- *If no response or refractory ascites*: Ensure that patient is not taking any salt or salt-containing diet or drugs. If serum albumin is low, diuretics may not respond. Then IV salt-poor albumin followed by IV frusemide may be given
- *Paracentesis (aspiration of ascitic fluid)*: Done in huge ascites with cardiorespiratory embarrassment or resistant ascites. 3–5 liters of fluid can be removed. After aspiration, IV albumin should be given. Dextran or haemaccel may be used
- Other modes of treatment (in resistant ascites). LeVeen shunt (peritoneovenous). TIPSS (transjugular intrahepatic portosystemic stent shunt)
- Liver transplantation may be considered, if all measures fail.

CIRRHOSIS OF LIVER

It is a chronic diffuse liver disease characterized by destruction of liver cells with fibrosis, distortion of normal liver architecture, and nodular regeneration due to proliferation of surviving hepatocytes. There are three types:
1. *Micronodular*: Regenerative nodule is usually small, 1 mm size, involving every lobule, also called Laennec's cirrhosis. It is common in alcoholics

2. *Macronodular*: Large nodules, common in postnecrotic cirrhosis, and found in HBV
3. Rarely, mixed type (micronodular and macronodular).

Causes:
- *Common*: Chronic viral hepatitis (B or C), chronic alcoholism and NAFLD
- *Others*: Primary biliary cirrhosis, secondary biliary cirrhosis, autoimmune hepatitis, primary hemochromatosis, genetic (Wilson's disease and α1-antitrypsin deficiency), Budd–Chiari syndrome, and drugs (methotrexate, idiopathic or cryptogenic).

Symptoms: May be asymptomatic. Weakness, fatigue, anorexia, nausea, vomiting, weight loss and upper abdominal discomfort. Others—Abdominal distension due to ascites and isolated hepatomegaly.

Signs: Due to hepatocellular failure and portal hypertension.

Signs of hepatocellular failure or stigmata of CLD:
- *In hands*: Palmar erythema (liver palm), Dupuytren's contracture, leukonychia, clubbing and flapping tremor. Others—spider angioma, xanthoma, pigmentation, jaundice and cyanosis
- *In face*: Parotid enlargement (bilateral), xanthelasma, spider angioma (also in neck, arm, forearm, hand and any part above the nipple line), pigmentation, hepatic facies, jaundice and cyanosis
- *In chest and abdomen*: Gynecomastia (also spider angioma), less hair in chest or body, scanty axillary (also pubic hair), engorged veins in chest, and also abdomen (due to portal hypertension)
- *In abdomen*: Splenomegaly, ascites, engorged veins, caput medusae, and testis is small and atrophied
- *Others*: Generalized pigmentation, purpura, bruise and ecchymosis.

Signs of portal hypertension: Splenomegaly, ascites, collateral circulation (esophageal varices, hemorrhoid, and venous hum between xiphisternum and umbilicus), portosystemic encephalopathy (PSE), and endoscopy shows esophageal varices.

Signs of decompensated cirrhosis: Ascites, increasing jaundice, hepatic encephalopathy, portal hypertension with variceal bleeding, and worsening liver function (prolonged PT and low albumin).

Complications of cirrhosis of liver: Portal hypertension with rupture of esophageal varices (causing hematemesis and melena), PSE (hepatic precoma), hepatic coma, hepatorenal syndrome, hepatopulmonary syndrome, hepatoma and SBP.

Investigations in CLD:
- Liver function test (serum total protein, A/G ratio, PT, serum bilirubin, SGPT and alkaline phosphatase)
- Ultrasonography of whole abdomen (in cirrhosis, liver may be small, shrunken, coarse, high echogenic texture, splenomegaly, ascites and dilated portal vein)
- Viral markers for HBV (HBsAg, HBeAg and anti-HBc) and for HCV (anti-HCV)
- Proctoscopy (to see hemorrhoid)
- Endoscopy (to see esophageal varices)
- Computed tomography scan of HBS
- Liver biopsy under USG control (confirmatory)

- *Other investigation according to cause*: For hemochromatosis, serum iron, total iron-binding capacity (TIBC) and ferritin. For PBC, AMA and other autoantibodies. For Wilson's disease, serum copper, ceruloplasmin and urinary copper. For α1 antitrypsin deficiency, serum α1 antitrypsin
- *If ascites*: Aspiration and test for cytology, biochemistry, and serum ascites albumin gradient (SAAG)
- *Other routine investigations*: CBC, ESR, serum urea, creatinine, electrolytes and blood sugar.

Treatment:
- *General treatment*: Avoidance of alcohol and hepatotoxic drugs. Good nutrition and vitamins
- Treatment of cause, if any
- Treatment of ascites (see in the previous page)
- Treatment of complication (such as SBP, encephalopathy and portal hypertension)
- Liver transplantation.

SPONTANEOUS BACTERIAL PERITONITIS

It means bacterial infection in peritoneum in cirrhosis with ascites in the absence of any primary source of infection (so it is called spontaneous). It is suspected in any patient with ascites with fever and deterioration of general condition. Infective organism gains access to peritoneum by hematogenous spread, most are *E. coli*, *Klebsiella* or enterococci.

Symptoms: Cirrhosis and ascites with fever, sudden abdominal pain, rebound tenderness and absent bowel sounds. Increasing ascites, not responding to diuretic.

Investigations: Ascitic fluid is cloudy with neutrophil >250/mm^3. Ascitic fluid C/S.

Treatment:
- *Broad-spectrum antibiotic*: Cefotaxime or piperacillin and tazobactam. *Or* ceftriaxone plus amoxyclav
- Recurrence of SBP is common, prevented by norfloxacin 400 mg daily or ciprofloxacin 750 mg weekly
- Liver transplantation may be needed.

PORTOSYSTEMIC ENCEPHALOPATHY OR HEPATIC PRECOMA

It is a state of neuropsychiatric syndrome due to biochemical disturbance of brain function caused by CLD, may progress from confusion to coma. It is due to involvement of brain by nitrogenous substances of gut origin. Normally, these substances are metabolized by healthy liver. In diseased liver, these are not metabolized and enter into the brain through portosystemic shunt. Nitrogenous substances are ammonia, gamma-aminobutyric acid (GABA), mercaptan, fatty acids and octopamine, which act as false neurotransmitters.

Factors precipitating PSE: High dietary protein, gastrointestinal (GI) bleeding, constipation, drugs (sedative, antidepressants and diuretics), infections including SBP, fluid and electrolytes imbalance (hypokalemia), trauma including surgery, portosystemic shunt operation, and transjugular intrahepatic portosystemic shunt (TIPS).

Clinical features of PSE (remember the formula DPIST-F):
- *D*: Disturbance of consciousness (confusion, disorientation, drowsiness, delirium, stupor and coma)
- Disorder of sleep (hypersomnia, inversion of sleep, and more sleep in daytime)
- *P*: Personality change (childish behavior, abnormal behavior, apathy and irritability)
- *I*: Intellectual deterioration, from simple mathematical calculation to organic mental function. Earliest is constructional apraxia (see below)
- *S*: Speech disturbance (slow, slurred, monotonous and dysphasia).
- *T*: Tremor (flapping tremor)
- *F*: Fetor hepaticus (sweet musty odor in breath).

Constructional apraxia: It means inability to perform a known act in the absence of any motor or sensory disturbance. It is tested in the following way (patient will be unable to do):
- Ask the patient to draw a star
- Writing disturbance (unable to write or disturbance of writing)
- Ask the patient to make triangle with three matchsticks or ask to light the cigarette by matchstick
- Reitan's trail making test (it is the ability to join or connect the numbers with a pen in a certain fixed time). It is prolonged in PSE.

Investigations: Diagnosis is clinical. LFT should be done.

Treatment:
- Precipitating factors should be avoided (drugs, constipation, electrolyte imbalance and bleeding)
- *No* sedative, *No* diuretic. *No* protein restriction is recommended. (3 No)
- Glucose (300–400 g/day) orally. If cannot take by mouth, IV should be given
- *Lactulose*: 15–30 mL 8 hourly. Lactitol is an alternative
- Low bowel wash (if no response to lactulose, then enema should be given)
- *Gut sterilizer*: Rifaximin (200–550 mg) 8 hourly orally. Metronidazole (200 mg 8 hourly)
- Correction of electrolytes. Control of infection by antibiotic
- *In chronic or refractory encephalopathy*: Liver transplantation
- Zinc deficiency should be corrected, if present
- If the patient is agitated, oxazepam (10–30 mg) may be given by mouth.

ACUTE (FULMINATING) LIVER FAILURE

It is a clinical syndrome of encephalopathy due to severe hepatic failure, occurring within 8 weeks in absence of previous liver disease. It may be hyperacute (<7 days), acute (within 8–28 days) or subacute (29 days to 12 weeks), between the onset of jaundice and encephalopathy. The two common causes are viral hepatitis (commonly B) and paracetamol toxicity. Other causes are acute fatty liver in pregnancy, Wilson's disease, following shock and rarely extensive malignancy of liver, unknown in 10 % cases.

Clinical features: Similar to PSE. Other features are
- Patient is restless with aggressive outburst
- Jaundice

- *Features of cerebral edema due to raised intracranial tension*:
  - Pupil: Unequal or abnormally reacting, fixed
  - Hyperventilation
  - Profuse sweating
  - Local or general myoclonus, focal fit or decerebrate posture
  - Rarely papilledema, a late feature.

Investigations:
- *Liver function test*: High bilirubin, high SGPT and SGOT, and prolonged PT
- Ultrasonography of HBS
- Viral screening for HBsAg, HAV, HEV and HCV
- *Others*: Blood glucose, serum electrolytes, calcium, magnesium, phosphate, urea, creatinine and arterial-blood gas (ABG). Other tests according to suspicion of cause (such as paracetamol toxicity).

Treatment: Similar to PSE. Others are
- *If raised intracranial pressure*: 20% mannitol 1 g/kg body weight IV, may be repeated
- Correction of hypoglycemia, hypokalemia, hypomagnesemia and hypocalcemia
- *Coagulopathy or bleeding*: IV vitamin K, fresh blood or fresh frozen plasma, and platelet
- Broad spectrum antibiotic to control infection
- Proton pump inhibitor (PPI) to prevent GI bleeding
- Liver transplantation may be considered.

ESOPHAGEAL VARICES

Complication is rupture, causing hematemesis and melena. Diagnosed by upper GI endoscopy. Barium swallow of esophagus (rarely done).

Treatment of rupture esophageal varices:
- Resuscitation (IV channel, blood transfusion and plasma transfusion)
- Endoscopy should be done to see source of bleeding (in 20% cases, bleeding is from gastric erosion)
- Variceal banding is the treatment of choice. Sclerotherapy is rarely done.
- *Other measures to reduce portal pressure*:
  - Vasopressin causes constriction of splanchnic arterioles and reduces portal blood flow. Glypressin or terlipressin IV 2 mg 6 hourly until bleeding stops, then 1 mg 6 hourly for 24 hours
  - Octreotide IV 50 µg followed by infusion of 50 µg/hr
  - Transjugular intrahepatic portosystemic stent shunting is used when all other measures fail.

Prevention of rebleeding: It can be prevented by following measures
- *Banding*: This is the treatment of choice
- *Sclerotherapy*: Sclerosing agent is injected at every 1–2 weeks interval, until varices are occluded. This may cause transient chest or abdominal pain, dysphagia, perforation and esophageal stricture
- *Drug therapy*:
  - β *blocker*: Propranolol. Pulse and blood pressure (BP) should be checked. Aim is to reduce pulse rate by 25%. Nadolol or carvedilol may be used

- *Other drugs (less effective)*: Isosorbide mononitrate, pentoxifylline and captopril.
- Balloon tamponade by Sengstaken–Blakemore tube may be used
- Transjugular intrahepatic portosystemic stent shunt
- *Surgery*: Portosystemic shunting (portocaval or selective splenorenal). Due to high mortality, it is not done nowadays
- Esophageal transection rarely done
- Liver transplantation should be considered.

Primary prevention of bleeding from varices: β blocker (propranolol, nadolol or carvedilol).

PORTAL HYPERTENSION

Portal vein is formed by superior mesenteric vein and splenic vein. Normal portal pressure is 5–8 mm Hg. Symptoms or complications develop when portal venous pressure is >12 mm Hg. Causes are:
- *Prehepatic*: Portal vein thrombosis (in neonatal sepsis, congenital absence of portal vein, umbilical vein transfusion, oral contraceptive use and idiopathic)
- *Intrahepatic*: Cirrhosis of liver (90%), schistosomiasis and congenital hepatic fibrosis
- *Posthepatic*: Budd–Chiari syndrome, veno-occlusive disease, cystic liver disease, rarely in right heart failure and chronic constrictive pericarditis.

Signs: Splenomegaly (cardinal sign, mild in adults and markedly enlarged in children). Ascites, collateral vessels in anterior abdominal wall and caput medusae (engorged veins radiating from the umbilicus), hemorrhoid, and endoscopy (shows esophageal varices).

Complications: Rupture of varices, causing hematemesis and melena. Congestive gastropathy, ascites, hypersplenism and hepatic encephalopathy.

HEMOCHROMATOSIS

In this disease, total body iron is increased, which is deposited in different organs causing damage of those organs. Normal body iron is 3–4 g. In hemochromatosis, it may be 20–60 g. Iron is deposited in liver, pancreatic islets, endocrine glands (pituitary and adrenal), heart, and skin. There are two types:
1. *Primary*
2. *Secondary*: In hemolytic anemia (β-thalassemia, sideroblastic anemia, and other chronic hemolytic anemias), exogenous iron overload (repeated blood transfusion causing transfusion siderosis and prolonged iron therapy), porphyria cutanea tarda, and alcoholic cirrhosis (in advanced stage).

Primary or hereditary hemochromatosis: This is a hereditary disorder, inherited as autosomal recessive. More in male. However, in postmenopausal women, it is equal in both sexes.

Clinical features: Common in male above 40 years.
- *Liver*: Hepatomegaly, features of CLD [about 30% may develop hepatocellular carcinoma (HCC)]
- Skin pigmentation (leaden grey or bronze-like)
- Diabetes mellitus (called bronze diabetes)

- Cardiac dysfunction (dilated cardiomyopathy, CCF and arrhythmia)
- Arthritis and chondrocalcinosis
- Hypogonadism (testicular atrophy may occur early).

Note: If CLD with cardiac disease, arthritis, skin pigmentation and diabetes, hemochromatosis is likely.

Investigations:
- Liver function tests (shows evidence of CLD)
- *Iron profile*: Serum iron (high), TIBC (>70% is saturated), and serum ferritin (high)
- Computed tomography scan or MRI of HBS
- Hepatic iron index (HII)
- Liver biopsy
- *Others*: Blood sugar, electrocardiogram (ECG), X-ray of chest, echocardiogram and X-ray of involved joint (shows chondrocalcinosis).

Treatment:
- *Venesection*: Weekly or twice weekly, 500 mL of blood until serum ferritin is normal
- *Chelating agent*: Desferrioxamine may be given. It is used if patient cannot tolerate venesection, especially those with cardiac disease or severe anemia
- Symptomatic treatment of cirrhosis, DM (usually by insulin), CCF, and cardiac arrhythmia
- Alcohol must be avoided
- Vitamin C must be avoided as it increases iron absorption
- Screening of family members.

Complication or cause of death: Death is usually due to cardiac failure (30%), hepatocellular failure or portal hypertension (25%), and HCC (30%).

HEPATOMA

It is the primary carcinoma of liver, also called hepatocellular carcinoma.

Causes:
- Chronic hepatitis B infection. 75–90% are associated with cirrhosis of liver
- Chronic hepatitis C infection. Risk is higher in HCV than HBV
- *Other causes of cirrhosis*: Alcoholic cirrhosis, NASH, hemochromatosis, Wilson's disease and PBC
- Aflatoxin produced by a fungus *Aspergillus flavus* (from contaminated ground nut grain)
- *Others*: Chronic arsenicosis, clonorchis sinensis (a parasitic infection), prolonged androgen therapy, anabolic steroid and oral contraceptive pill, and smoking (rare) may cause hepatoma.

Symptoms: May be asymptomatic. Features may be anorexia, nausea, vomiting, weight loss, heaviness in the right upper abdomen, abdominal distension, and features of metastasis.

Signs: Liver is enlarged, hard, surface is irregular and nodular, usually single nodule. Hepatic bruit.

Investigations:
- Ultrasonography (shows filling defects in 90% of cases)
- α-fetoprotein: High (in 60% cases)
- *Others*: Contrast-enhanced CT scan and CEA (high in secondaries)

- *Liver biopsy under USG control*: Confirmatory
- Viral markers (HBV and HCV).

Treatment:
- Surgical resection in noncirrhotic patient. Recurrence in 50% at 5 years
- *In cirrhotic patient*: Resection may be done in small tumor with good liver function
- Liver transplantation. Hepatitis B and C may recur in transplanted liver
- Percutaneous injection of ethanol. Recurrence in 50% at 3 years. May be repeated. It causes tumor necrosis
- Transcatheter radiofrequency ablation
- Transcatheter hepatic arterial embolization by Gelfoam and doxorubicin
- *Chemotherapy*: Sorafenib prolong survival up to 10 months.

SECONDARIES IN LIVER

Secondary carcinoma is more common in liver, due to relatively more blood flow and double blood supply (by portal vein and hepatic artery). Primary sites are:
- *In male*: Carcinoma of stomach, lung and colon
- *In female*: Carcinoma of breast, colon, stomach and uterus.

Investigations:
- Ultrasonography of whole abdomen (shows multiple space occupying lesions)
- Computed tomography or MRI of abdomen may be done
- *Liver function tests*: Usually alkaline phosphatase is high
- Other investigation to find out the primary source according to history. For example, X-ray of chest posteroanterior (PA) view, endoscopy of upper GI tract, and colonoscopy
- Fine needle aspiration cytology (FNAC) or USG-guided liver biopsy may be done.

Treatment:
- Treatment of primary cause, if possible
- *If single metastasis*: Surgery may be possible (in colorectal carcinoma)
- *If surgery is not possible*: Radiofrequency ablation of metastasis may be tried
- Majority requires palliative treatment.

Differences between primary and secondary carcinoma

Primary	Secondary
- History of hepatitis B or C infection or cirrhosis of liver	- History of primary carcinoma (GI tract, bronchus, breast, thyroid and kidney). No primary source in 50% cases
- Nodule usually single, may be more	- Usually multiple nodules
- No umbilication over the nodule	- There is umbilication (due to necrosis)
- Bruit present (due to increased vascularity)	- No bruit (because of necrotic lesion)
- Rub may be present	- Rub is more common
- Investigations: α-fetoprotein is high, alkaline phosphatase is slightly high, and CEA is normal	- Investigations: α-fetoprotein is not high, alkaline phosphatase is very high, and CEA is high

PRIMARY SCLEROSING CHOLANGITIS

It is a chronic cholestatic liver disease characterized by inflammatory destruction of intra- and extrahepatic bile ducts with fibrosis that causes obliteration of biliary tree, biliary cirrhosis, portal hypertension and hepatic failure.

Clinical features: Common in male. 75% is associated with inflammatory bowel disease, commonly ulcerative colitis. Anorexia, nausea, vomiting, fatigue, malaise and weight loss. Pain in right hypochondrium. Pruritus and features of malabsorption, cholestastasis (stool is clay or muddy-colored). Cholangiocarcinoma may occur in 10–30% cases.

Signs: Scratch marks in whole body, jaundice, and hepatomegaly. In advanced case, stigmata of CLD.

Investigations:
- Liver function tests (high alkaline phosphatase is common)
- Ultrasonography of HBS. MRCP is diagnostic. ERCP may be done
- Liver biopsy
- *Perinuclear anti-neutrophil cytoplasmic antibodies (p-ANCA)*: Positive in 60–80% cases in ulcerative colitis. Antinuclear antibodies (ANA) and anti-smooth muscle antibody may be positive.

Treatment:
- *Supportive*: Cholestyramine for pruritus, ursodeoxycholic acid and fat-soluble vitamin
- Immunosuppressive drugs such as prednisolone, azathioprine, cyclosporine, tacrolimus and methotrexate (MTX). Anti-TNF (tumor necrosis factor) agent (etanercept or infliximab) may be given
- Biliary stenting may improve biochemistry and symptoms
- Orthotopic liver transplantation is the definitive treatment.

ACUTE CHOLECYSTITIS

It is the acute inflammation of gallbladder, usually associated with gallstone.

Symptoms: Pain in right hypochondrium, colicky in nature, radiates to right shoulder tip or interscapular region. Fever, nausea and vomiting.

Signs: Tenderness in right hypochondrium with muscle guard or rigidity. Murphy's sign positive (if thumb is pressed over the tip of 9th costal cartilage and patient is asked to take deep breath, there is pain and arrest of breathing at the height of inspiration).

Investigations:
- Complete blood count (leukocytosis) and LFT (bilirubin, SGPT, alkaline phosphatase, all may be slightly high)
- Ultrasonography of HBS. CT scan may be done
- Plain X-ray shows gallstones in 10% cases.

Treatment:
- Bed rest. Nothing by mouth. Nasogastric suction may be necessary
- *Intravenous fluid*: 5% dextrose normal saline (DNS) and Ringer's lactate solution
- Analgesics to relieve pain
- *Antibiotic*: IV cefuroxime or piperacillin plus tazobactam plus metronidazole 500 mg IV 8 hourly

- Once acute attack subsides, oral feeding is started
- *Surgery*: Cholecystectomy may be done in acute attack or after 6 weeks.

CHRONIC CHOLECYSTITIS

It is the chronic inflammation of gallbladder usually associated with gallstone. Causes are gallstones (common cause), noncalculus, due to infection by *Salmonella typhi*. There is history of frequent attacks of biliary colic (like acute cholecystitis), flatulent dyspepsia with fatty food intolerance. Diagnosed by USG of HBS. During acute attack, treatment like acute cholecystitis. Cholecystectomy should be done.

CARCINOMA OF GALLBLADDER

It is common in elderly, more in females, over 70 years. Type is adenocarcinoma (90%). Rarely anaplastic, squamous cell carcinoma. Risk factors are gallstones, porcelain (calcified) gallbladder, gallbladder polyp >1 cm. Chronic infection with *S. typhi* is a risk factor.

Clinical features: May be asymptomatic, diagnosed incidentally during cholecystectomy. Other features are jaundice, recurrent attack of right upper abdominal pain, weight loss, anorexia and nausea. Right upper abdominal mass, which is hard and irregular.

Investigations:
- Ultrasonography abdomen. CT abdomen may be done
- Liver function test (high bilirubin and high alkaline phosphatase) and CBC
- X-ray of abdomen (may show gallbladder calcification).

Treatment: Surgical excision if possible. Chemotherapy may be given.

Endocrinology

THYROID GLAND

Diseases of the thyroid gland:
- *Hyperthyroidism*: Excess function by thyroid hormones (called thyrotoxicosis)
- *Hypothyroidism*: Insufficient secretion of thyroid hormones, so less function. When associated with mucopolysaccharide deposition in the skin, it is called myxedema. When hypothyroidism is present from birth, it is called "cretinism". If it occurs in early age, it is called "juvenile hypothyroidism"
- *Goiter*: It means enlargement of thyroid gland
- *Tumor*: May be benign (adenoma) and malignant
- *Infection or inflammation*: Subacute thyroiditis, also called De Quervain's thyroiditis. Pyogenic or bacterial thyroiditis (rare). Riedel's thyroiditis (unknown cause)
- *Autoimmune*: Hashimoto's thyroiditis and Graves' disease.

Hypothyroidism

It means hypofunction of thyroid gland due to decreased secretion of thyroxine (T4) and triiodothyronine (T3). There are two types:
1. *Primary hypothyroidism*: Cause in thyroid gland, usually associated with myxedema
2. *Secondary hypothyroidism*: Cause in pituitary (or rarely hypothalamus). In such case, myxedema is rare. Other features of hypopituitarism may be present.

Causes of primary hypothyroidism:
- *Autoimmune*: Spontaneous atrophic hypothyroidism (common), Hashimoto's thyroiditis and Graves' disease [associated with thyroid-stimulating hormone (TSH) receptor blocking antibody]
- *Iatrogenic*: Radioiodine therapy for thyrotoxicosis, post-thyroidectomy, postradiotherapy in neck and drugs (lithium, amiodarone and anti-thyroid drug)
- *Others*: Endemic iodine deficiency and postpartum thyroiditis. Rarely, dyshormonogenesis.

Causes of goitrous hypothyroidism: Hashimoto's thyroiditis, Graves' disease (there is also exophthalmos and diffuse goiter with dermopathy), endemic iodine deficiency (less common), and drugs (lithium, amiodarone, and iodide). Rarely, dyshormonogenesis.

Nongoitrous hypothyroidism: Autoimmune or idiopathic (spontaneous atrophic, common cause), after radioiodine therapy for thyrotoxicosis, postradiotherapy in neck, post-thyroidectomy, secondary to hypopituitarism, and hypothalamic disorders.

Myxedema

It is the severe form of hypothyroidism due to deposition of mucopolysaccharide substances in subcutaneous tissue.

Symptoms: Weight gain, swelling of whole body, cold intolerance, increased sleepiness, lethargy, anorexia, weakness, constipation, lack of concentration and poor memory. In female, menorrhagia.

Signs: The patient looks apathetic, whole body is swollen. Face is puffy with periorbital swelling, baggy eyelids and loss of outer one-third of eyebrows, and nonpitting edema. Skin is dry, rough, cold and thick. Bradycardia and high blood pressure (BP).

Other features of hypothyroidism:
- *Hematological*: Anemia
- *CVS features*: Sinus bradycardia, pericardial effusion, pericarditis, congestive cardiac failure (CCF), atherosclerosis, ischemic heart disease (IHD), and hypertension
- *Neurological features*: Voice is coarse, husky or croaky. Memory may be impaired or dementia. Slow relaxation of ankle jerks, carpal tunnel syndrome (or tarsal tunnel syndrome), psychosis (myxedema madness), myxedema coma and cerebellar syndrome.

Investigations:
- Serum FT3, FT4, and TSH (low FT3, low FT4, and high TSH)
- Autoantibody (for Hashimoto's thyroiditis—Antiperoxidase and antithyroglobulin antibody)
- *Others*: Ultrasonography (USG) of neck and electrocardiogram (ECG). X-ray of chest, serum cholesterol, low-density lipoprotein (LDL), and triglyceride (high).

Treatment: Thyroxine, started with low dose (50 µg), increases gradually after 3 weeks. Single dose is preferable, should be taken before breakfast. TSH should be repeated after 6–8 weeks. Once TSH is normal, maintenance dose should be continued lifelong.

Treatment of hypothyroidism in different conditions:
- *Ischemic heart disease*: Thyroxine in low dose (25 µg), increases slowly in 3–4 weeks interval, provided no anginal pain or ECG change. Beta-blocker (propranolol) should be added. Coronary dilator and calcium antagonist may be added
- *In elderly patient*: Treatment is same. But care should be taken in IHD. After thyroxine, it may precipitate angina and myocardial infarction (MI)
- *Hypothyroidism in pregnancy*: Thyroxine (100–150 µg daily). Requirement of thyroxine is relatively high (40–50%) in pregnancy.

Myxedema coma: It is characterized by depressed level of consciousness or even coma. Convulsion may occur. It is rare, may occur in severe hypothyroidism, in elderly. There is 50% mortality.

Treatment: Treated in intensive care unit (ICU). Before starting treatment, blood is taken for FT3, FT4, TSH and cortisol.
- Triiodothyronine (T3 and liothyronine) 20 µg, 8 hourly intravenous (IV). If T3 is not available, oral thyroxine through Ryle's tube should be given
- *Intravenous hydrocortisone*: 100 mg 8 hourly
- *Other treatment*: Slow rewarming, high-flow O_2 therapy, IV fluid and glucose, antibiotic and assisted ventilation may be necessary.

Cretinism: It is defined as hypothyroidism due to congenital deficiency of thyroid hormone, also called congenital myxedema. Clinical features are:
- *In neonate*: Prolonged physiological jaundice, hoarse cry, lethargy, constipation, feeding problem and hypotonia
- *In older baby*:
  - Characteristic facies: Dull, idiotic look, wrinkling of forehead, large head, sparse hair, broad flat nose with big nostrils, widely set eyes, thick everted lips with macroglossia, and protruded tongue. Fontanelles close later
  - Pot-belly with umbilical hernia, lethargy and hypotonia
  - Skin is dry, scaly, rough, cold and pale yellow. Hair is sparse, coarse and brittle
  - Delayed developmental milestones such as delayed dentition and delayed crawling
  - Mental development is retarded, imbecile. Genitalia are poorly-developed
  - Hoarse voice. Short stature, thick and short neck with presence of supraclavicular pad of fat.
- *In older children*: Typical features of hypothyroidism are present. Also called juvenile myxedema.

Investigations: Routine screening of neonates using blood spot for TSH.

Treatment: Thyroxine. If treatment is delayed, permanent brain damage may occur.

Hashimoto's Thyroiditis

It is an autoimmune thyroiditis characterized by destructive lymphoid infiltration of thyroid leading to atrophic change with regeneration and goiter formation. Common in middle-aged women. Goiter is usually diffuse, moderately enlarged, firm or rubbery. Usually associated with hypothyroidism.

Investigation: Antithyroid antibody (very high): Antimicrosomal (antiperoxidase) in 90% and antithyroglobulin antibodies.

Treatment: Thyroxine (it reduces the size of goiter also).

Thyrotoxicosis

It is the hyperfunction of thyroid gland due to excess production of thyroid hormones. Common in females.

Causes:
- *Graves' disease*: The most common cause
- Toxic multinodular goiter

- Toxic nodular goiter
- Thyroiditis (subacute thyroiditis, also called De Quervain's thyroiditis and postpartum thyroiditis. All are transient)
- Hashimoto's thyroiditis, also called Hashitoxicosis (later, hypothyroidism develops)
- Factitious thyrotoxicosis (self-intake of thyroxine)
- Iodine-induced (Jod-Basedow phenomenon) and drug (amiodarone).

Symptoms: Excessive sweating, heat intolerance, increased appetite, weight loss (in spite of good appetite), insomnia and restlessness.
- *Cardiovascular*: Palpitation, angina pain and breathlessness on exertion
- *Neurological*: Irritability, insomnia, nervousness and tremor
- *Gastrointestinal*: Increased appetite and diarrhea
- *Reproductive*: In female, amenorrhea or oligomenorrhea, and infertility.

Signs: In hand, pulse >100/min (tachycardia), warm and sweaty palm, and tremor of outstretched hand. Systolic BP may be high. Goiter and exophthalmos may be found.

Investigations:
- *To confirm thyrotoxicosis*: FT3, FT4, and TSH (low TSH, high T3, and T4), radioiodine uptake test, and thyroid scanning (shows rapid uptake and rapid turnover)
- *To find out causes*: USG of neck, thyroid autoantibody (in Graves' disease), and thyroid receptor antibody. Other tests—ECG, Chest X-ray (CXR), and blood sugar.

Treatment: There are three modes of treatment—drugs, radioiodine therapy and surgery.
- *Drugs*: Carbimazole, propylthiouracil and β blocker (such as propranolol).
    - *Carbimazole*: 45–60 mg daily. Dose is reduced when the patient is euthyroid, then maintenance dose of 5–20 mg daily for 18–24 months Periodic complete blood count (CBC), FT4, and TSH should be done
    - *Propylthiouracil*: 400–600 mg daily. Dose is reduced when the patient is euthyroid
    - β *blocker*: Propranolol (up to 160 mg/day).
- Radioiodine therapy
- *Surgery*: It is done in large or multinodular goiter, suspicion of malignancy, pressure effect and cosmetic purpose.

Graves' Disease

It is an autoimmune thyroid disease due to stimulating antibody against TSH receptor, characterized by triad of exophthalmos, diffuse goiter, and dermopathy (pretibial myxedema). M:F = 1:5. It may be hyperthyroid, euthyroid followed by hypothyroidism.

Investigations: As in thyrotoxicosis.

Treatment: If thyrotoxicosis, treat accordingly. If euthyroid, only symptomatic and supportive. If hypothyroid, thyroxine therapy.

Goiter

It is the enlargement of thyroid gland. More common in women, may be single nodular, multinodular and diffuse. Also may be simple or toxic.

Types:
- *Nodular goiter*: which may be single or multinodular
- Diffuse goiter
- *Neoplastic*: May be benign (adenoma) or malignant (papillary, follicular, anaplastic, medullary carcinoma of thyroid (MCT) and non-Hodgkin's lymphoma).

Also according to the features of toxicity, goiter may be:
- *Simple goiter*: No features of toxicosis
- *Toxic goiter*: Presence of features of toxicosis (resting tachycardia, tremor of outstretched hand, and warm and sweaty palm).

Investigations of goiter:
- Radioactive iodine uptake test
- Thyroid scan
- Ultrasonography of thyroid gland
- FT3, FT4, and TSH (all normal, TSH may be high, due to iodine deficiency)
- Fine-needle aspiration cytology (FNAC) of thyroid nodule.

Multinodular Goiter

Common in middle-aged and elderly, usually benign, malignancy is rare.

Simple multinodular goiter: May be due to iodine deficiency (common), drugs (lithium and amiodarone), and thiocyanate in diet.

Complications of multinodular goiter: May develop thyrotoxicosis (toxic multinodular goiter), compression such as dysphagia, hoarseness, stridor, and superior vena cava obstruction. Severe pain due to hemorrhage in nodule.

Investigations: As in goiter (above).

Treatment: If small, reassurance, follow-up annually. If large or mediastinal compression or cosmetic reason, partial thyroidectomy.

Toxic multinodular goiter: When associated with features of toxicosis, it is called toxic multinodular goiter.

Treatment: β-blocker (to reduce heart rate), radioiodine therapy is the treatment of choice. If severe toxicosis, antithyroid drug followed by radioiodine therapy. Occasionally, surgery, if large goiter.

Diffuse Goiter

Simple diffuse goiter: It is common in young 15–25 years, more in female.

Causes of diffuse goiter:
- Physiological (puberty and pregnancy) and iodine deficiency (endemic goiter)
- Autoimmune (Hashimoto's thyroiditis, Graves' disease and postpartum thyroiditis)
- *Drugs*: Amiodarone, lithium and iodide in large doses
- *Thiocyanate in diet*: Cabbage, cauliflower, turnips, soya beans and Brussels sprouts.

Treatment of simple diffuse goiter: If large goiter, surgery may be done. Otherwise, follow-up.

SOLITARY THYROID NODULE

Majority benign (80–90%) and may be malignant (5–10%).

Causes: Simple nodular goiter, palpable nodule on diffuse or multinodular goiter, thyroid cyst, thyroid adenoma or toxic adenoma, and malignancy (carcinoma and lymphoma).

Investigations: USG (to see whether cystic or solid), radioactive iodine uptake (RAIU) and thyroid scan, FT3, FT4, and TSH. FNAC and open biopsy (if suspected malignancy).

Fate of untreated thyroid nodule: May persist for long time. Spontaneous regression (30%), malignancy (5–10%), cystic changes due to hemorrhage within nodule, and secondary infection.

Suspicion of malignancy in a single thyroid nodule:
- History of recent and rapid growth and hoarseness of voice
- History of radiation therapy in childhood (in head and in neck)
- Family history (MCT)
- Gland is hard, irregular and fixed to underlying structures, and associated palpable lymph node.

Treatment of solitary thyroid nodule: Reassurance and follow-up. Surgery for cosmetic purpose or if suspicion of malignancy. If hot nodules, surgery or radioiodine therapy.

TUMORS OF THYROID GLAND

It may be benign or malignant.

Benign: Usually adenoma. There are three types—follicular, papillary and Hurthle cell type.

Treatment: If nonfunctioning, reassurance and follow-up. Surgery for cosmetic purpose or suspicion of malignancy. If toxic adenoma, radioiodine therapy or surgery.

Thyroid carcinoma: Common in females, except medullary carcinoma of thyroid, which occurs in both sexes equally. Types are papillary (70–80%), follicular (10%), anaplastic or undifferentiated (5%), MCT (5–10%), and others (5%, lymphoma and secondary in thyroid).

Papillary Carcinoma

The most common type, usually in young, 20–40 years. It is slowly growing and multifocal. Local lymph node metastasis is common and hematogenous spread is less. Usually, presents with thyroid nodule, but patient may present with cervical lymphadenopathy without thyroid enlargement. FNAC should be done for diagnosis.

Treatment and prognosis: Total thyroidectomy followed by high dose radioiodine therapy. Lifelong thyroxine. Prognosis is good. If distant metastasis, 40% survival up to 10 years.

Follow-up (following tests are done periodically): Serum thyroglobulin. If rises, indicates recurrence or metastasis. Periodic whole body scanning is done to see any metastasis. If recurrence, high-dose radioablation should be done.

Follicular Carcinoma

Common in middle-aged, 40–60 years of age. Usually, a single encapsulated lesion. Blood borne metastasis is common (to lung, brain and bone). Lymph node metastasis is rare. Diagnosis is done by open biopsy (FNAC is less specific). Treatment and follow-up is like papillary. Prognosis is good.

Anaplastic or Undifferentiated Carcinoma

Usually in elderly, >60 years, more in women, and highly malignant. Rapid thyroid enlargement, over 2–3 months. Goiter is hard and irregular. There may be hoarseness of voice due to recurrent laryngeal nerve palsy and stridor due to tracheal compression.

Treatment: If possible, total thyroidectomy followed by thyroxine therapy. Radiotherapy may be given. Median survival is 7 months, if surgery is not possible.

Medullary Carcinoma of Thyroid

It arises from parafollicular C cells, usually multifocal. May be inherited as autosomal dominant. Common in middle-aged and elderly, may occur in young, if family history. Patient usually presents with firm thyroid mass, cervical lymph node involvement is common but distant metastasis is rare initially. Associated with multiple endocrine neoplasia (MEN) type IIa (pheochromocytoma and hyperparathyroidism) and IIb (as in type IIa *plus* multiple neuroma and Marfanoid body). Serum calcitonin is high and useful in monitoring response to therapy.

Treatment: Total thyroidectomy with removal of affected lymph nodes and thyroxine therapy. External radiotherapy may be given after surgery. Does not take radioiodine, chemotherapy is not effective.

Prognosis: Relatively good. Some may survive up to 20 years, but some <1 year.

PARATHYROID GLAND

Diseases of parathyroid glands:

Hormone excess: Primary hyperparathyroidism (due to adenoma and hyperplasia), secondary hyperparathyroidism [in chronic kidney disease (CKD) and vitamin D deficiency], and tertiary hyperparathyroidism.

Hormone deficiency: Hypoparathyroidism (due to postsurgical and autoimmune).

Hormone resistance: Pseudohypoparathyroidism and pseudopseudo-hypoparathyroidism.

Hyperparathyroidism

It means hyperfunction of parathyroid gland associated with excess parathormone secretion. There are three types:
1. *Primary*: Excess secretion of parathyroid hormone (PTH) from parathyroid gland. Causes are adenoma (90%), hyperplasia or carcinoma of parathyroid. There is high calcium, low phosphate, and high PTH
2. *Secondary*: Due to compensatory hyperplasia of parathyroid gland secondary to hypocalcemia. Causes are CKD, malabsorption, and vitamin D deficiency (rickets or osteomalacia)

3. *Tertiary*: Continuous stimulation of parathyroid for long period due to secondary hyperparathyroidism causes adenoma that becomes autonomous. Features like primary.

Primary Hyperparathyroidism

Symptoms: Common in female, above the age of 50 years. May be asymptomatic. Most symptoms are due to hypercalcemia.

Features:
- *General*: Anorexia, nausea, vomiting, weakness, tiredness and drowsiness
- *Abdominal*: Pain, constipation, features of pancreatitis, peptic ulcer and reflux esophagitis
- *Renal*: Renal colic (due to stone or nephrocalcinosis) and polyuria
- *Musculoskeletal*: Bone pain, spontaneous fracture, features of gout and pseudogout
- *Neurological*: Headache, depression, impaired memory and psychosis
- *Ocular*: Cataract and band keratopathy
- *Cardiovascular*: Hypertension.

Note: Remember the formula regarding symptoms of hypercalcemia "Bones, Stones, Abdominal groans and Psychic moans".

Investigations:
- Serum Ca, PO4, alkaline phosphatase and parathormone assay
- *Hydrocortisone suppression test*: Hydrocortisone 100 mg 6–8 hourly for 10 days, there is failure of suppression of calcium (in other causes, there is fall of calcium)
- *X-ray of hand*: Shows subperiosteal erosion in medial side of phalanges and resorption of terminal phalanx
- *X-ray of skull*: Shows "pepper pot" appearance
- Ultrasonography or computed tomography (CT) scan of neck
- *Other tests*: Thallium/Technetium subtraction scan of thyroid and parathyroid.

Treatment of hyperparathyroidism:
- *Mild and asymptomatic case*: Follow-up
- *In adenoma or hyperplasia*: Surgery
- *Secondary hyperparathyroidism*: Causes should be treated
- *Tertiary hyperparathyroidism*: Surgery.

Hypocalcemia

Causes: Hypoalbuminemia, hypoparathyroidism, CKD, vitamin D deficiency, acute pancreatitis, psedohypoparathyroidism, and alkalosis (metabolic and respiratory).

Clinical features: May be asymptomatic.
- *Tetany*: Triad of carpopedal spasm, stridor and convulsion
- In adult, tingling in hands, feet and around the mouth
- *Other features*: Papilledema, calcification of basal ganglia, grand mal epilepsy, psychosis and cataract. If due to vitamin D deficiency, rickets in children and osteomalacia in adult
- Electrocardiogram shows prolongation of QT interval, may cause ventricular arrhythmia.

Treatment:
- *In acute case*: IV 10–20 mL 10% calcium gluconate slowly. IV infusion may be required for several hours. Magnesium deficiency should be corrected

- *In chronic case*: Oral calcium. Vitamin D analogue (alfacalcidol or calcitriol)
- Treatment of primary cause.

Tetany: It is characterized by muscle spasm due to increased excitability of peripheral nerves.

Causes: Hypocalcemia due to any cause (low serum ionized calcium) and alkalosis (due to repeated vomiting, hyperventilation and primary hyperaldosteronism).

Clinical features: As in hypocalcemia (above).

Treatment: As in hypocalcemia. In hyperventilation, reassurance and rebreathing in a paper bag. Correction of alkalosis by IV normal saline.

ADRENAL GLANDS

Disease of adrenal cortex: May be hyper- or hypofunction.

Hyperfunction: Cushing syndrome [non-ACTH (adrenocorticotropic hormone) dependent] and primary hyperaldosteronism (Conn's syndrome).

Hypofunction: Addison's disease and congenital adrenal hyperplasia (CAH).

Disease of adrenal medulla: Pheochromocytoma.

Cushing Syndrome

It is a syndrome caused by excess glucocorticoid for long duration that leads to constellation of symptoms and signs. Commonly due to prolonged use of steroid.

Causes:
- *Adrenocorticotropic hormone-dependent*:
  ○ Pituitary microadenoma <10 mm, called Cushing disease (in 80%). More in women
  ○ Ectopic ACTH syndrome: Due to oat-cell carcinoma of bronchus, bronchial adenoma, bronchial carcinoid and carcinoma of pancreas
  ○ Adrenocorticotropic hormone therapy.
- *Non-ACTH dependent*: Prolonged steroid therapy (common), adrenal adenoma, and adrenal carcinoma (common in women).
- *Others*: Pseudo-Cushing syndrome (due to alcohol, depression and obesity).

Symptoms:
- Weight gain but weakness. Proximal muscular weakness (characterized by difficulty in combing, raising the hands above the head, and standing from squatting)
- *In female*: Hirsutism, amenorrhea or oligomenorrhea
- Loss of libido and easy bruising
- Backache, pathological fracture (due to osteoporosis), and collapse of vertebra
- Frequent infection, especially fungal infection and slow wound healing
- *Mood disturbance*: Depression, insomnia, irritability and lethargy.

Signs:
- Moon face, buffalo hump, and increased fat above supraclavicular fossa
- Hirsutism with puffy and plethoric face, frontal baldness and acne

- Skin is thin, with multiple purpura, bruise with striae (pink or purple-colored)
- Growth retardation in children
- Truncal obesity with thin limbs (called "Lemon on a matchstick" appearance)
- Proximal myopathy, more marked in the lower limbs than upper limbs
- Spine tenderness (due to osteoporosis)
- Hypertension, diabetes mellitus (DM) (30%) or impaired glucose tolerance (IGT).

Difference between Cushing disease and Cushing syndrome:
- *Cushing disease*: Excess production of ACTH from pituitary that stimulates adrenals
- Cushing syndrome is caused by excess glucocorticoid due to any cause.

Investigations: First to confirm the diagnosis and then further tests to find out the cause.

Tests to confirm Cushing syndrome:
Screening test:
- 24 hours urinary free cortisol measurement
- *Or*, overnight dexamethasone suppression test (see below)
- *Or*, low dose dexamethasone suppression test (see below)
- *Or*, late night salivary cortisol
- *Or*, circadian rhythm (see below).

If normal, Cushing syndrome is unlikely. If anyone is abnormal, perform other tests and repeat the abnormal result. Cushing syndrome is confirmed by using two of three main tests:
1. Failure to suppress serum cortisol with low doses of oral dexamethasone
2. Loss of normal circadian rhythm of cortisol, with inappropriately elevated late night serum or salivary cortisol
3. Increased 24-hour urine free cortisol.

If confirmed, other tests to find out the cause (to localize the site of lesion):
- *Serum ACTH*:
  - If ACTH is low or undetectable: Adrenal cause is likely. Then USG, CT or magnetic resonance imaging (MRI) to find adrenal lesion (tumor or hyperplasia). If no mass is seen, adrenal vein sampling or adrenal scintigraphy should be done
  - If ACTH is high: Likely cause is pituitary (Cushing disease) or ectopic ACTH syndrome.
- *If Cushing disease is suspected*: MRI of skull, which shows pituitary microadenoma in 70% cases. If present (usually found if >6 mm), then:
  - Corticotropin-releasing hormone (CRH) test: 100 µg bovine CRH IV is given. Measure serum ACTH and cortisol for 2 hours. It increases in Cushing disease (ACTH >50%, cortisol >20%), but no response in ectopic ACTH
  - Then, high dose dexamethasone suppression test (HDDST, see below).
- If no pituitary mass is seen, or CRH test negative or HDDST shows <50% suppression:
  - Selective catheterization of inferior petrosal sinus to measure ACTH for pituitary lesion

- If negative, then likely cause is ectopic ACTH syndrome
- Then, CXR, CT scan of chest (to see carcinoma of bronchus or bronchial carcinoid), and CT scan of abdomen.

Other tests (to see effect): Electrolytes (hypokalemia), blood sugar, bone mineral density (BMD) to see osteoporosis.

Treatment: Depends on cause—
- *Cushing disease*: Transsphenoidal removal of microadenoma. If surgery is not possible, bilateral adrenalectomy (later, patient may develop Nelson's syndrome) or pituitary irradiation may be given. To reduce ACTH production, bromocriptine or cyproheptadine is rarely effective. Metyrapone and ketoconazole may be given
- *Adrenal tumor*: Adrenalectomy. Radiotherapy or chemotherapy or adrenolytic drugs like mitotane may be given. Metyrapone or ketoconazole may be used (inhibits synthesis of cortisol)
- *Ectopic ACTH*: Primary lesion should be treated. If not possible, medical therapy as above or bilateral adrenalectomy may be considered.

Addison's Disease

It is the primary adrenocortical insufficiency due to destruction of adrenal cortex resulting in deficiency of glucocorticoid and mineralocorticoid.

Causes:
- *Common causes*: Autoimmune (80%, more in female) and tuberculosis (TB) of adrenal gland (in 10%)
- *Other causes (less common)*: Amyloidosis, sarcoidosis, hemochromatosis, bilateral adrenal hemorrhage following meningococcal septicemia (Waterhouse–Friedrichsen syndrome) and trauma, secondary deposit in adrenals, human immunodeficiency virus (HIV) infection, bilateral adrenalectomy and lymphoma.

Symptoms: Weakness and weight loss, loss of appetite, nausea, vomiting, dizziness and vertigo, and pigmentation in different parts of body.

Signs: Hypotension may be postural. Patient is emaciated with pigmentation (may be generalized, more marked over face, neck, mucous membrane of mouth, palmar crease, knuckles, knees, elbows and recent scar), vitiligo may be present, and sparse (or less) axillary and pubic hair.

Diagnostic criteria in Addison's disease:
- Weakness or emaciation (100% cases)
- Pigmentation (90% cases)
- Hypotension (88%). Postural hypotension is common.

Investigations:
- *Routine tests*: CBC [shows high eosinophil, lymphocyte, and erythrocyte sedimentation rate (ESR)], blood glucose (low or lower limit), and serum electrolytes (hyponatremia and hyperkalemia). Other tests—Serum renin (high), aldosterone (low), and calcium (may be high).
- *Tests to confirm*:
  - Plasma ACTH and cortisol (high ACTH and low cortisol)
  - Short synacthen test. If cortisol level rises, it rules out Addison's disease. If it does not rise, it indicates primary or secondary adrenocortical deficiency.

- *Tests to find out cause*:
    - Chest X-ray (to diagnose TB), plain X-ray abdomen (to see adrenal calcification in TB)
    - Adrenal autoantibody
    - Ultrasonography or CT scan of adrenals (to look for calcification in TB or malignancy).

Treatment:
- *Replacement of hormones*:
    - Glucocorticoid: Hydrocortisone 15 mg in morning (after waking) and 5 mg in afternoon (6 pm). According to some authority, 10 mg after waking, 5 mg at 12 noon, and 5 mg at 6 pm. Or if hydrocortisone is not available, prednisolone 5 mg on waking in morning and 2.5 mg at 6 pm in evening
    - Mineralocorticoid: Fludrocortisone 0.05–0.15 mg (50–300 µg) daily
    - Androgen: Dehydroepiandrosterone (DHEA) 50 mg/day may be given in female. It increases libido and sense of well-being, but complications like acne and hirsutism may occur.
- Treatment of cause (antitubercular therapy in TB).

General advice to the patient:
- The patient should always carry a bracelet and steroid card, which should contain information regarding diagnosis, dose of steroid, and doctor's contact address
- Good nutrition, regular meal, high carbohydrate, and sufficient salt
- The patient should keep ampoules of hydrocortisone at home. If oral therapy is impossible, should take injection by himself, family members or GP
- The patient should know how to increase steroid dose. During intercurrent stress (fever, cold and trauma), dose should be doubled. If vomiting, IV hydrocortisone should be taken.

Following points are important:
- *During surgery*: Minor surgery, hydrocortisone 100 mg intramuscular (IM) or IV premedication. Major surgery, hydrocortisone 100 mg IM or IV 6 hourly for 24 hours, then 50 mg 6 hourly. Continued until the patient can take by mouth
- *If gastroenteritis*: IV or IM hydrocortisone should replace oral therapy.

Addisonian Crisis

It is the acute adrenocortical insufficiency characterized by shock with severe hypotension. Precipitated by disease, surgery or infection. Patient presents with muscle cramp, nausea, vomiting, diarrhea, acute abdomen, collapse and unconsciousness. May be unexplained fever.

Causes:
- Sudden withdrawal of steroid (common cause, if patient on steroid for long time)
- Stress (severe infection and operation)
- Bilateral adrenal hemorrhage (meningococcal septicemia, injury and anticoagulant)
- Thyroxine therapy in a patient with hypopituitarism without steroid therapy.

Laboratory findings: Hyponatremia, hyperkalemia, low cortisol, hypoglycemia and hypercalcemia.

Treatment: Blood is taken to measure cortisol, glucose and electrolytes. Three problems are present: Shortage of Salt, Sugar and Steroid (3S).
- Intravenous normal saline rapidly (1 L in 30–60 minutes). Later, several liters of normal saline may be required in 24 hours
- Intravenous 10% glucose
- Intravenous hydrocortisone 100 mg, then 100 mg IV 6 hourly, continued until the patient is stable and can take by mouth. Then, oral steroid is started
- Treatment of cause (infection, adrenal or pituitary pathology).

Pheochromocytoma

It is a neuroendocrine tumor, arising from adrenal medulla that secretes catecholamines (adrenaline and noradrenaline). Commonly occurs in adrenal medulla (90%), but may occur in any part of sympathetic chain (paraganglioma). Rule of "10"—*10%* malignant, *10%* extraadrenal (in sympathetic chain), and *10%* familial.

Symptoms: Hypertension, usually paroxysmal with headache, pallor, fear of death, anxiety or panic attack. Complications like MI, cardiovascular disease (CVD), and acute renal failure.

Investigations:
- Plasma and urinary catecholamines and metabolites (metanephrine)
- Abdominal ultrasound, CT scan or MRI
- Metaiodobenzylguanidine scan (MIBG) helpful for extraadrenal tumor
- *24-hour urinary vanillylmandelic acid (VMA)*: It is less done nowadays.

Treatment:
- Surgical resection
- *For hypertension*: α blocker (phenoxybenzamine 10–20 mg 6–8 hourly)
- *If tachycardia*: β blocker is added (only β-blocker is avoided, as it may cause crisis)
- During surgery hypertensive crisis may occur (from anesthetic induction or tumor mobilization). It is controlled by sodium nitroprusside or short-acting α antagonist phentolamine.

Primary Hyperaldosteronism (Conn's syndrome)

It is the tumor of adrenal cortex characterized by excess aldosterone secretion that causes sodium retention, hypokalemia and hypertension. It is also called Conn's syndrome.

Causes: Adrenal adenoma in 60% (Conn's syndrome) and 30% bilateral adrenal hyperplasia. Adrenal adenoma is usually small, common in young female. Adrenal hyperplasia is common in male, after the age of 40 years.

Symptoms: Hypertension in young. Muscular weakness, polyuria and polydipsia (due to hypokalemia). Tetany may occur.

Note: In any patient with hypokalemic alkalosis and hypertension, in the absence of diuretic use, it is highly suggestive of primary hyperaldosteronism.

Investigations:
- *Serum electrolytes*: High sodium, low potassium and high bicarbonate (metabolic alkalosis)
- Urine potassium >30 mmol in 24 hours
- Serum renin and aldosterone assay (low renin and high aldosterone)
- *Plasma aldosterone-renin ratio (ARR)*: High

- Ultrasonography of adrenal gland. High-resolution computed tomography (HRCT) scan or MRI of suprarenal gland.

Treatment: If adenoma, surgery. If hyperplasia, aldosterone antagonist such as spironolactone 100–400 mg daily. For hypertension, amiloride and calcium channel blocker may be used.

PITUITARY GLAND

Panhypopituitarism

It is a syndrome due to complete or near complete destruction of pituitary, causing deficiency of all pituitary hormones, characterized by asthenia, loss of sexual function and loss of target organ functions like thyroid, adrenal gland and gonads. First, loss of growth hormone (GH), luteinizing hormone (LH), and follicle-stimulating hormone (FSH), followed by ACTH and TSH.

Causes of hypopituitarism:
- *Pituitary cause*:
  - Pituitary adenoma, carcinoma (rare), secondaries, pituitary cyst and TB
  - Pituitary surgery (removal of tumor), irradiation, trauma, apoplexy and Sheehan's syndrome
  - *Infiltrative disease*: Hemochromatosis, sarcoidosis and amyloidosis
  - *Others*: Autoimmune hypophysitis, congenital, Langerhans cell histiocytosis and MEN-I.
- *Extrapituitary causes*: Craniopharyngioma, meningioma, germinoma, glioma, and pinealoma
- Secondary to hypothalamic disorder.

Common causes: Pituitary tumor, surgery, radiotherapy, head injury, craniopharyngioma and meningioma.

Symptoms: Weakness, lassitude, malaise, dizziness and giddiness. Loss of libido, absence of secondary sex characters, and amenorrhea. Weight loss, cold intolerance and constipation.

Signs: Patient is pale and emaciated, skin is fine and wrinkled, and loss of axillary and pubic hair.

Investigations:
- *Routine*: CBC, ESR, serum electrolytes, and random blood sugar
- *Serum hormone measurement*:
  - For adrenocortical insufficiency: Serum cortisol (low) and ACTH (low)
  - For thyroid: FT4 (low) and TSH (low)
  - For gonadotrophins: FSH and LH. Also, testosterone in male
  - Growth hormone assay is not routinely done
- Magnetic resonance imaging of brain to see pituitary gland.

Treatment:
- Hydrocortisone 15 mg in morning and 5 mg in afternoon. Or 10 mg after waking, 5 mg at 12 pm, and 5 mg at 6 pm. Or prednisolone 5 mg in morning and 2.5 mg at 6 pm
- *Thyroxine*: 50–150 µg in the morning before breakfast
- *In female*: Sex hormone replacement (to restore sexual function and to prevent osteoporosis)

- If the patient wishes for fertility: Human chorionic gonadotropin (hCG) + FSH or pulsatile gonadotropin-releasing hormone (GnRH) may be given
- *In male*: Testosterone IM, orally, transdermally or implant
- *In child with hypopituitarism*: GH should be given
- Steroid card should be maintained.

Sheehan's syndrome: It is a syndrome of hypopituitarism due to infarction of pituitary gland following prolonged postpartum hemorrhage.

Symptoms: Failure of lactation is the earliest symptom. Other symptoms such as breast atrophy, amenorrhea, loss of libido, reduction of secondary sex characters, weakness and asthenia appear over months or years.

Investigations: As in hypopituitarism.

Treatment: As in hypopituitarism.

ACROMEGALY

It is characterized by generalized enlargement of whole body due to excess GH secretion from pituitary macroadenoma after union of epiphysis. It is called gigantism if occurs before the union of epiphysis. If excess GH starts in adolescence and persists in adult life, both conditions may be present together.

Cause: Eosinophilic adenoma of pituitary (macroadenoma) causing excessive GH secretion.

Symptoms:
- Progressive increase body size (may be history of change in size of rings, shoes and hats)
- Weight gain but weakness
- Visual field defect due to pressure over optic chiasma (the patient gives history of collision with doors, person and car accident)
- *Others*: Features of raised intracranial pressure (ICP) (headache and vomiting), excessive sweating, features of hypertension, DM, change in voice and joint pain.

Signs:
- Large head with coarse facies, prominent supraorbital ridge, increased wrinkling of forehead, and baggy eyelids. Nose and ears are large
- Tongue, lips and jaw are enlarged. Lower jaw is protruded with malocclusion of teeth (prognathism)
- Hands are large, spade-like, warm and sweaty with doughy feeling. Feet are large
- Skin is thick, greasy and sweaty. Coarse body hair
- Voice is hoarse, husky and cavernous
- *Eye*: Visual field defect, usually bitemporal hemianopia, optic atrophy and papilledema
- *Cardiovascular system*: Cardiomegaly
- *Musculoskeletal system*: Joints (swollen and tender), may be kyphosis and scoliosis
- *Others*: Gynecomastia, thyroid is diffusely enlarged, and BP (may be high).

Investigations:
- *Radiology*: X-ray of skull, hands, feet, chest, knee joints or other joints, if needed
- *Growth hormone assay (radioimmunoassay)*: High
- *Glucose tolerance test (GTT) with simultaneous measurement of GH*: Normally during GTT, there is suppression of GH. But in acromegaly, failure of suppression of GH, may be paradoxical rise of GH
- Measurement of insulin-like growth factor 1 (IGF-1) (also called somatomedin-C): usually increased
- Computed tomography scan or MRI of skull
- *Others*: Assessment of other anterior pituitary hormones. Perimetry (to see bitemporal hemianopia), blood sugar (DM in 10% cases, IGT in 25% cases), ECG and serum calcium (increased in MEN-I).

Treatment:
- *Surgery*: Transsphenoidal removal of tumor is the treatment of choice. Occasionally, transfrontal surgery is done in large macroadenoma with suprasellar extension
- *Radiotherapy*: If surgery is not possible
- *Drugs*: If surgery is not possible or persistent acromegaly after surgery
  - Somatostatin analogue (injection octreotide or lanreotide), every 2-4 weeks
  - *Or*, Bromocriptine or cabergoline or quinagolide.
- *Other treatment*: Control of hypertension and DM.

DIABETES INSIPIDUS

It is characterized by persistent excretion of excessive quantities of dilute urine associated with thirst due to deficiency of antidiuretic hormone (ADH) or insensitivity ADH to renal tubules. There are two types:
1. *Cranial diabetes insipidus (DI)*: Decreased production of ADH by posterior pituitary
2. *Nephrogenic DI*: Renal tubules become insensitive to ADH.

Causes:

Cranial DI:
- Craniopharyngioma, head injury, histiocytosis X, sarcoidosis, pituitary tumor with suprasellar extension, meningitis, encephalitis and postsurgical
- *Others*: Idiopathic and genetic defect.

Nephrogenic DI: Genetic defect, drugs (lithium and demeclocycline), pyelonephritis, renal amyloidosis, multiple myeloma, Sjögren's syndrome, and sickle cell anemia.

Symptoms: Polyuria (patient may pass 5-20 L or more urine in 24 hours. Urine has low specific gravity and osmolality) and polydipsia.

Investigations:
- *Serum ADH*: May be undetectable
- Urine osmolality (low), may be below 600 mOsm/kg and plasma osmolality (high)
- Water deprivation test
- Hypertonic (5%) saline infusion and measurement of ADH secretion
- Serum electrolytes and serum calcium.

Treatment:
- *Cranial DI*: Desmopressin, DDAVP intranasally as spray. In very sick patient, DDAVP should be given as IM
- *Nephrogenic DI*: Thiazide diuretic (bendroflumethiazide 5–10 mg daily and amiloride 5–10 mg daily).

DIABETES MELLITUS

It is a clinical syndrome characterized by persistent hyperglycemia due to absolute or relative deficiency of insulin or resistance or both.

Clinical features:
- **3p's:** *Polyuria* (excessive urine), *Polydipsia* (excessive thirst), and *Polyphagia* (excessive hunger)
- *Others*: Weight loss, weakness, dryness of mouth, pruritus vulvae, balanitis and oral candidiasis. Patient may be asymptomatic, detected during routine examination.

Complications of DM:

Acute complications: Hypoglycemia, diabetic ketoacidosis (DKA), hyperglycemic hyperosmolar state (HHS) [previously called hyperosmolar nonketotic diabetic coma (HNDC)], and lactic acidosis.

Long-term complications:
- *Microvascular*:
  - Neuropathy: Peripheral neuropathy (sensory, motor or mixed), mononeuritis multiplex, mononeuropathy and autonomic neuropathy
  - Nephropathy (CKD)
  - Eye complications: Retinopathy and cataract
  - Foot complications: Ulcers, gangrene and arthropathy.
- *Macrovascular*:
  - Coronary circulation: Myocardial ischemia and infarction
  - Cerebral circulation: Transient ischemic attack (TIA) and CVD
  - Peripheral circulation: Ischemia and claudication
  - Foot complications: Ulcers, gangrene and arthropathy (Charcot's joint).
- *Others*: Boil, carbuncle, abscess, cellulitis and TB.

Investigations:
- Blood sugar (fasting and 2 hours after breakfast) and hemoglobin A1c (HbA1c)
- Urine routine/microbial examination
- Complete blood count, ESR, S. urea, creatinine, electrolytes and serum lipid profile
- *Others*: ECG, USG of whole abdomen, CXR posteroanterior (PA) view, and plain X-ray of abdomen (to see pancreatic calcification).

Criteria for diagnosis of DM: In symptomatic patients, diagnosis is made by any one of the following:
- Fasting plasma venous blood sugar level ≥7.0 mmol/L
- Random glucose or 2 hours after 75 g glucose, blood sugar ≥11.1 mmol/L
- HbA1c >6.5 (48 mmol/mol). HbA1c can be used as a diagnostic test for diabetes.

In asymptomatic patients, two diagnostic tests are required to confirm diabetes. Second test should be same as the first test to avoid confusion.

Prediabetes: It includes impaired fasting glucose (IFG) and IGT.
- *Impaired fasting glucose*: Fasting glucose level ≥6.1 and <7 mmol/L (110–126 mg/dL). Patients with IFG are prone to develop frank DM and CVD
- *Impaired glucose tolerance*: Fasting glucose is <7 mmol but 2 hours after 75 g glucose is 7.8–11.1 mmol/L. Patient with IGT may develop frank type 2 diabetes mellitus (T2DM) and macrovascular complications.

In both IFG and IGT, lifestyle modifications such as weight reduction, regular exercise, and follow-up. No drug is needed. Cardiovascular risk factors such as hypertension and dyslipidemia should be treated.

Latent diabetes or stress hyperglycemia: Blood glucose is usually normal, but may be high under certain stressful conditions such as pregnancy, infection, obesity and drugs like steroid and thiazide diuretics. Glucose is usually normal after stress is resolved.

Potential diabetes: Blood sugar usually is normal, but the patient has increased risk of developing DM in future due to genetic reasons like both parents are diabetic patient, one parent is diabetic patient and the other has family history of diabetes, has a diabetic sibling, in a twin, if one is diabetic patient.

Etiological classification of DM:

Primary:
- *Type 1*: IDDM (insulin-dependent diabetes mellitus)
- *Type 2*: NIDDM (noninsulin-dependent diabetes mellitus).

Secondary:
- *Pancreatic*: Chronic pancreatitis, pancreatectomy, hemochromatosis and cystic fibrosis
- *Endocrine*: Acromegaly, Cushing syndrome, glucagonoma, thyrotoxicosis and pheochromocytoma
- Chronic liver disease
- Drug-induced (corticosteroid and thiazide diuretics)
- *Gestational*: In pregnancy.

Gestational diabetes mellitus (GDM): It is defined as any degree of glucose intolerance with onset or first recognition during pregnancy. It constitutes 7% of women with pregnancy complicated by diabetes. More than 50% women develop T2DM in next 20 years, linked with obesity.

Oral glucose tolerance test (OGTT) with 75 g glucose is used as screening test for GDM between 24 weeks and 28 weeks of gestation. Blood glucose is measured at fasting, 1 hour and 2 hours after glucose load. GDM is diagnosed if blood glucose is:
- Fasting >5.1 mmol/L
- After 1 hour—10 mmol/L
- After 2 hour—8.5 mmol/L.

Management of GDM:
- Dietary modification
- *Monitoring of blood glucose regularly*: Premeal glucose should be <5.3 mmol/L and postmeal glucose < 6.4 mmol/L
- *Drug*: Mainly metformin or glibenclamide may be used in later pregnancy (both does not cross placenta). Insulin [if fasting blood sugar (FBS) >7 mmol/L]

- After delivery, glucose becomes normal. Follow-up is necessary
- There is risk of T2DM, 15–55% in 5 years. So, dietary and lifestyle advice are necessary to reduce the risk.

Management of diabetes in pregnancy:
- Diabetes mellitus must be well-controlled before planned pregnancy, otherwise there is more chance of complications of mother and fetus. Ketoacidosis, retinopathy and nephropathy may be more in pregnancy. Risk of fetal anomaly is also more
- Insulin is given usually. Oral drug should be avoided and metformin may be given
- Mother should measure blood glucose daily.

Complications of fetus in DM:
- *Teratogenicity*: Cardiac, renal, and skeletal malformations
- *Others*: Fetal macrosomia, neonatal hypoglycemia, hyaline membrane disease and stillbirth.

Types of neuropathy in DM: Sensory neuropathy (common), mixed motor and sensory neuropathy, asymmetrical motor neuropathy (diabetic amyotrophy), autonomic neuropathy, mononeuropathy and mononeuritis multiplex.

Causes of loss of vision in DM: Diabetic retinopathy, cataract, age-related macular degeneration, retinal vein occlusion, retinal artery occlusion, nonarteritic ischemic optic neuropathy and glaucoma.

Diabetic retinopathy: Occurs after 10–20 years. The most common cause of blindness. Types are simple or background retinopathy, maculopathy, preproliferative retinopathy and proliferative retinopathy.

Treatment:
- Good control of diabetes and hypertension. Avoiding smoking and regular check-up
- *Specific*:
  - Background and preproliferative retinopathy: Medical treatment
  - Maculopathy and proliferative retinopathy: Retinal photocoagulation (argon laser).

Diabetic Nephropathy: Common cause of CKD. About 30% patients with type 1 diabetes mellitus (T1DM) develop diabetic nephropathy 20 years after diagnosis, less common in T2DM (15–20%). Associated with poor glycemic control, long duration of diabetes, and pre-existing hypertension.

Treatment: Good control of blood glucose, hypertension, and salt restriction. Drugs [angiotensin-converting-enzyme (ACE) inhibitors or angiotensin II receptor blocker].

Microalbuminuria: It is defined as urinary albumin excretion 30–300 mg/day or 20–200 mcg/min. Normal albumin excretion is <30 mg/day. It is an important hallmark of early diabetic nephropathy and an indicator of underlying CVD and more in NIDDM.

Treatment: Good control of diabetes, hypertension, restriction of protein (40–60 mg/day). Drugs (ACE inhibitors).

Diabetic foot: May be ulcer, gangrene, osteomyelitis, arthropathy and sepsis. Causes are ischemia, neuropathy, combined ischemia and neuropathy and secondary infection.

Treatment: Good control of diabetes, local dressing, avoid weight-bearing, barefoot, tight shoes and smoking. Antibiotic to control secondary infection. Consult with chiropodist. Surgery may be required (amputation or angioplasty).

Diabetic Ketoacidosis

It is a metabolic complication of DM in which there is severe hyperglycemia with metabolic acidosis due to excess ketone bodies. Common in IDDM (type 1), rare in type 2.

Precipitating factors: Little or no insulin, intercurrent infection, severe stress like trauma and acute MI.

Symptoms: Polyuria, polydipsia, weakness, nausea, vomiting and abdominal pain. Acidotic deep sighing breathing (Kussmaul breathing), and altered consciousness. Coma may occur.

Signs: Severe dehydration (dry tongue and sunken eyes). Pulse (weak, tachycardia) and low BP. Air hunger, Kussmaul breathing, and acetone breath (sweetish). Others (reduced reflex and flexor planter response).

Investigations:
- Blood sugar and ketone bodies (high)
- Urine sugar and ketone bodies (present)
- Serum electrolytes (low sodium and potassium) and bicarbonate (low)
- *Arterial blood gas (ABG)*: Low pH
- *Others*: CXR, ECG, CBC, calcium, magnesium, etc.

Note: The three main problems in DKA are: hyperglycemia, hyperketonemia, and metabolic acidosis. Severe dehydration is common, average loss of fluid and electrolytes are:
- *Water*: 6 liters
- *Sodium*: 500 mmol
- *Chloride*: 400 mmol
- *Potassium*: 350 mmol
- Half of lost fluid is intracellular. If bicarbonate <12 mmol/L, it indicates severe acidosis.

Treatment:
- *Intravenous normal saline rapidly*: 1 liter in 30 minutes *then* 1 liter in 1 hour *then* 1 liter in 2 hours *then* 1 liter in 4 hours *then* 1 liter in 8 hours
- Intravenous soluble insulin with pump 0.1 IU/kg/hour *or* 20 units IM stat, then 6 units IM hourly
- Potassium correction with infusion depending on blood potassium
- When blood glucose is below 14 mmol/L, 5% glucose is added. Insulin dose is adjusted according to blood glucose
- Correction of acidosis by sodabicarb, if arterial pH is <7
- *Others*: Control of infection by broad spectrum antibiotic, catheterization, nasogastric feeding if needed, central venous (CV) line, and subcutaneous low-molecular-weight (LMW) heparin.

Complications: Cerebral edema, acute respiratory distress syndrome (ARDS), disseminated intravascular coagulation (DIC), thromboembolism, and acute circulatory failure. Mortality is 5–10%, more in elderly.

Hyperglycemic Hyperosmolar State

It was previously called hyperosmolar non ketotic diabetic coma (HNDC). As there may not be coma, this name is obliterated now. It is characterized by very high blood glucose (>30 mmol/L), high plasma osmolality (>320 mOsm/kg), and dehydration without ketosis. Insulin deficiency is partial and low endogenous insulin is present, sufficient to inhibit hepatic ketogenesis, but insufficient to control hyperglycemia. It may be the first presentation of DM, common in elderly with type 2 (NIDDM).

Precipitating factors: Consumption of glucose rich diet or fruits, concurrent medication like thiazide or steroid, MI and intercurrent illness [pneumonia and urinary tract infection (UTI)].

Symptoms: Onset is less insidious than DKA. Polyuria, polydipsia, altered consciousness and convulsion. Signs of severe dehydration are present.

Investigations:
- Blood glucose (very high)
- Serum and urinary ketone body (absent), and serum electrolytes (hypernatremia)
- Arterial blood gas (normal pH)
- Plasma osmolality >320 mOsm/kg.

Treatment:
- Intravenous 1/2 strength saline (0.45%) should be given. When osmolality is normal, 0.9% normal saline is given
- However, if hypovolemia is present (hypotension and oliguria), 0.9% saline may be given (1–3 liters over first 2–3 hours). Total 4–6 liters fluid may be required in first 8–10 hours
- Low dose soluble insulin with insulin pump, 2–6 units hourly. Insulin dose is adjusted to reduce glucose level by 50–70 mg/dL/hr
- When glucose is 250 mg/dL, 5% dextrose in either aqua or 0.45% saline or 0.9% saline. Rate of glucose infusion should be adjusted to maintain glucose level between 250 mg/dL and 300 mg/dL to reduce the risk of cerebral edema. When urinary output is 50 mL/hour or more, IV fluid may be stopped
- *Other treatment*: Nasogastric (NG) tube feeding, catheter if needed, antibiotic if infection, correction of electrolytes, low dose heparin (as thrombosis is common).

Clinical diagnosis of hypoglycemia and hyperglycemia:
- *Typical features of hypoglycemia*: Excessive sweating, tachycardia, tremor and others (jerks may be brisk, planter response bilaterally extensor)
- *Typical features of hyperglycemia*: Severe dehydration, weak pulse and low BP. Air-hunger is present (Kussmaul breathing and acetone breath). Others are reduced reflexes, flexor planter response.

Management of DM: It comprises general management and management of complications. In a newly diagnosed DM, adequate glucose control by diet and lifestyle changes are the key points. If not controlled, oral antidiabetic drugs or insulin may be needed or combination of both may be given depending on blood glucose, severity of symptoms and comorbid conditions. There are three modes of treatment:

1. Diet control and lifestyle modification
2. Diet control and oral antidiabetics
3. Diet control and insulin (*plus* occasional oral antidiabetics).

Diet: In 50–60% cases, DM can be controlled by diet control. Balanced diet comprising carbohydrate, fat and protein as follows:
- *Carbohydrate*: 45–60% (sucrose up to 10%)
- Total fat <35% (saturated <10% and monounsaturated 10–20%)
- *Protein*: 10–15% (not to be exceeded 1 g/kg body weight/day)
- Fruits and vegetables.

Lifestyle:
- Weight reduction, if obese. Aerobic exercise at least 30–45 minutes five times per week (walking, swimming and cycling). Rest period should not exceed more than 2 days
- Smoking should be stopped. Alcohol in moderate dose
- Low calorie, sugar free drinks may be given.

Drugs: Oral antidiabetics and insulin.

Oral Antidiabetics:
- *Biguanides*: Metformin in T2DM, if no contraindications (hepatic dysfunction and severe renal failure)
- *Sulfonylureas*: Gliclazide, glibenclamide, glimepiride and glipizide. Usually, added with metformin, when DM is not controlled with metformin alone, can be used in lean patient with T2DM
- *Meglitinide*: Repaglinides and nateglinides. They are also insulin secretagogues
- *Alpha-glucosidase inhibitors*: Acarbose and miglitols. They control postprandial glucose and delay carbohydrate absorption from the gut. This drug can be used with sulfonylurea
- *Incretin-based drugs*: Sitagliptin, vildagliptin, linagliptin, liraglutide and exenatide. Used in obese patients and can be used with metformin, sulfonylurea or insulin
- *Others*: Canagliflozin, dapagliflozin and empagliflozin (sodium/glucose transporter 2 inhibitors) may be used.

Insulin: It is used mainly for T1DM. In T2DM, it is used from the beginning if blood glucose is very high or patient is symptomatic.

Human insulin:
- *Short-acting*: Soluble and regular insulin
- *Intermediate-acting*: Isophane (NPH)
- *Premix formulations*: 30/70 (30% short-acting and 70% intermediate acting) and 50/50 (50% each type).

Insulin analogues:
- *Rapid-acting*: Lispro, aspart and glulisine. These are ultra-short-acting bolus insulin to control postmeal hyperglycemia
- Premix formulations of rapid acting *plus* intermediate acting (e.g. aspart 30% *plus* aspart-protamine 70% (e.g. NovoMix)
- *Long-acting*: Glargine and detemir. Used as basal insulin to control premeal hyperglycemia
- *Ultra-long-acting*: Degludec.

Absolute indications of insulin therapy: DKA, hyperosmolar hyperglycemic state, lactic acidosis, surgery, pregnancy, severe infection, hepatic failure, and severe renal failure.

Complications of insulin therapy: Hypoglycemia, weight gain and lipodystrophy at injection sites (lipoatrophy and lipohypertrophy). Development of insulin antibody (especially in animal insulin).

Treatment goal for DM: Treatment goal and plan should be individualized.
- *Preprandial capillary plasma glucose fasting blood glucose (FBG)*: <7.0 mmol/L
- *Postprandial capillary plasma glucose*: <10 mmol/L
- *HbA1C*: <7%
- *BP*: <140/80 mm Hg
- *Total cholesterol*: <200 mg/dL
- *Triglyceride*: <150 mg/dL
- *Low-density lipoprotein*: <100 mg/dL and <70 mg/dL, if overt CVD
- *High-density lipoprotein (HDL)*: >40 mg/dL for men and >50 mg/dL for women.

Hypoglycemia

It is defined as when blood glucose level is <3.5 mmol/L (63 mg/dL).

Causes in diabetic patient are: Missed, delayed or inadequate meal, unusual exercise, error in dose or schedule or administration. Malabsorption, comorbid conditions (Addison's disease and renal impairment), factitious, and strict glycemic control.

Causes of hypoglycemia in nondiabetic patient:
- *Endocrine*: Addison's disease and pituitary insufficiency
- *Postprandial*: Usually develops 2–5 hours after meal, and never during fasting. May occur after alcohol intake and gastric surgery (partial gastrectomy, gastrojejunostomy and pyloroplasty)
- *Neoplastic*: Insulinoma, hepatoma, retroperitoneal sarcoma, fibroma and mesothelioma
- *Others*: Acute hepatic failure, CKD, severe falciparum malaria (cerebral malaria), especially during quinine therapy, and factitious. Rarely, may be hypoglycemia in childhood (galactosemia and glycogen storage disease type I).

Symptoms: Usually develop when blood glucose level is <2.5 mmol/L, but in diabetic patient, symptoms may appear at a higher level.
- *Adrenergic*: Palpitation, sweating, tremor, hunger and anxiety
- *Neuroglycopenic*: Confusion, inability to concentrate, drowsiness, dizziness, speech difficulty, irritability, fits, even coma, if untreated. Persistent and prolonged hypoglycemia may cause irreversible brain damage.

Management:
- *If the patient is conscious*: Should take oral glucose or sugar or any sweet
- *If patient is semiconscious or unconscious*: IV 75 mL 20% dextrose is given. IM glucagon (1 mg) may be given, followed by glucose infusion till the patient can take by mouth.

Prevention of hypoglycemia:
- Patient's education is important about hypoglycemia. Should keep glucose or any sweet. If any symptoms, patient should take this immediately
- Food should be kept ready before taking insulin
- Avoid undue heavy exercise and excess alcohol

- Risk factors of hypoglycemia should be sorted and managed accordingly
- Relatives and friends of the patient should also be educated also.

OBESITY

It is defined as excessive accumulation of body fat, classically when body mass index (BMI) is >30 kg/m^2. It is associated with higher risk of morbidity and mortality. Obesity is diagnosed by the following:
- Measuring weight
- Body mass index
- Skinfold thickness over the middle of triceps. Normal—20 mm in male and 30 mm in female
- Waist or hip circumference ratio >1.0 in male and >0.9 in female.

Causes of obesity: Multiple factors may be responsible—
- Genetic
- Physical inactivity
- Excessive food intake
- Psychological factors
- *Drugs*: Steroid, oral contraceptive pill, sodium valproate and tricyclic antidepressant (TCA)
- *Secondary disease*:
  - Endocrine causes: Hypothyroidism, Cushing syndrome and insulinoma
  - Polycystic ovarian syndrome (PCOS) in female
  - Hypothalamic disorder (tumors and injury)
  - Metabolic syndrome
  - Genetic syndrome: Bardet-Biedl syndrome and Prader-Willi syndrome
  - Others: Pickwickian syndrome and Alstrom syndrome.

Complications of obesity:
- *Psychological*: Low self-esteem and depression
- *Mechanical*: Osteoarthrosis of knee and hips, back strain, varicose veins, urinary incontinence, hiatus hernia, abdominal hernia and flat foot
- *Hepatobiliary*: Nonalcoholic fatty liver disease, cirrhosis and gallstones
- *Respiratory*: Exertional dyspnea, obstructive sleep apnea and Pickwickian syndrome
- *Cardiovascular*: Hypertension, atherosclerosis, IHD, heart failure and thromboembolism
- Cardiovascular disease
- *Metabolic*: T2DM, hyperlipidemia, atherosclerosis, hyperuricemia and gout
- *Increased cancer risk*: Breast, uterus, colorectal, prostate and ovary
- *Others*: Groin and submammary candidiasis, menstrual abnormalities, postoperative problems, accident proneness and increased morbidity and mortality.

Investigations: Detailed history of patient (dietary history, physical activity or sedentary work, any drug, and alcohol) should be taken. Whether weight gain is recent or rapid (to exclude secondary disease like Cushing syndrome or hypothyroidism). Then following investigations should be done:
- Blood sugar, lipid profile, thyroid function test and liver function test
- Investigations for Cushing syndrome (if suspected)

- Ultrasonography of hepatobiliary system to see fatty liver. X-ray of chest, ECG, echocardiography to see cardiac status. Lung function test for sleep apnea. X-ray of individual joints in osteoarthrosis
- In female, if PCOS is suspected, investigations should be done accordingly (e.g. USG of ovary, serum FSH and LH).

Treatment: Multidisciplinary approach including—
- Low calorie diet, exercise, social support, avoidance of offending drug, smoking and alcohol
- Treatment of secondary cause
- *Drug treatment*: Sibutramine, orlistat, incretins, and metformin.
- *Surgical management*: Bariatric surgery to reduce the size of stomach and cosmetic surgery (liposuction).

Indication of surgery: In some cases of morbid obesity (BMI >40 kg/m^2) or BMI >35 kg/m^2 and obesity-related complications, after conventional treatments have failed.

SHORT STATURE

Causes:
- Constitutional (the most common cause)
- Familial or genetic
- Physiological growth delay
- Emotional deprivation and psychological factors
- Chronic systemic disease:
  - Cardiac: Congenital cyanotic heart disease like Fallot's tetralogy
  - Renal: Renal failure and renal tubular acidosis
  - Respiratory: Bronchiectasis and bronchial asthma
  - *Gastrointestinal tract (GIT)*: Small bowel disease like celiac disease and Hirschsprung's disease
  - Cystic fibrosis.
- *Endocrine diseases*: Hypopituitarism (pituitary dwarfism), isolated GH deficiency, cretinism (hypothyroidism), pseudohypoparathyroidism, pseudopseudohypoparathyroidism, Cushing syndrome and uncontrolled juvenile DM
- *Nutritional*: Protein–energy malnutrition (marasmus and kwashiorkor) and rickets
- *Chromosomal or genetic abnormalities*: Down syndrome, Turner syndrome, Noonan syndrome (male Turner), Prader–Willi syndrome, and Bardet–Biedl syndrome
- *Skeletal dysplasia*: If short limb and normal trunk, may be due to achondroplasia. If short limb and short spine, may be due to mucopolysaccharidoses (Hurler syndrome or Gargoylism)
- Gross kyphoscoliosis
- *Drugs*: Steroid.

Investigations: A detailed history, physical examination and investigation should be done.
- *History to be taken*:
  - Family history (parents and relatives)
  - Pregnancy record (growth retardation, weight at birth and any congenital disease)
  - Rate of growth, comparison with peers at school and siblings

- Systemic disease (respiratory, cardiac, GIT and renal)
- Nutrition (less intake and malabsorption)
- Age of appearance of secondary sexual characters (pubic hair, breast and menarche)
- Use of steroid during childhood
- Psychosocial deprivation.
- *Physical examination*:
  - Height and weight chart. Arm span and height (achondroplasia)
  - Short limbs compared to trunk (achondroplasia)
  - Reduction of weight and height (malnutrition and systemic disease)
  - More weight but short height indicates endocrine disease (hypothyroidism and Cushing syndrome) and genetic syndrome (Prader–Willi syndrome and Bardet-Biedl syndrome)
  - Grading of secondary sexual characteristics
  - Look for evidence of systemic disease (heart, kidney and respiratory)
  - Others (Turner syndrome, Noonan syndrome and pseudohypoparathyroidism).

After exclusion of systemic disease, proceed as follows:

- *Thyroid function test*: Serum TSH and FT4 to exclude hypothyroidism
- Growth hormone status
- *Bone age*: Nondominant hand and wrist X-rays for the assessment of bone age by comparison with standard charts
- Lateral skull X-ray (may show calcification—in craniopharyngioma)
- *Karyotyping in females*: To exclude Turner syndrome
- Other tests according to suspicion of causes.

Dwarfism: It means height of a person is much below than the normal according to age. Causes are like short stature. Causes according to body ratio in dwarfism:

- If upper and lower segments are equal, causes are hereditary, constitutional and pituitary dwarfism
- If upper segment is large than lower segment, causes are achondroplasia, cretinism and juvenile myxedema
- If upper segment is smaller than lower segment, cause is spinal deformity

Treatment: Any systemic disease should be treated. Nutritional supplementation and psychological support. In GH deficiency, recombinant GH (somatropin) is given.

REPRODUCTIVE SYSTEM

Delayed puberty: Puberty is considered to be delayed if onset of signs of puberty are not present at particular age (in boys, by 14 years of age and in girls 13 years).

Amenorrhea: It means failure of menstruation. May be primary or secondary.

Primary amenorrhea: It means no menstruation or absence of menarche by the age of 16 years.

Causes: Gonadal dysgenesis (e.g. Turner syndrome), endometrial hypoplasia and vaginal agenesis.

Secondary amenorrhea: It means previously had normal menstruation, but no menstruation for more than three cycles. In nonpregnant women,

Endocrinology **161**

secondary amenorrhea results from ovarian, pituitary or hypothalamic dysfunction.

Causes:
- *Physiological*: Pregnancy and menopause
- *Pathological*:
    - Hypogonadotropic hypogonadism (due to disease of pituitary or hypothalamus)
    - Ovarian dysfunction: PCOS, androgen-secreting tumor, and premature ovarian failure
    - Any systemic disease such as severe anemia, renal failure and hyperthyroidism

Investigations: Details of history, physical examination, and then investigations should be done.
- Pregnancy should be excluded
- Measurement of serum LH, FSH, estradiol, testosterone, prolactin, T4, and TSH
- Karyotype should be performed in Turner syndrome
- *Ultrasonography of abdomen*: To see uterus, ovary, adrenal glands, etc.

Management: Treatment should be given according to cause.

Turner Syndrome

It is a sex chromosomal abnormality characterized by absence of one X chromosomes (45, XO). Only affects females, all or part of one X chromosome is deleted, causing failure of ovarian development. Externally, patient appears female, but does not produce female sex hormones. So, the patient remains sexually immature.

Clinical features: Usually presents with amenorrhea and underdeveloped secondary sexual characters. Other features are:
- Short stature. Short, webbed neck, low hairline and redundant skinfold on the back of neck
- *Face*: Small lower jaw (micrognathia), small, fish-like mouth, high-arched palate and low set deformed ears
- *Chest*: Broad and wide apart nipples (shield-like chest)
- *Hand*: Short fourth metacarpal (other metacarpals may be short), lymphedema of hands (also feet), and hypoplastic nails
- *Elbow*: Increased carrying angles (cubitus valgus).

Investigations:
- *Karyotyping from buccal smear*: 45 (XO) is classical, occasionally 46 (XX) mosaics
- *Ultrasonography of abdomen*: Small uterus, fallopian tube and streak gonad
- *Hormone assay*: Low estrogen, high LH and FSH.

Treatment:
- Estrogen therapy at puberty. GH may accelerate height, but it is not yet established whether there is any effect on final height
- Gonadal tumor may occur rarely, especially in mosaic involving "Y" chromosome. So, it should be removed.

Associations or diseases that occur in Turner syndrome:
- *Heart*: Coarctation of aorta, atrial septal defect (ASD), ventricular septal defect (VSD), aortic stenosis and hypertension

- *Kidney*: "Horseshoe" kidney and hydronephrosis
- *Endocrine*: DM, Hashimoto's thyroiditis and hypothyroidism
- Lymphedema in infancy, red and green color blindness, strabismus and ptosis, premature osteoporosis, pigmented nevi and mental retardation (rare).

Noonan Syndrome: It is also called male Turner, characterized by short stature, mental retardation (common), downward slanting, wide-spaced eyes, low set ear, webbing of neck, low posterior hairline and pulmonary stenosis. It may affect both male and female. Female patients have Turner phenotype but with normal 46 XX, normal ovarian function, and normal fertility. Cardiac lesion is present more on the right side such as pulmonary stenosis. In Turner syndrome, left-sided cardiac lesion is more.

Polycystic Ovarian Syndrome

It is a syndrome in which there are multiple cysts in ovary and hyperandrogenemia characterized by amenorrhea or oligomenorrhea, obesity, hirsutism, infertility (due to anovulation), and virilization (in severe cases).

Diagnostic criteria of PCOS: Two of the following three features:
1. Menstrual irregularities (oligomenorrhea or amenorrhea)
2. Clinical or biochemical evidence of androgen excess
3. Multiple cysts in the ovaries (detected by USG).

Investigations:
- Ultrasonography of abdomen to see ovaries
- Serum testosterone (high), LH (high), FSH (normal or low, ratio of LH:FSH >2 or 3). Androgens (androstenedione and dehydroepiandrosterone are high), sex hormone-binding globulin (SHBG) (low), prolactin (slightly high, rarely greater than 1,500 mU/L), and estrogen (estradiol is usually normal)
- To exclude other cause, investigations should be done according to suspicion:
  - Serum 17-OH progesterone: High in late onset CAH
  - Computed tomography or MRI of adrenal (in suspected tumor)
  - Dexamethasone suppression test
  - Short ACTH stimulation test with measurement of 17-hydroxyprogesterone to diagnose CAH.

Treatment:
- *General measures*: Reduction of weight, regular exercise and diet control
- *For hirsutism*: Local therapy (plucking, bleaching, electrolysis, depilatory cream and shaving of hair). Drugs such as cyproterone acetate, spironolactone, finasteride and flutamide may be given
- *For fertility*:
  - Metformin: May improve ovulation and achieve conception
  - Clomiphene 50–100 mg/day, from days 2–6 of cycle. Dexamethasone 0.5 mg at bedtime with clomiphene may increase ovulation
  - If no response to clomiphene, metformin is added, 500 mg three times daily. May enhance ovulation
  - Prednisolone in reverse circadian rhythm (2.5 mg in morning and 5 mg at bedtime) may suppress pituitary ACTH and ovulatory cycle may become normal.

- *For menstrual disturbance*:
  - Metformin 500 mg three times daily. Improves hirsutism and obesity
  - Cyclical low dose estrogen or progesterone
  - If does not desire pregnancy, medroxyprogesterone 10 mg daily orally for first 10 days of each cycle
  - Menstrual irregularity can be improved by oral contraceptives
  - Wedge resection or laser surgery of ovary or laparoscopy ovarian drilling may be done.
- *For obesity*: Metformin may be used.

Complications of PCOS: Hyperinsulinemia and insulin resistance, glucose intolerance, T2DM, hypertension, dyslipidemia and cardiovascular risk.

Male Hypogonadism

It may be primary (due to disease in testes) or secondary (due to disease in pituitary or hypothalamus).

Causes:
- *Primary or hypergonadotropic hypogonadism*:
  - Testicular damage: Trauma, surgery, chemo or radiotherapy to testes, mumps orchitis, TB, hemochromatosis and leprosy
  - Developmental abnormality: Klinefelter syndrome and cryptorchidism.
- *Secondary or hypogonadotropic hypogonadism*: Hypopituitarism due to any cause, prolactinoma and Kallmann syndrome.

Clinical features:
- *If hypogonadism develops before puberty*: Presents with features of delayed puberty
- *If it starts after puberty*: Loss of libido, lethargy with muscle weakness, decreased frequency of shaving, infertility and osteoporosis.

Investigations:
- *Serum testosterone*: Low
- *Serum LH and FSH*: High in primary and low in secondary
- *Other investigations*: According to suspicion of cause (e.g. chromosomal analysis in Klinefelter syndrome).

Treatment: Testosterone should be given. It does not induce fertility. Treatment of cause, if any.

Infectious Disease and Tropical Medicine

MUMPS

It is an infection of parotid gland caused by mumps virus, common in children.

Incubation period: 2–3 weeks.

Symptoms: Fever, headache, malaise, myalgia, anorexia, sore throat, and earache on chewing and swallowing. Painful swelling of parotid gland (unilateral or bilateral), more on 3rd day, remains for 2–3 days and then subsides.

Signs: Parotid glands are enlarged and tender. Submandibular glands may be involved. Skin over parotid gland is red and shiny.

Investigation: Diagnosis is clinical. Investigations are unnecessary.

Complications: Orchitis, may be atrophy and sterility if both testes are involved, pancreatitis, epididymitis, oophoritis (in female), otitis media, myocarditis, aseptic meningitis and encephalitis.

Treatment:
- Rest and isolation in bed for 10 days. Maintenance of hydration, nutrition and oral hygiene
- Paracetamol for fever or pain. If orchitis or oophoritis, prednisolone 40 mg daily for 4 days.

Prevention: Live attenuated measles, mumps and rubella (MMR) vaccine.

MEASLES

It is caused by measles virus (RNA virus) and transmitted by infected droplet.

Incubation period: 10–14 days.

Clinical features:
- *Prodromal symptoms or catarrhal phase*: Fever, headache, sneezing, running nose, dry cough and redness of eyes. Patient looks miserable and irritable. Koplik's spots are present at this stage, which are small, irregular, and grayish white spots surrounded by erythema on buccal mucosa around the opening of parotid duct opposite the upper second molar

teeth. They appear 2 days before appearance of skin rash and disappear 1-2 days after the appearance of rash
- *Exanthematous stage*: Red maculopapular skin rash develops after 3-4 days of prodromal phase. Fever subsides after eruption of rash. Initially, rashes are pinhead-sized papules and coalesce to form red morbilliform rash, which fades after 4 days. Lymph nodes may be enlarged.

Investigations: Diagnosis is clinical. Investigations are unnecessary.

Complications: Bronchitis, bronchiolitis, bronchopneumonia, conjunctivitis, keratitis, retrobulbar neuritis, otitis media, myocarditis and thrombocytopenia. Subacute sclerosing panencephalitis (SSPE) and measles inclusion body encephalitis (MIBE) occur months to years after acute infection.

Treatment:
- Bed rest and isolation, until 5 days after rash has appeared. Adequate fluid, nutrition, oral hygiene and care of eyes. Paracetamol for fever. Antibiotic, if secondary infection
- Gamma globulin 0.25 mL/kg can modify the course of disease in immunocompromised patient
- Vitamin A (for children ≥12 months—200,000 IU/day for 2 days) is recommended by the World Health Organization (WHO) for all children with measles.

Prevention: Live attenuated measles vaccine.

RUBELLA (GERMAN MEASLES)

It is caused by rubella virus (RNA virus) and transmitted by infected droplet.

Incubation period: 2-3 weeks.

Symptoms: Fever, malaise, headache, anorexia, runny nose, sneezing, cough and arthralgia.

Signs: Maculopapular rash (appears first on the forehead, spreads to the trunk and limbs and fades after 3 days). Petechial rash may appear on the soft palate. Lymphadenopathy (postauricular, suboccipital and posterior cervical) and conjunctivitis.

Complications: Rubella is usually not serious and only harmful if it occurs in pregnancy.
- Thrombocytopenia, hepatitis, encephalitis, and spontaneous abortion
- *Congenital rubella syndrome*: If maternal rubella infection occurs in first trimester, there may be transplacental transfer of virus into the fetus causing congenital diseases such as cataract, microcephaly, mental retardation, deafness and congenital heart defects (patent ductus arteriosus and pulmonary stenosis).

Investigations: Diagnosis is clinical. Complete blood count (CBC) may show leukopenia. Serology (IgM antibody to rubella virus indicates recent infection).

Treatment: Bed rest, adequate fluid and nutrition. Paracetamol for fever and arthralgia.

Prevention: MMR vaccine.

DENGUE FEVER

It is a viral illness caused by dengue virus. Four serotypes—DEN-1, DEN-2, DEN-3, and DEN-4. It is transmitted by bite of *Aedes aegypti* and *A. albopictus* mosquito.

Manifestations of dengue viral infection:
- Asymptomatic
- *Symptomatic*:
  - Undifferentiated fever
  - Dengue fever with or without hemorrhage
  - Dengue hemorrhagic fever
  - Dengue shock syndrome.

Dengue fever: It is an acute febrile illness due to dengue virus.

Features:
- *Fever*: High, continuous, and persists for 2–7 days. After 4–5 days, fever may subside, may reappear after 2–3 days, called biphasic or saddleback fever
- After 4–5 days, fever usually subsides, and skin rash like petechiae, ecchymosis, and purpura appear. Also, platelet may fall, usually in 4–6 days. Bleeding and shock may occur. This time is called the "critical period"
- Severe headache, retro-orbital pain, nausea and vomiting
- Severe body ache, myalgia and arthralgia. So, it is called breakbone fever
- Acute abdominal pain may be confused with appendicitis and pancreatitis.

Dengue hemorrhagic fever: When associated with bleeding manifestations, it is usually due to fall of platelets, there may be—
- Petechiae, ecchymosis or purpura
- Epistaxis, gum bleeding, hematemesis, melena, bleeding from injection site, and menorrhagia or early onset of menstrual bleeding in female
- Positive tourniquet test.

Dengue shock syndrome: It is characterized by circulatory failure with one or more of the following features—
- Hypotension
- Cold clammy skin, restlessness, and rapid weak pulse
- Narrow pulse pressure
- Profound shock.

Investigations:
- *Complete blood count, platelet and packed cell volume (PCV)*: Shows leukopenia, thrombocytopenia, and raised PCV
- Dengue NS1 antigen (positive on 1st day of fever)
- Anti-dengue antibody (IgG and IgM, positive after 5–6 days)
- *Other tests*: Chest X-ray (CXR) (may be right-sided pleural effusion), USG of abdomen (ascites), serum protein (hypoproteinemia), and serum glutamic oxaloacetic transaminase (SGOT) and serum glutamic pyruvic transaminase (SGPT) (usually high).

Treatment:
- Rest
- *For fever*: Antipyretic (paracetamol) and tepid sponging

- Aspirin should be avoided especially in children, which may cause Reye's syndrome. Other nonsteroidal anti-inflammatory drugs (NSAIDs) should also be avoided
- Maintenance of fluid and electrolyte balance—oral rehydration therapy, plenty of fluid and fruit juice
- If the patient cannot take by mouth—IV infusion (normal saline and Ringer's lactate)
- Antibiotics, if secondary infection.

HERPES SIMPLEX VIRUS

Types: There are two types of herpes simplex virus (HSV) type 1 and 2. It is a DNA virus. Infection may be primary or recurrent. Primary infection is followed by episodes of reactivation throughout life.

Clinical features:
- Primary HSV-1 causes recurrent mucocutaneous infection commonly involving the head and neck such as gingivostomatitis, pharyngitis, herpes labialis (cold sore), keratoconjunctivitis, finger infection (herpetic whitlow), encephalitis, stomatitis, and genital infection. Primary attack may be associated with fever and regional lymphadenopathy
- HSV-2 usually causes genital infection or painful genital tract lesions, which may be recurrent
- Both can cause disseminated infection in immunocompromised.

Complications:
- Disseminated cutaneous lesions such as eczema (eczema herpeticum)
- Herpetic keratitis, dendritic ulcers, corneal scarring, and permanent visual impairment
- Primary HSV-2 can cause meningitis and transverse myelitis
- Encephalitis, usually with HSV-1
- Hemorrhagic necrotizing temporal lobe cerebritis produces temporal lobe epilepsy and altered consciousness
- Bell's palsy with lower motor neuron 7th nerve palsy
- Neonatal HSV is associated with primary infection during delivery
- Esophagitis, hepatitis, pneumonitis, encephalitis or retinitis in immunocompromised.

Investigations: Diagnosis is usually clinical.
- Anti-HSV antibodies 1 and 2
- Isolation of virus from vesicular fluid by direct immunofluorescence or polymerase chain reaction (PCR)
- *HSV encephalitis*: PCR for HSV in CSF, MRI or CT scan, and EEG.

Treatment:
- Acyclovir or valacyclovir or famciclovir is the treatment of choice
- Oral lesions in immunocompetent patient may be treated with topical acyclovir
- *If suspicion of HSV encephalopathy*: Immediate antiviral therapy
- *In acyclovir resistance (in immunocompromised)*: Foscarnet may be given.

Herpes Simplex Encephalitis

Herpes simplex type 1 may cause encephalitis and type 2 may cause benign recurrent lymphocytic meningitis. It usually involves the inferior aspect of frontal lobes and medial aspect of temporal lobe.

Clinical features:
- Flu-like illness, fever, severe headache, altered consciousness, behavior abnormality and speech disturbance
- Focal neurological deficit such as dysphasia, hemiparesis, and focal or generalized seizure, commonly temporal lobe seizure
- Olfactory and gustatory hallucinations, and impairment of memory
- There may be multiple cranial nerve palsy and ataxia. Untreated patient develops convulsion and coma. Mortality is high.

Investigations:
- Serum anti-HSV-1 antibody
- Lumbar puncture and CSF study—shows lymphocytic leukocytosis, normal protein, and sugar. HSV–DNA PCR is highly sensitive for rapid diagnosis
- EEG shows distinctive periodic pattern in some cases
- CT scan or MRI of brain.

Treatment:
- Acyclovir 10 mg/kg 8 hourly IV for 10 days
- Anticonvulsant may be necessary. Dexamethasone for raised intracranial pressure.

RABIES

It is caused by rhabdovirus, which infects central nervous system and salivary glands of mammals. Man is usually infected by saliva through bites of infected dog, rarely by cat, and also by licks on abrasions or on intact mucous membranes. Wild rabies is caused by bat and fox.

Incubation period: It varies in humans from 9 days to many months, usually 4–8 weeks. It depends on site of bites. Severe bites, especially on head or neck, are associated with shorter incubation period.

Clinical features:
- Initially, fever and paresthesia at the site of bite
- After 1–10 days, the patient becomes anxious and develops "hydrophobia" (fear of water). The patient is thirsty, but attempts at drinking provoke violent contractions of muscles of deglutition, diaphragm, and other inspiratory muscles. Even site or sound of water may cause spasm
- Delusions and hallucinations may develop. There is lucid interval in which the patient is more anxious. Cranial nerve lesions and terminal hyperpyrexia may develop
- Spitting, biting and mania. Secretion of large amount of thick saliva is common
- Death ensues, usually within a week.

Investigations: Diagnosis is usually clinical.
- Rapid immunofluorescent techniques can detect antigen in corneal impression smears or skin biopsies
- Infected animal is killed and brain is examined to see Negri bodies
- Isolation of virus from saliva or CSF.

Treatment:
Postexposure prophylaxis
- Wound should be thoroughly cleaned with running tap water and soap. Damaged tissues should be excised and the wound should not be sutured
- Rabies can be prevented if treatment is started within a day or two of biting
- Hyperimmune serum and vaccine should be given—human rabies immunoglobulin 20 U/kg, half is infiltrated around bite and half is given intramuscularly at different site
- Hyperimmune animal serum may be used but hypersensitivity reactions and anaphylaxis are common
- *Human diploid cell vaccine*: 1 mL IM on days 0, 3, 7, 14, 30 and 90
- Where human products are not available and when risk of rabies is slight (licks on skin, or minor bites of covered arms or legs), starting of treatment may be delayed while observing the biting animal or awaiting examination of its brain, rather than using the older vaccine
- Biting animal is observed for at least 10 days. If the animal dies within 10 days, then brain is examined for "Negri bodies". If it is normal after 10 days, probably there is no rabies.

Established disease: Treated in ICU, usually palliative. Sedation with diazepam, supplemented by chlorpromazine, if needed. Maintenance of fluid balance and nutrition.

Pre-exposure prophylaxis: Given in patients with high risk of contacting rabies, such as laboratory workers, animal handlers and veterinarians. Three doses (1 mL) of human diploid or chick embryo cell vaccine, deep subcutaneous or IM injection on days 0, 7 and 28. Booster dose is given after 1 year and every 3-5 years depending on the risk of exposure.

ENTERIC FEVER (TYPHOID AND PARATYPHOID)

It is an enteric infection caused by gram-negative bacteria *Salmonella typhi* and *paratyphi A, B* and *C*. Transmitted by feco-oral route through contamination of food, milk or water.

Typhoid Fever

Clinical features:
- 1st *week*: Fever, rises throughout the day, it is less in morning but gradually rises (called stepladder pattern). Headache, malaise, lassitude, weakness, body ache, constipation, cough and epistaxis
- 2nd *week*: Fever is continuous. At the end of 1st week, rash may appear on upper abdomen and back, called rose spots, which fade on pressure. It persists for 2-3 days, and then disappears. Diarrhea (pea soup stool) and hepatosplenomegaly. At the end of 2nd week, patient becomes very weak. There may be muttering delirium and coma vigil, with picking of bed clothes or imaginary object, called "typhoid state"
- 3rd-4th *week*: If not treated properly, there may be complications such as melena and perforation (at the terminal ileum).

Signs: Coated tongue, relative bradycardia (pulse rate does not proportionally rise with rise of temperature), spleen is enlarged (after 7-10 days), hepatomegaly, and cecal gurgling.

Complications: Perforation (in terminal ileum) and hemorrhage. Others are meningitis, pericarditis, myocarditis, endocarditis, bronchitis, cholecystitis and glomerulonephritis.

Investigations:
- Complete blood count—may be leukopenia
- Blood culture/sensitivity (C/S)
- Widal test, usually after 1st week
- Stool and urine culture in 3rd week.

Treatment: Rest, hydration, and adequate nutrition. For fever, paracetamol and tepid sponging. Correction of fluid and electrolytes imbalance.

Specific treatment:
- Ciprofloxacin (500 mg 12 hourly) or ofloxacin (400 mg 12 hourly) or pefloxacin (400 mg 12 hourly) or cefixime (400 mg 12 hourly) or azithromycin (500 mg 12 hourly) for 2 weeks
- Ceftriaxone (75 mg/kg/day) is an alternative
- Cotrimoxazole (160/800 mg) twice daily for 10–14 days
- *In pregnancy*: Ceftriaxone or amoxicillin 750–1,000 mg 6 hourly
- In severely ill patient, dexamethasone is given (3 mg/kg for initial doses, followed by 1 mg/kg every 6 h for 48 h)
- Surgical intervention, if perforation.

Carrier state: After recovery, 5–10% patients will continue to excrete *S. typhi* through stool for several months. This is called "convalescent carrier". About 1–4% patients will carry the organism for years, which is called "chronic carrier". Chronic carrier is common in >50 years, and more in female. Usual site is gallbladder and may be associated with gallstones. Chronic carriers should be treated with ciprofloxacin 750 mg 12 hourly for 4 weeks or norfloxacin 400 mg 12 hourly for 4 weeks. Cholecystectomy may be needed.

Paratyphoid fever: Course is shorter and milder than typhoid fever and onset is abrupt with acute enteritis. Rash may be more abundant and intestinal complications are less frequent. Treatment is done as in typhoid fever.

Prevention: Good sanitation and living conditions reduce the incidence of typhoid. Prevention of fecal contamination of food and milk. Hand washing is important. Travelers to the countries, where enteric infections are endemic, should take typhoid vaccines.

TYPHUS FEVER

Scrub Typhus Fever (Mite-borne)

It is caused by *Orientia tsutsugamushi* (formerly called *Rickettsia tsutsugamushi*), and transmitted by infected mites.

Incubation period: 10–12 days.

Clinical features:
- Mild or subclinical cases are common
- Initial lesion is eschar, surrounding cellulitis, enlargement of regional lymph nodes, and erythematous maculopapular rash, which appears on 5th–7th day and spreads to trunk, face, limbs, including palms and soles, and fades by 14th day

- May be headache (usually retro-orbital), fever, malaise, weakness, cough, and generalized painless lymphadenopathy. Fever is high, remittent with sweating, falls on 12th-18th day. In severe case, apathy, prostration, pneumonia, confusion and deafness. Cardiac failure, renal failure, and hemorrhage may develop
- Convalescence is often slow and tachycardia may persist for some weeks.

Investigations: Serology immunofluorescence assay (IFA) and PCR of eschars and blood is also effective.

Treatment: Doxycycline (100 mg 12 hourly) or chloramphenicol (500 mg qid) for 7-15 days, or 3 day course of azithromycin (500 mg qid) is effective.

Epidemic (Louse-borne) Typhus

It is caused by *R. prowazekii*, transmitted by infected feces of human body louse, through skin scratching.

Incubation period: of 12-14 days.

Clinical features:
- Onset is sudden with fever, rigors, frontal headache, confusion, pain in back and limbs, constipation, and bronchitis. Face is flushed and cyanotic, and eyes are congested
- Rash appears on upper trunk in 5th day of illness and spreads to involve whole body except face, palms and soles
- During 2nd week, symptoms increases and sores develop in lips. Tongue is dry, brown, shrunken and tremulous. May be stupor and delirium
- Spleen is palpable
- Temperature falls rapidly at the end of 2nd week and patient recovers gradually. In severe cases, the patient may die in 2nd week from toxemia, cardiac or renal failure or pneumonia.

Investigations: Serology and immunohistochemistry.

Treatment: Single dose of 200 mg doxycycline, repeated for 2-3 days to prevent relapse. Sometimes 100 mg 12 hourly given until 2-3 days after fever disappears.

Endemic (Flea-borne) Typhus

It is caused by *R. typhi*. It is transmitted by scratching the feces of rat flea at the biting site.

Incubation period: 8-14 days.

Symptoms: Resemble those of mild louse-borne typhus, and rash may be scanty and transient.

Investigations: Diagnosis is clinical.
- Complete blood count (thrombocytopenia), malaria parasite (to exclude malaria), and liver function test (LFT) (may be abnormal)
- Confirmed by antibody detection or PCR.

Treatment: Doxycycline (100 mg 12 hourly) or ciprofloxacin. Tetracycline 500 mg four times daily.

Q Fever

It is caused by *Coxiella burnetii*. Cattle, sheep, and goats are responsible for most human infection. They pass the bacteria through urine, feces, milk, and fluids, and the organism is transmitted to human by inhalation. Abattoir worker, veterinarians, farmers, and others who are in contact with these infected animals are at risk.

Incubation period: 3-4 weeks.

Clinical features:
- *Acute Q fever*: Symptoms and signs are nonspecific with fever, headache, chills, nausea, vomiting, diarrhea and cough. In 20% of cases, a maculopapular rash occurs. Pneumonia, hepatitis, pericarditis, and myocarditis may occur
- *Chronic Q fever*: Fever is usually absent or low grade, and may present with endocarditis commonly with previous valvular heart disease or in immunosuppressed person.

Investigations:
- *Acute*: CBC (thrombocytopenia) and CXR (pneumonia may be present)
- *Chronic*: Serological tests and IFA. Echocardiography (to see vegetation and also cardiac lesion).

Treatment:
- *Acute*: Doxycycline 100 mg bd for 14 days
- *Chronic*: Doxycycline 100 mg bd *plus* hydroxychloroquine 200 mg bd for 18 months *or* doxycycline 100 mg bd *or* ciprofloxacin 750 mg bd *plus* rifampicin 300 mg once daily may be used for 1 year. Valve surgery may be required for endocarditis.

BACILLARY DYSENTERY (SHIGELLOSIS)

It is an enteric infection caused by gram-negative rod *Shigella* that invades the colonic mucosa. It is transmitted by feco-oral route through contamination of food, milk or water.

Organisms: *S. dysenteriae, S. flexneri* (common in tropical country), *S. boydii* and *S. sonnei*.

Incubation period: 1-7 days.

Symptoms: Features develop due to release of endotoxin. Diarrhea mixed with fresh blood and mucus, nausea, vomiting, fever, malaise, weakness, and generalized body ache. Colicky abdominal pain and tenesmus, increased thirst, and dryness of mouth.

Signs: Patient may be toxic. Tenderness over left iliac fossa. Signs of dehydration (dry tongue, sunken eyes and hypotension).

Complications: Meningism, arthritis, iritis, hemolytic uremic syndrome (HUS) and Reiter's syndrome.

Investigations: Stool for R/M/E and C/S, CBC, serum electrolytes, and creatinine.

Treatment:
- Correction of dehydration [Oral rehydration solution (ORS) or, if diarrhea is severe, IV fluid] and maintenance of nutrition
- Ciprofloxacin 500 mg 12 hourly or norfloxacin 500 mg 12 hourly or azithromycin 500 mg 12 hourly for 5-7 days.

Prevention: Fecal contamination of food, milk or drink should be avoided. Hand washing is important.

AMOEBIASIS (AMOEBIC DYSENTERY)

It is an enteric infection caused by *Entamoeba histolytica* and transmitted by feco-oral route (ingestion of cysts) by contamination of uncooked food, milk or water.

Incubation period: Up to 2 weeks.

Symptoms: Diarrhea mixed with mucus and occasionally blood, colicky abdominal pain, nausea, vomiting, fever, malaise and weakness.

Signs: Abdominal tenderness mostly in right lower quadrant.

Investigations:
- *Stool for R/M/E*: May reveal motile trophozoites with red blood cells
- *Sigmoidoscopy*: Reveals typical flask-shaped ulcers in intestinal wall
- *Serological tests*: May detect anti-amoeba antibody.

Treatment:
- Correction of dehydration and maintenance of nutrition
- Oral metronidazole 400 mg 8 hourly for 5–7 days *or* tinidazole 1 g 12 hourly for 3–5 days *or* secnidazole 1 g 12 hourly for 3–5 days *or* nitazoxanide 500 mg 12 hourly for 3 days
- Diloxanide furoate 500 mg orally 8 hourly for 10 days to eliminate luminal cysts.

Complications: Amoebic hepatitis, amoebic liver abscess, chronic amoebiasis (may cause granulomatous lesion within the colonic wall called "ameboma", seen as a mass in right iliac fossa).

Prevention: Avoid eating uncooked vegetables or drinking unboiled water.

CHOLERA

It is an acute diarrheal illness caused by *Vibrio cholerae* (classic and El Tor serotype). New serotype O139 in Bangladesh is becoming a pandemic. Transmitted by feco-oral route by contaminated water, food and shellfish.

Incubation period: Few hours to 5 days.

Clinical features: The bacteria produce enterotoxin responsible for clinical manifestations.
- Profuse painless watery diarrhea known as "rice water stool", vomiting, fatigue and muscle cramps
- Signs of severe dehydration (pinched face, sunken eyes, poor skin turgor, dry tongue, tachycardia, thready pulse, hypotension, oliguria and shock)
- Death from acute circulatory failure, if not properly treated.

Complications: Hypovolemic shock, electrolyte imbalance and renal failure.

Investigations: Diagnosis is clinical.
- Serum electrolytes and creatinine
- *Stool R/M/E*: Shows the typical shooting star motility of *V. cholerae*
- Stool C/S or rectal swab for *V. cholerae*.

Treatment:
- Rest. Oral (ORS or rice ORS) or IV cholera saline or Ringer's lactate
- Oral tetracycline 250 mg 6 hourly for 3 days. *Or* doxycycline 300 mg single dose *or* ciprofloxacin 1 g single dose. Zinc supplement.

DIPHTHERIA

It is an acute infection of upper respiratory tract caused by *Corynebacterium diphtheriae*, and spreads by droplet infection from infected cases or carriers.

Incubation period: 2–4 days.

Sites: Tonsils, nose and larynx. Rarely occurs in skin, wound and conjunctiva.

Symptoms: Organism is localized at the site of infection but features are due to absorption of exotoxin, which typically damages heart muscle and nervous system.
- Sore throat. Low-grade fever, malaise and lethargy. Runny nose, may be blood stained, and sneezing (if nasal involvement)
- Croupy voice. In laryngeal diphtheria, husky voice, high-pitched brassy cough, and even respiratory obstruction requiring tracheostomy
- Excessive salivation, dysphagia, and neck swelling (bull neck).

Signs: The patient may be very toxic with tachypnea.
- There is pseudomembrane which is grayish-green, wash leather, elevated, thick, glistening, and firmly adherent with well-defined erythematous edge on tonsils and pharynx
- In severe case, there may be cervical tender lymphadenopathy and marked edema of submandibular space, giving rise to "bull neck appearance". It is also called "malignant diphtheria".

Complications:
- *Effects due to diphtheria exotoxin*:
  - *Myocarditis*: In 1st or 2nd week, causing arrhythmia and cardiac failure. Death may occur due to acute circulatory failure within first 10 days. Most cases recover with no permanent damage
  - *Neurological*: Paralysis of soft palate and posterior pharyngeal wall causing bulbar and pseudobulbar palsy (nasal voice and nasal regurgitation), peripheral neuropathy, and paralysis of accommodation, manifested as difficulty in reading small print. Also cranial nerve palsy and rarely encephalitis.
- *Effects due to pseudomembrane*: Laryngeal obstruction or paralysis.

Investigations: Diagnosis is clinical and therapy should be started, if diphtheria is suspected.
- CBC may show leukocytosis
- Throat swab smear for Albert's stain (to see club-shaped organism)
- Throat swab culture in Loeffler's serum.

Treatment: Rest and isolation of patient. Maintenance of adequate hydration and nutrition.
- Diphtheria antitoxin should be given immediately (no role, once the toxin is fixed to the tissue). It neutralizes the circulatory toxin
- Intravenous benzylpenicillin, 1,200 mg 6 hourly or amoxicillin 500 mg 8 hourly for 2 weeks. If the patient is allergic to penicillin, erythromycin can be given
- Rifampicin and clindamycin may be given, if resistance to penicillin or erythromycin
- If myocarditis or severe neck swelling—corticosteroid
- If laryngeal obstruction—emergency tracheostomy.

Prevention: Active immunization should be given to all children. If diphtheria occurs in a closed community, contacts should be given erythromycin. All contacts should also be immunized or given a booster dose of toxoid.

WHOOPING COUGH

It is an infectious disease caused by *Bordetella pertussis*, a gram-negative *Coccobacillus*. Transmission is through contaminated droplets.

Incubation period: 7–16 days.

Clinical features: Three stages—
1. *Catarrhal stage*: Infectivity is high during this stage. Cough, runny nose, congested eyes, lacrimation, fever and malaise
2. *Paroxysmal stage*: Paroxysm of cough, ending with a high-pitched deep inspiratory "whoop". Vomiting and cyanosis may occur. "Whoop" may not be present in infants. Episodes of choking and apnea may occur. May be engorged conjunctiva, periorbital edema, and petechial hemorrhage
3. *Convalescent stage*: Patient's symptoms improve and cough becomes less.

Complications: Convulsion, subconjunctival hemorrhage, bronchopneumonia, bronchiectasis and rectal prolapse.

Investigations: Diagnosis is clinical.
- *CBC*: Lymphocytosis. Culture of nasopharyngeal swab or sputum in Bordet-Gengou media
- X-ray of chest may show enlarged mediastinal nodes and patchy atelectasis
- Polymerase chain reaction and direct immunofluorescent antibody test may be done.

Treatment:
- Erythromycin 50 mg/kg/day, 6 hourly for 14 days, or clarithromycin 10 mg/kg/day 12 hourly for 7 days, or azithromycin 10 mg/kg/day once daily for 5 days
- Co-trimoxazole, 12 hourly for 2 weeks, if patient cannot tolerate other drugs
- Short-course prednisolone may shorten the clinical course
- Antispasmodics, antitussives, and sedatives are of no proven value
- Close contacts should be treated with erythromycin for 14 days. Children should be isolated for 5 days after initiation of erythromycin therapy.

Prevention: Prevention by active immunization with triple vaccine [diphtheria, pertussis and tetanus (DPT)].

TETANUS

It is an infection caused by *Clostridium tetani*, an anaerobic gram-positive bacilli. It produces exotoxin "tetanospasmin", responsible for clinical manifestations. The toxin affects the anterior horn cells, which causes rigidity and convulsion.

Mode of transmission: Organism is found in soil and the disease is due to contamination of cuts, wounds or umbilical stump.

Incubation period: 7–8 days.

Clinical features:
- Fever, malaise and irritability
- *Lockjaw or trismus*: Due to spasms and stiffness of masseter muscles. It is painless
- *Risus sardonicus*: Due to sustained contraction of facial muscles (occipitofrontalis)
- *Opisthotonos*: Due to contraction of neck and back muscles, produces arching of back
- Board-like abdominal rigidity. Difficulty in swallowing due to esophageal spasm
- In severe case, generalized muscular spasm, which may be spontaneous, lasting for several minutes, triggered by loud noise, light or handling the patient
- Patient remains conscious and experiences severe pain during spasm
- *Autonomic dysfunction*: Hypertension or hypotension, tachycardia or bradycardia, hyperpyrexia, profuse sweating and peripheral vasoconstriction
- Retention of urine due to urethral spasm.

Complications: Spine or bone fracture due to spasm, laryngeal spasm causing upper airway obstruction, and apnea.

Treatment: Patient should be admitted in an isolated, quiet, and well-ventilated dark room.
- Wound should be identified, cleaned, and debridement of necrotic materials should be done
- Adequate ventilation, hydration and nutrition
- Single IM tetanus immunoglobulin 3,000–5,000 units, with part of dose infiltrated around wound
- *Or* human tetanus immunoglobulin (injection TIG 500 IU IM) *plus* IM tetanus toxoid at a different site. If there is no history of primary tetanus toxoid vaccination, then patient should receive a second dose 1–2 months after the first dose and a third dose 6–12 months later
- Diazepam 5 mg IV or infusion. Alternative drugs are midazolam and propofol. Injection magnesium sulfate may also be used
- Intravenous metronidazole, 500 mg 6 hourly. Benzyl penicillin 600 mg IV four times daily for 10 days
- If airway is obstructed, intubation and mechanical ventilation may be necessary
- Treatment of secondary infection.

Prevention: By active immunization with DPT vaccine. In contaminated wounds, immediate danger can be prevented by 1,200 mg penicillin IM, followed by oral penicillin for 7 days. If allergic to penicillin, erythromycin may be used. IM 250 IU human tetanus antitoxin with tetanus toxoid, should be repeated at 1 and 6 months later. If already immunized, only a booster dose of toxoid is required.

Neonatal tetanus: It occurs due to infection of umbilical stump with *C. tetani*. Features are—failure to thrive, poor sucking, irritability, grimacing, rigidity and spasm. Diagnosis is clinical. Treatment as tetanus.

CHICKEN POX

It is caused by varicella-zoster virus and transmitted through contaminated respiratory droplets.

Incubation period: 10–21 days.

Clinical features:
- Fever, malaise, generalized body ache, headache, anorexia, nausea and vomiting
- Itchy skin rash develops in crops at first, on back then chest, abdomen, face and limbs. Distribution is centripetal, more on upper arms and thighs, and upper part of face. Initially macule, then papule, and then multiple vesicles develop, and turn to pustules in 24 hours. Scabs in 2–5 days.

Investigation: Diagnosis is clinical. Investigation is rarely necessary.

Treatment:
- Rest and isolation of patient. Maintenance of adequate hydration and nutrition
- *Oral acyclovir*: In children, 20 mg/kg 6 hourly. In adults, 800 mg five times daily *or*, valacyclovir 1 g 8 hourly *or*, famciclovir 250 mg 8 hourly for 5–7 days.
- Antihistamine for itching and also calamine lotion.
- *In severe case or immunocompromised*: IV acyclovir 5 mg/kg 8 hourly until patient is improving, then oral therapy.

Complications: Pneumonia, post-varicella encephalitis, secondary skin infection, and herpes zoster or shingles (due to reactivation of dormant varicella virus).

Prevention: Active immunization with varicella vaccine and passive immunization with varicella immunoglobulin.

Small pox: It was caused by small pox virus. Two variants—variola major and variola minor. Clinical features are high fever and development of characteristic rash. The disease is now eradicated.

BRUCELLOSIS

It is a zoonotic disease caused by *Brucella*, a gram-negative *Bacillus*, transmitted from cows, goats, pigs or sheep. Person-to-person transmission is rare. Four species:
1. *B. abortus* (cattle or buffalo)
2. *B. melitensis* (goat, sheep and camels)
3. *B. suis* (pigs or swine)
4. *B. canis* (dogs).

Mode of transmission: Infection occurs usually orally, by consuming contaminated dairy product (especially unpasteurized milk) or uncooked meat. It may also spread through cuts or abrasion by contact with infected animal and their products (mainly in slaughterhouse worker, butcher and farmer). From gastrointestinal tract, bacilli travel to lymphatics and infect lymph nodes, and then there is hematogenous spread to other organs.

Incubation period: 2–4 weeks.

Symptoms:
- Onset is insidious. Malaise, headache, myalgia, arthralgia, back pain, weakness, and night sweats are common. There is an undulant high fever
- Lymphadenopathy and hepatosplenomegaly may occur
- There may be arthritis, orchitis, endocarditis, osteomyelitis and meningoencephalitis
- It may be chronic, associated with fatigue, myalgia, depression, and occasionally fever. Splenomegaly is characteristic. Infection may be localized to specific organs such as bone, heart or central nervous system. In such cases, systemic features are absent in 60% cases and antibody titers are low.

Investigations:
- *CBC*: May reveal pancytopenia. Blood C/S
- *Brucella agglutination test*: Positive within 4 weeks of onset. Serum IgG (may be raised)
- Species-specific PCR test.

Treatment:
- *Nonlocalized disease*: Doxycycline 100 mg orally twice daily for 6 weeks *plus* gentamicin 5 mg/kg for 7 days or streptomycin 0.75–1 g IM daily for 2–3 weeks. *Or* Doxycycline 100 mg orally twice daily *plus* rifampin 600–900 mg orally daily for 6 weeks
- *Bone disease*: Doxycycline 100 mg orally twice daily *plus* rifampin 600–900 mg orally once daily for 6 weeks *plus* gentamicin 5 mg/kg daily for 7 days or ciprofloxacin 750 mg twice daily *plus* rifampin 600–900 mg orally once daily for 3 months
- *Neurobrucellosis*: Doxycycline 100 mg orally twice daily *plus* rifampin 600–900 mg orally once daily for 6 weeks *plus* IV ceftriaxone 2 g twice daily for 3–6 months
- *Endocarditis*: Almost always needs surgery *plus* doxycycline 100 mg orally twice daily *plus* rifampin 600–900 mg orally once daily for 6 weeks *plus* trimethoprim 5 mg/kg for 6 months *plus* gentamicin 5 mg/kg IV for 2–4 weeks.

Complications: Uveitis, retinal thrombophlebitis, cranial nerve palsies, pneumonia or abscess, paravertebral or psoas abscess, osteomyelitis, meningitis, stroke, intracranial or subarachnoid hemorrhage, myocarditis, endocarditis, and splenic abscess.

Prevention: Careful handling of infected animals, vaccination of animals, and pasteurization of milk.

MALARIA

It is a protozoal disease caused by *Plasmodium* species. Four species of *Plasmodium*: (1) *P. vivax*, (2) *P. falciparum*, (3) *P. malariae*, and (4) *P. ovale*.

Mode of transmission: Bite by infected female anopheles mosquito, rarely by blood transfusion and transplacentally.

Types: Three types of malaria—
- *Benign tertian*: Caused by *P. vivax* and *P. ovale*. Classical bouts of fever occur on alternate days
- *Benign quartan*: Caused by *P. malariae*. Symptoms are mild and bouts of fever every 3rd day

- *Malignant tertian*: Caused by *P. falciparum*. No typical paroxysm of fever, may be continuous, remittent or irregular. Widespread organ damage occurs due to capillary blockage. It is more serious.

Symptoms: Typical paroxysm of fever has three stages. Usually found in *P. vivax*.

1. *Cold stage*: Fever, temperature rises rapidly up to 104°F or more with chills and rigor. Patient feels intense cold, shivers vigorously, teeth chatter, and needs warm clothes or blanket. This stage lasts for 15–60 minutes
2. *Hot stage*: Temperature is very high, with headache, flushing and tachycardia. Patient feels very hot, and throws blanket. Pulse is full and bounding. Respiration is rapid. Nausea and vomiting may be present. This stage lasts for 2–6 hours
3. *Wet or sweating stage*: There is profuse sweating, temperature falls, and patient feels comfortable. This stage lasts for 2–4 hours.

Signs: Appears after some days. Anemia, jaundice, hepatomegaly and splenomegaly.

Falciparum malaria (malignant malaria): Infected RBCs develop knob-like surface projection, which causes adhesion of RBC to endothelium of blood vessel causing vascular occlusion with severe organ damage.

- Fever. No particular pattern, may be continuous, typhoid like, sometimes prolonged, and irregular. Typical three stages are absent
- Headache, malaise, vomiting, cough and diarrhea
- *In cerebral type*: Headache, confusion, seizure, and even coma
- *Other features*: Hypoglycemia, pulmonary edema, renal failure, severe anemia, disseminated intravascular coagulation (DIC), gastrointestinal tract (GIT) features like diarrhea, bleeding and jaundice.

Complications:
- *CNS*: Cerebral malaria
- *Hematological*: Severe hemolytic anemia and DIC
- *Renal*: Oliguria, acute renal failure, and immune complex glomerulonephritis
- *Respiratory*: Pulmonary edema
- *GIT*: Diarrhea and jaundice
- *Metabolic*: Hypoglycemia and metabolic acidosis
- *Others*: Shock.

Investigations:
- Complete blood count and peripheral blood film for malaria parasite (both thick and thin)
- Rapid diagnostic test [immunochromatographic test (ICT) for falciparum]
- QBC for malaria (fluorescence microscopy-based test).

Treatment: Treatment for *P. vivax*, *P. ovale* and *P. malariae* (non-falciparum)—

- *Chloroquine (150 mg base)*: Four tablets on 1st day, four on 2nd day, and two on 3rd day (24 hours apart)
- *Or another regime*: Four tablets stat on 1st day, two tablets after 6 hours. From next day, one tablet twice daily for 2–3 days
- *Then, for radical cure*: Primaquine 15 mg daily for 14 days (0.25–0.5 mg/kg/day).

Or, if known resistance to chloroquine or dual infection with *P. falciparum*—Artemisinin-based combination therapy. Coartemether (artemether *plus* lumefantrine) for 3 days. Then, for radical cure, primaquine 15 mg daily for 14 days (0.25–0.5 mg/kg/day).

Treatment for falciparum malaria: Many cases are resistant to chloroquine.
- *Mild or uncomplicated case*:
    - Coartemether (artemether *plus* lumefantrine): 1st day, four tablets stat, then four tablets after 8 hours. From next day, four tablets 12 hourly for 2 days (total 24 tablets). After this, primaquine (0.75 mg/kg/day) single dose
    - *Or*, oral quinine 600 mg (10 mg/kg) 8 hourly for 7 days *plus* doxycycline 100 mg 12 hourly for 7 days *plus* primaquine (0.75 mg/kg/day) single dose. If quinine toxicity develops, give 12 hourly
    - *Or* single dose of sulfadoxine 1.5 g *plus* pyrimethamine 75 mg (Fansidar 3 tablets).
- *Complicated or severe falciparum infection or cerebral malaria:*
    - *Injection artesunate*: 2.4 mg/kg IV at 0, 12 and 24 hours, then once daily for 7 days. It should be replaced by oral therapy (2 mg/kg once daily) when patient can swallow. Total dose is 17–18 mg/kg (avoid in pregnancy unless strongly indicated)
    - *Or, artemether*: 80 mg IM twice daily on 1st day, then 80 mg daily for 4 days
    - *Or*, IV quinine initially 20 mg/kg, with 500 cc 5% dextrose in aqua over 4 hours, then 10 mg/kg 8 hourly for 7 days, until patient can take orally
    - *Pre-referral treatment*: In remote places with less facilities, rectal artesunate 10 mg/kg single dose. *Or*, IM quinine, diluted in normal saline, 20 mg/kg divided in two thigh (in anterior part).

Radical cure: It is the eradication of hypnozoite of malarial parasite from liver. *P. vivax* and *P. ovale* persist in liver cell as dormant form called hypnozoite, which may develop into merozoite months or years later, causing relapse of malaria. So, after treatment of malaria, primaquine is given, 15 mg daily for 14 days to eradicate exoerythrocytic cycle. *P. falciparum* and *P. malariae* have no exoerythrocytic cycle.

Treatment during pregnancy: In *P. vivax* and *P. ovale* infections, chloroquine is given as usual dose. If there is no response, quinine 600 mg 8 hourly for 1 week is given. For radical cure, no primaquine is given during pregnancy and lactation. So, chloroquine 600 mg weekly should be given, continued until delivery and breastfeeding are completed. Then, glucose-6-phosphate dehydrogenase (G6PD) should be measured. If normal, primaquine is given to prevent relapse.

In *P. falciparum* malaria:
- *Uncomplicated*:
    - First trimester: Quinine *plus* clindamycin, or quinine 600 mg 8 hourly for 1 week
    - Second and third trimester: Coartemether may be given.
- *In severe malaria*: IV artesunate. If it is not available, IM artemether or, IV quinine is given (until artesunate is obtained).

KALA-AZAR (LEISHMANIASIS)

Organisms: *Leishmania donovani* (India and Southeast Asia), *L. infantum* (Middle East and Mediterranean area) and *L. chagasi* (South and central America).

Source or reservoir: Human (Indian kala-azar).

Incubation period: 1–2 months (may be months to years, even 10 years).

Modes of transmission: Bite by infected female sandfly (common), rarely transplacentally and blood transfusion.

Note: *Following points are important—*
- Human is the only reservoir in Indian subcontinent
- Other reservoirs are dog, jackal, fox, and wild rodents in other countries
- Leishmania has two forms—amastigote and promastigote. Amastigote form (oval) is found in human, and Leishmania donovani body is found in monocyte/macrophage system.

Symptoms: Fever, usually intermittent, double or triple rise, may be continuous, loss of weight but good appetite, heaviness in left upper abdomen, and blackening of skin.

Signs: Cachexia, anemia, abdominal distension (due to hepatosplenomegaly), lymphadenopathy (common in African and Chinese kala-azar, rare in Indian kala-azar). Skin is pigmented, dry, thin, and scaly, and bleeding spots may be found.

Complications: Secondary infection (pneumonia and tuberculosis), bleeding, anemia, gastroenteritis, bacillary dysentery, cirrhosis of liver, post kala-azar dermal leishmaniasis (PKDL). Rarely, cancrum oris occurs. If not treated, patient may die within 1–2 year due to secondary infection or bleeding.

Investigations:
- *CBC*: Leukopenia, high lymphocyte and monocyte, neutropenia, thrombocytopenia, and high erythrocyte sedimentation rate (ESR). If CBC is repeated after some days, there is "progressive leukopenia"
- *Immunological tests, based on antibody*:
  - Direct agglutination test (DAT): It may be positive after 2 weeks (usually within month)
  - Immunochromatographic test (ICT): Rapid rK39 test is highly sensitive and specific
  - Indirect hemagglutination assay (IHA)
  - Indirect fluorescent antibody test (IFAT)
  - ELISA
  - Complement fixation test (CFT): It is nonspecific and positive after 3 weeks
  - Aldehyde test: It is still helpful where there is no facility.
- *Detection of antigen*: Done by latex agglutination test (KAtex) in urine
- *Definitive diagnosis*: Isolation of LD body from bone marrow and spleen puncture, also from liver, lymph node, and skin lesion. Culture is done in NNN media (Nicolle-Novy-MacNeal)
- Polymerase chain reaction (from lymph node or bone marrow aspiration)
- Blood for total protein and A/G ratio (high total protein, low albumin and high globulin).

Treatment:
- *First-line therapy*: Liposomal amphotericin B, miltefosine, paromomycin, or combination
  - Liposomal amphotericin B: Single IV infusion 10 mg/kg
  - Oral miltefosine for 28 days. Age >12 years (50 mg daily if <25 kg and 50 mg twice daily, if >25 kg). Age 2–12 years (2.5 mg/kg in two divided

doses, not exceeding 50 mg/day). Avoided in pregnancy due to fetal toxicity
  - Paromomycin: 15 mg/kg/day IM in gluteal muscles for 21 days.
- *Second-line therapy*: Amphotericin B deoxycholate (conventional) or sodium stibogluconate
  - Conventional amphotericin B: 1 mg/kg for 15 doses, slow infusion in 5% dextrose solution 500 cc for 4–6 hours daily or on alternate days. It is nephrotoxic, given after a test dose
  - Sodium stibogluconate: 20 mg/kg for 30 days IV or IM. It can be given in infusion with normal saline. IM injection is very painful, given only if ECG abnormality (arrhythmia or long QT interval). *Or*, meglumine antimoniate (50 mg/kg) is an alternative.
- *General treatment*: Maintenance of nutrition, correction of anemia, and control of secondary infection.

Note: Liposomal amphotericin B is expensive and not widely available. Sodium stibogluconate is mostly used. Following points are important while treating with sodium stibogluconate:
- Before starting, perform renal and liver function tests, ECG (to see dysrhythmia, prolonged QT and ischemia) and CXR (latent TB and pneumonia)
- During IV injection, if patient complains of chest pain or cough, stop the drug
- Monitor ECG, CBC including platelet, and hepatic and renal functions
- The drug should be stopped, if there is bleeding, ECG change
- No limitation of dose (previously it was thought that dose should not exceed 1 g/day).

Post Kala-azar Dermal Leishmaniasis

It is a nonulcerative cutaneous lesion that occurs after treatment and apparent recovery from visceral leishmaniasis. It initially starts as macules, then erythematous lesion followed by wart-like nodules. It mainly involves the face, the chin, and ear lobules. Hypopigmented macules can occur in any part of body.

Types: There are two types—

Indian: It occurs in few patients, 6 months to 3 years or more after initial infection, creating a persistent human reservoir. The patient usually presents with macules, papules, nodules (most common) and plaques on face, mainly around the chin. Hypopigmented macules can occur all over the body. No systemic symptoms and no spontaneous healing.

African: In Sudan, about 50% develop skin manifestations of PKDL with visceral leishmaniasis or within 6 months. Skin features are as above. There may be measles like micropapular rash all over the body. Children are affected more frequently. Spontaneous healing occurs in about 75% cases within 1 year.

Investigations: Biopsy from nodular lesion and PCR (detects parasites in 80% cases).

Treatment:
- *First-line treatment*: Usually miltefosine is given. In adult, 50 mg twice daily for 12 weeks. In children, 2.5 mg/kg daily in two divided doses for 12 weeks (not exceeding 50 mg/day).

- *Second-line treatment*:
  - Liposomal amphotericin B
  - Amphotericin B deoxycholate
  - Sodium stibogluconate
  - In Sudan, sodium stibogluconate for 2 months is considered adequate.

Complications: Apart from disfigurement, PKDL patients are important source of infection. Treatment should be given for the benefit of the community.

FILARIASIS

Filariasis is a parasitic infection caused by thread-like nematode *Filariae*. The disease is transmitted by bite of infected *Culex* and sometimes *Anopheles* mosquito.

Organisms: *Wuchereria bancrofti, Brugia malayi* and *B. timori*.

Clinical features:
- *Acute lymphangitis*: Fever, pain, and redness along inflamed lymphatic vessels. Lymphadenitis of regional lymph nodes (axillary or inguinal), local edema, epididymitis and orchitis
- *Chronic lymphatic disease*: Skin of affected area becomes coarse, corrugated and fissured. Subcutaneous edema, thickening, hydrocele, massive scrotal enlargement, chyluria, and chylous effusion may occur. Progressive enlargement of skin and subcutaneous tissue causes "elephantiasis" due to lymphatic obstruction.

Investigations:
- Complete blood count (shows eosinophilia) and serum IgE (high)
- Immunochromatographic test for filaria, indirect fluorescence, ELISA and PCR
- Blood film at night to see microfilariae. It can also be detected from chylous urine or scrotal swelling.

Treatment:
- *Diethylcarbamazine (DEC)*: 6 mg/kg daily for 12 days
- Albendazole (400 mg 12 hourly for 21 days)
- Albendazole and DEC both daily for 7 days
- Doxycycline (100 mg bid) for 3 weeks *plus* DEC is alternative regimen
- A single dose of albendazole (400 mg) combined with DEC (6 mg/kg) or ivermectin (200 µg/kg) for eradication campaign
- Treatment of *Wolbachia* with doxycycline (200 mg/day) for 4–8 weeks provides additional benefit by eliminating the bacteria
- *Other treatment*: Crepe bandage, elastic stockings, and elevation of the limbs may be helpful. Plastic surgery and surgical removal of tissues of elephantiasis may be done in some cases.

Tropical pulmonary eosinophilia: In this condition, microfilariae is trapped in pulmonary capillaries and destroyed by allergic inflammation. The patient usually complains of cough, wheeze, and fever, associated with high eosinophil count. If untreated, it may progress to chronic interstitial lung disease. Serological test is strongly positive and serum IgE level is very high. CXR shows miliary mottling.

Treatment: DEC 6 mg/kg in three divided doses for 14 days.

ANCYLOSTOMIASIS (HOOKWORM INFESTATION)

It is caused by *Ancylostoma duodenale* or *Necator americanus*. Usually occurs by filariform larva that penetrates through the skin during walking barefoot over contaminated soil.

Symptoms:
- *By the larva*: Creeping eruption usually on the feet (ground itch)
- *By adult worm*: Upper abdominal pain, anorexia, nausea, vomiting, diarrhea, and features of anemia.

Signs: No specific sign except anemia.

Investigations: Stool R/M/E (ovum may be found). CBC (may show anemia and eosinophilia).

Complications: Iron deficiency anemia, protein losing enteropathy, and hypoproteinemia. Mental and physical retardation in children.

Treatment:
- Mebendazole 100 mg 12 hourly for 3 days
- *Or* albendazole 400 mg or pyrantel pamoate 11 mg/kg, maximum 1g as a single dose
- *For anemia*: Iron therapy.

Prevention: Personal hygiene and regular washing of hands. All members of the family should be treated simultaneously. Night clothes and bed linens of patient should be washed thoroughly.

ASCARIASIS (ROUNDWORM)

It is caused by *Ascaris lumbricoides* by eating food contaminated with mature ova.

Clinical features: Usually asymptomatic. May be abdominal pain, intestinal obstruction in children, and Loeffler's syndrome (during migration of larva to lungs, there may be cough, wheeze, and breathlessness. It is also called *Ascaris* pneumonia).

Investigations: Stool for R/M/E (ova may be found). CBC (may show eosinophilia).

Treatment: Mebendazole 100 mg orally 12 hourly for 3 days *or* albendazole 400 mg orally single dose *or* pyrantel pamoate 11 mg/kg, maximum 1 g as a single dose orally.

Complications: Intestinal obstruction, intussusception, volvulus, hemorrhagic infarction or perforation, obstruction of common bile duct causing obstructive jaundice, and acute appendicitis.

Prevention: Personal hygiene and regular washing of hands. All members of the family should be treated accordingly. Night clothes and bed linens of the patient should be washed thoroughly.

ENTEROBIUS VERMICULARIS (THREADWORM)

It is caused by *Enterobius vermicularis* by eating food contaminated with mature ova.

Clinical features: Itching around anus, especially at night. The ova are often carried to mouth by fingers, so reinfection may occur. In females, the genitalia may be involved. Adult worms may be seen moving on the buttocks or in stool.

Investigation: Ova can easily be detected. Investigation is rarely necessary.

Treatment: A single dose of mebendazole 100 mg or albendazole 400 mg orally. It may be repeated after 2 weeks to control autoinfection.

Prevention: Personal hygiene and regular washing of hands. All members of the family should be treated accordingly. Night clothes and bed linens of the patient should be washed thoroughly.

TAENIASIS

It is an infestation caused by *Taenia* species.

Organisms: *T. saginata*, *T. solium* and *T. asiatica*.

Modes of infection:
- *T. solium* infection occurs by eating undercooked beef contaminated with larva
- *T. saginata* and *T. asiatica* infections occur by eating undercooked pork contaminated with larva.

Clinical features: Usually asymptomatic. May be upper abdominal pain, anorexia, nausea, diarrhea, weakness, lassitude, hunger and giddiness. Subcutaneous nodules may develop over lips, neck, chest, masseter muscles, back and groin.

Investigations:
- *Stool R/M/E*: Ova or adult segments may be found
- *CBC*: Shows eosinophilia
- *X-ray of muscles and soft tissue*: Shows calcification
- *CT or MRI of brain*: May show circular or ring-shaped shadow of calcified larva.

Treatment:
- *T. saginata*: Praziquantel 5–10 mg/kg or niclosamide 2 g both as a single dose or nitazoxanide 500 mg twice daily for 3 days
- *T. solium*: Niclosamide followed by laxative.

Complication: Cysticercosis.

Cysticercosis

It is caused by larval stage of *T. solium*. The larvae penetrate the intestinal mucosa, carried to many parts of the body, where they develop and form cysticerci, 0.5–1 cm cysts that contain the head of young worm. Common locations are subcutaneous tissue, skeletal muscles and brain. Neurocysticercosis may cause epileptic seizures, personality changes, staggering gait, and signs of hydrocephalus.

Investigations: CBC (shows eosinophilia), X-ray (shows calcification), and CT or MRI of brain.

Treatment:
- Albendazole 15 mg/kg daily for 8 days or praziquantel 50 mg/kg in three divided doses for 10 days
- Prednisolone 10 mg 8 hourly is started 1 day before starting above drugs for 14 days
- Antiepileptics, if brain is involved.

STRONGYLOIDIASIS

It is caused by *Strongyloides stercoralis*.

Mode of infection: Penetration of human skin by filariform larva. Sometimes, larval form can penetrate directly the perianal skin and reinfect host (autoinfection).

Clinical features:
- Itchy rash at the site of penetration
- Upper abdominal pain, anorexia, nausea, diarrhea and weight loss
- Migration of larva through lungs may cause cough, wheezing, respiratory distress and pneumonia
- Urticarial plaques and papules due to allergic reaction. Migratory linear wheel around the buttock and lower abdomen called "Cutaneous Larva Currens" may also occur.

Complication: Meningoencephalitis.

Investigations:
- *Stool R/M/E*: Motile larvae may be found. Excretion is intermittent, so repeated examination is required
- *CBC*: Shows eosinophilia
- *Serology*: ELISA.

Treatment: Two doses of ivermectin 200 µg/kg on successive days. Alternatively, albendazole orally 15 mg/kg twice daily for 3 days.

GIARDIASIS

It is an infection caused by *Giardia lamblia* by ingestion of contaminated water by cyst, which remains viable up to 3 months in water.

Incubation period: 1–3 weeks.

Symptoms: Incubation period is 1–3 weeks. Frequent diarrhea, abdominal pain, distension, bloating, weakness, anorexia, nausea and vomiting.

Signs: Abdominal distension and tenderness.

Investigation: Stool R/M/E (shows cyst).

Treatment: Single dose of tinidazole 2 g *or* metronidazole 400 mg three times daily for 10 days *or* nitazoxanide 500 mg orally twice daily for 3 days.

ANTHRAX

It is a zoonotic disease caused by *Bacillus anthracis,* which produces number of toxins, responsible for clinical manifestation of the disease. Anthrax is a disease of sheep, goat and cattle. Infectious form is spore, which is transmitted to human from contaminated animal, animal products or soil by inhalation or rarely by ingestion. Three types of infection—Cutaneous anthrax, gastrointestinal anthrax and inhalational (pulmonary) anthrax.

Clinical features:
- *Cutaneous anthrax*: There is single skin lesion, associated with occupational exposure to anthrax spores during processing of hides and bone products, or with bioterrorism. Lesion is single papule on a hemorrhagic edematous base, which progresses to a depressed black eschar

- *Gastrointestinal anthrax*: It develops after ingestion of contaminated or incompletely cooked meat. There are nausea, vomiting, anorexia, fever followed by abdominal pain and bloody diarrhea. Death may occur
- *Inhalational anthrax*: Fever, dyspnea, cough, headache, and septicemia may develop 3–14 days after exposure. CXR may show widening of mediastinum and pleural effusion.

Complications: Meningitis, septicemia and respiratory failure.

Investigations: CBC, culture from skin swab, and CXR.

Treatment:
- Ciprofloxacin 500 mg bd or benzylpenicillin 2.4 g IV 4 hourly or phenoxymethylpenicillin 500–1,000 mg 6 hourly for 10 days. Aminoglycoside can be used in severe disease
- Ventilatory assistance may be needed in inhalational disease.

Prevention: Prophylaxis with ciprofloxacin (500 mg 12 hourly) is recommended for anyone at high risk of exposure to anthrax spores.

LEPROSY (HANSEN'S DISEASE)

It is a chronic granulomatous disabling disease caused by *Mycobacterium leprae*. It involves peripheral nerves, skin, mucous membrane, bone and viscera. *M. leprae* is a gram-positive, acid-fast, and alcohol-fast *Bacillus*, also called Hansen's *Bacillus*. Man is the only reservoir of infection.

Route of transmission: By droplet infection from nasal mucosa of leprosy patient, and sometimes by skin contact (if ulcerated).

Types (or classification) of leprosy: Five types—
1. Tuberculoid leprosy (TT)
2. Borderline tuberculoid (BT)
3. Borderline leprosy (BB)
4. Borderline lepromatous leprosy (BL)
5. Lepromatous leprosy (LL).

Depending on cell-mediated immunity, leprosy is divided into two polar forms and a borderline form (Flowchart 1).

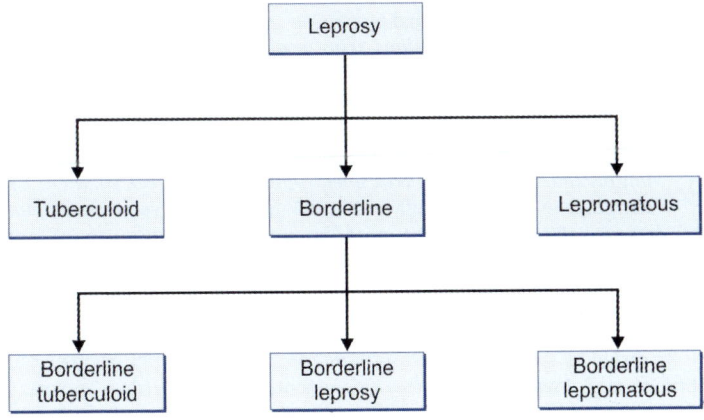

FLOWCHART 1: Types of leprosy.

Also classified into two types:
1. *Paucibacillary*: Few organisms in the tissue. Skin smear for *M. leprae* bacilli is negative or few (found in TT and BT)
2. *Multibacillary*: Large number of organisms in tissue. Skin smear for *M. leprae* bacilli is positive (found in BT, all BB, BL and LL).

Symptoms:
- *Lepromatous type*: Initially hypopigmented erythematous macules. Later multiple nodular lesions appear on ear lobe, face, forearm and legs. In the face, it is called "Leonine facies". There is no loss of sensation
- *Tuberculoid type*: Hypopigmented small macules in different parts of the body with loss of sensation. Skin lesions are dry and scaly with anhydrosis. Supraorbital, great auricular, median, ulnar, radial, and lateral popliteal and posterior tibial nerves are thickened bilaterally, but are nontender.

Investigations:
- Slit skin smear, nasal scraping or biopsy from skin or thickened nerve (shows acid-fast bacilli)
- Skin biopsy for histopathology
- *Histological findings*:
  - In tuberculoid type: Epithelioid granuloma may be found
  - In lepromatous leprosy: *M. leprae* may be found in skin macrophage.

Nerves commonly involved in leprosy:
- *Supraorbital*: Over the forehead, lateral to midline
- *Facial nerve*: Crossing the zygomatic arch
- *Great auricular nerve*: Posterior triangle of neck
- *Radial nerve*: In the radial groove of humerus and at the insertion of deltoid muscle
- *Radial cutaneous nerve*: In the wrist
- *Ulnar nerve*: In elbow, in between the medial epicondyle and olecranon process
- *Median nerve*: Middle of the front of wrist
- *Lateral popliteal or common peroneal nerve*: Around the neck of fibula
- *Posterior tibial nerve*: Ankle, a little below and posterior to medial malleoli.

Treatment: WHO recommended protocol—
- *Paucibacillary (3–5 skin lesions, skin smear negative or few, tuberculoid, and BT)*: Rifampicin 600 mg monthly (supervised) *plus* dapsone 100 mg daily (self-administered) for 6 months
- *Paucibacillary single lesion*: Rifampicin 600 mg *plus* ofloxacin 400 mg *plus* minocycline 100 mg, in single dose (ROM therapy)
- *Multibacillary (>5 lesions, skin smear positive, BT, all BB, BL and LL)*: Rifampicin 600 mg and clofazimine 300 mg monthly (supervised) *plus* dapsone 100 mg and clofazimine 50 mg daily (self-administered) for 12 months or until smear negative (may be up to 24 months).

LEPTOSPIROSIS (WEIL'S DISEASE)

It is caused by spirochete *Leptospira interrogans*. Main types occurring in human are *L. icterohemorrhagica* (from rodents), *L. canicola* (dogs and pigs), *L. hardjo* (cattle) and *L. pomona* (pigs and cattle). Rodents, particularly rats, are the most important reservoir of infection. The organism is excreted in urine, may survive in soil for several weeks. It enters in human host through cuts and abrasions on skin, or through intact mucous membranes or contaminated water.

Incubation period: 1–2 weeks.

Occupations: Sewerage workers, fishermen, vets and farmers.

Clinical features:
- *Initial or septicemic phase*: Persists for 4–7 days, characterized by fever, headache, myalgia, abdominal pain, vomiting, and skin rash (macular, maculopapular or hemorrhagic), and conjunctival ingestion (bloodshot eyes). Proteinuria, hematuria, and impaired liver and renal function or renal failure may occur. Hepatosplenomegaly may be present; lung involvement may cause dry cough, hemoptysis, and confluent shadow in CXR
- *Second or immune phase*: Lasts for 3–10 days. No fever. Antibody to *Leptospira* rises. Symptoms resolve, meningism may be present, and recovery occurs from this stage.

Combination of hepatitis, renal failure, and carditis is highly suggestive of leptospirosis.

Complications: DIC, acute hepatic failure, and carditis.

Investigations:
- *CBC*: Shows leukocytosis and thrombocytopenia
- Blood culture in special media is positive in first 10 days. Urine culture is positive in 2nd week
- Anti-*Leptospira* antibody (or microscopic agglutination test, MAT)
- Liver function tests—High SGPT, prothrombin time (PT) may be prolonged, and high creatine phosphokinase. PCR in blood and urine.

Treatment:
- Doxycycline 100 mg 12 hourly for 1 week. IV benzylpenicillin (1.5 megaunit 6 hourly) or IV ceftriaxone 1 g daily is equally effective
- Renal failure may require dialysis. Blood transfusion, if bleeding.

POLIOMYELITIS

It is caused by polio virus and is spread by feco-oral route as it is excreted in feces. The virus affects nervous system, mainly anterior horn cells of spinal cord and cranial nerve neurons. It causes lymphocytic meningitis and infects gray matter of spinal cord, brainstem and cortex.

Incubation period: 7–14 days.

Types: Three types of virus—
1. *Type I*: Brunhilde (common type, 80% of paralytic illness)
2. *Type II*: Lansing
3. *Type III*: Leon.

Clinical features: It is common in childhood, but rare in adulthood.

Three types of poliomyelitis:
1. *Abortive*: Characterized by mild fever, myalgia, sore throat, headache and weakness. It persists for 24–48 hours, with spontaneous cure
2. *Nonparalytic*: After a week of well-being, there is recurrence of fever, headache, myalgia and meningism. This stage may persists for 24–48 hours and recovery is complete

3. *Paralytic poliomyelitis (0.5–1%)*:
   - Spinal form: In some cases, paralytic form may occur 4–5 days after initial illness. Meningeal irritation and muscle pain recur, followed by asymmetrical flaccid paralysis without sensory loss, involving the lower limbs. It is found below 5 years of age, and upper limbs are involved in older children. In adult, there may be paraplegia or quadriplegia
   - Bulbar poliomyelitis: Characterized by cranial nerve (IX and X) involvement and respiratory muscle paralysis. Soft palate, pharyngeal, and laryngeal muscle palsies are common. The patient complains of facial weakness, dysphagia, dysphonia, and nasal voice and nasal regurgitation.

Stage of residual disability: Muscular wasting leads to persistent contracture, deformity, and shortening of limb may occur usually in one limb.

Investigation: Diagnosis is clinical. CSF shows high lymphocytic, high protein, and normal sugar. Virus may be cultured from CSF and stool.

Treatment:
- Complete bed rest
- *If respiratory paralysis*: Ventilatory support and tracheostomy may be needed
- *After recovery*: Physiotherapy, occupational therapy, and orthopedic measures
- Prevention by live (Sabin) vaccine.

Types of vaccine for poliomyelitis: Two types—
- Oral live attenuated polio virus (OPV) or Sabin vaccine
- Inactivated polio virus (IPV) or Salk vaccine (less used because OPV is cheaper and easily administered).

Complication of OPV (also called provocation poliomyelitis): It can cause vaccine-associated paralytic poliomyelitis (VAPP) in a small percentage of recipients, particularly in immunodeficient patients. In such cases, individuals and their family members should take IPV.

Provocation poliomyelitis: It is caused by administration of IM injection during the incubation period of wild poliovirus or shortly after exposure of OPV.

SEPSIS AND SEPTIC SHOCK

Sepsis: It is defined as life-threatening organ dysfunction caused by a dysregulated host response to infection. Patient with suspected infection who have two or more of:
- Low blood pressure (SBP ≤100 mm Hg)
- High respiratory rate (≥22/min)
- Altered mental status (Glasgow coma scale <14).

It is also diagnosed by suspected infection and >2 points on SOFA (Sequential Organ Failure Assessment) score. A score of 1–4 is allocated to six organ systems (respiratory, cardiovascular, liver, renal, coagulation and neurological) to represent the degree of organ dysfunction.

Septic shock: It is a subset of sepsis with underlying circulatory or cellular or metabolic abnormalities associated with increased mortality. Sepsis and both of the following (after fluid resuscitation):

- Persistent hypotension requiring vasopressors to maintain a mean arterial pressure >65 mm Hg
- Serum lactate >2 mmol/L (18 mg/dL).

Risk factors: Diabetes mellitus, immunodeficiency (cytotoxic drug, chemotherapy and radiotherapy), trauma, burn, alcohol, substance abuse, chronic illness (heart, lung, kidney and liver), hematological disease, recent surgery, and invasive procedures like IV lines, urinary catheter, and nasogastric tube.

Causes:
- *Bacteria*: *Staphylococcus aureus*, *Neisseria meningitidis*, *Escherichia coli* and other gram-negative organisms, *Pseudomonas aeruginosa*, *M. tuberculosis*, and *M. avium* complex (MAC)
- *Fungal*: *Histoplasma capsulatum* and *Candida*
- *Parasitic*: Falciparum malaria.

Clinical features:
- *Evidence of severe infection plus signs of systemic inflammatory response syndrome (SIRS), which is defined by the presence of two or more of:*
  - Fever (oral temperature >38°C or <36°C)
  - Tachycardia (pulse rate >90/min)
  - Tachypnea (respiratory rate >24/min)
  - Leukocytosis (WBC >12,000 cells/mm^3) or leukopenia (WBC <4,000 cells/mm^3)
  - $PaCO_2$ <32.5 mm Hg.
- *Others*:
  - Generalized erythroderma (toxic shock syndrome by *S. aureus*), petechial or hemorrhagic rash (*N. meningitidis*)
  - Confusion, delirium and coma
  - Acute respiratory distress syndrome (ARDS) and acute renal failure may occur
  - Hepatic dysfunction: Jaundice and high enzymes
  - GIT: Anorexia, nausea, diarrhea and ileus
  - Features of DIC, bleeding due to coagulopathy
  - Vasodilatation, warm peripheries, bounding pulse, and rapid capillary refill
  - Hypotension, low diastolic pressure, and wide pulse pressure
  - Hyperglycemia or hypoglycemia
  - Damage to different organs (multi-organ failure).

Investigations:
- Complete blood count, ESR shows polymorphonuclear leukocytosis and thrombocytopenia
- Culture of blood, urine, sputum, wound secretion, IV line, tracheal aspirate
- Urea, creatinine and electrolytes
- Liver function test, coagulation profile (prothrombin time, activated partial thromboplastin time (APTT), D-dimer and fibrin degradation products)
- Arterial blood gas (ABG) analysis
- Chest X-ray (to see consolidation, ARDS) and USG of abdomen
- Other investigations according to suspicion of cause.

Treatment:

"Sepsis Six" recommendations are:
1. High flow oxygen via face mask
2. Blood culture (before antibiotic therapy). Source control should be established (drainage of an abscess or removal of an infected intravenous access device)
3. Intravenous antibiotic (e.g. imipenem, meropenem, cefepime, piperacillin-tazobactam and vancomycin)
4. Intravenous fluid resuscitation, e.g. 30 mL/kg of crystalloid (0.9% saline)
5. *Hemoglobin and serial lactate measurement*: Blood transfusion when hemoglobin is <70 g/L.
6. *Hourly urine output measurement*: Aim for a urine output of >0.5 mL/kg/h.

Other therapies: Vasopressor agents for hypotension (noradrenaline, dopamine or dobutamine), IV corticosteroid may be given (hydrocortisone or methylprednisolone).

HYDATID DISEASE (CYST)

It is a parasitic infestation due to *Echinococcus* species mainly *Echinococcus granulosus*. Cyst has three layers. Outer layer, derived from host (pericyst), intermediate laminated layer (ectocyst), and inner germinal layer (endocyst) that buds off brood capsule to form daughter cyst. May be single or multiple cysts, may calcify.

Definitive host: Dog, also fox and jackal.

Intermediate host: Human.

Mode of infection: Close contact with infected dogs or eating undercooked vegetables or drinking water contaminated with feces of infected dog.

Organisms: *E. granulosus* of dogs. *E. multilocularis* (life cycle between fox and vole). Man is infected accidentally.

Sites of hydatid cyst: Liver (60%, right lobe), lungs (30%), kidneys (3%), brain (1%), and other organ (spleen, heart, muscles, and biliary tree).

Clinical features: Infection occurs in childhood, grows slowly. Usually asymptomatic.
- *Hepatomegaly*: Occasionally, jaundice occurs due to obstruction in bile duct. Rarely, rupture into the abdominal cavity, pleural cavity or biliary tree occurs
- *Features of cyst in other organs*: Cyst in lung, may be infected causing lung abscess. Cyst in brain may cause seizure. Renal cyst may cause hematuria
- Calcification of cyst occurs in 40% cases.

Complications: Pressure effect to surrounding tissue, rupture causes anaphylactic shock and secondary infection.

Investigations:
- *CBC*: Shows high eosinophil
- *USG and CT scan*: Shows cyst and daughter cysts within the parent cyst
- *Serology*: CFT, hemagglutination test, flocculation test, indirect fluorescent antibody test, immunoelectrophoresis (Arc 5 test), and ELISA
- *Plain X-ray of abdomen*: Calcification may be seen.

Treatment:
- Surgical resection. Praziquantel 20 mg/kg for 14 days kills protoscolices perioperatively
- *Medical treatment*: Albendazole 400 mg twice daily for 3–6 months may be repeated
- *PAIR therapy (puncture, aspiration, injection and reaspiration)*: Percutaneous aspiration of cyst, followed by injection 100% ethanol into the cyst, then reaspiration of cyst contents. Albendazole 400 mg twice daily before the procedure and 4 weeks afterward should be given or mebendazole may be combined with PAIR
- Calcified cyst may be left untreated.

INFECTIOUS MONONUCLEOSIS

It is characterized by pharyngitis, lymphadenopathy, fever, and lymphocytosis, caused by Epstein–Barr virus (EBV).

Mode of transmission: Oral contact via saliva, either by droplet infection or environmental contamination in childhood or by kissing among adolescents and adults.

Incubation period: 7–10 days.

Clinical features:
- Fever, headache, and malaise, sore throat or tonsillitis
- Lymphadenopathy, mostly cervical, nontender. May be generalized
- Palatal petechiae, periorbital edema, macular, petechial rash or erythema multiforme may occur. Rash aggravates by taking "ampicillin"
- Hepatitis with or without jaundice and splenomegaly
- Fever resolves after 2 weeks, and fatigue and other abnormalities settle after few weeks.

Complications: Chronic fatigue syndrome, hepatitis, hemolytic anemia, thrombocytopenia, myocarditis, pericarditis, cranial nerve palsy, transverse myelitis, meningoencephalitis, glomerulonephritis, and rupture of spleen.

Investigations:
- *CBC*: Leukopenia, high lymphocytes, also atypical lymphocytes
- Paul-Bunnell or "Monospot" test
- *Specific EBV serology*: IgM antibody.

Treatment: Usually symptomatic.
- Rest. Paracetamol for fever. Ampicillin or amoxicillin should be avoided
- *If pharyngeal edema is severe*: Prednisolone 30 mg daily for 5 days. Steroid is also indicated in airway obstruction, hemolytic anemia or severe thrombocytopenia
- Current antiviral drugs are not effective against EBV.

TOXOPLASMOSIS

Organism: *Toxoplasma gondii*, an intracellular parasite. Cat is the definitive host and parasite lives in gut of definitive host and produces oocysts, which are shed in feces on soil. Spread to intermediate hosts (human, cattle, sheep, pigs and rabbit), occurs by ingestion of oocysts. Once ingested, cysts are transformed to rapidly developing tachyzoites and remain dormant in host tissue.

Mode of infection:
- Human are infected by contamination of foods with cat feces or eating raw or undercooked infected meats. Outbreaks of toxoplasmosis may occur due to consumption of unfiltered water
- Transplacental transfer from mother to fetus
- Blood transfusion from infected person.

Clinical features: Toxoplasmosis may be congenital or acquired. Most acquired primary infections are subclinical. In HIV-1 infection, toxoplasmosis occurs as opportunistic infection.
- Common presenting feature is painless lymphadenopathy, local or generalized. Cervical nodes are commonly involved, but mediastinal, mesenteric or retroperitoneal groups may be affected
- Spleen may be palpable
- Most patients have no systemic symptoms; some may have malaise, fever, fatigue, muscle pain, sore throat and headache. Some may develop myocarditis, polymyositis, pneumonitis or hepatitis
- In immunocompromised or in HIV patients, acute toxoplasmosis may occur due to reactivation of latent infection in 95% cases, new infections occur in few cases. Fever, encephalopathy, meningitis or meningoencephalitis, cerebral abscess, seizure or convulsion.

Congenital toxoplasmosis: Seropositive females infected 6 months before pregnancy have no risk of fetal transmission. Congenital disease affects fetus in early gestation. Many fetal infections are subclinical at birth, but CNS is mainly affected. If the infant survives, parasites disappear from all organs except brain. Long-term sequelae are choroidoretinitis, microcephaly and hydrocephalus.

Investigations:
- *Indirect fluorescent antibody test (Sabin–Feldman dye test)*: It detects IgG antibody
- *Toxoplasma*-specific IgM antibody indicates acute infection
- Isolation of *Toxoplasma* organisms in lymph node biopsy
- PCR detects *Toxoplasma*-specific DNA
- X-ray of skull may show calcification
- CT scan or MRI of brain shows single or multiple ring-enhancing lesions
- Ophthalmoscopy for chorioretinitis.

Treatment:
- *In immunocompetent asymptomatic case*: No treatment is necessary
- *In symptomatic case or progressive disease or in immunocompromised*: Pyrimethamine (25 mg) *plus* sulfadiazine (2–4 g) and folinic acid for 4 weeks. Cotrimoxazol one tablet daily is an alternative
- *In HIV with cerebral abscess*: Pyrimethamine *plus* sulfadiazine and folinic acid for 6 weeks. Clindamycin and pyrimethamine is an alternative
- *Pregnant woman with recent infection*: Spiramycin (3 g daily in divided doses) should be given until term
- If fetal infection is present, sulfadiazine and pyrimethamine *plus* folinic acid (spiramycin does not cross placental barrier)
- *Ocular toxoplasmosis*: Pyrimethamine *plus* sulfadiazine or clindamycin (sometimes prednisolone for 1 month).

FOOD POISONING

Food poisoning is defined as gastroenteritis caused by consumption of food or water contaminated with bacteria or their toxins or chemical. Diagnosis is likely when more persons are affected after eating same food.

Causes:
- *Infective*:
  - Toxin producing: *S. aureus*, *B. cereus*, and *E. coli* (ETEC), *E. coli* 0157:H7, *C. perfringens*, *C. difficile*, and *V. parahaemolyticus*
  - Invasion of mucosa: *Campylobacter jejuni, Yersinia enterocolitica, B. anthracis, Salmonella* and *Shigella* species.
  - Others: Without invasion such as rotavirus and novovirus (Norwalk virus).
- *Noninfective*: Shellfish, strawberry, phallotoxin, amatoxin, scombrotoxin (fish) and ciguatoxin (tropical fish).

Clinical features:
- Bloody mucous diarrhea, vomiting, cramping abdominal pain, fever, and headache
- *Features of dehydration*: Dry tongue, low BP, low volume pulse, cold and clammy extremities, scanty urine, pinched face, and shrunken eyes
- *In more serious cases*: Life-threatening neurologic, hepatic, and renal dysfunction, leading to permanent disability or death.

Investigations: CBC (leukocytosis), serum electrolytes, creatinine, blood urea nitrogen, stool (R/M/E and C/S), and blood C/S.

Treatment:
- Correction of dehydration and electrolyte imbalance. ORS should be given
- *If vomiting*: IV fluid (e.g. normal saline, cholera saline, and Ringer's lactate)
- Avoid milk, dairy products, and other lactose-containing foods during acute diarrhea
- *Antibiotics*: Ciprofloxacin, norfloxacin and rifaximin.

Prevention: Maintenance of strict personal hygiene. Food should be cooked adequately. Avoid cross-contamination of raw and cooked foods. Keep all foods at appropriate temperature.

Nephrology

USUAL INVESTIGATIONS

Chemical examination of urine:
- *Reaction*: Normal urine is acidic (pH 4.6–6.3)
- *Proteins*: Normally 150 mg protein is excreted in 24 hours. Presence of excess protein in urine is called proteinuria
- *Sugar*: Present in diabetes mellitus (DM) (called glycosuria)
- *Ketone bodies (acetone, acetoacetate and beta-hydroxybutyric acid)*: Appear in urine in ketosis due to diabetic ketoacidosis, persistent vomiting and prolonged starvation
- *Bilirubin*: Normally no bilirubin. Conjugated bilirubin is found in obstructive, also some cases of hepatocellular jaundice
- *Bile salt*: Absent in normal urine. May be present in obstructive jaundice
- *Blood*: Hematuria means presence of red blood cells (RBCs) in urine. Hemoglobinuria means presence of hemoglobin in urine, which indicates intravascular hemolysis. Myoglobinuria means presence of myoglobin in urine, due to rhabdomyolysis
- *Chyle*: Milky urine due to fat particles in urine. Causes are filariasis and fistula between urinary tract and lymphatic system.

Microscopic examination of urine:
- *Epithelial cells*: Found in normal urine, no significance
- *Red cells*: >2/mm^3 in urine is abnormal, indicates bleeding from urogenital tract. Presence of dysmorphic red cells suggests nephritis
- *Pus cells*: >10/mm^3 is abnormal, called pyuria. It indicates urinary tract infection (UTI)
- *Casts*: Formed in kidney tubules by coagulation of proteins. Common casts are—
    - Epithelial casts: Found in acute glomerulonephritis (AGN), degeneration of renal tubules
    - Red blood cell casts: Found in AGN. It indicates glomerular lesion
    - White blood cell (WBC) casts: Suggestive of pyelonephritis. Also found in interstitial nephritis
    - Granular casts: Found in inflammation and degeneration of renal tubules, indicates chronic renal disease

- Hyaline casts: May be present in normal urine. Also found in chronic glomerulonephritis, hypertension, fever, after exercise, due to loop diuretics
  - Tubular cell casts: Found in acute tubular necrosis.

Causes of red urine: Ingestion of beet root, senna, some dyes used to color sweets, hematuria, hemoglobinuria, myoglobinuria, drugs (rifampicin, usually orange color, clofazimine, phenindione, purgative like phenolphthalein).

Causes of black urine (fresh urine is normal, but when kept for hours, it turns dark): Acute intermittent porphyria and alkaptonuria.

HEMATURIA

Passage of blood in urine.

Types:
- *Initial hematuria*: Presence of blood at the beginning of micturition (due to penile urethral cause)
- *Terminal hematuria*: Presence of blood at the end of micturition (due to bladder neck or prostatic urethral cause)
- *Total hematuria*: Presence of blood throughout micturition, due to bladder or urinary tract disease (renal cell carcinoma, papilloma of urinary bladder, UTI and renal stone) or blood dyscrasias or excess anticoagulant.

Causes of hematuria:
- *Prerenal*: Bleeding disorder [hemophilia, Christmas disease and immune thrombocytopenic purpura (ITP)], anticoagulant or antiplatelet drug, malignant hypertension and infective endocarditis
- *Renal*: Glomerulonephritis (GN), commonly immunoglobulin A (IgA) nephropathy, renal tuberculosis (TB), trauma, renal calculi, polycystic kidney disease (PKD) (clot colic), renal cell carcinoma and interstitial nephritis
- *Postrenal*: Ureter (stone and neoplasm), urinary bladder (cystitis, papilloma, transitional cell carcinoma, stone, bilharziasis or schistosomiasis), urethra (urethritis), prostate [benign enlargement of prostate (BEP), and carcinoma of prostate], trauma and hemorrhagic cystitis due to cyclophosphamide.

Causes of painless hematuria: GN, commonly IgA nephropathy, renal TB, PKD, renal cell carcinoma or hypernephroma, papilloma of urinary bladder, BEP, bilharziasis (schistosomiasis), interstitial nephritis, anticoagulant or antiplatelet drug, and bleeding disorder (hemophilia, Christmas disease and ITP).

Causes of painful hematuria: Urethritis, cystitis, renal calculi, trauma, PKD (clot colic), renal papillary necrosis, loin pain hematuria syndrome and hemorrhagic cystitis due to cyclophosphamide.

PROTEINURIA

Presence of protein in urine above normal limit (>150 mg in 24 h).

Causes:
- *Physiological*: Orthostatic or postural proteinuria
- *Nephrotic proteinuria (>3.5 g/24 h)*: Nephrotic syndrome (NS) due to any cause

- *Non-nephrotic proteinuria (<3.5 g/24 hr)*: GN due to any cause
- *Nonrenal cause*: Toxemia of pregnancy (eclampsia and pre-eclampsia), malignant hypertension, high fever and severe exercise.

Orthostatic proteinuria: Presence of proteinuria in a person with prolonged upright position (e.g. traffic police). It is absent in morning specimen of urine after getting up from sleep.

MICROALBUMINURIA

Urinary albumin excretion 30–300 mg in 24 hours or 20–200 µg/min is called microalbuminuria. Not detected by urine dipstick test. It is a predictor of early diabetic nephropathy.

It occurs both in insulin-dependent diabetes mellitus (IDDM) and noninsulin-dependent diabetes mellitus (NIDDM), but common in NIDDM, more in male. 30–40% develop irreversible nephropathy. Patient with microalbuminuria has 20 times greater incidence of nephropathy than normal people. It is associated with atherosclerosis, peripheral vascular disease, hypertension and ischemic heart disease (IHD), also proliferative diabetic retinopathy and increased incidence of blindness.

Treatment: Good control of diabetes. Control of hypertension [by angiotensin-converting-enzyme (ACE) inhibitor or calcium antagonist]. Restriction of protein—Intake should be 40–90 g/day.

Few common definitions:
- *Anuria*: Passage of urine <50 mL in 24 hours
- *Oliguria*: Passage of <400 mL of urine in 24 hours
- *Polyuria*: Passing of large volume (>3 L of urine) in 24 hours
- *Nocturia*: Need to get up during the night to pass urine
- *Frequency of micturition*: Repeated scanty urination without increase in volume
- *Dysuria*: Pain or discomfort during micturition
- *Pyuria*: Presence of pus in urine.

Incontinence of urine: Involuntary passage of urine. There are four types—
1. *Stress incontinence*: Leakage of urine with activity such as coughing, sneezing, lifting any object and exercise. Found in women after childbirth and in man after prostate operation
2. *Urge incontinence*: Uncontrolled leakage of urine preceded by strong urge to void urine. It is due to UTI, enlargement of prostate, and stone in urinary bladder
3. *Overflow incontinence*: It occurs when the bladder is chronically overdistended. Found in benign prostatic enlargement and pelvic surgery leading to pelvic nerve damage
4. *Continual incontinence*: Patient voids urine at any time, at any position due to loss of sphincter control. Found in vesicovaginal fistula and ureterovaginal fistula.

Causes of oliguria or anuria: Any cause of acute renal failure, may be reversible.
- *Prerenal cause*:
  - Fluid loss due to diarrhea, vomiting, and dehydration
  - Blood loss due to hemorrhage and plasma loss in burn

- Hypotension due to myocardial infarction, shock, vasodilator drugs and heart failure
  - Other causes of acute renal failure: Rhabdomyolysis, hemolytic uremic syndrome, hepatorenal syndrome and renal artery stenosis.
- *Renal (intrinsic renal disease)*:
  - Acute tubular necrosis or toxic or septic renal failure (85%)
  - Rapidly progressing glomerulonephritis (RPGN) due to: Primary GN [e.g. mesangiocapillary glomerulonephritis (MCGN) and IgA nephropathy]
  - Systemic disease: Systemic lupus erythematosus (SLE), rheumatoid arthritis, systemic sclerosis, multiple myeloma and vasculitis
  - Tubulointerstitial disease by drugs [nonsteroidal anti-inflammatory drug (NSAID), ciprofloxacin, allopurinol, sulfonamide and cyclosporine].
- *Postrenal*:
  - Urethral: Phimosis, paraphimosis, stricture, stone, blood clot and sloughed papilla
  - Bladder neck: Prostatic hypertrophy, malignancy and stone
  - Bilateral: Ureteric calculus, following surgery, pelvic tumor, uterine prolapse and retroperitoneal fibrosis (due to radiation and idiopathic).

Cause of polyuria:
- *Physiological*: Excess intake of fluid, alcohol, tea and coffee
- *Pathological*: DM, diabetes insipidus, hypercalcemia due to any cause and chronic kidney disease (CKD)
- Psychogenic polydipsia
- *Drug*: Diuretic.

Causes of nocturia: CKD, BEP, congestive cardiac failure (CCF) and insomnia.

Causes of frequency of micturition: Excessive fluid intake, DM, diabetes insipidus, cystitis, BEP, stone and tumor of urinary bladder.

NEPHROTIC SYNDROME

It is characterized by generalized edema, massive proteinuria (>3.5 g/day) and hypoalbuminemia, with or without hyperlipidemia.

Causes:

Primary renal disease: GN due to any cause—
- Minimal change glomerular disease (common in children)
- Membranous GN (common in adult)
- Mesangiocapillary and proliferative GN
- Focal and segmental glomerulosclerosis
- Immunoglobulin A nephropathy.

Secondary to other disease:
- Diabetic nephropathy
- *Collagen disease*: SLE and rheumatoid arthritis (by amyloidosis)
- Amyloidosis
- *Drugs*: Penicillamine (common) and captopril
- *Neoplastic*: Carcinoma (bronchial carcinoma) and lymphoma

- *Infection*: Quartan malaria, bacterial endocarditis, hepatitis B virus (HBV), hepatitis C virus (HCV), human immunodeficiency virus (HIV), secondary syphilis and leprosy
- *Hereditary*: Congenital NS and Alport syndrome
- *Allergies*: Bee stings, snake bite, anti-snake venom and pollens.

Note: Common cause in children is minimal change and in adult membranous GN.

Symptoms: Generalized body swelling. At first, periorbital edema, then becomes generalized and massive (anasarca). Scanty urine, which may be frothy.

Signs: Bilateral pitting leg edema, generalized body swelling, may be ascites and bilateral pleural effusion.

History to be taken in nephrotic syndrome:
- Diabetes mellitus
- Malignancy (lymphoma and leukemia)
- *Drugs*: Captopril, NSAID and penicillamine
- Skin rash, arthritis, arthralgia and alopecia (SLE)
- History of other diseases like malaria, leprosy, syphilis, HBV, HCV, amyloidosis and vasculitis
- Family history of sickle cell disease, Alport syndrome and Nail–patella syndrome.

Investigations:
- *Urine routine microscopic examination (RME)*: Shows gross proteinuria
- 24 hours urinary protein (>3.5 g/day is suggestive of NS)
- Serum total protein, serum albumin and A:G ratio (hypoalbuminemia)
- Serum lipid profile (high cholesterol and high triglycerides may be present)
- Blood sugar, blood urea, serum creatinine and serum electrolytes should be done
- Ultrasonography (USG) of whole abdomen to look for renal pathology
- *Other investigations*: According to history and suspicion of cause—
  - Blood sugar (to exclude diabetic nephropathy)
  - Chest X-ray (CXR) (to see bronchial carcinoma, lymphoma, bilateral pleural effusion and pericardial effusion)
  - Antinuclear antibody (ANA), anti-double stranded deoxyribonucleic acid (anti-dsDNA) (in SLE), perinuclear antineutrophil cytoplasmic antibodies (p-ANCA), and cytoplasmic antineutrophil cytoplasmic antibodies (c-ANCA) (in vasculitis)
  - HBsAg and anti-HCV screening and complement C3 and C4
  - Renal biopsy (to see type of GN).

Complications of nephrotic syndrome:
- Hypercoagulability leading to venous thrombosis or pulmonary embolism
- *Infections*: Pneumococcal, streptococcal, meningococcal and cellulitis
- Hyperlipidemia leading to atherosclerosis
- Oliguric renal failure
- Bilateral pleural effusion and pericardial effusion
- Loss of thyroxin binding globulin that causes low FT3 and FT4
- Loss of transferrin and iron, resulting in iron deficiency anemia
- Loss of vitamin D binding protein, leading to osteomalacia

Treatment:
- *Fluid restriction*: Average 500–1,000 mL/day. Salt restriction (avoid extra salt)
- *Diuretics*: Furosemide, bumetanide and spironolactone
- Normal protein diet. High protein is not necessary, it increases proteinuria
- Intravenous (IV) salt poor albumin may be given if diuretic resistance
- *If infection*: Antibiotic. Pneumococcal vaccine is recommended
- *Venous thrombosis*: To prevent, prolonged bed rest should be avoided. Prophylactic heparin in immobile patient (enoxaparin may be given), followed by oral anticoagulant
- *For hyperlipidemia*: Statin may be added
- Angiotensin-converting enzyme inhibitor or angiotensin II receptor antagonist is used in all types of GN (reduce proteinuria).

Specific measures:
- *In minimal change disease (MCD)*:
  - Prednisolone: 60 mg/m^2 (maximum 80 mg/day) for 4–6 weeks, then 40 mg/m^2 every alternate day for 4–6 weeks. *Or*, prednisolone 1 mg/kg/day for 3 months, then taper in next 3 months
  - If relapse after withdrawal of steroid, it should be given again with gradual withdrawal. Some patients may require low maintenance dose (5–10 mg/day) for 3–6 months
  - If frequent relapse or high dose steroid is needed or less response to steroid: Cyclophosphamide (1.5–2 mg/kg/day for 8–12 weeks) and prednisolone 7.5–15 mg/day should be given
  - Rituximab may be used in frequent relapse.
- For other treatment, see below in GN.

GLOMERULONEPHRITIS

It means inflammation of glomeruli, mostly immunologically mediated with deposition of antibodies in glomerulus. There are two types:
1. Primary glomerulopathy
2. Secondary to systemic diseases.

Primary: Histologically, it is divided into—
- Minimal change disease
- Focal segmental glomerulosclerosis (FSGS)
- Focal segmental glomerulonephritis (FSGN)
- Membranous GN
- Immunoglobulin A nephropathy
- Mesangiocapillary GN
- Postinfectious GN.

Secondary: SLE, Goodpasture syndrome, polyarteritis nodosa, Wegener's granulomatosis, microscopic polyangiitis, amyloidosis, bacterial endocarditis, DM and mixed essential cryoglobulinemia.

Minimal change disease: Common cause of NS in children, more in boys, may occur in all ages. On light microscopy, no abnormality. On electron microscopy, fusion of podocyte foot process. Progression to renal failure is rare, good response to steroid and cytotoxic drugs.

Focal segmental glomerulosclerosis: There is segmental scar in glomeruli with C3 and IgM deposition. Cause is unknown, may be related to HIV, heroin abuse, morbid obesity, reflux nephropathy, secondary to other GN. Present as idiopathic NS with massive proteinuria, hematuria and hypertension, may progress to renal failure.

Treatment:
- Prednisolone 0.5-2 mg/kg/day for 6 months. If no response, mycophenolate mofetil 1-2 g/day or cyclosporine 5-6 mg/kg/day for 3 months, then dose is reduced and maintained up to 15 months. Cyclophosphamide, chlorambucil and azathioprine may be used
- Renal transplantation, if renal failure.

Membranous glomerulopathy: Common cause of NS in adult, more in male. Causes are idiopathic, also secondary to SLE, bronchial carcinoma, penicillamine, HBV and HCV. Renal vein thrombosis is a common complication, may progress to CKD. Renal biopsy may be done for diagnosis. Treated by high dose steroid and cyclophosphamide.

IgA nephropathy: It is a nephropathy of unknown cause characterized by mesangial IgA deposition with increased mesangial matrix and cells. Usually presents with recurrent macroscopic hematuria and hypertension. No specific treatment.

Mesangiocapillary glomerulonephritis: Also called membranoproliferative glomerulonephritis (MPGN), characterized by increase in mesangial cells, thickening of glomerular capillary walls, and subendothelial deposition of immune complex and complement. Causes are idiopathic, also infection (hepatitis C), autoimmune, subacute bacterial endocarditis and cryoglobulinemia. Usual presentations are proteinuria and hematuria.

Treatment:
- In idiopathic MCGN with normal renal function and non-nephrotic range proteinuria, no specific therapy is required. Control of blood pressure (BP) with ACE inhibitor
- In children with nephritic syndrome and/or impaired renal function, alternate day prednisolone 40 mg/m^2 for 6–12 months
- Aspirin or dipyridamole may be given.

Rapidly progressing glomerulonephritis: Also known as "crescentic glomerulonephritis" characterized by rapid loss of renal function over days to weeks. Causes are Goodpasture disease, small vessel vasculitis, SLE, IgA and other nephropathies. Rapid onset disease may be associated with relatively little proteinuria. Renal biopsy shows crescentic, necrotizing lesions within the glomerulus. Treatment depends on underlying cause. In Goodpasture disease, plasma exchange with steroid and immunosuppressant. In ANCA-associated vasculitis and SLE, steroid and immunosuppressant.

Postinfectious glomerulonephritis: Usually after streptococcal infection, may be due to other infections. There is diffuse proliferation of endothelial and mesangial cells, infiltration of neutrophils and macrophage with or without crescent formation. Patient usually presents with severe sodium and fluid retention, hypertension, hematuria and oliguria. Usually resolves spontaneously.

ACUTE GLOMERULONEPHRITIS/ACUTE NEPHRITIC SYNDROME

It means acute inflammation of glomeruli characterized by hematuria, hypertension, edema (periorbital, leg or sacral), and oliguria. Urine shows proteinuria and red cell cast.

Causes:
- *Infection*: Poststreptococcal (common), infective endocarditis, infectious mononucleosis and HBV
- *Primary glomerular disease*: Diffuse proliferative GN, IgA nephropathy, membranous GN and FSGS
- *Systemic disease*: SLE, Henoch–Schönlein purpura, Goodpasture syndrome, vasculitis and cryoglobulinemia
- Shunt nephritis.

Symptoms: Puffiness of face, scanty, high-colored, smoky or red urine. Anorexia, nausea, vomiting, fever, lethargy and weakness. Features of hypertension. Features of complication such as breathlessness and cough [due to left ventricle function (LVF)].

Signs: Periorbital swelling, puffy face, edema and high BP. Skin infection or healing skin lesion.

Investigations: Routine—
- *Urine RME*: Looks smoky, mild-to-moderate proteinuria, RBC, RBC cast, and granular cast (RBC cast is suggestive of AGN)
- 24 hours urinary total protein (high, but <3 g/L) and volume is less
- Complete blood count (leukocytosis may be present), blood urea, serum creatinine and serum electrolytes
- Antistreptolysin O (ASO) titer and throat swab for culture/sensitivity (C/S) (to see streptococcal infection)
- Ultrasonography of whole abdomen (to look for renal pathology)
- Chest X-ray (cardiomegaly or pulmonary edema, if LVF)
- *Serum C3*: Reduced.

Other investigations, according to suspicion of cause:
- Antinuclear antibody, anti-dsDNA (in SLE), p-ANCA and c-ANCA (in vasculitis)
- HbsAg, anti-HCV, and renal biopsy may be done in some cases.

Complications: Acute renal failure, hypertension and its complications such as acute LVF, cerebrovascular disease, and hypertensive encephalopathy, electrolyte imbalance, NS and chronic glomerulonephritis.

Treatment:
- *Rest*: Fluid (500–1,000 mL/day), salt and protein restriction (if urea and creatinine are high)
- *Diuretic (furosemide)*: To relieve edema
- *If hypertension*: Antihypertensive
- *Antibiotic*: Oral phenoxymethylpenicillin or erythromycin for 7–10 days, especially in poststreptococcal glomerulonephritis (PSGN)
- *Management of complication*: Pulmonary edema, hypertensive encephalopathy and acute kidney injury (AKI) (dialysis may be needed)
- *If recovery is slow*: Steroid may be given.

POSTSTREPTOCOCCAL GLOMERULONEPHRITIS

It is a common cause of acute nephritis, caused by group A beta-hemolytic streptococci, which can occur due to other infection. Common in children. There is a latent period of about 10 days (1–3 weeks) after throat infection or longer after skin infection (infected scabies, impetigo and furunculosis), suggesting an immune mechanism. Streptococcal otitis media or cellulitis can cause PSGN. Common with poor personal hygiene, overcrowding, and skin infection like scabies. Clinical features are periorbital puffiness and reduced urinary volume. Anorexia, nausea, vomiting, fever, malaise and hypertension.

Investigations:
- *Urine RME*: Red or smoky, proteinuria and hematuria
- Blood urea and serum creatinine and serum electrolytes
- Evidence of streptococcal infection (high ASO and culture of throat swab)
- Serum C3 and C4 (both low) and USG of renal system

Treatment: Complete rest. Salt and fluid restriction. Diuretic (frusemide). Antibiotic (oral phenoxymethylpenicillin for 7–10 days). Spontaneous cure may occur in 7–10 days.

IMMUNOGLOBULIN A NEPHROPATHY

Common in children and young males, 20–35 years of age. Most patients are asymptomatic. May present with recurrent microscopic or gross hematuria following viral respiratory or gastrointestinal tract (GIT) infection. Hematuria is universal, proteinuria is usual and hypertension is common. 5% may develop NS. In some cases, progressive loss of renal function, leading to end-stage renal failure, 20% in 20 years.

Investigations:
- *Urine RME*: Shows RBC
- Urea, creatinine and electrolytes
- Serum IgA and immune complex estimation
- Ultrasonography of renal system, plain X-ray of kidney, uterus and bladder (KUB), and computed tomography (CT) scan of renal system
- Kidney biopsy may be done.

Treatment: Episodic attack resolves spontaneously. Steroid is indicated if patient has proteinuria over 1–3 g/day, mild glomerular change, and good renal function. In progressive renal disease, prednisolone plus cyclophosphamide for 3 months, then prednisolone plus azathioprine. Combination of ACE inhibitor and angiotensin-receptor blocker (ARB) should be given to all cases. Tonsillectomy may be helpful, if recurrent tonsillitis.

POLYCYSTIC KIDNEY DISEASE

It is an inherited cystic disease of kidney. There are two types:
1. *Adult polycystic kidney disease (APKD)*: It is inherited as autosomal dominant (AD), common type, and male and female are equally affected
2. *Infantile polycystic kidney disease (IPKD)*: It is inherited as autosomal recessive (AR), rare, associated with cyst in other organs and hepatic fibrosis. Fatal in first year due to hepatic or renal failure.

Clinical features: May be asymptomatic (renal mass, detected during routine examination).
- Discomfort, pain or heaviness in loin. Recurrent painful hematuria and recurrent UTI. Acute loin pain or renal colic and features of renal failure
- Features of hypertension (usually after 20 years of age) and its complications
- Cerebrovascular accident (CVA) (usually subarachnoid hemorrhage, due to rupture of berry aneurysm)

- *Other features*: Polycythemia, renal stone in 10% cases and renal neoplasm rarely.

Investigations:
- Ultrasonography of whole abdomen, high resolution CT or MRI
- Urine routine microscopic examination (RME) (shows hematuria and proteinuria)
- Complete blood count (polycythemia), blood urea, serum creatinine and electrolytes
- Intravenous urogram (IVU).

Causes of death in polycystic kidney disease: Chronic renal failure (CRF), subarachnoid hemorrhage and myocardial infarction.

Treatment of polycystic kidney disease: Usually management is symptomatic and supportive.
- Control of hypertension and control of UTI
- Plenty of fluid and also extra salt in some cases (in salt loser)
- *Large cyst*: May be aspirated under USG guidance. In some cases, laparoscopic cystectomy
- Treatment of renal failure (either dialysis or renal transplantation)
- Genetic counseling, family screening (anyone above 20 years of age, USG is done to detect cyst).

ACUTE RENAL FAILURE

It is characterized by sudden deterioration of renal function occurring within days or weeks, associated with reduced urine volume, biochemically detected by high urea and creatinine level. Usually reversible. It is also called acute kidney injury.

Causes:
- *Prerenal*:
  - Fluid loss: Due to diarrhea, vomiting and excessive sweating
  - Blood loss: Due to hemorrhage
  - Plasma loss in burn
  - Hypotension or less cardiac output: In myocardial infarction, shock, vasodilator drug and heart failure
  - Others: Rhabdomyolysis, hemolytic uremic syndrome and hepatorenal syndrome.
- *Renal (intrinsic renal disease)*:
  - Acute tubular necrosis: Due to toxin (contrast material) or septic renal failure (85%)
  - Glomerular disease: MCGN and IgA nephropathy
  - Renal artery occlusion or stenosis
  - Systemic disease: SLE, rheumatoid arthritis, systemic sclerosis, multiple myeloma and vasculitis
  - Tubulointerstitial disease: Due to NSAID, ciprofloxacin, allopurinol, sulfonamide and cyclosporine.
- *Postrenal*:
  - Urethral: Phimosis, paraphimosis, stricture, stone, blood clot, and sloughed papilla
  - Bladder neck obstruction: Prostatic hypertrophy, malignancy, and stone

- Bilateral ureteric calculus, following surgery, pelvic tumor, uterine prolapse, and retroperitoneal fibrosis (due to radiation, idiopathic).

Clinical features: Scanty or no urination. Features of electrolyte imbalance (hyperkalemia and hyponatremia), metabolic acidosis, anorexia, nausea, vomiting, drowsiness, confusion, hiccough, fit or convulsion and coma.

Investigations:
- Urine RME
- Complete blood count, erythrocyte sedimentation rate (ESR), serum urea, creatinine and electrolytes
- Plain X-ray of KUB, CXR and USG of abdomen
- *Complement*: C3 and C4
- *Others*: According to suspicion of cause.

Treatment: Restriction of fluid and salt. Avoid excess protein intake. Maintenance of nutrition by carbohydrate and fat. Electrolytes correction (especially hyperkalemia) and acidosis correction (IV sodium bicarbonate). Treatment of primary cause. Dialysis, if necessary.

CHRONIC KIDNEY DISEASE/CHRONIC RENAL FAILURE

It is the irreversible deterioration of renal function classically developing over months to years.

End-stage renal disease or failure (ESRD): It is the stage when renal replacement therapy is compulsory either dialysis or renal transplantation, without which death is likely.

Causes of chronic kidney disease:
- Diabetes mellitus (20–40%)
- Interstitial diseases (20–30%)
- Glomerular diseases (10–20%). IgA nephropathy is common
- Hypertension (5–20%)
- Systemic inflammatory diseases (5–10%, e.g. SLE and vasculitis)
- Renovascular disease (5%)
- Congenital and inherited (5%), e.g. PKD and Alport syndrome
- Unknown (5–20%).

Clinical features:
- May be asymptomatic, until glomerular filtration rate (GFR) falls below 30 mL/min/1.73 m^2 of body surface area. High urea and creatinine may be found on routine investigation
- There may be hypertension, anemia and proteinuria on routine urine examination
- *General features*: Early features may be nocturia, polyuria, anorexia, nausea, vomiting, diarrhea, weakness, malaise, insomnia, breathlessness on exertion, paresthesia, bone pain, edema, amenorrhea in woman and sexual dysfunction in man
- *In ESRD*: General features are severe, central nervous system (CNS) symptoms may be more. Features like hiccough, pruritus, deep respiration (Kussmaul respiration), muscular twitching, fit and drowsiness, even coma may occur
- *Other features*: Due to involvement of different systems of the body described below.

Bone diseases (renal osteodystrophy):
- Osteomalacia (or rickets, called renal rickets)
- Osteoporosis
- Osteosclerosis (in vertebral body, giving rise to *Rugger Jersey spine*)
- Osteitis fibrosa cystica.

Skin disease: Dryness, hyperpigmentation, ecchymosis and pruritus.

Gastrointestinal: Anorexia, nausea, vomiting, peptic ulcer, acute pancreatitis and constipation.

Metabolic abnormalities:
- Hyponatremia, hyperkalemia, hypokalemia, hypocalcemia and hyperphosphatemia
- Metabolic acidosis
- Hyperuricemia, gout, hypercholesterolemia and hypertriglyceridemia.

Endocrine abnormalities:
- Secondary hyperparathyroidism, may be tertiary
- *Insulin*: Half-life is prolonged and requirement decreases. In advanced CKD, resistance may occur
- *Others*: Increased luteinizing hormone (LH), decreased testosterone, oligo or amenorrhea (in female), growth retardation in children, abnormal thyroid hormone levels (hypothyroidism) and hyperprolactinemia.

Muscle dysfunction: Generalized myopathy, muscle cramps and restless leg syndrome.

Nervous system:
- *Peripheral nervous system*: Polyneuropathy and median nerve compression in carpal tunnel
- *Central nervous system*: Clouding of consciousness, convulsion, coma, flapping tremor, myoclonus, dialysis disequilibrium syndrome, dementia, anxiety, depression, phobia and psychosis
- *Autonomic dysfunction*: Postural hypotension, fixed heart rate, urinary retention or incontinence, constipation and impotence.

Cardiovascular: Hypertension, cardiac failure, pericardial effusion, constrictive pericarditis, uremic cardiomyopathy, atherosclerosis and coronary artery calcification.

Respiratory: Pulmonary edema (uremic lung) due to fluid overload.

Malignancy: Incidence of renal cell carcinoma is increased.

Stages of chronic kidney disease:

Stage	Features	GFR (mL/min/1.73 m^2)
1	Kidney damage with normal or ↑ GFR	≥90
2	Kidney damage with mild ↓ GFR	60–89
3	Moderate ↓ GFR A and B	30–59 (A: 45–59, B: 30–44)
4	Severe ↓ GFR	15–29
5	Kidney failure	<15 (or dialysis)

Investigations:
- Urine RME (to see pus cell, RBC or WBC cast, proteinuria and hematuria)

- Complete blood count and peripheral blood film (PBF) (show normocytic and normochromic anemia)
- *Renal function tests*: Blood urea, serum creatinine (high) and creatinine clearance
- Serum electrolytes. Serum calcium (low), phosphate (high) and serum uric acid (high)
- Plain X-ray of abdomen (renal stone and kidney size)
- Ultrasonography of KUB
- CT scan of abdomen
- Intravenous urogram (rarely needed) and isotope renogram
- *Renal biopsy*: To find out the cause
- *Other investigation according to suspicion of cause*: ANA and anti-dsDNA for SLE, screening for hepatitis B and C, and HIV.

Treatment:

General measures: Fluid restriction, salt restriction and protein restriction (0.5 g/kg/day). Severe protein restriction is avoided. Smoking should be stopped. Social and psychological support.

Symptomatic and supportive:

- *Hypertension*: Target of BP is 130/80 mm Hg [if urine total protein (UTP) <1g/day] and 125/75 mm Hg (if UTP >1 g/day). ACE inhibitor or ARB and diuretics may be added. Calcium channel blocker (verapamil or diltiazem) is added, if goal is not achieved
- *Dyslipidemia*: Statin
- *Hyperkalemia*:
  - Dietary restriction of potassium (fruits like banana, orange and coconut)
  - Drugs causing potassium retention should be stopped (e.g. spironolactone)
  - Injection 10% calcium gluconate 10 cc over 5 minutes, may be repeated
  - Glucose and insulin (50 mL of 50% glucose IV *plus* injection insulin 10 units), may be repeated
  - Correction of acidosis
  - Occasionally, calcium resonium powder 15 g in 1 cup water to be taken orally
  - If all measures fail or hyperkalemia is severe, hemodialysis or peritoneal dialysis may be needed.
- *Acidosis*: Sodium bicarbonate (1.26% IV) or calcium carbonate (up to 3 g/day). Bicarbonate should be maintained above 22 mmol/L
- *Calcium and phosphate control and suppression of parathyroid hormone (PTH)*:
  - For hypocalcemia: Calcitriol or alfacalcidol and calcium supplementation.
  - For hyperphosphatemia: Dietary restriction of phosphate containing food (milk, cheese and eggs). Phosphate-binding drugs like calcium carbonate, aluminum hydroxide and lanthanum carbonate may be used with food to prevent phosphate absorption.
- *Anemia*: Erythropoietin (side effects are hypertension and thrombosis). Blood transfusion in severe anemia

- *Male erectile dysfunction*: Testosterone deficiency should be corrected. Phosphodiesterase inhibitors like sildenafil may be used
- *Treatment renal osteodystrophy*: Calcium supplement. 1-α-hydroxylated synthetic analogue of vitamin D
- Treatment of primary cause (DM, hypertension, APKD, and removal of obstruction in obstructive uropathy).

Definitive treatment: Renal replacement therapy such as hemodialysis, hemofiltration, peritoneal dialysis and renal transplantation.

Indications of renal replacement therapy:
- Serum creatinine >600–800 μmol/L (7–9 mg/dL)
- Hyperkalemia (plasma potassium >6 mmol/L despite medical treatment)
- Metabolic acidosis pH <7.25, HCO3 <10 mmol/L
- Fluid overload and pulmonary edema
- Uremic pericarditis or encephalopathy.

Indications of urgent dialysis:
- Severe hyperkalemia
- Pulmonary edema or severe fluid overload
- Severe metabolic acidosis
- Uremic pericarditis and uremic encephalopathy
- Toxicity with a dialyzable poison (methanol and barbiturate)
- Recurrent vomiting due to uremia.

Contraindications of renal transplantation:
- *Absolute*:
  - Active malignancy: A period of at least 2 years of complete remission recommended for most tumor
  - Active vasculitis or recent anti-GBM (glomerular basement membrane) disease
  - Severe heart disease or any severe comorbid condition
  - Severe occlusive aortoiliac vascular disease.
- *Relative*:
  - Age: Not routinely done in very young children (<1 year) or older people (>75 years)
  - High risk of disease recurrence in transplant kidney
  - Disease of lower urinary tract: In impaired bladder function and stricture urethra
  - Significant comorbidity.

To prevent rejection: Combination of cyclosporine or tacrolimus *plus* azathioprine or mycophenolate mofetil/sirolimus or everolimus *plus* prednisolone.

ACUTE INTERSTITIAL NEPHRITIS

It is an acute inflammation of tubulointerstitium of kidney commonly due to drugs, but may also be due to systemic infection and toxin.

Causes:
- *Drugs (70%)*: Penicillin and NSAID (common), sulfonamide, allopurinol, cephalosporin, rifampicin, phenytoin and diuretic (frusemide)
- *Others*: Autoimmune, infection [acute pyelonephritis, TB, *cytomegalovirus (CMV)*, *hanta virus*, leptospirosis], multiple myeloma and idiopathic.

Symptoms: Fever, arthralgia, skin rash and body ache. Oliguria, anuria and features of renal failure.

Investigations:
- Urine RME (shows RBC, proteinuria and leukocyte. Eosinophil count is high in 70% cases)
- Complete blood count (very high eosinophil), serum creatinine, electrolytes and urea
- Ultrasonography of KUB and CT scan
- Intravenous urogram, if needed
- Renal biopsy may be done.

Treatment: Offending drug should be stopped. Prednisolone 1 mg/kg/day. Taper the dose when clinical improvement. Correction of electrolytes. Dialysis may be required if renal failure.

ANALGESIC NEPHROPATHY

It is a chronic tubulointerstitial nephritis with papillary necrosis after prolonged use of NSAID.

Symptoms: It is twice as common in women and is an important cause of CRF.
- *Hypertension*: 60% of patients are hypertensive at presentation
- Sloughing of renal papillae can cause urinary tract obstruction, which may precipitate acute renal failure. Recurrent UTIs are common. There may be sterile pyuria
- Also, occasionally salt-losing nephropathy.

Diagnosis can be made by history and characteristic appearances on IVU. There is risk of tumors of uroepithelium. Total recovery of renal function occurs in 25% patients.

Investigations:
- Urine RME
- Blood urea, creatinine and electrolytes
- Ultrasonography of KUB and CT scan of abdomen
- Intravenous urogram
- Renal biopsy is sometimes done, which shows interstitial fibrosis and tubular atrophy.

Treatment: Withdrawal of offending drug. Maintain a fluid intake of 2–3 liters per day. Control of hypertension and biochemical correction.

RENAL TUBERCULOSIS

Genitourinary TB develops in approximately 5% cases after pulmonary TB. It is usually due to hematogenous spread to renal cortex during primary infection.

Symptoms:
- *General features of TB*: Fever, malaise, night sweat and weight loss
- Hematuria, frequency of micturition, burning and urgency
- *Features of complication*: Retention of urine due to urethral stricture
- Features of CKD.

Investigations:
- Urine RME (shows pus cells and RBC). Urine for C/S (shows sterile pyuria)
- Urine for acid-fast bacillus (AFB) and mycobacterial C/S
- Mantoux test
- Chest X-ray, USG of KUB and CT scan of renal system
- Intravenous urogram.

Treatment: Standard anti-Koch's therapy, to be continued for 9 months to 1 year. Steroid may be added. Surgery (if obstructive uropathy or if kidney is severely damaged).

URINARY TRACT INFECTION

It is the infection involving the urinary tract.

Types:
- *Upper UTI*: Involving renal pelvis called pyelonephritis
- *Lower UTI*: Acute urethritis and cystitis.

Causative organisms: *Escherichia coli*, *Proteus*, *Pseudomonas*, *Streptococci*, *Staphylococcus epidermidis* and *Klebsiella*.

Some common definitions:
- *Cystitis*: Infection of urinary bladder
- *Urethritis*: Infection of urethra
- *Prostatitis*: Infection of prostate
- *Pyelonephritis*: Infection of renal pelvis
- *Sterile pyuria*: Presence of pus cell in urine, but no organism is detected in routine culture
- *Asymptomatic bacteriuria*: Presence of organism in urine on culture, but no symptom
- *Significant bacteriuria*: Presence of bacteria in urine >100,000/mL.

Spectrum of presentations of urinary tract infection:
- Asymptomatic bacteriuria
- Symptomatic acute urethritis and cystitis
- Acute pyelonephritis
- Acute prostatitis
- Septicemia (usually Gram-negative bacteria).

Predisposing factors for urinary tract infection:
- *Incomplete bladder emptying*: Bladder outflow obstruction (due to benign prostatic enlargement, prostate cancer and urethral stricture), vesicoureteric reflux, uterine prolapse and neurological problems (multiple sclerosis, spina bifida and diabetic neuropathy)
- *Foreign body*: Urethral catheter, ureteric stent and urolithiasis
- *Loss of host defense*: Atrophic urethritis and vaginitis in postmenopausal women and DM
- Instrumentation of bladder may also introduce organisms.

Clinical features: Features of lower UTI (cystitis and urethritis)—
- Frequency of micturition
- Urgency and scalding pain in urethra during micturition (dysuria)
- Suprapubic pain during and after voiding

- Intense desire to pass more urine after micturition, due to spasm of inflamed bladder wall (strangury). Urine may appear cloudy and have an unpleasant odor. Hematuria, microscopic or visible. Systemic symptoms are usually slight or absent
- Prostatitis is suggested by perineal or suprapubic pain, pain on ejaculation and prostatic tenderness on rectal examination.

Investigations:
- Urine RME and C/S (midstream urine)
- Complete blood count, ESR and blood sugar
- Serum urea, creatinine and electrolytes
- Ultrasonography of KUB. In some cases, CT scan or MRI, IVU and micturating cystourethrogram may be needed.

Management:
- Antibiotic should be given. Urine for C/S is sent, antibiotic is started, may be changed after report
- *Antibiotic*: Trimethoprim 200 mg 12 hourly *or* nitrofurantoin 100 mg 6 hourly *or* ciprofloxacin 500 mg 12 hourly *or* cephalexin 250 mg 6 hourly *or* co-amoxiclav 625 mg 8 hourly *or* amoxicillin 500 mg 8 hourly. Continued for 7–14 days
- Seriously ill patients may require IV cephalosporin, quinolone or gentamicin or amikacin
- *General measures*: Plenty of fluid, at least 2 L/day. Regular complete emptying of bladder. Good personal hygiene. Emptying of bladder before and after sexual intercourse. Cranberry juice may be effective.

Asymptomatic bacteriuria: It is defined as >100,000 organisms/mL of urine in apparently healthy asymptomatic patients. Approximately 1% of children under 1 year of age, 1% of school girls, 0.03% of school boys and men, 3% of nonpregnant women, and 5% of pregnant women have asymptomatic bacteriuria. It is increasingly common in those over 65 years. Usually no treatment is necessary. 30% will develop infection in 1 year. Treatment is required in infants, pregnant woman, and those with urinary tract abnormality. Antibiotic should be given as described in UTI.

Urethral syndrome: In some patients, commonly females, there are symptoms of urethritis and cystitis, but no bacteria in culture. It is called urethral syndrome. It may occur in postcoital bladder trauma, vaginitis, atrophic vaginitis or urethritis in elderly. In sterile pyuria, chlamydia and TB should be excluded.

Persistent or recurrent UTI: If the causative organism persists on repeated culture despite antibiotic or if there is reinfection with any organism after an interval, then an underlying cause is more likely to be present (see predisposing factors of UTI written above) and more detailed investigation should be done. In women, recurrent infections are common. Recurrent UTI may cause permanent renal damage.

Treatment: Underlying cause should be treated. Suppressive antibiotic therapy should be given continuously for several months (trimethoprim 100 mg at night or nitrofurantoin 50 mg at night or co-amoxyclav, 250/125 mg at night).

Sterile pyuria: It means presence of pus cells in urine, but no organism on routine culture. Causes are renal TB, partially treated UTI with antibiotic, nongonococcal urethritis, schistosomiasis, tubulointerstitial nephritis, papillary necrosis and renal calculi.

ACUTE PYELONEPHRITIS

It is the infection of renal pelvis and surrounding parenchyma. Small abscesses are often evident in renal parenchyma. Predisposing factors are:
- Diabetes mellitus
- Chronic urinary tract obstruction
- Analgesic nephropathy
- Sickle cell disease
- Renal cyst or scarring
- A necrotizing form of pyelonephritis with gas formation, "emphysematous pyelonephritis" is occasionally seen in patients with DM.

Cause: Usually ascending infection from urinary bladder. Organisms are same as lower UTI (see above).

Clinical features: Classic *triad* of loin pain, fever and tenderness over kidneys. Systemic symptoms are fever with chill and rigor, nausea, vomiting, and hypotension. May be dysuria, frequency and urgency.

Investigations:
- Urine RME and C/S (midstream urine)
- Complete blood count, ESR, blood sugar, serum urea, creatinine and electrolytes
- Ultrasonography of KUB. In some cases, CT scan or MRI, IVU and micturating cystourethrogram may be needed.

Treatment: Antibiotic (as in UTI). Plenty of fluid, if needed and IV infusion. Treatment of primary cause. If obstruction is present, percutaneous nephrostomy or ureteric stenting may be done.

Complications: Pyonephrosis or abscess formation, emphysematous pyelonephritis, chronic pyelonephritis and septic shock.

Differential diagnoses: Acute appendicitis, diverticulitis, cholecystitis, salpingitis, ruptured ovarian cyst or ectopic pregnancy.

CHRONIC PYELONEPHRITIS

It occurs from recurrent urinary infection due to vesicoureteric reflux and infection acquired in infancy or early childhood. It is called reflux nephropathy.

Vesicoureteric reflux: Normally, vesicoureteric junction acts as a one-way valve. No urine enters during voiding as the urinary bladder contracts. If the valve is incompetent, there is reflux of urine into the ureter during voiding of urine. As a result, there is infection and reflux of infected urine that leads to kidney infection and damage. In kidney, there is gross scarring, reduction of size, narrowing of cortex and medulla and atrophy with impaired kidney function.

Investigations:
- Urine RME and C/S
- Serum urea, creatinine and electrolytes

- Ultrasonography of KUB. CT scan (shows irregular renal outline, clubbed calyces and reduction of renal size)
- Intravenous urogram or micturating cystourethrogram.

Treatment: Antibiotic according to C/S for prolonged period (3–6 months). Removal of any obstruction. If pyonephrosis in one kidney, nephrectomy may be needed.

RENAL ARTERY STENOSIS

It is a rare disorder, in which the patient usually presents with hypertension.

Causes:
- Atherosclerosis in elderly
- Fibromuscular dysplasia in young, aged 15–30 years. Commonly presents with hypertension, more in women
- Rarely, vasculitis, thromboembolism and aneurysm of renal artery.

Pathophysiology: Renal artery stenosis causes reduction in renal perfusion, which activates the renin-angiotensin system, leading to increased circulating levels of angiotensin II. This causes vasoconstriction and increases aldosterone secretion from adrenals, which causes sodium retention by renal tubules.

- In atherosclerosis, there is small vessel disease which affects the kidneys. If stenosis is severe, global renal ischemia leads to shrinkage of affected kidney and may cause renal failure. Patients with peripheral vascular disease, coronary artery disease, CCF and aortic aneurysm are at high risk of developing renal artery stenosis
- In fibromuscular dysplasia, there is hypertrophy of media (medial fibroplasia), which narrows the artery but rarely leads to total occlusion. Irregular narrowing may occur in distal renal artery and also intrarenal branch
- Rarely, may occur in large vessel vasculitis, such as Takayasu's arteritis and polyarteritis nodosa.

Clinical features: May be asymptomatic. May be hypertension. Renal failure in bilateral disease. Deterioration in renal function when ACE inhibitor or ARB are used or acute pulmonary edema.

Signs: Renal bruit present on auscultation.

Investigations:
- *Doppler USG*: Shows asymmetrical size (>1.5 cm) of two kidneys
- CT angiography
- Magnetic resonance (MR) angiography reveals a characteristic string of beads appearance in fibroplasia
- Serum urea, creatinine and electrolytes (hypokalemia due to hyperaldosteronism)
- Elevated plasma renin activity
- Rapid sequence IVU may be done.

Treatment:
- *If due to fibromuscular dysplasia*: Angioplasty, sometimes with stenting *plus* antihypertensive
- *If due to atherosclerosis*: Antihypertensive drug, supplemented with statins and low dose aspirin. Angioplasty and stenting may be tried.

NEPHROCALCINOSIS

It means diffuse deposition of calcium within renal parenchyma. Commonly, it involves medulla and rarely cortex.

Causes:
- Distal renal tubular acidosis (RTA)
- Chronic pyelonephritis
- Hypercalcemia (due to hyperparathyroidism, multiple myeloma, sarcoidosis and hypervitaminosis D)
- Medullary sponge kidney
- Healed renal TB.

Clinical features: May be asymptomatic. Frequency of micturition, hematuria, polyuria, recurrent renal colic or pain in loin, and recurrent UTI.

Investigations:
- Urine routine examination and C/S
- Serum creatinine, electrolytes, calcium, phosphate, blood urea, creatinine clearance and uric acid
- Plain X-ray of KUB and USG of KUB
- Intravenous urogram
- Other investigations according to suspicion of causes.

Treatment: Treatment of primary cause. Plenty of fluid.

RENAL CALCULUS

It may occur in any part on urinary tract like kidney, ureter and bladder.

Causes:
- Dehydration (in hot environment)
- Hypercalcemia due to any cause
- Hypocalciuria
- Hyperoxaluria
- Hyperuricemia and hyperuricosuria
- Infection by proteus mirabilis (causes magnesium ammonium phosphate stone)
- Cystinuria
- Renal tubular acidosis
- Primary renal disease (APKD and medullary sponge kidney)
- *Bladder stone*: Usually due to bladder outflow obstruction, e.g. urethral stricture, BEP and presence of foreign body (e.g. catheter and nonabsorbable suture).

Types: Oxalate stone, phosphate stone, mixed stone and magnesium ammonium phosphate. Rarely, cystine, uric acid and xanthine stone.

Clinical features:
- *Renal stone*: May be asymptomatic. Renal colic, hematuria and UTI may occur
- *Ureteric stone*: Severe pain radiating from loin to groin (toward right iliac fossa or testes in male or labia in female). Sweating, vomiting, pallor and restlessness
- *Vesical calculus*: Frequency, dysuria and hematuria. Anuria and painful bladder distension, if bladder outflow obstruction.

Staghorn calculus: It is so called because calculi fill all or most of the collecting system, giving it a staghorn-like appearance. It is a phosphate stone, formed in alkaline urine.

Investigations:
- Urine RME and C/S
- Serum urea, creatinine, electrolytes, serum uric acid calcium, and phosphate
- Plain X-ray of KUB, USG of KUB and CT of KUB
- Intravenous urogram
- Sometimes retrograde pyelography.

Radiolucent stones: Uric acid and xanthine stone. All other stones are radiopaque.

Treatment:
- *During pain*: Diclofenac 75 mg intramuscular (IM) or pethidine IM
- Plenty of fluid, if needed IV infusion
- Small stone <0.5 cm may pass out spontaneously
- *Stone >1 cm*: Surgical interference.
    - ESWL (extracorporeal shock wave lithotripsy)
    - Ureteroscopy with YAG laser can be used for large stone
    - Percutaneous nephrolithotomy may be used
    - Pyelolithotomy for pelvic stone
    - Ureterolithotomy for ureteric stone
    - Open surgery is rarely needed.
- Treatment of primary cause.

RENAL CELL CARCINOMA

The tumor is adenocarcinoma, arising from proximal tubular epithelial cells. Common in elderly, 65–75 years. Males affected twice more than females.

Symptoms: Commonly presents with *triad* of painless hematuria, loin pain or heaviness, and palpable mass in loin. In 10% cases, tumor may be bilateral. In 20% cases, pyrexia of unknown origin (PUO) may be the only manifestation, due to secretion of pyrogen by the tumor. Hypertension and features of metastasis (by lymphatic to para-aortic lymph node. By blood-borne metastasis to lung, brain and bone). General features are malaise, anorexia, weight loss and features of polycythemia.

Investigations:
- Urine for RME (shows RBC) and urine for malignant cells
- Complete blood count, blood urea, creatinine, electrolytes (hypokalemia may occur), and serum calcium
- Ultrasonography of renal system is the investigation of choice
- Intravenous urogram and CT scan
- *Biopsy*: USG or CT-guided.

Treatment:
- *Nephrectomy*: Radical (includes perirenal fascial envelope and ipsilateral para-aortic lymph nodes is done, if possible). Or, partial (may be done if tumor is small, <4 cm)
- Radiotherapy is not helpful

- *Chemotherapy*: Interferon and interleukin-2 may be used in metastasis. Sunitinib, pazopanib (tyrosine kinase inhibitor), temsirolimus and everolimus may be used.

Wilms' Tumor (Nephroblastoma): It is the malignant tumor of kidney in childhood. It occurs within first 3 years, usually unilateral, but may be bilateral. May be asymptomatic. Abdominal mass may be found. Rarely, hematuria.

Investigations: Ultrasonography, CT or MRI.

Treatment: Combination of nephrectomy, radiotherapy and chemotherapy. 5-year survival is 90%.

TUMORS OF URINARY BLADDER

There are two types—Benign (papilloma) and malignant (carcinoma, usually transitional cell).

Papilloma: Patient usually presents with painless hematuria. Diagnosis is confirmed by cystoscopy. Treatment is also cystoscopic removal.

Carcinoma: Tumor usually arises from transitional epithelium causing transitional cell carcinoma. It is rare under the age of 40 years, common in males.

Causes: Exposure to industrial carcinogens like aromatic amines, aniline dyes and aldehydes, smoking, chronic inflammation or irritation due to stones or schistosomiasis.

Clinical features: Painless and macroscopic hematuria. Symptoms of obstruction, depending on the site of involvement, dysuria, urinary frequency and urgency. Features of metastasis.

Investigations:
- Urine for RME (shows RBC)
- Ultrasonography and CT urogram is gold standard. Cystoscopy is mandatory
- Intravenous urogram and CT scan of abdomen, pelvis and chest for staging.

Treatment:
- Transurethral resection of tumor by endoscope
- *Intravesical chemotherapy*: Mitomycin C is given after resection to prevent recurrence, or may be given as prolonged course to treat multiple low-grade bladder tumors
- Patient with carcinoma in situ have a high risk of progression to invasive cancer. This responds well to intravesical BCG (Bacillus Calmette-Guérin), but radical treatment may also be needed if unsuccessful
- Regular check cystoscopies are required to look for evidence of recurrence
- *If recurrences with superficial disease*: Further resection and diathermy. If unsuccessful, cystectomy may be needed
- *In invasive bladder tumor*: Radical cystectomy with urinary diversion into an incontinent ileal conduit or a continent catheterizable bowel pouch.

BENIGN ENLARGEMENT OF PROSTATE

It is common in men over the age of 60 years, cause is unknown. Enlargement of the gland stretches and distorts the urethra, obstructing bladder outflow.

Clinical features:
- Frequency of urination, usually first noted as nocturia
- Urgency of micturition, urge incontinence and hematuria
- Difficulty in voiding urine due to obstruction of the urethra by prostate and postvoid dribbling
- Hesitancy, poor urinary flow, reduction of flow after straining, and sensation of incomplete emptying
- Sometimes acute urinary retention with painful distended bladder
- *Per rectal examination*: Shows gland is smooth and soft in consistency with prominent median sulcus.

Investigations: USG with PVRV (post voidal residual volume).

Treatment:
- Patients with moderate prostatic symptoms can be treated medically
- *Drugs*: Alpha-blocker (tamsulosin 0.4 mg daily at night), finasteride or dutasteride
- *Surgery*: If deterioration in renal function or upper tract dilatation.
  - TURP (transurethral resection of prostate)
  - Other therapy: Holmium laser enucleation
  - Open prostatectomy, if suspicion of malignancy.

Prostatic Carcinoma

It is common in elderly, accounts for 7% of all cancers in men, 6th common cancer in the world. Histologically, it is an adenocarcinoma. Hormonal factors may be responsible for this.

Clinical features: May be asymptomatic.
- Frequency of micturition, nocturia, hematuria, weight loss or anemia
- *Features of metastasis*: Common in pelvic lymph node, lumber spine, pelvis, liver and lung. Per-rectal examination shows stony hard irregular gland with loss of median sulcus
- Incidental histological finding after prostatectomy.

Investigations:
- Ultrasonography, preferably TRUS (transrectal ultrasound scan)
- *Serum prostate-specific antigen*: PSA >4 ng/mL is abnormal, but between 4 ng/mL and 10 ng/mL can be due to benign hypertrophy and cancer
- Transrectal ultrasound-guided needle biopsy
- *Other investigations to see metastasis*: Isotope bone scan, CT or MRI scan of involved organ and USG of abdomen
- Endorectal coil MRI helps to detect extraprostatic extension
- X-ray of dorsolumbar spine or pelvis to see metastasis.

Treatment:
- *If confined to gland*: Radical prostatectomy, external beam radiotherapy or brachytherapy (implantation of small radioactive particles into the prostate)
- *Locally extensive disease*: Radiotherapy with or without androgen ablation therapy

- *Hormonal therapy*:
  - Orchidectomy and gonadotrophin-releasing hormone (GnRH) analogues, such as buserelin, goserelin and leuprorelin are equally effective. An alternative is gonadorelin antagonist, degarelix
  - Androgen receptor blockers: Bicalutamide, cyproterone acetate or enzalutamide
  - Androgen synthesis inhibitors such as abiraterone (act by inhibiting CYP17)
  - Corticosteroid and estrogen may also be helpful in disease refractory to castration.
- Nonhormonal chemotherapy is usually unhelpful
- *For metastases*: Orchidectomy with androgen therapy is used.

RENAL TUBULAR ACIDOSIS

It is characterized by severe metabolic acidosis associated with failure to acidify urine either due to defect in excretion of hydrogen ion by distal tubule or due to failure of absorption of bicarbonate by proximal tubule. There is failure of acidification of urine despite severe metabolic acidosis. There are four types:

Type-1 or distal tubular acidosis (DTA): It is due to failure of hydrogen ion excretion in distal tubule. There is acidosis, hypokalemia and inability to lower urine pH <5.3, despite severe acidosis and low urinary ammonium production. Causes are:
- *Congenital*: AD or AR or sex-linked
- *Autoimmune*: Sjögren's syndrome, chronic active hepatitis, primary biliary cirrhosis and SLE
- *Drugs*: Amphotericin B, lithium, NSAID and lead
- *Others*: Amyloidosis, cryoglobulinemia, obstructive uropathy and renal transplant rejection.

Treatment: Sodium bicarbonate, potassium supplement and treatment of underlying cause.

Type-2 or proximal tubular acidosis (PTA): It is due to failure of sodium bicarbonate reabsorption in proximal tubule. Common in children. Causes are congenital (AD), cystinosis, Wilson's disease, tyrosinemia, glycogen storage disease type 1, multiple myeloma, hyperparathyroidism and drugs (degraded tetracycline and carbonic anhydrase inhibitor).

In PTA, there is proximal tubular defect resulting in aminoaciduria, glycosuria and phosphaturia, called "Fanconi syndrome".

Treatment: Sodium bicarbonate in high dose, potassium supplement and treatment of underlying cause.

Type-3: Combined proximal and DTA (rare).

Type-4: It is also called hyporeninemic hypoaldosteronism. Main features are hyperkalemia and acidosis in a patient with mild CKD usually caused by tubulointerstitial disease or DM. Plasma renin and aldosterone are low.

Treatment: Fludrocortisone (0.1 mg daily) and sodium bicarbonate. Diuretic or ion exchange resin to remove potassium.

Clinical features of renal tubular acidosis:
- *Distal RTA*: May present at any age. Children presents with failure to thrive. Adult presents with renal colic, muscular weakness due to hypokalemia and osteomalacia
- *Proximal RTA*: Features of acidosis. Polydipsia, polyuria, hypokalemia, myopathy, rickets or osteomalacia.

Note: Diagnosis is suspected in any patient with hyperchloremic acidosis and can be confirmed by early morning urinary pH >5.3. If suspected, but no acidosis is present, an acid load test using ammonium chloride is done. Following this test, if urinary pH remains >5.3 despite a plasma bicarbonate of 21 mmol/L, diagnosis is confirmed.

CHAPTER 9

Rheumatology

INTRODUCTION
- Arthralgia means painful joint without swelling
- Arthritis means painful joint with swelling
- *Seropositive arthritis*: Means RA test is positive (e.g. rheumatoid arthritis)
- *Seronegative arthritis*: Means RA test is negative (e.g. ankylosing spondylitis, psoriatic arthritis, Reiter's syndrome and enteropathic arthritis)
- *Monoarticular*: Single joint involved
- *Oligoarticular or pauciarticular*: Two to four joints involved
- *Polyarticular*: Five or more joints involved
- *Migratory or fleeting*: Arthritis involving one joint and then another
- Acute arthritis means <6 weeks duration and chronic means >6 weeks duration
- *Features of inflammatory arthritis*: Pain at rest, increases with activity or exercise. Morning stiffness, joint inflammation, and loss of function
- *Noninflammatory (mechanical) arthritis*: More painful with activity and improves with rest.

Causes of monoarthritis: (Remember the mnemonic: GRASP-TH)—
- *G*: Gout
- *RA*: Reactive arthritis
- *S*: Septic arthritis (pyogenic)
- *P*: Pseudogout
- *T*: Trauma and tuberculous
- *H*: Hemophilia (in early age).

Note: In children, septic arthritis and juvenile idiopathic arthritis (JIA) are common. Hemophilic arthritis, leukemia, and osteomyelitis may occur.

Causes of polyarthritis:
- Infective (bacterial and viral)
- *Inflammatory*: Rheumatic fever, RA and its variants, seronegative arthritis, JIA (<16 years), and collagen disease [systemic lupus erythematosus (SLE), dermatomyositis, systemic sclerosis and polyarteritis nodosa]

- Degenerative (osteoarthrosis)
- Metabolic (gout and pseudogout)
- Neuropathic arthropathy (Charcot's joint)
- *Hematological*: Hemophilic arthritis and Henoch–Schönlein purpura
- *Others*: Polymyalgia rheumatica, sarcoidosis, hemochromatosis, acromegaly and hypertrophic.

SPONDYLOARTHROPATHY OR SPONDARTHRITIS

Group of inflammatory arthritis characterized by:
- Seronegative rheumatoid factor (RA test is negative)
- Sacroiliitis and inflammatory spondylitis
- Asymmetrical inflammatory oligoarthritis (lower > upper limbs and bigger joints are involved)
- Inflammatory enthesitis
- Absence of nodules and other extra-articular features of RA
- *Typical overlapping extra-articular features*: Mucosal inflammation (conjunctivitis, buccal ulceration, urethritis, prostatitis and bowel ulceration), pustular skin lesions, nail dystrophy, anterior uveitis, aortic root fibrosis (AR and conduction defects) and erythema nodosum
- Familial association (high in HLA-B27).

Diseases in spondyloarthropathy: Ankylosing spondylitis, Reiter's syndrome or reactive arthritis, enteropathic arthritis (Crohn's disease and ulcerative colitis), and psoriatic arthritis.

Ankylosing Spondylitis

It is a chronic inflammatory arthritis characterized by progressive stiffening and fusion of axial skeleton. Common in young adults, 20–40 years, Male:Female = 3:1. Cause is unknown, probably autoimmune.

Symptoms: Low back pain with morning stiffness, worse in the morning and with inactivity. Pain improves after exercise. Peripheral arthritis occurs in 10% cases.

Signs: Loss of lumbar lordosis, thoracic kyphosis and compensatory hyperextension of neck. In advanced stage, *question mark "?"* or stooped posture. The patient is unable to look up and turn to any side without movement of whole body. Restricted movement of spine in all directions. Standing against the wall, the patient is unable to make contact between occiput of head and wall. Sacroiliitis, Achilles tendinitis and plantar fasciitis are present.

Extra-articular manifestations of ankylosing spondylitis:
- *Eyes*: Anterior uveitis (iritis) and conjunctivitis
- *Heart*: Aortic regurgitation, mitral regurgitation and conduction defect
- *Lungs*: Upper lobe fibrosis, cavitation, chest pain (pleuritic), reduced chest expansion, pulmonary hypertension and cor pulmonale
- *Neurological*: Cauda equina syndrome (weakness of lower limbs, loss of sphincter, and rectal control with saddle sensory loss)
- *Others*: Plantar fasciitis, Achilles tendinitis, amyloidosis, osteoporosis and prostatitis.

Investigations:
- X-ray of sacroiliac (SI) joints and spine (lumbosacral, dorsal and cervical)
- Complete blood count (CBC) with erythrocyte sedimentation rate (ESR) (may be high)
- C-reactive protein (CRP) (may be high), rheumatoid factor is negative, and human leukocyte antigen (HLA) B27 (positive in 90%).

X-ray shows:
- *Sacroiliitis*: Irregularities, marginal sclerosis and later fusion of SI joint
- *In lumbodorsal spine*: Squaring of vertebrae, syndesmophyte formation, ossification of anterior longitudinal ligament and bamboo spine appearance.

Treatment:
- Exercise (swimming is the best). Prolonged sitting or inactivity should be avoided
- Nonsteroidal anti-inflammatory drug (NSAID) to relieve pain
- Physiotherapy
- *Disease modifying anti-rheumatic drug (DMARD)*: Sulfasalazine or methotrexate (MTX)
- *In persistent active inflammation*: Anti-TNF (tumor necrosis factor) drug therapy (etanercept and infliximab)
- Local steroid injection for persistent plantar fasciitis, other enthesopathies, and peripheral arthritis. High dose steroid may be needed for acute uveitis
- *Orthopedic measures*: For severe hip, knee or shoulder restriction.

Rheumatoid Arthritis

It is a chronic autoimmune, inflammatory, destructive and deforming polyarthritis characterized by bilateral symmetrical involvement of small and large joints with systemic and extra-articular features with exacerbations and remissions. Common in female, 30–50 years. Before menopause, three times more in female. After menopause, sex ratio is almost equal.

Symptoms: Polyarthritis, mainly involving small joints of hands and feet. Morning stiffness lasting >1 hour, improves with activity. There may be extra-articular manifestations.

Signs in hand: Spindle-shaped swelling of proximal interphalangeal joints. Swan neck deformity, boutonniere deformity, Z-deformity of thumb, ulnar deviation and dorsal subluxation of ulnar styloid. Wrist joints may be swollen. Generalized wasting of small muscles of hands with dorsal guttering [distal interphalangeal (DIP) joint is not involved].

Signs in other joints: In foot, loss of arch causing flat foot, dorsal subluxation of metatarsophalangeal joints. In knee, swelling, tenderness, Baker's cyst in popliteal fossa.

Extra-articular manifestations in RA:
- *Eye*: Episcleritis, scleritis, scleromalacia, scleromalacia perforans and keratoconjunctivitis sicca
- *Respiratory*: Pleurisy, pleural effusion, fibrosing alveolitis and lung nodule (Caplan's syndrome)

- *Cardiac*: Pericarditis, pericardial effusion (rare), and chronic constrictive pericarditis (rare)
- *Vasculitis*: Digital arteritis, nailfold infarct, Raynaud's phenomenon, visceral arteritis, mononeuritis multiplex and pyoderma gangrenosum
- *Neurological*: Entrapment neuropathy, commonly carpal tunnel syndrome (median nerve compression), and tarsal tunnel syndrome (posterior tibial nerve compression), peripheral neuropathy, mononeuritis multiplex, and cervical cord compression (due to atlantoaxial subluxation)
- *Hematological*: Anemia, thrombocytosis and pancytopenia
- *Others*: Lymphadenopathy, splenomegaly, osteoporosis, general features (malaise, fever, weakness, loss of weight and wasting), and amyloidosis.

Investigations:
- Complete blood count with ESR (ESR is high and pancytopenia in Felty's syndrome)
- Rheumatoid arthritis test, ACPA (anti-citrullinated protein antibody), and CRP (high)
- X-ray of hands and other involved joints, and chest X-ray
- Urine analysis (proteinuria, may occur in amyloidosis).

Treatment:
- *Relief of symptoms*: Rest and NSAID, and physiotherapy
- *Suppression of activity and progression*: DMARD
- Surgical treatment may be needed.

Disease modifying anti-rheumatic drugs:
- *First choice*: Sulfasalazine and MTX
- *Other drugs*: Chloroquine, hydroxychloroquine, leflunomide, azathioprine and cyclosporine
- Disease modifying anti-rheumatic drug should be started, may take 4–12 weeks for response. If no effect in 6–12 weeks, combination may be given. Prednisolone 7.5–10 mg may be added
- *Biological therapy*: Anti-TNF-a, anti-interleukin-1 (IL-1), and rituximab are more effective than other DMARDs in preventing joint erosions. If disease activity persists after use of two DMARDs, biological therapy should be considered.

Methotrexate: 7.5–10 mg, in a fixed day weekly (up to 25 mg). Folic acid 5 mg/day should be given on the next day. Folinic acid is more preferable.

Sulfasalazine: Started with low dose, increase the dose every week. Initially, 250 mg (half tablet) twice daily for 1 week. Then 500 mg (one tablet) twice daily for 1 week. Then 1,000 mg (two tablets) twice daily to be continued (maximum dose 2–3 g daily).

Chloroquine: 250 mg daily as a single dose. Or hydroxychloroquine, 200–400 mg daily. Alone in mild disease or with other DMARD.

Leflunomide: 100 mg daily for 3 days, then 10–20 mg daily.

SJÖGREN'S SYNDROME

It is an autoimmune disorder characterized by dryness of eye (keratoconjunctivitis sicca) and dryness of mouth (xerostomia) with nonerosive arthritis. Fibrosis and atrophy of salivary glands occur. There is infiltration of lymphocytes and plasma cells in lacrimal and salivary glands.

Types: There are two types—
1. *Primary*: Not associated with collagen disease (sicca syndrome)
2. *Secondary*: Associated with collagen disease (commonly RA).

Clinical features of primary Sjögren's syndrome: Common in female, F:M = 9:1, 40–50 years.
- Dryness of mouth and eyes. Arthralgia and nonprogressive arthritis
- Raynaud's phenomenon and dysphagia
- *In lung*: Pulmonary diffusion defect and fibrosis
- Renal tubular acidosis and nephrogenic diabetes insipidus
- Vasculitis, fever, weakness, lymphadenopathy, neuropathy, convulsion, and depression
- High incidence of non-Hodgkin's B cell lymphoma
- May be associated with other autoimmune disease [thyroid disease, myasthenia gravis, primary biliary cholangitis (PBC) and autoimmune hepatitis].

Investigations:
- Complete blood count (high ESR)
- Schirmer's test (a strip of filter paper is placed inside lower eyelid. If it is <10 mm in 5 minutes, it indicates defective tear production)
- Biopsy of lip or salivary gland (shows lymphocytic and plasma cell infiltration)
- Rose Bengal staining of eyes shows punctate or filamentary keratitis
- *Antibody test*: RA test (positive in 90%), antinuclear antibody (ANA) (positive in 80%), anti-Ro (SSA, positive in 60–90%. It can cross placenta causing congenital complete heart block in newborn baby). Anti-La (SS-B) and antimitochondrial antibody (positive in 10%).

Treatment: Treat the primary cause, if any.
- Artificial tear (hypromellose), contact lens, oral hygiene, artificial saliva and oral gel. Stimulation of saliva flow by sugar-free chewing gum or lozenge may be helpful
- Oral candidiasis should be treated promptly
- Vaginal dryness is treated with lubricants such as K-Y jelly
- Hydroxychloroquine (2–3 mg/kg daily, may improve the flow of tear)
- Steroid may be needed. Immunosuppressive drugs can be added.

SYSTEMIC SCLEROSIS (SCLERODERMA)

It is a connective tissue disease characterized by fibrosis and degenerative changes in skin, blood vessels and internal organs.

Types: There are two types—
1. *Diffuse cutaneous systemic sclerosis (DCSS, 30%)*: Skin involvement of trunk and extremities above the knee and elbow
2. *Limited cutaneous systemic sclerosis (LCSS, 70%)*: Skin involvement only at the extremities, hands, feet or forearm. Pulmonary hypertension is common.

Other varieties (localized):
- *Scleroderma sine scleroderma*: Involves internal organ without skin lesion
- *Morphea*: Localized, plaque with central hypopigmentation and tethering of skin
- *Linear*: Skin involvement usually in lower limbs.

Clinical features: Common in female (F:M = 4:1), age 30–50 years.
- *Raynaud's phenomenon*: 90–97% cases. May occur before other symptoms
- Tightening and thickening of skin of hands and other parts of the body
- Arthralgia and arthritis (nonerosive inflammatory)
- Heartburn (reflux esophagitis), dysphagia and odynophagia. Occasionally, diarrhea and constipation (blind loop syndrome)
- Shortness of breath and cough [diffuse parenchymal lung disease (DPLD)]

Investigations: Diagnosis is usually clinical.
- Complete blood count and ESR (high)
- *Serology*: RA test, ANA, anti-topoisomerase I or anti-Scl-70 and anti-centromere antibody
- Skin biopsy for histopathology
- *Others*: Urine routine examination (may be proteinuria), serum urea, creatinine, electrolytes, X-ray of hands and chest, lung function tests, barium swallow, barium follow through, electrocardiogram (ECG) and immunoglobulin G (IgG) level (raised).

Treatment:
- *For Raynaud's phenomenon*:
  - Avoidance of cold, smoking should be stopped, regular exercise and cleanliness of digital ulcer
  - *Drugs to be avoided*: Beta-blocker, ergotamine and oral contraceptive
  - *Antiplatelet*: Aspirin or clopidogrel, calcium antagonist (nifedipine), angiotensin-converting enzyme (ACE) inhibitor, and angiotensin receptor blocker (ARB) (valsartan) may be effective
  - *If no response or severe*: Prostacyclin analog epoprostenol infusion intermittently. If still no response—surgical treatment. If gangrene—amputation of fingers or toes.
- *For arthritis*: NSAIDs and physiotherapy
- *Other treatment*: MTX (weekly 7.5–15 mg), cyclosporine and penicillamine.

Limited cutaneous systemic sclerosis (CRST or CREST): It is a syndrome characterized by—
- *C*: Calcinosis
- *R*: Raynaud's phenomenon
- *E*: Esophageal involvement (dysphagia)
- *S*: Sclerodactyly
- *T*: Telangiectasia

Anticentromere antibody is present in 70–80% cases.

MIXED CONNECTIVE TISSUE DISEASE

It is the combination of systemic sclerosis, SLE and polymyositis (or other collagen disease, e.g. RA). It is also called overlap syndrome. Common in female, 30–40 years.
- Patient usually presents with Raynaud's phenomenon, muscular pain or weakness, and swollen, edematous hands and fingers. Later, features like sclerodactyly, calcinosis and cutaneous telangiectasia. Skin rash of SLE or dermatomyositis. Sjögren's syndrome may develop later
- May be lung, heart, kidney and gastrointestinal tract (GIT) involvement.

Investigations: Anti-RNP (ribonucleoprotein) antibody (high), ANA (positive), anti-Scl 70 (may be positive), and creatine phosphokinase (CPK) (high). Other investigations—CBC and ESR (high), and X-ray of chest.

Treatment: Prednisolone, which responds quickly. 10 years survival in 80% cases.

GOUT

It is a disorder of purine metabolism characterized by hyperuricemia associated with deposition of monosodium urate monohydrate (MSUM) crystals causing arthritis, tenosynovitis, bursitis and tophaceous deposit. There are two types—primary (cause is unknown) and secondary (due to underlying disease).

Secondary causes of gout:
- *Defect in renal excretion*:
    - Renal failure
    - Drugs diuretic (thiazides), low-dose aspirin, pyrazinamide, ethambutol, nicotinic acid, ethanol, cytotoxic drug and cyclosporine
    - Others: Hyperparathyroidism, myxedema, chronic lead poisoning and Down syndrome.
- *Excess production of uric acid*: Myeloproliferative disease, lymphoproliferative disease, psoriasis, idiopathic (common) and tumor lysis syndrome.

Symptoms: In typical acute attack, severe pain mainly metatarsophalangeal joint of great toe, usually in early morning or late night, awaking the patient from sleep. Other joints are also involved.

Signs: Joint is red, swollen and tender. In chronic tophaceous gout, repeated attack may cause deformity with swelling of joints, commonly DIP joints. There may be tophus.

Investigations: Diagnosis is clinical and investigations are done for secondary causes:
- Complete blood count, ESR (high), and leukemia should be excluded. CRP (high)
- Urea and creatinine [to exclude chronic kidney disease (CKD)]
- Blood sugar and lipid profile. X-ray of joint
- *To confirm*: Aspiration of joint fluid to see MSUM crystal (needle shaped).

Treatment:
- *For pain*: NSAID (indomethacin, naproxen, and diclofenac, oral or suppository)
- *If no response*: Colchicine 0.5 mg 2 or 3 times daily till relief of symptoms
- *In severe arthritis and effusion*: Aspiration and intra-articular steroid may be given
- *Other treatment*:
    - Dietary restriction: Avoid uric acid containing diet (liver, kidney, brain, red meat, cabbage, cauliflower, carrot and spinach)
    - Avoid alcohol and starvation, slow reduction of weight, if obese. Avoid precipitating drugs
    - Allopurinol: 100 mg/day, 50 mg in elderly and renal failure. Doses increase slowly. Febuxostat is also helpful
    - Allopurinol or febuxostat should not be given in acute attack, start after several weeks.

OSTEOARTHRITIS

It is a degenerative disease of joint characterized by degeneration of articular cartilage with proliferation of new bone and remodeling of joint contour. Commonly involves weight bearing joints (knee and ankle).

Type: There are two types—
1. *Primary*: Unknown cause
2. *Secondary*: To some other diseases, usually asymmetrical. Causes are—
   - Trauma
   - Congenital or developmental
   - Inflammatory: RA, septic arthritis, gout and hemophilic arthritis
   - Neuropathic joints (Charcot's joint)
   - Endocrine diseases: Acromegaly and hyperparathyroidism
   - Metabolic: Hemochromatosis, alkaptonuria, Wilson's disease and chondrocalcinosis.

Symptoms: Pain of affected joints, increases with activity and diminishes with rest. Commonly knee and hip joints are involved. Limitation of movement.

Signs: Joints are swollen with restricted movement. Later on joint deformity may occur. Crepitus on movement of joints. In hand, bony swelling at the proximal (Bouchard's node) and distal (Heberden's node) interphalangeal joints. DIP joints are commonly involved.

Investigation: X-ray of joints.

Treatment:
- Explanation and reassurance, patient's education, regular exercise, and weight reduction, if obese. Use of appropriate footwear and walking stick
- *For pain*: Paracetamol and NSAID. Intra-articular steroid may be needed
- Chondroitin sulfate and glucosamine sulfate may be helpful. Intra-articular hyaluronic acid is also helpful
- *Others*: Physiotherapy. Surgery in some cases (osteotomy and joint replacement).

OSTEOPOROSIS

It is a metabolic bone disease characterized by reduction of bone mass with increased risk of fracture. Ratio of osteoid tissue to calcium and phosphate is normal (calcium, phosphate and alkaline phosphatase are normal). Bone matrix is decreased, but mineralization is normal.

Causes:
- Postmenopausal
- Senile
- *Secondary*:
  - Endocrine: Hypogonadism, hyperparathyroidism, hyperthyroidism and Cushing's syndrome
  - Inflammatory disease: Ankylosing spondylitis and RA
  - Drugs: Corticosteroid, anticonvulsant and alcohol excess
  - Gastrointestinal tract: Malabsorption and chronic liver disease
  - Genetic disease: Osteogenesis imperfecta, homocystinuria and Ehlers–Danlos syndrome
  - Others: Smoking, prolonged immobilization, CKD, multiple myeloma and anorexia nervosa

Symptoms: Usually asymptomatic, may present with spontaneous fracture (neck of femur), back pain, collapse of a vertebrae (with loss of height), and kyphoscoliosis.

Signs: No specific sign.

Investigations:
- *X-ray of bone*: Shows reduction of bone density (osteopenia)
- Serum calcium, phosphate and alkaline phosphatase (all are normal)
- Serum 25-hydroxy vitamin (low)
- Bone mineral density by dual-energy X-ray absorptiometry (DEXA) is gold standard.

Treatment:
- *General*: Smoking must be stopped, alcohol restriction and weight reduction. Exercise and physiotherapy. Adequate calcium and vitamin D in diet. Calcium 800–1,000 mg/day and vitamin D 400–800 IU/day. Calcitriol may be given
- *Drug therapy*:
    - *Bisphosphonate*: Alendronate (10 mg/day or 70 mg weekly), risedronate (5 mg/day or 30 mg weekly), zoledronic acid [5 mg intravenous (IV) yearly], and ibandronate (150 mg monthly)
    - Denosumab (60 mg subcutaneous every 6 months)
    - Hormone replacement therapy in early menopause, if no contraindication (risk of breast cancer and cardiovascular disease).

PSORIATIC ARTHRITIS

It is a seronegative arthritis associated with psoriasis, occurs in 7–20% of patients with psoriasis.

Types: There are five types of arthritis in psoriasis—
1. Asymmetrical inflammatory oligoarthritis—40%
2. Symmetrical seronegative polyarthritis (like rheumatoid)—25%
3. Sacroiliitis or spondylitis—15%. More among males
4. Predominant DIP joint arthritis—15% (typical), and nail dystrophy is invariable
5. Arthritis mutilans—5%.

Symptoms: Mainly pain and swelling in the affected joints with history of psoriasis.

Signs: Patch of psoriatic lesions. Joint may be swollen and tender.

Extra-articular features: Typical psoriatic patch, nail change (nail pitting, horizontal ridging, thickening of nail, onycholysis and subungual hyperkeratosis), and eye (conjunctivitis and uveitis).

Investigations: CBC, ESR (may be high), CRP (high), RA, antinuclear factor (negative), and serum uric acid (may be high). X-ray of the joint.

Treatment:
- For psoriasis: General measures, local therapy and systemic therapy (see in dermatology)
- *Treatment of arthritis*:
    - Nonsteroidal anti-inflammatory drug for pain
    - In persistent and progressive: MTX, sulfasalazine and azathioprine (helpful in both skin lesion and arthritis). Cyclosporine is also helpful

- Biological agents: Monoclonal antibody (infliximab and etanercept, if other drugs fail)
- Acitretin 20 mg daily, effective in arthritis and skin lesion (avoid in young female, it is teratogenic). Steroid may be needed (sometimes, given intra-articularly)
- Psoralen and ultraviolet A (PUVA) for skin lesion.

Note: Drugs to be avoided in psoriasis—chloroquine, hydroxychloroquine, beta blocker, ACE inhibitor, lithium and alcohol.

SYSTEMIC LUPUS ERYTHEMATOSUS

It is an autoimmune chronic multisystem disease characterized by production of multiple autoantibodies, immune complexes, and multiple immune-mediated organ damage. Common in young females, F:M = 9:1, 20–40 years. Sex ratio is equal in children and elderly.

Symptoms:
- Fever, arthritis and arthralgia, butterfly photosensitive rash, oral ulcer and alopecia
- *In female*: History of repeated abortion
- Other features according to involvement of multiple organs.

Different systems involved in SLE:
- *Heart*: Pericarditis, pericardial effusion, myocarditis and mitral regurgitation. Noninfective endocarditis called Libman–Sacks endocarditis
- *Vascular*: Raynaud's phenomenon, vasculitis, and arterial and venous thrombosis
- *Lungs*: Pleural effusion (may be bilateral) and pneumonitis
- *Eyes*: Episcleritis, scleritis, optic neuritis, Sjögren's syndrome and retinal vasculitis
- *Gastrointestinal tract*: Mouth ulcer, mesenteric vasculitis causing small bowel infarction or perforation.
- *Hematological*: Thrombocytopenia, leukopenia and autoimmune hemolytic anemia
- *Neurological*: Epilepsy, migraine, cerebrovascular disease (CVD), psychosis, depression, transverse myelitis, lymphocytic meningitis, cerebellar ataxia, cranial nerve palsy and peripheral neuropathy
- *Kidney*: Glomerulonephritis, nephrotic syndrome and renal vein thrombosis
- *Others*: Lymphadenopathy, splenomegaly, hepatomegaly, fever and weight loss.

Drugs causing SLE: Hydralazine, procainamide, anticonvulsant (carbamazepine and phenytoin), phenothiazine, isonicotinylhydrazide (INH), oral contraceptive pill, ACE inhibitor, penicillamine, methyldopa and minocycline. Drugs causing SLE usually do not aggravate primary SLE.

Features of drug-induced SLE: Sex ratio is equal. Lung involvement is common, but renal and neurological involvement is rare. ANA is usually positive, but anti-double-stranded deoxyribonucleic acid (anti-dsDNA) is negative. Complements are normal. Antihistone antibody is positive in 95%.

Treatment: Withdrawal of drugs. Short course of prednisolone.

Investigations in SLE:
- Complete blood count (thrombocytopenia) and ESR (high)
- Urine [proteinuria, hematuria, red blood cell (RBC) or granular cast] and 24 hour urinary protein
- *C-reactive protein*: Normal (if CRP is high, it indicates infection)
- Antinuclear antibody is positive in 95%. Anti-dsDNA-positive in 30–50%
- Anti-Sm (Smith) antibody is positive in 10–25%
- *Complements*: C3 and C4 (low in active disease)
- Serum antiphospholipid antibody
- *If renal or central nervous system (CNS) involvement*: Investigate accordingly.

Treatment:
- *General measures*: Explanation, reassurance and psychological support
- *Drug therapy*:
  - Mild cases: NSAID (if fever, arthralgia and headache). Chloroquine or hydroxychloroquine (in skin lesion, arthritis, arthralgia, and serositis without organ involvement). Short course of prednisolone (in skin rash, synovitis and pleuropericarditis)
  - In severe and active disease: Prednisolone should be given
  - Acute life-threatening SLE: High dose steroid and immunosuppressive drug. Pulse methylprednisolone (500 mg to 1 g IV) daily for 3–5 days, followed by oral prednisolone. Cyclophosphamide (2 mg/kg IV) may be given.

Pregnancy with SLE: Not contraindicated. The disease should be in remission and pregnancy should be avoided, if there is neurological, renal, and cardiac abnormality. Repeated abortion (due to presence of antiphospholipid antibody), stillbirth, and intrauterine growth retardation may occur. Relapse may occur in the first trimester and in puerperium. If the mother has "anti-Ro antibody" (SSA), there may be congenital complete heart block of the baby due to transplacental transfer of antibody. Treatment—Prednisolone should be continued.

POLYMYOSITIS AND DERMATOMYOSITIS

It is nonsuppurative and noninfective inflammation of skeletal muscle of unknown cause, characterized by necrosis, fibrosis and regeneration of muscles. When associated with skin rash, it is called dermatomyositis.

Types: There are five types—
1. Primary idiopathic polymyositis
2. Primary idiopathic dermatomyositis
3. Dermatomyositis or polymyositis associated with neoplasia
4. Childhood dermatomyositis or polymyositis associated with vasculitis
5. Dermatomyositis or polymyositis associated with collagen vascular disease.

Causes of dermatomyositis: Unknown. May be autoimmune, associated with malignancy (commonly bronchial carcinoma in male and ovarian carcinoma in female).

Clinical features: Common in female, F:M = 2:1, age 50–60 years. Progressive muscular weakness and wasting of proximal muscles (shoulder and pelvic girdle). Skin rash, typically affects upper eye lids with erythema called "heliotrope rash", erythematous rash in different parts of body. Pharyngeal, laryngeal, and respiratory muscle involvement may cause dysphagia, dysphonia, and respiratory failure. Arthralgia, arthritis, myalgia, Raynaud's phenomenon and acute renal failure may occur.

Investigations:
- Complete blood count and ESR (high). CPK (very high, most sensitive test)
- Electromyography (EMG)
- Muscle biopsy
- *Other tests*:
    - To exclude malignancy [chest X-ray, ultrasonography (USG), computed tomography (CT) scan, magnetic resonance imaging (MRI), positron emission tomography (PET) scan, mammogram, GIT imaging]
    - Rheumatoid arthritis test and ANA (positive in 50% cases). Anti-Jo-1 antibody is more specific.

Treatment:
- Prednisolone 0.5–1 mg/kg daily. Continue for 1 month, then taper slowly. Maintenance dose 5–7.5 mg daily, may be required for months, even years
- *If severe case*: Methylprednisolone 1 g daily for 3 days. Then, prednisolone
- *If no response*: MTX *or* azathioprine *or* cyclosporine *or* cyclophosphamide *or* mycophenolate mofetil may be given. High dose IV Ig may help in some cases
- Treatment of underlying malignancy may improve the condition
- Physiotherapy.

TUBERCULOSIS OF BONE OR JOINT

Any joint or bone may be involved, commonly knee and hip. Organism is *Mycobacterium tuberculosis*. In children, it occurs as primary disease. In adult, it is due to hematogenous spread from lung.

Symptoms: Pain and swelling of involved joint with deformity. General features like fever, night sweating and weight loss may be present.

Signs: Joint is swollen and tender, may be stiff with deformity and limitation of movement. Joint effusion may be present.

Investigations:
- Complete blood count (ESR is high usually)
- X-ray of chest posteroanterior (PA) view and X-ray of involved joints
- Mantoux test (MT)
- CT scan or MRI of joint
- Fine-needle aspiration cytology (FNAC) (CT or USG-guided)
- Arthroscopy and biopsy may be needed. If effusion is present, aspiration and analysis of the fluid may be done
- Sometimes open biopsy.

Treatment:
- Standard anti-Koch's therapy comprising four drugs, continued for at least 1 year
- Prednisolone may be added.

TUBERCULOSIS OF SPINE (POTT DISEASE)

It is also called tuberculous spondylitis, usually due to reactivation of dormant hematogenous focus. Rarely, spread from local paravertebral lymph node. Infection starts at intervertebral disc (diskitis), then spread along the spinal ligaments to involve the adjacent margins of vertebral body, causes erosion and destruction of disc and vertebral body. There is collapse of vertebra, causing anterior wedging of one or more adjacent vertebrae and "gibbus" formation. Also, paravertebral abscess formation.

Symptoms: Usually back pain, mainly lower thoracic and lumbar spine. Swelling (due to gibbus) with restriction of movement. General features of tuberculosis (TB) such as fever, malaise, night, sweating and loss of weight. Features of complications (e.g. paraplegia).

Signs: Local tenderness over spine, gibbus (swelling over spine), and paravertebral abscess. If spinal cord compression, spastic (if lesion is above L1) or flaccid (if lesion is below L1) paraplegia.

Investigations:
- Complete blood count (ESR is high usually)
- X-ray of chest PA view (primary focus may be seen). X-ray of spine shows collapse of vertebrae, may be paravertebral shadow
- MT
- CT scan or MRI of spine
- Fine-needle aspiration cytology (CT or USG-guided)
- Occasionally, open biopsy may be needed.

Treatment:
- Standard anti-Koch's therapy comprising four drugs for 2 months. Then, INH and rifampicin continued for another 10 months, even more
- Prednisolone may be added
- *If spastic paraplegia*: Standard anti-Koch's therapy. Neurosurgical intervention (decompression and drainage of abscess).

REITER'S SYNDROME

It is a seronegative arthritis characterized by arthritis, conjunctivitis and urethritis. Reactive arthritis means when only arthritis follows after an attack of diarrhea or dysentery or sexual exposure (pathology in one site, but affecting the joints), and no conjunctivitis. It is actually a variety of Reiter's syndrome. Organisms are *Salmonella, Shigella, Campylobacter, Chlamydia* and *Yersinia*. It is common in male (M:F = 15:1), 16–35 years of age.

Triad of Reiter's syndrome: Arthritis, conjunctivitis and urethritis (nonspecific).

Features:
- History of urethritis, diarrhea or dysentery and sexual exposure. After 1–3 weeks, asymmetrical oligoarthritis involving the bigger joints (knee and ankle), conjunctivitis, and urethritis
- *Extra-articular features*: Conjunctivitis and iritis, skin rash (macular, vesicular or pustular), Achilles tendinitis, plantar fasciitis, circinate balanitis, keratoderma blennorrhagica (in palm, sole or toes), nail dystrophy, and buccal erosion.

Investigations:
- Complete blood count and ESR (high). CRP (high)
- *Urine*: Shows pus cells, sterile on routine culture (sterile pyuria)
- Rheumatoid arthritis test and ANA (negative)
- X-ray of the joints involved and SI joint
- *If joint effusion is present*: Aspiration of fluid and analysis
- HLA-B27 positive in 70% cases
- Serology and cultures (blood, urine, stool, cervix and urethra), particularly for chlamydia.

Treatment:
- Rest and NSAID for pain. Sometimes, intra-articular steroid injection
- Antibiotic (tetracycline or azithromycin for nongonococcal urethritis)
- Short course prednisolone may be given
- *In recurrent and remitting arthritis*: Sulfasalazine *or* MTX *or* azathioprine
- In severe case, high dose steroid may be given. Anti-TNF may be helpful
- Physiotherapy.

ACUTE OSTEOMYELITIS

It is the primary infection in bone. Any part of bone may be involved. The infection causes localized areas of osteonecrosis (bone death). A separated part of dead is called "sequestrum". Perforation of cortex by pus stimulates local new bone formation ("involucrum") by the subperiosteum and periosteum, often with sinuses that discharge through the skin.

Causes:
- Hematogenous, direct infection may complicate a compound fracture, penetrating injury or orthopedic surgery
- *Organisms are*: *Staphylococci* (90%), *Streptococci*, *Haemophilus influenzae*, and *Salmonella*
- *Risk factors*: Childhood and adolescence, diabetes mellitus, acquired immunodeficiency syndrome (AIDS), and sickle cell disease.

Clinical features: Pain at the site of infection, swelling and redness, and child may limp. High fever with chill and rigor. Sinus tract with discharge of pus may be present. Chronic infection may be associated with abscess within the bone (Brodie abscess).

Investigations:
- Complete blood count and ESR. Blood for culture/sensitivity
- *X-ray of involved bone*: After 1–2 weeks, shows radiolucent lesion and periosteal elevation. Reactive sclerosis will be absent
- CT or MRI.

Treatment:
- *For pain*: NSAID
- Intravenous broad-spectrum antibiotic for at least 2 weeks, then oral antibiotic for at least 4 weeks
- Surgical decompression and removal of any dead bone
- Rehabilitation.

HEMOPHILIC ARTHRITIS

Hemarthrosis occurs, if plasma factor VIII is <1%. Arthritis may be spontaneous without trauma or may follow even minor trauma.

Symptoms: Commonly knee, elbow, ankle and hip joints are involved. Joint is red, hot, swollen and painful. Progression of arthritis may cause ankylosis of joint.

Treatment:
- Complete rest, if needed splinting of joint
- *Factor VIII transfusion*: 20–30 IU/kg, repeated after 12 hours, 24 hours and 36 hours
- Analgesic may be given (paracetamol or acetaminophen or codeine). Aspirin or other NSAIDs are avoided
- After acute stage, the patient should be mobilized and physiotherapy should be started
- Arthrocentesis (aspiration from joint) is rarely necessary
- To prevent recurrent bleeding into the joint, patient with severe hemophilia is given factor VIII infusions regularly three times per week.

JUVENILE IDIOPATHIC ARTHRITIS

When arthritis develops before 16 years of age and persists for more than 3 months.

Types:
- *Systemic onset (Still's disease)*: Characterized by fever, skin rash, arthritis, hepatosplenomegaly and serositis
- *Oligoarthritis (pauciarticular)*: Four or less joints are affected
- *Polyarthritis*: More than four joints are affected
- *Others*: Enthesitis-related JIA, psoriatic arthritis and atypical JIA.

Investigations:
- Complete blood count with ESR (leukocytosis, may be lymphocytosis, thrombocytosis and high ESR)
- C-reactive protein (high), ACPA (negative), and RA test (usually negative, positive in 10% cases)
- Antinuclear antibody and anti-dsDNA (if SLE is suspected)
- X-ray of involved joint. Other investigations to exclude other diseases.

Features of systemic onset JIA (Still's disease):
- *Arthritis*: Involving knee, wrist and ankle. Other joints may be involved
- *Fever*: High and intermittent, and may be continuous
- *Skin rash*: Appears with fever and disappears when fever subsides. These are macular or maculopapular, salmon pink color rashes (Salmon rash)
- *Extra-articular features*: Hepatosplenomegaly and lymphadenopathy (common). May be pericardial effusion, pleural effusion, and disseminated intravascular coagulation (DIC)
- *In chronic case*: Small mandible, fusion of cervical spine, and growth retardation.

Treatment:
- *General measures*: Explanation and reassurance to the parents. NSAID for pain. Rest and passive movement of limb to prevent contracture and physiotherapy
- *In severe case*: Prednisolone. Pulse methylprednisolone may be given and followed by MTX
- *Disease modifying drugs*: MTX (5 mg weekly, increase gradually), sulfasalazine (30–50 mg/kg daily). If no response, anti-TNF may be given.
- Orthopedic surgery, if needed.

CHAPTER 10

Dermatology

INTRODUCTION

Layers of skin: Consists of three layers
- *Epidermis*: It has five layers from top to bottom, they are
  - Stratum corneum (horny layer)
  - Stratum lucidum
  - Stratum granulosum (granular layer)
  - Stratum spinosum (prickle cell or malpighian layer)
  - Stratum basale (basal layer).
- Dermis
- Hypodermis or subcutis.

Epidermis is an avascular stratified squamous epithelium, attached to dermis by basement membrane. Basal cells move outward toward superficial horny layer, time taken is 4 weeks. Of the total, 95% cells of epidermis are keratinocytes, and 5% are Langerhans cells and melanocytes. Also, few Merkel cells. Dermis contains blood and lymphatic vessels, nerves, muscle, appendages and immune cells such as mast cells and lymphocytes. Also, collagen, elastin, and ground substance.

Appendages of the skin: Nail, hair, sebaceous gland and sweat gland.

ITCHING OR PRURITUS

Itching is due to skin disease and systemic (or medical) disease.

Skin diseases: Eczema, scabies, dermatitis herpetiformis, lichen planus and urticaria.

Systemic disease:
- *Liver disease*: Obstructive jaundice and primary biliary cirrhosis
- *Renal*: Chronic kidney disease
- *Hematological*: Polycythemia rubra vera (after hot bath), lymphoma (Hodgkin's disease), leukemia, multiple myeloma and iron deficiency anemia
- *Endocrine*: Hypothyroidism, thyrotoxicosis and diabetes mellitus (DM) (associated with candidiasis)

- *Others*: Any internal malignancy, human immunodeficiency virus (HIV), psychogenic and senile pruritus.

Dermatological manifestations of internal malignancy:
- *Dermatomyositis*: Found in bronchial carcinoma, malignancy of gastrointestinal tract (GIT) and genitourinary
- *Acanthosis nigricans*: Found in malignancies of GIT, lung and liver
- *Paget's disease of nipple*: Found in ductal carcinoma of breast
- *Erythroderma*: Found in lymphoma and leukemia
- *Tylosis*: Found in esophageal carcinoma
- *Ichthyosis*: Found in lymphoma
- Erythema gyratum repens (found in malignancy of lung and breast)
- Necrolytic migratory erythema (found in glucagonoma).

SCABIES

It is caused by *Sarcoptes scabiei*. The common sites are interdigital area, fingers, ulnar edge of hand and wrist. Other sites are antecubital fossa, elbow joint, axilla, areola, around umbilicus, lower abdomen, genitalia, buttock and dorsum of foot (face and scalp are never involved except in infants, children and immunocompromised). Transmitted by direct skin contact from affected individual and from bed sheet and clothing.

Symptoms: Intense itching, mostly at night, usually all family members are affected.

Signs: "Burrow" which is short, wavy, dirty line, found in edge of fingers, toes or sides of hand and foot. It contains female mites, eggs and feces of mite.

Diagnosis: Clinical (hand lens is used to see burrow and mite).

Complications: Secondary bacterial infection, eczema, lichenification, poststreptococcal glomerulonephritis, urticaria and exfoliative dermatitis.

Treatment: Simultaneous treatment of affected family members. Washing of clothes, bed sheet and control of secondary infection. Antihistamine for itching. Drugs are:
- *Permethrin 5% cream*: Applied once from neck to toe, may be repeated after 1 week
- 1% gamma benzene hexachloride lotion (for consecutive three nights)
- Benzyl benzoate 25% lotion (for consecutive three nights)
- Monosulfiram 5–8% emulsion (for consecutive three nights)
- 10% precipitated sulfur in white petrolatum (for consecutive three nights)
- Crotamiton 10% lotion or cream
- Ivermectin in immunocompromised, crusted or Norwegian scabies (200 mg/kg in single dose).

PSORIASIS

It is chronic inflammatory disease of skin characterized by well-defined erythematous plaque with silvery white scales, associated with recurrence and remission. There are four types:
1. *Chronic plaque psoriasis (the most common)*: Characterized by well-demarcated, red, covered with dry silvery white scale. Commonly involves elbow, knee and lower back

2. *Guttate psoriasis*: Characterized by raindrop-like red small circular or oval plaques, over trunk about 2 weeks after streptococcal sore throat. Common in children and young adults
3. *Pustular psoriasis*: May be localized in palm and sole, and rarely generalized
4. *Erythrodermic psoriasis*: >90% of body surface becomes red, scaly and generalized.

Pathology: Rapid proliferation and abnormal differentiation of epidermis.

Sites: Extensor surfaces of knee, elbow, wrist, back of ear, scalp, hairline and submammary fold.

Clinical features:
- *Skin*: Red, dry, and well-demarcated, with silvery scales
- *Nails*: Pitting, thickening, subungual hyperkeratosis, onycholysis, oil spot and cracking of free edges
- *Joints*: Psoriatic arthropathy
- *Eye*: Iritis, blepharitis, keratitis and conjunctivitis
- *Auspitz's sign*: On removing the scales forcibly, capillary bleeding points may be seen
- *Koebner phenomenon*: Appearance of psoriatic lesion after scratching normal skin. May also occur in surgical scar.

Types of arthritis: There are five types (see in chapter 'Rheumatology').

Investigations: Diagnosis is clinical.
- *Routine*: Complete blood count (CBC), serum creatinine, electrolytes, uric acid, lipid profile, liver function tests, X-ray of chest, serum immunoglobulin E (IgE) and urine routine examination (R/E) (to see proteinuria)
- *Specific tests*: Skin biopsy for histopathology (definitive)
- *Others*: Antistreptolysin O (ASO) titer and throat swab C/S (in guttate psoriasis), and X-ray of affected joints.

Drugs that aggravate psoriasis: Chloroquine, hydroxychloroquine, lithium, beta-blocker, angiotensin-converting enzyme (ACE) inhibitor (lisinopril and captopril), alcohol and systemic steroid.

Treatment: Explanation and reassurance, avoid trauma, precipitating drugs and anxiety. Specific treatment—Local therapy, systemic therapy and combination therapy.

Local therapy (topical therapy on lesion):
- *Emollient*: Petroleum, paraffin, urea (up to 10%) and olive oil
- Salicylic acid (≥5%) or crude tar (3–5%) or dithranol or calcipotriol (vitamin D3 analogue). Topical steroid and tazarotene
- *Others*: Ultraviolet radiation (UVR) therapy [narrow band ultraviolet B (UVB)], tacrolimus, pimecrolimus and excimer laser.

Systemic therapy:
- PUVA (psoralen and ultraviolet A): Long-term use may cause squamous cell carcinoma, basal cell carcinoma and melanoma
- Retinoid (acitretin). Avoided in young female (teratogenic)
- *Others*: Methotrexate, azathioprine and cyclosporine
- *Biologic agents*: Anti-TNF (tumor necrosis factor) α (infliximab, etanercept, adalimumab and eculizumab) may be given when all other drugs fail.

EXFOLIATIVE DERMATITIS OR ERYTHRODERMA

It is characterized by generalized exfoliation, scaling and erythema involving different parts of the skin.

Causes:
- Primary or idiopathic
- *Secondary to*:
  - Skin disease: Psoriasis, atopic dermatitis, dermatomyositis, systemic lupus erythematosus (SLE), pemphigoid and pemphigus foliaceus
  - Systemic disease or malignancy: Leukemia, lymphoma, carcinoma of lung and rectum, multiple myeloma and graft versus host disease
  - Drugs: Allopurinol, carbamazepine, sulfonamide and barbiturates.

Clinical features: More in males.
- *Cutaneous manifestations*: Skin exfoliation, scaling, pruritus and widespread erythema. Loss of hair, nails may be dystrophic, brittle, subungual hyperkeratosis and distal onycholysis. Mucous membranes are usually spared
- *General features*: Anorexia, nausea, diarrhea, anemia, edema and tachycardia.

Investigations:
- *Routine*: CBC, chest X-ray posteroanterior (PA) view, urine R/E, serum total protein, albumin:globulin (A:G) ratio, serum electrolytes, blood urea, serum creatinine, uric acid and IgE
- *Definitive*: By skin biopsy for histopathology
- Others to exclude any primary cause.

Treatment:
- *General measures*: Maintenance of fluid and electrolyte balance, good nutrition and frequent bathing. Offending drug should be stopped
- *Topical*: Lubricant and emollient (e.g. liquid paraffin), and hydrocortisone ointment
- *Symptomatic*: Antihistamine (cetirizine and loratadine), antibiotic (if secondary infection), iron, vitamin and folic acid supplement
- Treatment of primary causes (such as psoriasis, lymphoma and leukemia).

BULLA AND BULLOUS DISEASES

Bulla is a circumscribed, fluid-filled elevation of skin >1 cm.

Causes:
- *Common causes*: Erythema multiforme, pemphigus vulgaris, bullous pemphigoid and dermatitis herpetiformis
- *Others*: Bullous impetigo, insect bite, congenital (epidermolysis bullosa), porphyria cutanea tarda, staphylococcal scalded skin syndrome (SSSS), toxic epidermal necrolysis (TEN), diabetic bullous lesions of skin and herpes gestationis.

PEMPHIGUS VULGARIS

It is an autoimmune blistering disease characterized by thin-walled, flaccid, and easily ruptured bullae in skin and mucous membrane. There are four types: pemphigus vulgaris, pemphigus foliaceus, paraneoplastic pemphigus and IgA pemphigus.

Causes: Unknown. Probable factors are autoimmunity, genetic predisposition, drugs (penicillamine, captopril, rifampicin and cephalosporin), UV light, PUVA and ionizing radiation.

Clinical features: Common in middle age, 50–60 years, equal in both sexes.
- Multiple thin-walled, flaccid bullae over scalp, face, neck, axilla, groin and genitals. Some may rupture forming denuded areas with crusts
- Multiple painful and irregular ulcerations in the oral mucous membrane
- Nikolsky and Asboe-Hansen signs are positive.

Nikolsky's sign: Rubbing of unaffected skin causes separation of epidermis.

Asboe-Hansen sign: Pressure on intact bullae gently forces the fluid to wander under the skin away from pressure site.

Investigations:
- *Routine*: CBC, blood sugar, urine R/E, liver and renal function tests
- *Specific*: Skin biopsy for histopathology and immunofluorescence test. Cytological (Tzanck test), to see acantholytic cell
- *Direct immunofluorescence*: Shows intercellular deposition of IgG throughout epidermis.

Treatment:
- *General measures*: Bed rest, daily bath to remove thick crusts, and foul odor. Maintenance of fluid, electrolyte balance and nutrition. Antibiotic and blood transfusion (if necessary). Antiseptic mouth wash and care of eye
- *Topical*: 1% silver sulfadiazine
- *Systemic*: Prednisolone, 100–200 mg daily, taper when remission occurs. Maintenance dose is given for long time (even lifelong). If new blister occurs, dose should be increased
  - Intravenous (IV) methylprednisolone 1 g/day for 5 days
  - Other treatment: Mycophenolate mofetil, azathioprine, cyclophosphamide, methotrexate, cyclosporine and dapsone. In resistant case, IV Ig. Biologic agent (infliximab, rituximab and etanercept).

Complications: Secondary bacterial infection (pneumonia and septicemia) and hypoproteinemia.

BULLOUS PEMPHIGOID

It is characterized by tense bullae with less tendency to rupture, in trunk, limbs and flexures.

Site of lesion: Basement membrane between epidermis and dermis (subepidermal). So, less tendency to rupture.

Clinical features: Common in elderly, >60 years. Multiple large tense bullae over different parts of body. Intact blisters contain clear fluid. Mouth involvement is rare.

Investigations:
- *Routine*: CBC, blood sugar and urine R/E
- *Specific*: Tzanck test. Skin biopsy (shows subepidermal bullae and no acanthocyte). Direct immunofluorescence (DIF) (shows deposition of IgG and complement C3 at basement membrane in linear pattern).

Treatment:
- *General*: Bed rest, maintenance of electrolytes, adequate nutrition and antihistamine
- *Specific*: Prednisolone 0.5–0.75 mg/kg daily, taper slowly over few weeks after improvement. Potent topical steroid can be given. In severe cases, IV methylprednisolone 1 g/day for 5 days
- *Other drugs*: Dapsone, azathioprine, methotrexate, cyclophosphamide, cyclosporine, mycophenolate mofetil and IV Ig.

ERYTHEMA MULTIFORME AND STEVENS–JOHNSON SYNDROME

It is an acute inflammatory reaction in skin and mucous membrane characterized by multiple erythematous skin lesions, such as macules, papules, vesicles, bullae and target lesions involving the extensor surfaces of limbs.

Stevens–Johnson syndrome (SJS): It is a severe form of erythema multiforme with involvement of mouth, eyes, and genitalia, associated with severe constitutional symptoms.

Causes:
- *Infections*: Herpes simplex virus type-1, *mycoplasma pneumoniae*, *Streptococcus* and *Histoplasma*
- *Drugs*: Sulfonamides, carbamazepine, barbiturate, penicillin and phenytoin
- Idiopathic (50% cases)
- *Others*: Malignancy (carcinoma and lymphoma), collagen disease (SLE and dermatomyositis), Wegener's granulomatosis, and sensitivity to vaccination [polio and BCG (Bacillus Calmette–Guérin)].

Clinical features: Multiple erythematous, maculopapular, urticarial, vesicular and bullous lesions involving the skin of whole body with few target lesions. Mouth ulcer is present in SJS. Typical lesion is target lesion (also called *iris lesion* or *Bull's eye lesion*, characterized by central pallor or dusky purpura with edema and peripheral redness).

Investigations: CBC, ASO titer, antibody to herpes simplex type-1 and anti-mycoplasma antibody. Other investigations according to suspicion of causes.

Treatment: Treatment of primary cause; offending drugs should be stopped. Local care of eyes and mouth. Symptomatic (IV fluid, antipyretic and antibiotic).
- Aciclovir (for recurrent herpes simplex infection)
- Intravenous steroid (hydrocortisone or dexamethasone). When improved, oral prednisolone
- In severe cases, especially in SJS, IV Ig can be given.

ERYTHEMA NODOSUM

It is an inflammatory disorder characterized by nonsuppurative, painful, palpable, tender and red nodular lesion in skin, common in shin below the knee.

Causes:
- Acute sarcoidosis
- Streptococcal β-hemolyticus infection (in throat)

- Primary pulmonary tuberculosis (TB)
- *Drugs*: Sulfonamide, penicillin, estrogen-containing oral pill, salicylates and barbiturates
- Inflammatory bowel disease (Crohn's disease and ulcerative colitis)
- Fungal infections (histoplasmosis, coccidioidomycosis and blastomycosis common in USA)
- Leprosy (erythema nodosum leprosum)
- *Others*: Cat-scratch disease and Behçet's syndrome. Idiopathic (in 50% cases).

Clinical features: More in female. Multiple red painful lesions in front of legs with fever and arthralgia. Nodules are 2–6 cm, occur in crops over 2 weeks, then resolves over months, leaving stain in skin, never ulcerates, and may be recurrent. Features of primary disease.

Investigations:
- Complete blood count, erythrocyte sedimentation rate (ESR), and peripheral blood film (PBF) (leukocytosis in streptococcal infection and high ESR in TB)
- Antistreptolysin O titer, throat swab and blood for C/S (in streptococcal infection)
- Chest X-ray (TB and sarcoidosis)
- *Other investigations*: According to suspicion of cause.

Treatment: Rest. Nonsteroidal anti-inflammatory drug (NSAID) for pain. Treatment of primary cause. If severe, prednisolone should be given. In some case, dapsone 100 mg daily or hydroxychloroquine or colchicine 500 µg twice daily.

ACNE VULGARIS

It is characterized by excessive sebum secretion with obstruction of pilosebaceous duct. Common sites are face, nose, back, shoulders and upper chest.

Clinical features: Common in young, <25 years, often familial, found in oily skin. Comedone is the primary lesion. It may be open comedones (black heads) and closed comedones (white heads). Also papule, pustules or cyst. Seborrhea (greasy skin), presents on face and scalp. Scarring may occur on skin.

Treatment: Explanation and reassurance. Face should be washed with soap and water 2–3 times daily. Avoid cosmetics, squeezing or scratching of the lesion.
- *Drugs treatment*: Depending on severity
  - Mild:
    - Topical retinoid, azelaic acid, salicylic acid or topical benzoyl peroxide
    - If inflammatory: Topical retinoid or topical antimicrobial or azelaic acid or topical antimicrobial (erythromycin or clindamycin).
  - Moderate:
    - Oral antibiotic (see below) and topical retinoid and/or topical benzoyl peroxide
    - For females: Oral antiandrogen and topical retinoid/azelaic acid and/or topical antimicrobial.

- Severe:
  - Oral isotretinoin. High-dose oral antibiotic and topical retinoid and topical benzoyl peroxide
  - For females: Oral antiandrogen and topical retinoid and/or topical antimicrobial, and topical benzoyl peroxide.

Note: Oral antibiotics such as tetracycline (250–500 mg 1–4 times daily) or doxycycline (50–100 mg once or twice daily) or erythromycin (250–500 mg 2–4 times daily) for 3–6 months. Minocycline or clindamycin may be given.

- *Other measures*: Cryotherapy, chemical cauterization and laser therapy. Surgical removal of comedone or pustule or cyst. Intralesional triamcinolone acetonide in inflamed nodules.

Complications: Scarring, hyperpigmentation, keloid, pyogenic granuloma and folliculitis.

LUPUS VULGARIS

It is the TB of skin, usually occurs as a post primary infections. Common sites are skin of head, neck, face, around the nose and also in arms and legs.

Clinical features: Reddish-brown plaque (or nodules) or ulcerated area with irregular margin with smooth and glistening fine scaling over it. Lesions heal with scarring and new lesions slowly spread to form chronic solitary erythematous plaque.

Investigations: CBC, ESR, mantoux test, chest X-ray and skin biopsy for histopathology.

Treatment:
- *Standard anti-TB therapy*: Rifampicin, isonicotinylhydrazide (INH), ethambutol and pyrazinamide for 2 months
- *In continuation phase*: Rifampicin and INH for 4–10 months.

LEG ULCER

Causes:
- Traumatic
- Diabetes mellitus
- *Infection*: Pyogenic, TB, leprosy, cutaneous leishmaniasis and fungal infection
- *Arterial causes*: Atherosclerosis, peripheral vascular disease, Buerger's disease and Raynaud's disease
- *Venous ulcer*: Usually due to varicose vein
- *Neuropathic ulcer*: Due to DM, tabes dorsalis, syringomyelia, leprosy and polyneuropathy
- *Collagen disease*: SLE, rheumatoid arthritis (RA), Felty's syndrome, cryoglobulinemia and polyarteritis nodosa
- *Hematological diseases*: Sickle cell disease, thalassemia, hereditary spherocytosis and paroxysmal nocturnal hemoglobinuria
- *Neoplastic*: Squamous cell carcinoma, basal cell carcinoma and Kaposi's sarcoma
- *Others*: Pyoderma gangrenosum, dermatitis, artefact and drugs.

Investigations:
- Complete blood cell, ESR and PBF, blood sugar, and lipid profile. Pus for C/S, acid-fast bacillus (AFB), and Leishmania donovani (LD) bodies

- X-ray of leg (calcification in artery), Doppler USG of lower limb vessels and arteriography
- Biopsy
- *Others*: According to suspicion of causes—Antinuclear antibody (ANA), cold agglutinin and RA test.

Treatment:
- Smoking must be stopped. Control of DM, hypertension and obesity. Treatment of primary cause. Local care (cleaning and dressings)
- *Specific measures*: Antibiotic, if any infection. Low-dose aspirin. In some cases, surgery (balloon dilatation) and amputation. Consultation with chiropodist.

LICHEN PLANUS

It is characterized by flat-topped, pruritic, and polygonal violaceous papules on the flexors of wrist, trunk, medial aspect of thighs and shins. Oral mucosa shows reticulated whitish (or violaceous) plaques consisting of pinhead papules on the inner aspect of cheeks.

Clinical features:
- *Skin*: Bilateral symmetrical multiple flat-topped violaceous papules. Koebner phenomenon and Wickham striae are present
- *Oral mucosa*: Violaceous reticular lesions in inner side of cheeks with silvery-white papules
- Nails show grooving, onycholysis, ridging and splitting.

Investigations:
- *Routine*: CBC, viral marker for hepatitis B and C, and liver and renal function tests
- *Specific*: Skin biopsy for histopathology and DIF.

Treatment:
- Protection from trauma. Precipitating drugs like diuretic, beta blocker, and antimalarial should be avoided
- *For skin lesion*: Topical steroid, tacrolimus, pimecrolimus, psoralen and UV light. Oral prednisolone 30–80 mg/day. Etretinate, acitretin, and isotretinoin may be given. If no response, cyclosporine, dapsone, hydroxychloroquine, azathioprine and mycophenolate mofetil may be given
- *For oral lesion*: Topical steroid, nystatin with clobetasol, topical tretinoin with steroid, and 0.1% topical tacrolimus. Oral hydroxychloroquine or thalidomide.

ARSENICOSIS

Prolonged ingestion of tube well water contaminated with arsenic produced arsenicosis. May involve any system of the body.

Clinical features:
- *Melanosis*: Hyperpigmentation (generalized or localized) with few scattered hypopigmented areas giving rise to "raindrop" appearance
- Hyperkeratosis of palm and sole. May be multiple, punctate, hard, discrete, papule and verrucous plaque
- *Nails*: Brittle, may show transverse white striae of finger nails (Mees' line)

- *Hair*: Dry, sparse and may fall off
- *Eye*: Conjunctivitis
- *Nose*: Rhinitis, epistaxis, nasal obstruction and septal perforation.

Investigations:
- *Routine*: CBC, urine for R/E, chest x-ray, and liver and renal function tests
- *Specific*: Measurement of arsenic in hair, nail, urine and serum
- *Others*: According to the organ involved.

Systemic effects of chronic arsenic toxicity:
- *Gastrointestinal tract*: Anorexia, nausea and vomiting
- *Hepatic*: Hepatomegaly, cirrhosis of liver, noncirrhotic portal hypertension and hepatoma
- *Nervous system*: Peripheral neuropathy, seizure, confusion and encephalopathy
- *Hematological*: Anemia, leukopenia and thrombocytopenia
- *Musculoskeletal*: Myalgia, arthralgia, wrist drop or foot drop
- *Renal*: Dysuria, anuria and renal tubular necrosis
- *Heart*: Cardiomyopathy, arrhythmia and heart failure
- *Vascular*: Peripheral vascular insufficiency causing blackfoot disease
- *Endocrine*: DM may be precipitated
- *Malignancy*: Skin (squamous cell carcinoma, basal cell carcinoma and Bowen's disease), and carcinoma of lung, kidney, urinary bladder, liver, prostate and colon.

Treatment: Drinking of arsenic contaminated water must be stopped. High protein diet with vegetable and fresh fruit.
- Antioxidant (vitamin A 50,000 IU, vitamin C 500 mg and vitamin E 200 mg daily for 3 months). Other vitamin and mineral supplements
- Spirulina (an algae), rich in high protein, may help to clear arsenic
- *For skin lesion*: Keratolytic emollients (salicylic acid, urea and retinoic acid), cryotherapy, electrocautery and laser therapy
- *Drugs (chelating agent may be used)*: D-penicillamine or dimercaprol (BAL), dimercaptosuccinic acid (DMSA) and dimercaptopropane sulfonate (DMPS).

Prevention: Drinking water should be safe.

TINEA VERSICOLOR (PITYRIASIS VERSICOLOR)

It is benign superficial skin infection caused by malassezia furfur. Common in warm months also in immunocompromised. Upper trunk is mostly involved. Lesions are small white spots on trunk, neck, upper arm, and face. May be velvety, faintly brown macules, may fuse together forming bigger area of depigmentation. On scratching, fine scales may be separated from the patch.

Investigations: Diagnosis is clinical.

Treatment: Personal hygiene.
- *Local therapy*: Selenium sulfide (2.5%) lotion may be applied from neck to waist for 5–15 minutes or, ketoconazole shampoo over chest and back for 5 minutes or Azole creams (ketoconazole, econazole, miconazole and clotrimazole) or terbinafine 1% solution
- *Systemic therapy*: Oral ketoconazole (200 mg daily for 1 week or 400 mg single dose), may be repeated at monthly intervals or oral itraconazole

(200 mg once daily for 7 days). Also, fluconazole (400 mg once, can be repeated at monthly intervals).

DERMATOPHYTE INFECTION (RINGWORM)

It is caused by different types of dermatophytes that infect the skin and appendages (hair and nail). Lesion is ring-like and annular. According to the site of involvement, types are:
- *Tinea capitis*: In scalp and hair
- *Tinea corporis*: In trunk and limbs (body)
- *Tinea cruris*: In groin
- *Tinea pedis*: In foot, called athlete's foot
- *Tinea unguium*: In nails
- *Tinea barbae*: In beard hair.

Tinea Capitis or Scalp Ringworm

It is common in children, may be any age, more in boys.

Clinical features: Broken stumps of hairs, surrounded by or contain fungus with rounded patches, crusts or pustules, scaling, diffuse or circumscribed alopecia.

Investigations: Wood's lamp. Also, direct microscopy and fungal culture.

Treatment:
- *Topical*: Clotrimazole, miconazole, ketoconazole, econazole and terbinafine
- *Systemic antifungal*: Griseofulvin, itraconazole, terbinafine and fluconazole
- Selenium sulfide shampoo or ketoconazole shampoo on scalp for 5 minutes three times a week. It can be used with oral antifungal agents.

Tinea Cruris

It is common in adults, more in males, caused by *Trichophyton rubrum* and *Trichophyton mentagrophytes*.

Clinical features: Large, scaling or plaques with central clearing. Papules and pustules may be present at margins. Commonly in groin and thighs, and may extend to buttocks.

Diagnosis: Usually clinical. Skin scrapings for fungus and culture on a suitable medium.

Treatment: Same as above.

Tinea corporis: *T. rubrum*, involves trunk, legs, arms and neck. Common in animal worker.

Clinical features: Scaling, peripheral enlargement with central clearing, produce ring-like lesions, single or scattered multiple.

Diagnosis: Clinical.

Treatment: Same as above.

Tinea Unguium (Onychomycosis): Infection of nail plate by *T. rubrum*.

Clinical features: Starts at distal corner of nail, involves the junction of nail and its bed, becomes rough, friable, and discolored, and nail plate is fragmented with subungual hyperkeratosis. Entire nail becomes brittle and separated with branny scaling and erythema.

Diagnosis: Clinical.

Treatment: Topical ciclopirox and amorolfine nail lacquers are modestly effective. Oral itraconazole or terbinafine or fluconazole.

Tinea Barbae: It is characterized by red inflammatory papules, vesicles or pustules surrounding the hair root of beard. Oozing and crust formation may occur. Involved hairs are usually shed off. Treatment like *T. corporis*. Griseofulvin may be given for about 1 month.

MELASMA (CHLOASMA)

It is an acquired light or dark brown hyperpigmentation that occurs on cheeks. It may be associated with pregnancy, sun exposure, drugs [oral contraceptive pill (OCP) and diphenyl hydantoin] or idiopathic.

Clinical features: Common in young. Macular hyperpigmentation, sharply defined in the malar and frontal areas of face. Usually, uniform but also blotchy.

Treatment: Avoid exposure to sunlight. Sunblock with broad-spectrum UVA coverage should be used daily. Topical hydroquinone (2–4%) or tretinoin cream may be added. Combination of hydroquinone, tretinoin and steroid (called "Kligman's formula") can be used once daily. Mequinol, azelaic acid, kojic acid and vitamin E cream may be used.

ECZEMA

It is defined as pruritic inflammatory disease of skin, characterized by papules, vesicles, scaling, crusting and lichenification. It may be exogenous and endogenous.

Clinically, it is classified as:
- *Acute*: There is itching with erythema, papulovesicular eruption and scab formation
- *Subacute*: There is scab and crust formation
- *Chronic*: Scratch mark and fissure, lichenification or hyperpigmentation.

Clinical features: Depend on type. In endogenous eczema, atopic and seborrheic dermatitis are common.

Investigation: Diagnosis is clinical. Routine: CBC, ESR, serum IgE, skin scraping microscopy, and culture to exclude fungal infection. Skin biopsy for histopathology. Patch test may be done in some cases.

Treatment: Patient's education and psychological support. Avoid excessive rubbing, vigorous bathing, tight clothing, scratching, excessive soap, extreme heat and cold, sweating, stress and external irritants. Use of petrolatum after bath.

- Topical or systemic antibiotic, if infection. Antihistamine for itching.
- *Specific treatment*:
  - Topical steroid (in infants, low potency steroid ointment like hydrocortisone, in older children and adult, medium potency steroid like triamcinolone). In refractory case and thick plaques, betamethasone, clobetasol or halobetasol are used. Tacrolimus and pimecrolimus may be used. 1% to 5% crude coal tar in white petrolatum or hydrophilic ointment is sometimes used
  - Phototherapy: Narrow band UVB therapy when topical therapies fail

- Systemic therapy: Systemic steroid to control acute exacerbation. Cyclosporine, azathioprine, mycophenolate mofetil, methotrexate and omalizumab may be used.

Seborrheic Dermatitis

It is characterized by yellow greasy scale on an erythematous base, involves where sebaceous glands are most active. Sites are scalp, eyebrows, eyelids, nasolabial crease, lips, ears, axillae, submammary folds, umbilicus, groin and gluteal crease.

Clinical features: Common in males. May occur in any age.
- *In skin*: Orange red or greyish-white skin, often with "greasy" or white dry scaling macules and papules of varying size or patches
- On the scalp marked scaling (dandruff), diffuse involvement
- On the face—lesions are scattered, discrete, nummular, polycyclic and annular.

Diagnosis: Usually clinical. Laboratory investigations may be done to isolate dermatophyte.

Treatment: Topical and systemic therapy.

Topical:
- *Scalp*: In adults—shampoo-containing selenium sulfide, zinc pyrithione or tar. 2% ketoconazole shampoo, glucocorticoid solution, lotion or gels after medicated shampoo (ketoconazole or tar) may be used for severe cases, and pimecrolimus 1% cream. In infants—removal of crusts with warm olive oil, followed by 2% ketoconazole shampoo and 1% to 2.5% hydrocortisone cream or 2% ketoconazole cream and 1% pimecrolimus cream
- *Face and Trunk*: Ketoconazole shampoo, 2% glucocorticoid cream and lotions. In resistant case, clobetasol propionate, 2% ketoconazole, 1% pimecrolimus cream, 0.03% or 0.1% tacrolimus ointment
- *Eyelids*: Gentle removal of crusts. Apply 10% sodium sulfacetamide in 0.2% prednisolone and 0.12% phenylephrine, 2% ketoconazole, 1% pimecrolimus cream or 0.03% tacrolimus ointment.

Systemic: In severe case, retinoic acid orally, 0.5-1 mg/kg. Contraception should be used in females of childbearing age. In mild case, itraconazole 100 mg twice daily for 2 weeks.

CONTACT DERMATITIS

It is defined as acute or chronic inflammatory reaction of skin that occurs after contact with any substance. Types are:
- *Irritant contact dermatitis*: Caused by chemical irritant
- *Allergic contact dermatitis*: Caused by antigen (allergen).

Irritant contact dermatitis: Common agents are soap, detergent, acids and alkali, industrial solvent (coal tar solvent, petroleum and chlorinated hydrocarbon), fiberglass, wool and rough synthetic clothing. Also, occupational exposure such as housekeeping, hairdressing, food preparation and catering, printing, painting and construction.

Acute irritant contact dermatitis: Features are burning, stinging and smarting. There is sharply demarcated erythema, vesicle and superficial edema. In severe case, blisters, erosions and frank necrosis. Later, crusting, shedding of crusts and scaling, and then healing.

Chronic irritant contact dermatitis: It occurs after repeated exposure to mild irritants (water, soap and detergent) usually on hands.

Treatment of contact dermatitis:
- *Acute*: Removal of causative agent. Wet dressings with Burrow's solution, changed every 2–3 hour. Larger vesicles may be drained, but tops should not be removed. Topical glucocorticoid may be used. In severe case, prednisolone 40–60 mg initially, then taper
- *Chronic*: Removal of causative agent. Potent topical steroid (betamethasone or clobetasol). Adequate lubrication. As healing occurs, continue with lubrication.

Systemic treatment: Acitretinoin 0.5 mg/kg for 6 months.

Treatment of occupational contact dermatitis: Avoid irritating and sensitizing substances, use of protective measures (cloth and barrier cream), clothing changes and cleansing showers. Topical steroid or tacrolimus ointment or pimecrolimus cream may be used.

URTICARIA

It is a vascular reaction of skin characterized by formation of wheals, surrounded by red halo or flare, associated with severe itching. It is due to allergen.

Causes:
- *Physical agent*: Trauma, heat and cold
- *Drugs*: Sulfonamide, penicillin and NSAID
- *Food allergen*: Shell fish, crab and egg
- *Other*: Grass pollen, house dust, mites, feathers, animal dander, cosmetics and aerosols
- *Infection*: In upper respiratory tract (streptococcal), infection in tonsil, tooth and sinuses
- *Parasitic*: Ascariasis, giardiasis and strongyloidiasis
- *Neoplasm*: Carcinoma, Hodgkin disease and chronic lymphocytic leukemia
- *Others*: Autoimmune, vasculitis, emotional stress and idiopathic.

Classification:
- *Acute urticaria*: Lasting <6 weeks
- *Chronic urticaria*: Lasting >6 weeks. Common in women.

Clinical features: Wheals of variable size and shape, fused together forming bigger wheal (called angioedema), and itching. Angioedema may occur in lips, mouth and tongue. If involves larynx and trachea, may cause respiratory obstruction.

Investigations: CBC (eosinophilia), serum IgE (high), and stool for R/E (to exclude parasitic infection). Other investigations according to suspicion of cause.

Treatment:
- *Acute urticaria*: Avoidance of allergen and treatment of primary cause. Antihistamine (chlorpheniramine, loratadine and fexofenadine). If no response, systemic corticosteroid. In angioedema, parenteral

dexamethasone and antihistamine. If respiratory obstruction, intubation or tracheostomy may be needed
- *Chronic urticaria*: Antihistamine (cetirizine, levocetirizine and loratadine). Doxepin may be added. Dapsone and colchicine may be helpful in neutrophil rich urticaria. If fails, systemic steroid. In severe case, immunosuppressive therapy, plasmapheresis or IV Ig.

ALOPECIA

It is defined as loss of hair. There are three types:
1. Alopecia areata (localized loss of hair in scalp)
2. Alopecia totalis (hair loss of entire scalp)
3. Alopecia universalis (total loss of body hair).

Causes of alopecia totalis: May be nonscarring and scarring or cicatricial.

Alopecia areata: It is the localized loss of hair in scalp, may be due to autoimmune mechanism. It is found in SLE, associated with other autoimmune diseases, such as Hashimoto's thyroiditis, Graves' disease, pernicious anemia, DM and vitiligo.

Diagnostic points:
- Patches are 1-5 cm in diameter. Complete, patchy loss of hair, round or oval shape
- At the periphery of bald patches, there are loose hairs that may be broken off leaving short stumps. When they are pulled out, a tapered attenuated bulb is seen called exclamation point hair. Skin is smooth and shiny without inflammation and scaling
- There may be nail pitting.

Investigations:
- Skin scraping for fungus (to exclude tinea capitis)
- Antinuclear antibody and anti-dsDNA (SLE)
- Serological test for syphilis.

Treatment:
- Topical steroid, 1% anthralin cream and topical minoxidil (2-5%)
- Intralesional injection triamcinolone
- Photochemotherapy using topical or systemic methoxsalen and UVA (PUVA)
- 308 nm xenom chloride excimer LASER helps to produce regrowth after 11-12 sessions (9-11 weeks)
- Analogous hair transplantation.

Vitiligo

It is the area of localized depigmentation, probably due to autoimmune mechanism due to focal loss of melanocyte. Generalized vitiligo may occur, usually symmetrical, involving hand, wrist, knee, neck, around the eyes, mouth, dorsum of feet, sites at friction or trauma. Equally affects both sexes and familial in 30%.

Diseases associated in vitiligo: May be associated with autoimmune diseases, such as systemic sclerosis, Addison's disease, pernicious anemia, Graves' disease, Hashimoto's thyroiditis, premature ovarian failure, DM and primary biliary cirrhosis.

Investigations: Diagnosis is clinical.
- Woods light examination shows chalky or ivory white fluorescence
- Skin scraping for malassezia furfur
- Blood sugar. Other tests according to suspicion of causes.

Treatment: Reassurance, use sunscreen, and self-tanning cream containing dihydroxyacetone.
- *Topical*: Steroid (betamethasone and clobetasol propionate). Topical calcipotriene can be added to topical steroid and 0.1% tacrolimus ointment in facial vitiligo
- *Phototherapy*: Narrow band UVB and topical 8-methoxypsoralen followed by UVA
- Surgical in some case.

CHAPTER 11

Sexually Transmitted Diseases

GONORRHEA

It is a sexually transmitted disease (STD) caused by *Neisseria gonorrhoeae*, a gram-negative diplococcus.

Incubation period: 2–14 days.

Mode of transmission: Sexually from partner and neonate exposed to infected secretions in birth canal.

Clinical features:
- *In male*: Dysuria, frequency and burning micturition, lower abdominal pain. Mucopurulent or purulent urethral discharge, which may profuse and stain underwear. It may cause prostatitis and epididymo-orchitis. In chronic case, chronic prostatitis and urethral stricture may be observed
- *In female*: Same as above. Also vulvovaginitis, cervicitis, salpingitis, salpingo-oophoritis, and Bartholin's abscess
- *Other features*: According to site of involvement
  - *Anorectum*: Proctitis with pain and purulent discharge
  - *Pharynx*: Pharyngitis with erythema secondary to orogenital sexual exposure
  - Disseminated gonococcal infection or septicemia may occur causing arthritis of one or more joints, tenosynovitis, pustular erythematous skin lesions and fever
  - *In neonate*: Ophthalmia neonatorum characterized by conjunctivitis, swollen eyelids, severe hyperemia, chemosis, profuse purulent discharge. Rarely, corneal ulcer and perforation.

Investigations:
- *Gram stain*: Gram-negative diplococci are seen on microscopy of smear from infected site
- Culture (in chocolate agar media, Thayer-Martin media). Urethral swab in men and endocervical swab in women. Also, swab from rectum, oropharynx in both
- Nucleic acid amplification test (NAAT) is the investigation of choice. In men, first-voided urine (FVU) or urethral swab and in female, vulvovaginal swab or endocervical swab are taken for this test.

Treatment:

Uncomplicated
- Single dose intramuscular (IM) ceftriaxone 500 mg plus azithromycin 1 g orally. *Or* cefixime 400 mg stat. *Or* ciprofloxacin 500 mg orally stat. *Or* ofloxacin 400 mg orally stat
- *In pregnancy and breastfeeding*: Ceftriaxone 500 mg plus azithromycin 1 g IM stat *or* spectinomycin 2 g IM stat.

Complicated
- *Epididymitis*: Ceftriaxone (250 mg IM once) with doxycycline (100 mg bd for 10 days)
- *Conjunctivitis in adult*: Ceftriaxone, 1 g IM, single dose
- *Ophthalmia neonatorum*: Ceftriaxone [25–50 mg/kg intravenous (IV), single dose, not to exceed 125 mg]
- *Meningitis*: Ceftriaxone 1–2 g IV bd for 10–14 days
- *Endocarditis*: Ceftriaxone 1–2 g IV bd for ≥4 weeks
- *Disseminated infection*: Ceftriaxone 1 g IM or IV daily or cefotaxime 1 g IV 8 hourly or ceftizoxime 1 g IV 8 hourly. Spectinomycin 2 g IM 12 hourly if allergic to above drugs. It should be continued for 24–48 hours after improvement. Then, oral cefixime 400 mg 12 hourly for 1 week.

Note: Abstinence from sex for at least 7 days should be advised. All sexual contacts should be examined and treated.

NONGONOCOCCAL URETHRITIS

It is an STD caused by organism other than *N. gonorrhoeae*, also called nonspecific urethritis. It is caused by *Chlamydia trachomatis* and *Ureaplasma urealyticum*. Others—*Trichomonas vaginalis*, Herpes simplex virus, and *Candida albicans*.

Incubation period: 2–3 weeks.

Clinical features: Discomfort or burning during micturition with purulent or mucoid urethral discharge occurs mainly in early morning. Dysuria, discomfort or itching in urethra may be present.

Diagnosis: Urine routine microscopic examination shows pus cells. Isolation of organism in a special culture media is carried out. NAAT for *N. gonorrhoeae* and *C. trachomatis* should be performed in all men with symptoms of urethritis on either an FVU sample or urethral swab.

Treatment: Abstinence from sex for at least 7 days should be advised. All sexual contacts should be examined and treated. Doxycycline 100 mg 12 hourly for 7 days or erythromycin 500 mg 6 hourly for 7 days or azithromycin 1 g single dose orally.

LYMPHOGRANULOMA VENEREUM

It is a venereal disease caused by *Chlamydia trachomatis*, an obligate intracellular bacterium.

Mode of transmission: Through sexual contact.

Incubation period: 3 days to 3 weeks.

Clinical features: Three stages
1. *First stage or primary lymphogranuloma venereum (LGV)*: Within few days after sexual contact, small painless vesicle or ulcer or papule is

found in the genitalia that heals in few days. Infection can spread from primary site to regional lymph nodes through lymphatics
2. *Second stage or secondary LGV*: Painful inguinal lymphadenopathy. Initially, nodes are discrete, but later matted, large, and suppurative with discharge of yellow pus. Painful and swollen lymph nodes coalesce to form buboes, which may rupture. Scarring with formation of multiple sinuses
3. *Third stage or tertiary LGV*: It is also called genito-anorectal syndrome. It is common in female and homosexual male. In rectum, it can cause fistulae, stricture, and fibrosis, mimicking Crohn's disease. There is discharge of blood, mucus, and pus through anus. There may be lymphedema of vulva, penis and scrotum.

Diagnosis: It is usually clinical. NAAT is performed from cervical swab, male urethral swab, rectal swab, and urine specimen.

Treatment: Oral doxycycline 100 mg twice daily for 21 days or oral erythromycin 500 mg four times daily for 21 days.

CHANCROID

It is caused by *Haemophilus ducreyi*, a gram-negative coccobacillus.

Incubation period: About 4–7 days.

Mode of transmission: Transmitted through sexual contact.

Clinical features: Primary lesion is small red papule or pustule on genitalia and surrounding skin. Within a few days, single or multiple ulcers develop which is painful with sharp and undermined border. Painful inguinal lymphadenopathy may suppurate (bubo).

Diagnosis: Painful ulcer with tender lymphadenopathy is suggestive of chancroid. Microscopy and culture is done on special culture media. Polymerase chain reaction is most sensitive but not widely available.

Treatment: Azithromycin 1 g single dose or IM ceftriaxone 250 mg in single dose. Ciprofloxacin 500 mg twice daily for 3 days or erythromycin 500 mg three times daily for 7 days.

SYPHILIS

It is caused by *Treponema pallidum*.

Mode of transmission: Sexual contact, transplacental or perinatal transmission. It is classified as congenital and acquired.

Congenital Syphilis

Features develop in 4 months of gestation, when fetus becomes immune competent. Miscarriage or stillbirth. May be premature delivery. It may be early (diagnosed within first 2 years) and late (diagnosed after 2 years of life).
- *Early congenital syphilis (neonatal period)*: Maculopapular rash, condylomata lata, mucous patches, fissures around the mouth, nose, and anus, rhinitis with nasal discharge (snuffles), hepatosplenomegaly, osteochondritis or periostitis, generalized lymphadenopathy, choroiditis, meningitis, anemia and thrombocytopenia

- *Late congenital syphilis*: Benign tertiary syphilis, periostitis, paroxysmal cold hemoglobinuria, neurosyphilis, 8th nerve deafness, interstitial keratitis, and Clutton's joints (painless effusion into knee joints).

Acquired Syphilis

Types may be primary, secondary and tertiary.

Primary Syphilis

Incubation period—10–90 days. Average 21 days.

Clinical features: Genital or extragenital lesions at sites of inoculation called "Chancre", which is a painless ulcer and is usually single with raised border and scanty serous exudate. Extragenital chancre occurs at any site of inoculation, anus or rectum, mouth, lips, tongue tonsils, fingers (painful), toes, breast and nipple. Chancre heals in 4–6 weeks, even without treatment.

Diagnosis: Clinical suspicion. Confirmed by
- Detection of *T. pallidum* by dark ground illumination from chancre
- *Serological tests*:
   - Nontreponemal (nonspecific) tests: Venereal Disease Research Laboratory (VDRL) test or rapid plasma reagin (RPR) test
   - Treponemal (specific) antibody tests: Treponemal antigen by ELISA, treponemal hemagglutination assay (TPHA), *T. pallidum* particle agglutination assay (TPPA), and fluorescent treponema antibody absorption test (FTA-ABS).

Secondary Syphilis

Appears 6–10 weeks after primary infection.

Clinical features: General features are fever, sore throat, weight loss, malaise, arthralgia, anorexia, headache and meningism.
- *Skin lesions*: Maculopapular rash, copper or roseola in color, may be generalized on the trunk, limb, palms and soles. Diffuse hair loss, patchy, moth-eaten alopecia on the scalp and beard area. Loss of eyelashes and lateral third of eyebrows
- *Condylomata lata*: Warty lesion is common in anogenital region and also in moist areas
- *In mucous membrane of mouth*: Painless grayish ulcer is called "snail track ulcer"
- *Generalized lymphadenopathy*: It involves cervical, suboccipital, inguinal, epitrochlear, axillary which are small, discrete and nontender
- *Other features*: Periostitis of long bones (tibia), arthralgia, iritis, optic neuritis, uveitis, hepatitis, ulcerative colitis, glomerulonephritis, nephrotic syndrome, cystitis, prostatitis and splenomegaly.

Investigations: As in primary. Cerebrospinal fluid (CSF) study—abnormal in 40% cases. Spirochetes are found in CSF in 30%.

Diagnosis: Clinical suspicion is confirmed by laboratory tests. Dark-ground illumination (DGI) is positive in all secondary syphilis lesions except for macular exanthem.

Treatment: As in primary syphilis.

Tertiary or Late Syphilis

This stage can occur at any time after secondary syphilis, even after many years. It may involve any organ. No organism is detected, so it is not infective. Typical lesion is formation of "gumma". It may be of following types:

Benign Tertiary Syphilis

It develops between 3 and 10 years after infection. Single or multiple nodular or papulosquamous plaques (called gumma) that occur at any site of skin, especially on scalp, face, chest, mucus membranes, bone, muscle, and viscera (larynx, liver and stomach) that may ulcerate and form circles.

Neurosyphilis

It may be asymptomatic or symptomatic which may present as features of tabes dorsalis or general paresis of insane (GPI). In eye, there is Argyll Robertson pupil.

Meningeal or Meningovascular Syphilis

It is characterized by headache, nausea, vomiting, neck stiffness, cranial nerve palsy, seizure, and change in mental status.

Cardiovascular Syphilis

It is caused due to endarteritis obliterans of vasa vasorum. It occurs in 10% of late untreated syphilis, 10-40 years after infection. Aortitis, aortic regurgitation, aortic aneurysm, and coronary ostial stenosis may occur.

Treatment:

- *Primary, secondary, and early latent*: Injection benzathine penicillin 2.4 million units in single dose IM or, oral doxycycline 100 mg twice daily for 14 days
- *Late latent, cardiovascular and gummatous*: Injection benzathine penicillin 2.4 million units IM once a week for 3 weeks. If allergic to penicillin, doxycycline 100 mg 12 hourly for 28 days
- *Neurosyphilis*: Injection procaine penicillin 2.4 million units IM daily plus probenecid 500 mg daily for 14-17 days. If allergic to penicillin, doxycycline 100 mg 12 hourly for 28 days. Prednisolone may be given to prevent reaction
- *Pregnancy*: Penicillin is safe. If allergic to penicillin, erythromycin may be given. Ceftriaxone for 10 days may be given.

Latent Syphilis

There is no clinical feature and no organism is detected. Only serological tests are positive. This stage may persist for many years or for life with little or no ill-health. Treatment as above.

CHAPTER 12

Neurology

INFECTION OF CENTRAL NERVOUS SYSTEM
- *Meningitis*: It means infection of meninges
- *Encephalitis*: It means infection or inflammation of brain parenchyma
- *Meningoencephalitis*: It means infection of meninges and brain
- *Myelitis*: It means infection or inflammation of spinal cord
- *Myelopathy*: It is the disease of spinal cord
- *Encephalomyelitis*: It means infection or inflammation of brain and spinal cord
- *Radiculopathy*: It means disease of spinal nerve root.

Meningitis
It is the infection or inflammation of meninges.

Types:
1. *Acute meningitis*: Clinical features lasting less than 4 weeks
2. *Chronic meningitis*: Clinical features lasting for 4 weeks or more.

Causes:
- *Bacterial*: Pyogenic (*Meningococcus*, pneumococcus, *Haemophilus influenzae* type B in children, *Listeria monocytogenes* and *Staphylococcus aureus*), and *Mycobacterium tuberculosis*
- *Viral*: Coxsackie B virus, echovirus, poliovirus, mumps virus, Epstein-Barr virus (EBV), herpes simplex virus (HSV), and human immunodeficiency virus (HIV)
- *Fungal*: *Cryptococcus neoformans*, *Candida albicans*, *Coccidioides* and *Histoplasma capsulatum*
- *Protozoal*: Toxoplasmosis and cysticercosis
- *Noninfective*: Carcinomatous meningitis, systemic lupus erythematosus (SLE), sarcoidosis and Behcet's disease.

Acute Bacterial Meningitis
Causative organism according to age:
- *Neonate*: Gram-negative bacillus (*Escherichia coli* and *Proteus*), *Streptococcus* group B. Also *L. monocytogenes*

- *Small child*: H. influenzae, Neisseria meningitidis and Streptococcus pneumoniae. Also M. tuberculosis
- *Older children and adult*: N. meningitidis and S. pneumoniae. Also L. monocytogenes, M. tuberculosis, S. aureus (skull fracture) and H. influenzae. Listeria is common in immunosuppressed, diabetic, alcoholic and pregnant women.

Symptoms: High fever with chill and rigor. Headache, nausea, vomiting, photophobia, drowsiness, impaired consciousness and convulsion. Pneumococcal meningitis may be associated with pneumonia, common in elderly and alcoholics.

Signs: Neck rigidity, positive Kernig sign, positive Brudzinski sign, and petechial or nonspecific blotchy red rash in skin (in meningococcal meningitis with septicemia).

Complications of meningitis:
- *Central nervous system*: Cranial nerve palsy, hydrocephalus, focal neurological deficit, epilepsy, mental retardation and behavioral disturbance
- *Others*: Disseminated intravascular coagulation (DIC), septicemic shock, renal failure, peripheral gangrene, arthritis and pericarditis.

Investigations:
- Complete blood count (CBC) (shows neutrophilic leukocytosis), and blood Culture/Sensitivity (C/S)
- Lumbar puncture and cerebrospinal fluid (CSF) study (before doing lumbar puncture, fundoscopy should be done to see papilledema to exclude raised intracranial pressure). Looks purulent or turbid with high polymorphs, high protein and low sugar. Gram staining shows organism
- Computed tomography (CT) scan of head and Chest X-ray.

Treatment: Hospitalization, adequate nutrition and hydration.
- *If Meningococcus is suspected*: Benzylpenicillin 2.4 g IV 6 hourly *or* cefuroxime 1–2 g IV 6 hourly *or* ceftriaxone 2 g IV 12 hourly *or* cefotaxime 2 g IV 6 hourly
- *If S. pneumoniae or H. influenzae is suspected*: Ceftriaxone 2 g IV 12 hourly or cefotaxime 2 g IV 6 hourly for 10–14 days
- *If Listeria is suspected*: Ampicillin 2 g IV 4 hourly *plus* gentamicin IV 5 mg/kg daily
- Antibiotic can be changed depending on C/S result
- Dexamethasone 0.4 mg/kg every 12 hours can also be used.

Treatment of pyogenic meningitis of unknown cause:
- *Adult 18–50 years*: Ceftriaxone 2 g IV 12 hourly or cefotaxime 2 g IV 6 hourly. If penicillin resistance is suspected—vancomycin 1 g twice daily should be added
- *Adult >50 years with suspected Listeria*: As above *plus* ampicillin 2 g IV 4 hourly
- Dexamethasone 0.15 mg/kg 6 hourly or 2–4 days.

Viral meningitis

Common organisms are enterovirus, echovirus, coxsackievirus, poliovirus, mumps virus and HIV.

Clinical features: Common in children or young adult. Severe headache, fever, and other features of meningitis. Lumbar puncture and CSF study shows high lymphocyte, protein and sugar are usually normal (however, this picture is found if treated with antibiotic).

Treatment: Symptomatic and supportive. Usually benign, self-limiting, and improves in 4–10 days.

Tuberculous Meningitis

It commonly occurs after primary infection in childhood or as a complication of miliary tuberculosis.

Symptoms: Low-grade fever, night sweat, weight loss, headache, vomiting, confusion and abnormal behavior. History of of tuberculosis may be present.

Signs: Signs of meningeal irritation (neck rigidity and Kernig sign), cranial nerve palsy (commonly 3rd and 6th cranial nerve), and focal neurological signs. Fundoscopy shows choroid tubercle.

Complications: Cranial nerve palsy, hydrocephalus, focal neurological deficit, epilepsy, mental retardation and behavioral disturbance.

Investigations:

- Complete blood count, erythrocyte sedimentation rate (ESR) (high), chest X-ray (to see any tuberculous focus), and Mantoux test (MT), CT scan or magnetic resonance imaging (MRI) of brain
- *Lumbar puncture and CSF study*: Shows increased pressure and straw color. When kept for some hours, it shows cobweb appearance. Biochemistry shows high protein and low sugar. Cytology shows increased lymphocytes. Adenosine deaminase (ADA) is high. Acid-fast bacillus (AFB) may be positive. Polymerase chain reaction (PCR) may be done.

Treatment:

- Standard antituberculosis therapy with isonicotinylhydrazide (INH), rifampicin, pyrazinamide and ethambutol is given for 2 months. Then INH and rifampicin is given for 7–10 months depending on clinical response. If there is eye complication, ethambutol may be replaced by streptomycin
- Pyridoxine 20 mg/day to prevent INH-induced peripheral neuropathy
- Prednisolone 60 mg daily for 3 weeks is given, and then tapered
- Neurosurgical intervention is performed, if hydrocephalus is suspected.

Encephalitis

It is the inflammation of brain parenchyma. It is mostly by virus, may be bacterial or other infection.

Causes: Herpes simplex type I, *Enterovirus* (poliovirus, coxsackievirus and echovirus), mumps, influenza, Japanese B encephalitis, togavirus, rabies virus, HIV and lymphocytic choriomeningitis.

Clinical features: Fever, headache, nausea, vomiting, photophobia, drowsiness, impaired consciousness and even coma. Convulsion and focal neurological signs (aphasia, hemiplegia and cranial nerve palsy). Abnormal behavior, agitation and hallucination.

Investigations:

- *CT scan or MRI*: Shows area of edema and low-density lesion in temporal lobe in herpes simplex encephalitis
- *Lumbar puncture and CSF study*: Shows clear fluid, high lymphocyte, and normal glucose but protein may be slightly high

- Viral serology in blood and CSF
- Electroencephalogram (EEG).

Treatment: IV acyclovir 10 mg/kg 8 hourly for 2–3 weeks. IV dexamethasone 6–8 hourly. Others—IV fluid, nutrition, and care of eyes, bowel, and bladder.

Herpes Simplex Encephalitis

Herpes simplex type 1 may cause encephalitis and type 2 may cause benign recurrent lymphocytic meningitis. It affects the inferior part of frontal lobe and medial part of temporal lobe.

It is characterized by flu-like illness followed by fever, severe headache, altered consciousness, behavior abnormality and speech disturbance. There may be focal neurological deficit, such as dysphasia, hemiparesis, and focal or generalized seizure, commonly temporal lobe seizure. Olfactory and gustatory hallucinations, and impairment of memory may be present. There may be multiple cranial nerve palsy and ataxia, convulsion, and coma. Mortality is high.

Investigations:
- Serum anti-HSV antibody
- Cerebrospinal fluid study shows high lymphocyte, and normal protein and sugar. PCR is performed for rapid diagnosis
- EEG shows distinctive periodic pattern in some cases
- CT scan shows low-density lesion in temporal lobes that enhances with contrast
- MRI shows orbitofrontal and medial temporal lobe involvement (not found in other virus).

Treatment: Acyclovir 10 mg/kg 8 hourly IV for 2–3 weeks. Anticonvulsant may be necessary. Dexamethasone IV 8 hourly.

BRAIN ABSCESS

Causes:
- It directly spreads from head injury, penetrating injury and trauma
- It spreads from infection of ear, nose, paranasal sinus and tooth
- Hematogenous in septicemia
- *Others*: HIV infection, immunocompromised case and Fallot's tetralogy.

Causative organisms: *S. anginosus*, *Bacteroides*, *Staphylococcus*, anaerobes and fungus. Mixed infections are common. Multiple abscesses are common in septicemia and also in HIV.

Clinical features: Fever may be very high with chill and rigor. Headache, drowsiness, confusion, nausea and vomiting. Convulsion and focal neurosurgical signs (hemiparesis, aphasia and hemianopia). Signs of meningism.

Investigations:
- CBC (leukocytosis), and blood for C/S
- CT scan or MRI of brain (will show ring-like shadow in brain).

Treatment:
- *Broad-spectrum antibiotic*: Cefotaxime 2 g IV 6 hourly or cefuroxime 1.5 g IV 8 hourly *plus* metronidazole 500 mg IV 8 hourly. Vancomycin should be added in neurosurgical case

- Injection dexamethasone IV 8 hourly
- Surgery may be necessary, if drug fails (burr-hole aspiration)
- Mortality is 25%. Epilepsy may occur in survivor.

HEADACHE

Causes:
- *Tension headache*: It occurs in anxiety, stress, and depression, functional
- *Vascular headache*: It occurs in migraine, cluster headache, transient ischemic attack (TIA), cardiovascular disease (CVD), subarachnoid hemorrhage, temporal arteritis and uncontrolled hypertension
- Traumatic
- *Infection*: Meningitis, encephalitis, sinusitis and cerebral abscess
- *Neoplastic*: Brain tumor
- Raised intracranial pressure due to any cause
- Referred pain from cervical spondylosis, eye, sinus, teeth and temporo-mandibular joint
- *Cranial neuralgia*: Trigeminal and glossopharyngeal
- *Drug*: Nitroglycerine
- *Others*: Postlumbar puncture headache and any acute febrile illness.

Migraine

It is characterized by paroxysmal, unilateral headache associated with nausea, vomiting and visual disturbance.

Types: Classic (with aura), common (without aura), migraine variants (retinal, ophthalmologic, hemiplegic and basilar). It is precipitated by stress, food (chocolate and cheese), alcohol, menstruation, oral contraceptive pill (OCP) and caffeine.

Clinical features: It is more in women, from puberty to middle age. Attacks occur at intervals and persists for hours to days. Initially prodromal symptoms such as malaise, irritability, aura (silvery zigzag lines and shimmering light), tingling, and numbness in one part of the body to other. Then, unilateral, throbbing headache, nausea, vomiting and visual disturbance. Patient prefers to stay in quiet and dark room.

Treatment: During acute attack, reassurance, and rest in quiet and dark room. Analgesics and antiemetics (prochlorperazine and metoclopramide). Also triptans (sumatriptan, zolmitriptan and rizatriptan).

Prevention: Avoid precipitating factors. One or combination of the following drugs can be used—propranolol (80–160 mg daily), amitriptyline (10–50 mg at night), topiramate (80–150 mg daily), pizotifen (1.5–3 mg at night), sodium valproate (300–600 mg daily), verapamil (80–160 mg), and flunarizine (5–10 mg).

Pregnancy with migraine: Usually during pregnancy, migraine is improved.

Cluster Headache

It is also called "migrainous neuralgia", characterized by recurrent episodes of unilateral headache usually associated with periorbital pain and autonomic features. It typically lasts for 4–12 weeks, followed by pain-free period for month or even 1–2 years before another cluster begins.

Clinical features: It can occur at any age, but is common in 30–40 years; occurs more in males. Headache occurs repeatedly in clusters over weeks.
- Severe unilateral headache, usually around one eye, lasts for 15 minutes to 3 hours, and radiates to frontotemporal region, jaw, neck or shoulder
- Autonomic features like lacrimation, facial flushing, nasal or conjunctival congestion, and meiosis
- Ipsilateral eye is red and watery, rhinorrhea occurs or ipsilateral nostril is blocked
- Typically, patient develops these symptoms at a particular period of day, usually in early morning or late hours at night, or after awakening the patient from sleep.

Treatment:
- *During acute attack*: High-flow oxygen (10–12 L/min for 15–20 min) or sumatriptan [6 mg subcutaneous (SC) or 20 mg nasal spray] is useful for the acute attack. Drugs used in migraine are not effective
- It can be prevented by verapamil, sodium valproate or short-course prednisolone (60 mg daily for 7 days, then taper over 21 days). In severe case, lithium can be used.

Causes of unilateral headache: Migraine, cluster headache, giant cell or temporal arteritis, intracranial space occupying lesion, unilateral sinusitis and unilateral glaucoma.

Headache of raised intracranial tension: Diffuse, dull, more on waking from sleep, improves throughout the day; it worsens on bending forward, coughing and straining. It is associated with morning vomiting without nausea.

BELL'S PALSY

It is a lower motor neuron (LMN) type of facial palsy associated with Bell's phenomenon. It is idiopathic in 95% cases, and may be due to viral infection.

Site of lesion: Facial canal, in petrous part of temporal bone.

Symptoms (in affected side): Pain around or behind ear, followed by weakness of face. Numbness and stiffness of cheek. Dribbling of saliva and liquid, food may accumulate between cheek and teeth. Watering from eye, loss of taste sensation (if chorda tympani branch is involved), and hyperacusis (if nerve to stapedius is involved).

Signs (in affected side): Facial asymmetry and inability to wrinkle forehead. Affected eye cannot be closed and on attempting to close, Bell's phenomenon occurs (eyeball is rolled upward and outward). Nasolabial fold is less pronounced, drooping of corner of mouth, weakness of affected side of face on puffing the cheek, and failure to whistle and smile. If asked to show teeth, affected part of face cannot be opened and face is pushed to normal side.

Investigation: Diagnosis is clinical. Blood sugar should be done.

Treatment: Prednisolone 60–80 mg daily is given for 5 days, and then tapered over 5 days. Physiotherapy (facial muscle exercise, massage and electrostimulation). Protection of eye during sleep (shut with tape or even tarsorrhaphy) and artificial tears or ointment. Residual paralysis may occur in 10% cases. Cosmetic surgery may be helpful. Antiviral (acyclovir or valaciclovir) has no role.

Causes of bilateral facial palsy: Guillain–Barré syndrome (GBS), sarcoidosis, bilateral Bell's palsy (rare), bilateral parotid disease, Lyme disease, and any cause of mononeuritis multiplex (rare).

SIXTH NERVE PALSY

Causes:
- Raised intracranial pressure (common) due to stretching of nerve in its intracranial course (a false localizing sign)
- Brainstem lesion (vascular, neoplastic and multiple sclerosis)
- Cavernous sinus lesion (tumor, thrombosis, infection and aneurysm)
- Trauma
- Any cause of mononeuritis multiplex
- Idiopathic (common)
- *Others*: Acoustic neuroma and nasopharyngeal carcinoma.

Clinical features: Convergent squint at rest. No lateral movement of affected eye and on attempting to look on that side, there is diplopia (outermost image comes from the affected eye).

Causes of bilateral 6th nerve palsy: Trauma, Wernicke's encephalopathy, mononeuritis multiplex and raised intracranial pressure (6th nerve palsy often associated with 7th nerve lesion also).

Treatment: According to cause.

THIRD NERVE PALSY

Causes:
- Nuclear lesion (infarction, hemorrhage, neoplasm and multiple sclerosis)
- *Midbrain CVD (Weber syndrome)*: Ipsilateral 3rd nerve palsy with contralateral hemiplegia due to thrombosis of a branch of posterior cerebral artery
- Unruptured aneurysm of posterior communicating artery (painful ophthalmoplegia)
- *Others*: Mononeuritis multiplex [causes are diabetes mellitus (DM), SLE, polyarteritis nodosa (PAN), sarcoidosis, amyloidosis and leprosy], subacute meningitis (carcinomatous, lymphomatous, fungal, tuberculous and meningovascular syphilis), raised intracranial pressure (due to long tortuous course so, likely to be compressed by any displacement of brainstem), ophthalmoplegic migraine, and Guillain–Barré syndrome.

Signs of 3rd nerve lesion: Complete ptosis, external squint, inability to move the eye upward, downward and medially, pupil (dilated, loss of direct and consensual light reflex), and loss of accommodation reflex.

Investigations: CBC (high ESR in vasculitis) and blood sugar. CT or MRI of brain. Occasionally, cerebral arteriography (if aneurysm is suspected).

Treatment: According to cause.

PTOSIS

It means drooping of upper eyelid. It may be unilateral or bilateral.

Causes of unilateral ptosis: Congenital, traumatic, senility, 3rd nerve palsy, Horner's syndrome (partial ptosis), myasthenia gravis (may cause unilateral or bilateral ptosis), and hysterical conversion reaction.

Causes of bilateral ptosis: Myasthenia gravis, tabes dorsalis, myopathy (myotonic dystrophy and facioscapulohumeral myopathy), ocular and oculopharyngeal myopathy, congenital (rare), and bilateral Horner's syndrome (rare, may occur in syringomyelia).

Treatment: Refer to ophthalmologist.

PAPILLEDEMA

It is the swelling of optic nerve head.

Causes:
- *Raised intracranial pressure due to any cause*: Brain tumor, brain abscess, meningitis, encephalitis and subarachnoid hemorrhage
- Central retinal vein occlusion
- Benign intracranial hypertension
- Hypertensive retinopathy (stage IV).

OPTIC NEURITIS

It is the inflammation of optic nerve.

Causes:
- *Demyelinating disease*: Multiple sclerosis
- *Drugs*: Ethambutol, quinine and chloroquine
- *Toxins*: Methanol poisoning, and lead, arsenic, and cyanide poisoning
- Neurosyphilis
- *Nutritional amblyopia*: Vitamin B12 deficiency, tobacco and alcohol.

OPTIC ATROPHY

It is the degeneration of optic nerve head, sometimes due to optic neuritis.

Types:
1. *Primary*: Due to involvement of optic nerve (optic neuritis, compression in optic nerve and glaucoma)
2. *Secondary*: Due to chronic papilledema
3. *Consecutive*: Secondary to disease of retina (retinitis pigmentosa, choroidoretinitis and Tay-Sachs disease). The term consecutive is controversial; it is actually secondary optic atrophy (OA).

Features:
- *Primary*: Disk is pale with clear margin and no change in retina
- *Secondary*: Disk is greyish white and margin is indistinct. Retinal exudate or hemorrhage may be present.

Causes: Raised intracranial pressure due to ICSOL (intracranial space occupying lesion) (neoplasm, abscess and cyst), chronic papilledema, secondary to optic neuritis, hereditary [Friedreich's ataxia, Leber's OA and DIDMOAD (diabetes insipidus, diabetes mellitus, optic atrophy, and deafness) syndrome], ischemic optic neuropathy (in giant cell arteritis). Others—trauma in optic nerve, Paget's disease and retinal artery occlusion.

Investigations:
- *CBC and peripheral blood film (PBF)*: Shows macrocytic anemia in vitamin B12 deficiency

- *Serological test for syphilis*: Venereal disease research laboratory (VDRL) and treponema pallidum hemagglutination (TPHA)
- X-ray of skull and CT or MRI of brain
- Other investigations according to suspicion of causes.

PUPIL

It may be constricted (miosis) or dilated (mydriasis).
- *Causes of constricted pupil*: Horner's syndrome, Argyll Robertson pupil, pontine hemorrhage, senility (pupil in old age tends to be small and may be irregular), morphine, miotic drugs (pilocarpine and physostigmine), and poisoning (organophosphorus and opium)
- *Causes of dilated pupil*: 3rd nerve palsy, Holmes-Adie pupil, optic nerve lesion (optic neuritis or retrobulbar neuritis), mydriatics (atropine and homatropine), other drugs (tricyclic antidepressant and amphetamine), datura poisoning, and fixed dilated pupil (in brain death, deep coma).

TRIGEMINAL NEURALGIA

It is characterized by lancinating pain along the distribution of trigeminal nerve, commonly along 2nd and 3rd division territory.

Clinical features: Usually above 50 years. Severe, paroxysmal unilateral facial pain of short duration (few seconds), knife like or electric shock like. Precipitated by touching the trigger zone within trigeminal territory by cold wind, eating, touching, washing and shaving. No physical sign. Diagnosis is clinical.

Treatment:
- *Carbamazepine*: Start with low dose (may cause severe Stevens–Johnson syndrome)
- Oxcarbazepine or phenytoin or gabapentin or pregabalin may be used
- *If no response*: Injection alcohol or phenol into the peripheral branch of nerve may be given
- *If still no response*: Radiofrequency lesion in the nerve near gasserian ganglion
- *Surgery*: Decompression of vascular loop encroaching on trigeminal root.

MULTIPLE SCLEROSIS

It is a demyelinating disorder of CNS characterized by multiple plaques of demyelination within the brain and spinal cord, gliosis, and varying degree of inflammation. Presence of two neurological lesions in anatomically unrelated sites or at different times indicates multiple sclerosis.

Causes: Unknown.

Sites of lesion: Optic nerve, brainstem, cerebellum, periventricular region and spinal cord (posterior column and corticospinal tract).

Symptoms: More in female, 20–45 years of age, rare before puberty and after 60 years.
- Weakness of one or more limbs and blurring of vision (due to optic neuritis)
- Features of spastic paraplegia and features of cerebellar signs (ataxia and tremor)

- Features of brainstem dysfunction (vertigo, diplopia, nystagmus, facial numbness or weakness, dysarthria, dysphagia and pyramidal signs in limbs)
- Bladder dysfunction (incontinence, dribbling and hesitancy)
- *Sensory disturbance*: Tingling of extremities and light banding sensation around the trunk or limbs (due to posterior column involvement)
- Euphoria despite disability
- *Temperature sensitivity*: Worsening of symptoms or weakness with rise of body temperature such as after exercise or hot bath
- *Others (rarely)*: Epilepsy, trigeminal neuralgia, recurrent facial palsy, 6th nerve palsy, dementia, neuropsychiatric dysfunction and depression.

Clinical courses (or types) of multiple sclerosis:
- *Relapsing and remitting (80–90%)*: Episodes of acute attack with recovery and remains stable between relapses
- *Primary progressive (10–20%)*: Gradual neurological deterioration from the onset. It usually begins after 40 years
- *Secondary progressive*: Some cases of relapsing and remitting course show gradual neurological deterioration
- Fulminating or relapsing progressive (<10%).

Signs and symptoms of multiple sclerosis (remember the formula WATSON):
- *W*: Weakness
- *A*: Ataxia (cerebellar)
- *T*: Tremor (cerebellar)
- *S*: Speech (scanning)
- *O*: Optic neuritis
- *N*: Nystagmus.

Investigations:
- *MRI of brain and spinal cord*: Investigation of choice as CT scan is not sensitive
- Lumbar puncture and CSF study
- *Others*: To exclude other diseases.

Treatment:
- *During acute attack*: IV methylprednisolone 1 g for 3–5 days, then oral prednisolone 40 mg daily for 10 days, then 20 mg for 2 days, then 10 mg for 2 days. Or prednisolone 40–60 mg daily for 10 days, then taper over 2 days (no role for long-term use for prevention). Plasmapheresis is helpful in severe case, unresponsive to corticosteroid
- *To prevent relapse, disease-modifying drugs may be given*: Azathioprine, β interferon (1a or 1b) or pegylated β1a, and glatiramer acetate. Monoclonal antibody (natalizumab and alemtuzumab). IV immunoglobulin may be helpful in aggressive cases
- *Symptomatic treatment*: For complication and disability
- *Others*: Control of infection, prevention of pressure sore, rehabilitation, occupational therapy, walking aids, visual aids, counseling and patient education.

Pregnancy in multiple sclerosis: Mild protective effect during pregnancy. Exaggeration may occur in puerperium.

SYRINGOMYELIA

It is a developmental anomaly in which there are cavities (syrinx) filled with fluid within the spinal cord, mostly originating at C8 and T1 segment, but may occur anywhere in spinal cord. Expanding cavity in the spinal cord gradually destroys anterior horn cells of spinal cord, lateral spinothalamic tract, corticospinal tract, and may involve brainstem (called syringobulbia).

Symptoms: Usually in 20–40 years, rarely in early age. Wasting of muscles of hands, forearms, shoulder girdles, loss of pain and temperature sensation, may be painless burn, and difficulty in walking.

Signs: Dissociated sensory loss in neck, shoulder and arm (loss of pain and temperature but intact light touch, vibration and position sense). LMN lesion signs in upper limb (wasting of muscles in hand and forearm with loss of reflex), and upper motor neuron (UMN) lesion signs in lower limbs.

Investigations: X-ray of neck to see congenital anomaly and MRI (investigation of choice).

Treatment: No specific treatment. Surgical decompression may be necessary. Supportive (regular activity, physiotherapy, avoid burn, trauma or hot water).

POLYNEUROPATHY

It is a clinical syndrome characterized by disturbance of function of peripheral nerves either motor or sensory or mixed or autonomic. It starts affecting the distal part and then gradually progresses proximally.

Causes:
- Diabetes mellitus
- Nutritional deficiency (B1, B6, B12, folic acid, pantothenic acid, and vitamin E)
- Malignancy (bronchial carcinoma, lymphoma and multiple myeloma)
- Drugs (isoniazid, vincristine, phenytoin, amiodarone, statins, cisplatin and dapsone)
- Infections (leprosy, HIV, typhoid and diphtheria)
- Collagen disease [SLE, PAN and rheumatoid arthritis (RA)]
- *Others*: Alcoholism, GBS, chronic kidney disease (CKD), chronic inflammatory demyelinating polyneuropathy (CIDP), idiopathic, industrial toxin (lead, arsenic, organophosphate), and genetic neuropathy (Charcot-Marie-Tooth disease, and hereditary sensory and autonomic neuropathy).

Note: Common causes of neuropathy—DM, leprosy, alcohol, GBS, CKD, drugs (INH and vincristine), and deficiency (vitamin B12, B1, nicotinic acid and B6).

Symptoms:
- *Sensory*: Tingling, numbness, burning sensation or pins and needles in glove and stocking pattern
- *Motor*: Weakness, heaviness and wasting of muscles (starting in hands or feet). Patient may complain of difficulty in walking
- *Autonomic*: Vertigo, disturbance of sweating, palpitation, gastrointestinal, and bladder and sexual dysfunction.

Signs:
- *Sensory system*: Both superficial and deep sensation (diminished or lost), and vibration and position sense (absent)
- *Motor system*: Wasting of muscle, muscle tone (diminished), muscle power (diminished), reflexes (diminished or absent), and coordination (impaired).

Investigations:
- CBC, PBF [macrocytosis indicates subacute combined degeneration (SCD) of spinal cord due to vitamin B12 deficiency], blood sugar, and chest X-ray (to exclude bronchial carcinoma)
- Serum B12 and folate assay, serum urea and creatinine, and liver function tests (LFT)
- Bone marrow (if suspicion of B12 deficiency)
- Other investigations according to suspicion of causes [antinuclear antibody (ANA) and RA test]
- Nerve conduction studies (axonal or demyelinating).

Causes of predominantly sensory neuropathy: DM, leprosy, deficiency of vitamins B1, B6 and B12, CKD, paraneoplastic neuropathy (in bronchial carcinoma), drugs (INH and vincristine), hereditary sensory neuropathy, HIV and multiple myeloma.

Causes of predominantly motor neuropathy: GBS, CIDP, Charcot–Marie–Tooth disease, acute intermittent porphyria, chronic lead poisoning, diabetic amyotrophy, diphtheria and paraneoplastic syndrome.

CARPAL TUNNEL SYNDROME (MEDIAN NERVE PALSY)

It is a type of entrapment neuropathy due to compression of median nerve under flexor retinaculum of wrist.

Causes: Pregnancy, obesity, RA, acromegaly, myxedema, CKD on long-term dialysis, tuberculous tenosynovitis, primary amyloidosis, tophaceous gout, drug (OCP), osteoarthrosis of carpus (related to old fracture), idiopathic (common in female, middle aged and obese).

Clinical features: It is common in female. Symptoms are tingling, numbness, nocturnal pain, and paresthesia in palm and fingers, which often occur at night after awakening the patient from sleep, may be referred to whole arm and shoulder.

Signs:
- Wasting along the distribution of median nerve and sensory loss of radial three and half digit
- *Tinel's sign*: Percussion over flexor aspect of wrist (flexor retinaculum) or tap the median nerve in forearm, patient may experience paresthesia along the distribution of nerve
- *Phalen's sign*: Flexion or extension of wrist for 1 minute produces paresthesia along the distribution of nerve (lateral three and half fingers).

Investigation: Nerve conduction study.

Treatment: Treatment of primary cause. Splint of wrist at night and ultrasound therapy. Local steroid injection proximal to the carpal tunnel (not into the tunnel, as it may damage the nerve). Diuretic may help. In severe cases, surgical decompression of carpal tunnel may be required.

ULNAR NERVE PALSY

Causes: Fracture of ulna or dislocation of elbow, injury at the wrist or palm, and mononeuritis multiplex due to any cause (DM, PAN, RA, SLE, amyloidosis and leprosy), osteoarthrosis of elbow, and occupation with constant leaning of elbows (clerk) or constant flexion or extension at elbow (carpenter, painter and decorator) and wrist (screw driver and drills).

Clinical features: Generalized wasting of small muscles of hands (except thenar) with dorsal guttering. Ulnar claw hand (extension of MCP and flexion of IP joint of 5th and 4th fingers), loss of sensation along 5th and half of the 4th finger, weakness of abduction and adduction of fingers, and wasting of medial side of forearm (due to involvement of flexor carpi ulnaris and medial half of flexor digitorum profundus). Froment's sign is positive.

RADIAL NERVE PALSY

Causes:
- *Axilla*: Trauma, radiation, compression by improper use of crutch and axillary growth
- *Spiral groove or mid shaft of humerus*: Trauma and compression (e.g. Saturday night palsy)
- *Proximal forearm*: Trauma, subluxation of radius and repetitive forearm supination
- *Wrist*: Trauma and compression by tight bracelet or handcuff
- Chronic lead poisoning
- Mononeuritis multiplex (due to any cause).

Clinical features: Wrist drop. Also, inability to straighten the fingers, if wrist is passively extended, patient is able to straighten the fingers at interphalangeal joint (due to action of interossei and lumbricals). There is weakness of extension of wrist and elbow, wrist flexion is normal. Triceps reflex is absent and loss of sensation of anatomical snuff box.

Saturday night palsy: Patient is heavily sedated with alcohol, sleeps with arms hanging over back of chair, and radial nerve is compressed at middle 3rd of humerus, causing paralysis of nerve. Brachioradialis and supinator and extensors of forearm are involved. Usually, complete recovery occurs within weeks.

SUBACUTE COMBINED DEGENERATION

It is a clinical syndrome due to B12 deficiency in which there are degeneration of posterior and lateral column of spinal cord and peripheral nerve. It is called combined degeneration, because there are peripheral neuropathy (due to demyelination of peripheral nerve), posterior column lesion (loss of vibration and position sense), and signs of pyramidal lesion (plantar is extensor, knee jerk is brisk and ankle jerk is absent).

Clinical features: Age 40–60 years, equally involved in both sexes.
- *Sensory*: Paresthesia and tingling or numbness, starting in toes and fingers. Lower limbs are more commonly affected than upper limbs
- *Motor*: Weakness, ataxia and loss of all reflexes. It may be exaggerated knee reflex with loss of ankle jerk, but extensor plantar

- *Bladder involvement*: Urinary incontinence and dribbling (usually in late stage)
- *Eye*: Optic atrophy
- *Mental change*: Dementia, impaired memory, confusion and depression
- *Others*: Anemia and glossitis.

Investigations:
- CBC and PBF (macrocytosis and hypersegmented neutrophil), bone marrow (to see megaloblast). Macrocytosis in blood and megaloblastic marrow are invariable in SCD
- Serum B12 assay
- Other investigations according to cause (Addisonian pernicious anemia and Crohn's disease).

Treatment:
- Injection of vitamin B12 1,000 µg IM, 6 doses 2–3 days apart, then maintenance therapy 1,000 µg every 3 months (lifelong in Addisonian pernicious anemia)
- After therapy, iron deficiency may occur. So, oral iron therapy should be given
- After B12 therapy, there may be hypokalemia, which should be corrected
- B12 orally 2 mg/day may be given. 1–2% is absorbed by diffusion without intrinsic factor. Sublingual B12 may be effective
- Treatment of primary cause.

Note: If folic acid deficiency is present with B12 deficiency, folic acid should not be given alone without B12, otherwise neurological features are aggravated.

PARKINSONISM

It is a syndrome characterized by tremor, rigidity and hypokinesia due to involvement of basal ganglia.

Parkinson's disease (paralysis agitans): Primary or idiopathic parkinsonism. There is deficiency of dopamine with relative increase in cholinergic transmission, so imbalance between dopamine and acetylcholine occurs.

Parkinsonian plus: Features of Parkinsonism with other degenerative disease like progressive supranuclear palsy (Steele–Richardson–Olszewski syndrome), olivopontocerebellar degeneration, nigrostriatal degeneration, primary autonomic failure (Shy-Drager syndrome), and Creutzfeldt–Jakob disease.

Causes: Unknown and multiple factors are responsible—
- Paralysis agitans (idiopathic, also called Parkinson's disease). Common in middle aged or elderly
- Postencephalitic
- *Drugs*: Phenothiazines (chlorpromazine and prochlorperazine), butyrophenones (haloperidol), metoclopramide, and tetrabenazine
- Neurosyphilis
- *Poisoning*: Carbon monoxide, manganese and MPTP (1-methyl-4-phenyl-1,2,3,6-tetrahydropyridine)
- Herbicide (paraquat)
- Trauma (punch-drunk syndrome and repeated head injury)
- Genetic (Wilson's disease and Huntington's disease)

- Cerebral tumor (involving basal ganglia)
- Parkinsonian plus
- Normal pressure hydrocephalus (triad of urinary incontinence, gait apraxia and dementia)
- Atherosclerotic parkinsonism (stepwise progressive broad-based gait and pyramidal signs).

Clinical features:
- Unilateral resting tremor in hand. Initially, pill-rolling movement between thumb and index finger, flexion and extension of fingers, abduction and adduction of thumb, and pronation and supination of forearm. Later, tremor may affect arms, legs, feet, jaw and tongue. Tremor disappears or reduces during voluntary activity, sleep, and holding something and increases with emotion or anxiety
- Difficulty in initiating movement, slowness of movement (bradykinesia or hypokinesia). Patient is unable to fasten button. Inability to touch tip of all fingers with thumb successively, if asked to count, there is slow initiation, unable or can do slowly. If asked to do rapid fine finger movement, it becomes indistinct, slurred and tremulous. Micrographia (handwriting is tremulous and untidy)
- *Rigidity*: Lead pipe or cogwheel
- *Others*: Titubation of head. Mask-like and expressionless face with less blinking of eyes, staring look and dribbling of saliva. Speech (slow initiation, husky, slurred, indistinct, lacking intonation, low volume and monotonous or mutism)
- *Glabellar tap*: Taping in forehead above the bridge of nose repeatedly. In normal person, blinking will stop after 3–5 blinks. In Parkinsonism, patient continues to blink. This sign is unreliable
- *Gait*: Rapid small shuffling step (festination) with stooping forward and narrow base to avoid falling, hardly raises foot from ground and feet may scrap the ground. During walking, less swinging of arms with flexed attitude. Difficulty in rapid turning (fractionated gait), turns "en bloc".

Investigations: Diagnosis is clinical. Investigations are done to find out cause or to exclude other disease.
- CT scan or MRI (done if pyramidal, cerebellar or autonomic involvement or doubtful diagnosis)
- *In patient <50 years, screening for Wilson's disease*: Serum ceruloplasmin (low), serum copper (high), and 24 hour urinary copper (high). Liver function tests may be done.

Treatment: Drug is not given in mild case due to side effects. Only given if disability and symptoms.
- *Drug therapy*:
  - Combination of levodopa and dopa-decarboxylase inhibitor is usually given. Available combinations are levodopa and carbidopa (110 or 275 mg), and levodopa and benserazide (62.5 mg). It starts with low dose and gradually increases as needed
  - For tremor, trihexyphenidyl, benztropine, orphenadrine, benzhexol and biperiden (less used because of side effects)
  - Other drugs: Amantadine, monoamine oxidase (MAO-B) inhibitor (selegiline and rasagiline), and catechol-O-methyltransferase (COMT) inhibitors (entacapone and tolcapone) may be used.

- *General measures*: Physiotherapy, speech therapy, occupational therapy and rehabilitation
- *Other measures*: Cognitive impairment and psychiatric symptoms may be helped by rivastigmine
- *Surgery*: Surgery is rarely done. Stereotactic thalamotomy or pallidotomy, deep brain stimulation, and fetal midbrain or adrenal tissue implantation in basal ganglia.

INVOLUNTARY MOVEMENTS

Types: Tremor, chorea, athetosis, hemiballismus, myoclonus, tic, torsion and dystonia.

Tremor: It is the involuntary, oscillatory and rhythmical movement of one or more parts of the body due to alternate contraction of a group of muscles and their antagonists.

Causes:
- *Functional*: Anxiety, nervousness and hysterical conversion reaction
- *Endocrine*: Thyrotoxicosis, pheochromocytoma and hypoglycemia
- Parkinsonism
- Cerebellar tremor (also called intention tremor)
- Benign essential tremor
- Senile tremor
- *Drugs*: Salbutamol and other beta-agonist, phenothiazine, butyrophenone, methyldopa, lithium intoxication and anticonvulsant (phenytoin, carbamazepine and sodium valproate)
- Alcohol (chronic alcoholism and alcohol withdrawal)
- *Others*: Toxin (mercury, arsenic and lead), general paresis of insane (GPI), and flapping tremor.

Types of tremor: Usually three types—
1. Resting tremor (typical of parkinsonism)
2. Action tremor or postural tremor (present on outstretched hands)
3. Intention tremor (it comes on voluntary movement but disappears on rest, caused by cerebellar lesion due to any cause).

According to the amplitude or nature, tremor may be fine or coarse:
- *Causes of action tremor*: Anxiety, thyrotoxicosis, senile tremor, benign essential tremor, cerebellar tremor, familial and idiopathic
- *Causes of fine tremor*: Anxiety, thyrotoxicosis, senile tremor, benign essential tremor, drugs (salbutamol and terbutaline), familial and GPI
- *Causes of coarse tremor*: Parkinsonism, intention tremor, flapping tremor in hepatic precoma, Wilson's disease, and sometimes in senile tremor.

Benign Essential Tremor

It is a familial tremor inherited as autosomal dominant, present in outstretched hands, also when holding a glass or spoon. Occasionally, present at rest, worse in upper limbs, and common in elderly (but may occur at any age). It is slowly progressive and rarely produces severe disability. No rigidity and no hypokinesia, and not aggravated by movement.

Treatment: Propranolol in small dose. Alcohol may relieve tremor, but may cause addiction. Primidone and also in severe case, injection botulinum toxin may be helpful. In intractable case, stereotactic thalamotomy or thalamic deep brain stimulation.

Chorea

It is involuntary, nonrepetitive, quasi-purposive, irregular and jerky movements of one or more parts of body due to extrapyramidal lesion. It may be unilateral or generalized. It worsens with anxiety or activity and disappears during sleep (chorea means dance, a Greek word). Lesion is in caudate nucleus of basal ganglia.

Causes:
- Rheumatic chorea (poststreptococcal, called Sydenham's chorea or St Vitus' dance)
- Senile chorea
- *Hereditary*: Huntington's chorea, Wilson's disease and benign familial chorea
- *Drug induced*: Phenothiazine, butyrophenone and OCP
- Pregnancy (chorea gravidarum)
- Encephalitis lethargica
- After stroke.

Treatment: Reassurance and treatment of primary cause. Phenothiazine, butyrophenones (haloperidol), tetrabenazine and sodium valproate may be given.

Sydenham's Chorea

It is one of the major criteria of rheumatic fever. History of rheumatic fever may be present in one-third cases. Common in children and adolescents, and more in female, 5–15 years.

Features:
- Chorea, associated with emotional instability, irritability, inattentiveness, confusion and fidgety. Speech is often affected
- Other evidences of rheumatic fever may be absent when chorea is present
- Carditis may be the first manifestation and rheumatic heart disease may occur
- Fever is unusual. ESR, antistreptolysin (ASO) titer and C-reactive protein (CRP) are usually normal
- It is usually self-limiting and recovers within weeks or 1 month. Recurrence may occur in 20% cases. Occasionally, it may relapse during pregnancy (called chorea gravidarum) or in those who use OCP.

Treatment: No treatment is given in most cases as recovery is spontaneous. In severe chorea, benzodiazepine, haloperidol, tetrabenazine or valproate may be given. Penicillin prophylaxis is given as in rheumatic fever.

Huntington's Chorea

It is inherited as autosomal dominant, in which chorea is associated with progressive dementia. Gene responsible is on the short arm of chromosome 4.

Symptoms: Common in adult, during third to fourth decade. Lower limbs are more involved than upper limbs. It is diagnosed by family history and chorea is followed by progressive dementia. There may be dancing gait. Occasionally, there is juvenile onset where parkinsonism is the main feature.

Investigations: CT scan or MRI (atrophy of caudate nucleus and cerebrum) and DNA analysis.

Treatment: Haloperidol or phenothiazine for dyskinesia. Tetrabenazine may be given. Psychological support, institutional care for dementia, and genetic counseling.

Athetosis: It is the involuntary, slow, coarse, and writhing movement of limbs, face or trunk. Causes are basal ganglia lesion (due to cerebral palsy and kernicterus), drugs (phenothiazine), and metabolic (Wilson's disease).

Hemiballismus: It is the involuntary, flinging or swinging movement of limbs. Causes are hemorrhage or infarction of contralateral subthalamic nucleus.

Myoclonus: It is the sudden, involuntary, and jerky movement of a single muscle or group of muscles. Causes are benign essential myoclonus and epilepsy.

Tics: These are repetitive, jerky or twitching movement of face, neck or hands such as shrugging of shoulder, sniffing and grimacing.

Dystonia: It is the involuntary movement of limb or head with abnormal posture. It may be generalized or localized such as spasmodic torticollis, writer's cramp, oromandibular dyskinesia, blepharospasm and hemiplegic dystonia. Cause—drugs such as phenothiazine (prochlorperazine) and metoclopramide.

MOTOR NEURON DISEASE

It is a progressive disease of unknown cause, characterized by degeneration of motor neurons in spinal cord, cranial nerve nuclei and pyramidal neurons in motor cortex. Common in middle aged and elderly male, rare before 30 years. No remission, fatal within 3–5 years.

Symptoms: Weakness and inability to walk, weight loss, and wasting of limb muscles, and occasional twitching of muscles.

Signs:
- *Motor system*: Wasting of muscles, muscle tone (may be increased), muscle power (may be diminished), reflexes (may be diminished or exaggerated), patellar and ankle clonus may be present; coordination may be impaired. Multiple fasciculations may be present
- *Sensory*: No change.

Types: According to the site of lesion—
- *Spinal cord lesion*:
  - LMN lesion: Progressive muscular atrophy
  - Combined UMN and LMN lesion (LMN lesion in upper limbs and UMN lesion in lower limbs): Amyotrophic lateral sclerosis
  - Pure UMN lesion (rare): Primary lateral sclerosis.
- *Cerebral lesion*: Medullary lesion (progressive bulbar palsy) and cortical lesion (pseudobulbar palsy).

According to type of lesion:
- *Pure UMN lesion*: Primary lateral sclerosis (PLS) and pseudobulbar palsy
- *Pure LMN lesion*: Primary muscular atrophy (PMA) and bulbar palsy
- *Mixed lesion*: Amyotrophic lateral sclerosis (ALS).

Progressive muscular atrophy: Weakness, wasting and fasciculation of distal limb muscles, usually starts in small muscles of one or both hands. Tendon reflex is lost (due to involvement of anterior horn cell).

Amyotrophic lateral sclerosis: Weakness, wasting, fasciculation, and loss of all reflexes (LMN lesion) in upper limbs *plus* spastic weakness with exaggerated reflexes and extensor plantar response in lower limbs (UMN lesion) or generalized hyper-reflexia. Bulbar and pseudobulbar palsy may occur.

Primary lateral sclerosis: Only UMN lesion (both in upper and lower limbs). Progressive tetraparesis with terminal pseudobulbar palsy may occur.

Progressive bulbar palsy: Lesion is in nucleus of lower cranial nerves in medulla (IX, X, XI and XII). Lesion is bilateral and LMN type. Causes are motor neuron disease (MND), GBS, syringobulbia, brainstem infarction, poliomyelitis, neurosyphilis and neurosarcoid.

Clinical features:
- *The patient presents with 3 "D"s:* Dysarthria, Dysphonia and Dysphagia. There is nasal regurgitation and dribbling of saliva. Speech is nasal, indistinct and slurred
- Tongue is wasted, wrinkled and fasciculating. There is palatal palsy and gag reflex is absent.

Pseudobulbar palsy: Bilateral UMN lesion (supranuclear) involving the pyramidal tract (supranuclear lesion of lower cranial nerves-IX, X, XI and XII). Causes are bilateral repeated CVD involving internal capsule (multi-infarct dementia), demyelinating disease (multiple sclerosis), and motor neuron disease.

Clinical features: It is common in women. The patient is emotionally labile (crying and laughing).
- *Speech*: Nasal, slurred, indistinct and high pitched (called *Donald Duck* or *hot potato* dysarthria due to tight immobile tongue)
- *Tongue*: Small and tight, spastic, unable to protrude, but no wasting or fasciculation
- Jaw jerk is exaggerated, palatal movement is absent, and gag reflex is present.

Investigations in MND: Diagnosis is clinical. Investigations are done to exclude other disease—
- Blood sugar (to exclude diabetic amyotrophy)
- VDRL or TPHA (to exclude neurosyphilis)
- Chest X-ray (to exclude bronchial carcinoma) and X-ray of cervical spine
- Ultrasonogram of whole abdomen (to see any neoplasm)
- Electromyography (EMG), nerve conduction velocity (NCV) test, and CT or MRI of brain and spinal cord may be done.

There are some "No's" in MND:
- No sphincter disturbance (rarely involved in late case)
- No sensory involvement
- No loss of awareness till death
- No dementia
- No ocular involvement
- No cerebellar or extrapyramidal lesion
- No abnormality of CSF usually.

Treatment of MND: No curative treatment. Only symptomatic and supportive treatment—
- Psychological support

- *Nutritional care. If needed*: Enteral feeding and percutaneous endoscopic gastrostomy
- Speech and communication therapy, respiratory therapy and palliative care
- Physical rehabilitation and occupational rehabilitation
- *Neuroprotective agents*: Riluzole, vitamin E and coenzyme Q10. Riluzole is a glutamate antagonist, which may retard progression and prolong survival.

Prognosis: MND is a progressive disorder; remission is unknown, and is fatal within 3–5 years. Younger patient with early bulbar syndrome tend to show a more rapid course.

STROKE (CVD OR CEREBROVASCULAR ACCIDENT)

It may be defined as sudden development of focal neurological deficit due to nontraumatic vascular cause.

Subvarieties:
- *Transient ischemic attack (TIA)*: Sudden neurological dysfunction caused due to cerebral ischemia lasts for less than 24 hours and recovers completely within 24 hours
- *Stroke in evolution*: Symptoms worsen gradually or in a stepwise pattern over hours or days, neurological deficit persists for more than 24 hours
- *Complete stroke*: Clinical signs of neurological deficit are persistent
- *Reversible ischemic neurological deficit (RIND)*: Neurodeficit persists for more than 24 hours, but recovers within 3 weeks
- *Partial nonprogressive stroke (PNS)*: Neurodeficit persists for more than 3 weeks, but is either partial or with minimal residual deficit.

Diseases included in CVD: Cerebral hemorrhage, cerebral thrombosis, cerebral embolism, subarachnoid hemorrhage, hypertensive encephalopathy, cerebellar hemorrhage and cerebellar infarction.

Risk factors:
- *Nonmodifiable*: Age, gender (more in male), ethnicity or race, genetics and family history
- *Modifiable*: Hypertension, DM, smoking, alcohol, lifestyle, obesity, heart disease (atrial fibrillation, ischemic heart disease and cardiomyopathy), dyslipidemia, OCP, carotid vessel atherosclerosis and atheromatous aortic arch.

Symptoms: Weakness of one side of the body, difficulty in speech and swallowing, urinary incontinence, and semiconsciousness or unconsciousness.

Signs:
- Patient may be semiconscious or unconscious. Slurring of speech may be present
- *Motor system (signs of UMN lesion)*: Usually hemiplegia
  - In one-half of body, muscle tone may be increased, and muscle power may be reduced
  - Reflexes: Exaggerated on the affected side. Patellar and ankle clonus may be present
  - Coordination: Impaired. Hemiplegic gait.
- *Sensory system*: May be intact.

Investigations:
- CT scan of head (first investigation to be done)
- *Routine*: CBC with ESR, blood sugar, urea, serum creatinine, electrolytes, serum lipid profile, chest X-ray P/A view and electrocardiogram (ECG)
- *To find source*: Doppler study of carotid vessels, echocardiography, MRA (magnetic resonance angiography) of cerebral vessels, and DSA (digital subtraction angiography) of cerebral vessels
- *Other tests*: According to suspicion of cause.

Treatment:
- *General measures*: Oropharyngeal suction, IV channel, nasogastric (NG) tube feeding, maintenance of nutritional status and regular change of posture (2 hourly) to prevent bed sore. Care of bladder (catheterization), bowel, mouth and eyes
- *Control of risk factors*: Hypertension, DM and hyperlipidemia
- *If cerebral edema*: Dexamethasone or mannitol
- *Specific treatment according to type of stroke (after CT scan)*:
  - Cerebral infarction: Antiplatelet drugs (aspirin and clopidogrel). Cerebral vasodilator like vinpocetine. If atrial fibrillation occurs, heparin followed by warfarin should be considered
  - Cerebral hemorrhage: For massive hemorrhage, neurosurgical intervention may be required. Other treatment is symptomatic and supportive
  - Subarachnoid hemorrhage: Nimodipine, neurosurgical intervention is essential.
- *Others (to improve quality of life)*: Physiotherapy, speech therapy and occupational therapy.

Prevention: Risk factors (hypertension, DM and obesity) should be identified and controlled. Smoking and alcohol should be stopped. Antiplatelet drug (aspirin) should be given in ischemic stroke. Statin should be given to all patients. Lifestyle modification (regular physical exercise and dietary modification). Treatment of primary cause.

Causes of CVD in young patient:
- Mitral stenosis with atrial fibrillation. Other cardiac causes [patent foramen ovale, ventricular septal defect (VSD) and tetralogy of Fallot (TOF)]
- Antiphospholipid syndrome, SLE and vasculitis
- *Hematological disease*: Sickle cell anemia, polycythemia rubra vera (PRV), inherited deficiency of naturally occurring anticoagulant (protein C, protein S, antithrombin III and factor V Leiden)
- Behcet's disease
- *Vascular malformation*: Arteriovenous malformation (AVM) and berry aneurysm causing subarachnoid hemorrhage (SAH)
- *In female*: OCP and eclampsia
- Homocystinuria
- Premature atherosclerosis may occur in familial hyperlipidemia.

Investigations in young patient with stroke:
- Chest X-ray, ECG and echocardiography (to exclude cardiac cause)
- CBC and ESR (to exclude polycythemia rubra vera)
- Serum lipid profile (in juvenile hyperlipidemia)

- For collagen disease (ANA, anti-dsDNA, anticardiolipin and anti-phospholipid antibodies)
- Coagulation screening, serum antithrombin III, and protein C and protein S levels
- *Others*: Red cell mass (in PRV), chromatographic test in serum and urinary level of homocystine or methionine (homocystinuria), TPHA, and VDRL (syphilis).

Brief Description in Different Types of Cerebrovascular Disease

Cerebral infarction or ischemic stroke: It is a common cause of CVD in middle aged or elderly (85%). The site is internal capsule, involvement of middle cerebral artery. Onset is insidious with stepwise progression. It usually occurs during sleep or soon after waking. Loss of consciousness is rare, but there may be headache and convulsion.

Cerebral embolism: Onset is very acute or stormy (develops quickly in seconds), during exertion or activity, and no warning signs of TIA. Left-sided vascular lesion is common as left common carotid artery arises directly from aorta. Left middle cerebral artery is commonly involved. There is usually a source of embolus or valvular heart disease with atrial fibrillation. Features may be diminished or disappear due to dislodgement of embolus. Shifting hemiplegia may occur. Rapid recovery may occur.

Cerebral hemorrhage: It is common in elderly with uncontrolled hypertension, and occurs in 15% cases of CVD. Onset is sudden. Common site is internal capsule. Other sites are pons, thalamus, cerebellum and cerebral white matter. Commonly lenticulostriate branch of middle cerebral artery is involved.

Subarachnoid hemorrhage: It usually occurs in young adults. The common cause is rupture of congenital berry aneurysm. Also in head injury, leaking from arteriovenous malformation. Features are severe thunderclap headache, which usually occurs in occipital region. There may be vomiting, convulsion, and rapid loss of consciousness. Neck rigidity and Kernig sign are present. Fundoscopy shows subhyaloid hemorrhage with upward concavity (boot shaped). Lumbar puncture and CSF study shows raised CSF pressure, which is frankly hemorrhagic. If CSF is kept for hours, xanthochromia may occur. CT scan is diagnostic. CT angiogram may be done. Treatment—control of hypertension, nimodipine and surgical treatment.

MYASTHENIA GRAVIS

It is an autoimmune disease of skeletal muscle characterized by weakness or fatigue, especially ocular, facial, neck, and bulbar muscles following activity. It is due to autoantibody (IgG) against postsynaptic nicotinic acetylcholine receptor. It is common in women aged 15–50 years. It is common in men over 50 years associated with thymic atrophy or thymic tumor.

Symptoms: Muscular weakness or fatigue after activity occurs usually at the end of the day. Drooping of upper eyelid and double vision, and difficulty in chewing, swallowing and speaking.

Signs:
- Ptosis, usually bilateral, may be unilateral; frontalis overactivity

- *Counting test*: When the patient is asked to count 1 to 50, voice becomes gradually indistinct
- *Ceiling test*: If patient is asked to look at the ceiling for some time, ptosis occurs
- Muscle power is initially normal, but with activity becomes weak
- *Reflexes*: Normal.

Investigations:
- CBC and ESR
- Chest X-ray (to exclude bronchial carcinoma and thymoma), and CT scan of chest (to exclude thymoma)
- Edrophonium (Tensilon) test
- Vital capacity
- Serum acetylcholine receptor antibody and serum anti-MuSK
- Single-fiber EMG shows progressive decremental response. Repetitive nerve stimulation test
- *To see other associations*: Thyroid function test, anti-skeletal muscle antibody (suggest presence of thymoma), ANA, rheumatoid factor, serum creatine phosphokinase (CPK), and antibody against intrinsic factor.

Treatment:
- Anticholinesterase, e.g. pyridostigmine 60 mg tablet (4–16 tablets in divided doses up to 5 times daily)
- *Others*:
  - Thymectomy: In all patients with thymoma and thymic hyperplasia
  - Steroid: Low-dose prednisolone initially 5 mg/day, increase 5 mg/week up to 1 mg/kg. Continued for 1–3 months, then alternate day regimen over 1–3 months. On remission, reduce the dose (may take months). Azathioprine may be added (2.5 mg/kg daily) or weekly methotrexate may be given. Sometimes, IV methylprednisolone or mycophenolate mofetil may be used
  - Plasmapheresis: In severe myasthenia or myasthenic crisis or preoperative preparation
  - IV immunoglobulin: An alternative to plasma exchange in severe myasthenia.

Drugs to be avoided in myasthenia gravis: Aminoglycoside, penicillamine, ciprofloxacin, quinine and antiarrhythmic.

TRANSVERSE MYELITIS

It is an acute inflammatory and demyelinating disorder of spinal cord causing paraparesis or paraplegia or sometimes quadriplegia. Commonly post-infectious. It is the common cause of noncompressive spinal cord syndrome. Mid-thoracic region is the common site.

Causes:
- *Postinfectious or postvaccinal inflammation*: Viral (coxsackievirus, poliovirus, EBV, herpes virus and HIV), bacterial (pyogenic, tuberculous and syphilitic). Others (parasitic, fungal and schistosomiasis)
- Traumatic
- Vascular (arteritis and anterior spinal artery occlusion)
- Nutritional myelopathy
- *Collagen vascular disease*: SLE, Sjögren's syndrome and mixed connective tissue disease (MCTD)

- *Miscellaneous*: Acute disseminated encephalomyelitis (ADEM), multiple sclerosis, sarcoidosis and neuromyelitis optica
- Idiopathic.

Symptoms: It usually follows viral illness or vaccination. Fever may be present, acute or subacute onset of paralysis or paraparesis associated with back pain. At the level of lesion, girdle constriction with hyperesthesia just above the lesion may be present. Usually there is no root pain, spinal tenderness or spinal deformity. Urinary problem like retention, incontinence as bladder involvement is early.

Signs:
- *Motor system*: Muscle tone (may be increased), and muscle power (may be diminished), reflexes (may be normal or exaggerated). Coordination (may be normal)
- *Sensory*: Partial or complete sensory loss with a definite upper level.

Investigations:
- CBC (leukocytosis in systemic infection)
- X-ray of dorsolumbar spine (to exclude other cause)
- CSF study (high protein and lymphocyte)
- CT scan and MRI of brain and spinal cord.

Treatment:
- Reassurance and psychological support. Care of bowel, bladder (catheterization), eyes and skin. Passive physiotherapy. For spasticity, baclofen, diazepam and tinazidine. Rehabilitation
- Treatment of specific cause, if any
- In patient with severe and rapidly progressive disease, high-dose IV methylprednisolone and IV acyclovir. Plasmapheresis may be done.

CEREBELLAR LESIONS

Signs: Titubation of head, tilting of head toward site of lesion, nystagmus (horizontal), scanning speech, intention tremor, incoordination, dysdiadochokinesis, past-pointing (dysmetria), ataxia, hypotonia and diminished tendon reflex (knee jerk may be pendular).

Causes of cerebellar lesion:
- *Vascular*: Hemorrhage, infarction, arteriovenous malformation and brainstem vascular lesion
- *Demyelinating*: Multiple sclerosis
- *Alcohol and Drugs*: Phenytoin, carbamazepine and lithium
- *Neoplasm*: Hemangioblastoma, medulloblastoma, acoustic neuroma and secondary deposit
- *Infection*: Cerebellar abscess and HIV infection
- *Inherited*: Friedreich's ataxia, ataxia telangiectasia and other hereditary ataxias
- Cerebellar syndrome of malignancy (paraneoplastic syndrome), due to carcinoma of ovary, uterus, breast and small cell carcinoma of the lung
- *Cerebellar syndrome*: Shy-Drager syndrome, Steele-Richardson-Olszewski syndrome, Creutzfeldt-Jakob disease and Wilson's disease
- *Others*: Hypothyroidism, Arnold-Chiari lesion and trauma (punch-drunk syndrome).

Investigation: MRI.

FRIEDREICH'S ATAXIA

It is the common type of hereditary ataxia, inherited as autosomal recessive trait and in some cases, autosomal dominant. Sites of lesion are cerebellum, spinocerebellar tract, posterior column lesion, and dorsal root ganglia, degeneration of peripheral sensory fibers, corticospinal tract (lateral column lesion), and eye (primary OA). There is progressive degeneration.

Symptoms: Usual onset at 8–16 years. There may be difficulty in walking due to weakness of lower limbs, hearing loss and dysarthria.

Signs:
- Cerebellar signs (dysarthria, nystagmus, intention tremor and ataxic gait)
- *Posterior column lesion*: Absent vibration and position sense and positive Romberg sign
- *Corticospinal tract sign lesion*: Extensor plantar response and weakness
- *Peripheral nerve*: Absent reflexes in lower limb and wasting of muscles
- *Other features*: DM (common), kyphoscoliosis, pes cavus, cocking of toes, OA, spina bifida and hypertrophic cardiomyopathy. Normal mentation (may have mild dementia).

Investigations: Diagnosis is clinical.
- CBC, ESR, blood sugar (high), chest X-ray (cardiomegaly) and ECG (arrhythmia)
- MRI of brain and spinal cord (shows atrophy of cerebellum and spinal cord), and NCS.

Treatment: Symptomatic and supportive.

BENIGN (IDIOPATHIC) INTRACRANIAL HYPERTENSION

It is defined as symptoms of raised intracranial pressure without space occupying lesion or ventricular dilatation or focal neurological sign. Actual cause is unknown, may be due to reduced or defect of CSF reabsorption by arachnoid villi. It is common in young females aged 18–40 years, obese, and rarely familial. It may be associated with pregnancy, obesity, OCP, hypo- or hyperthyroidism, adrenal insufficiency, steroid use or withdrawal, drugs (sulfur, nitrofurantoin, nalidixic acid, and tetracycline), and hypervitaminosis A.

The patient usually presents with frequent headache, visual disturbance (transient obscurations of vision mainly with change in posture), and 6th nerve palsy (false localizing sign). Fundoscopy shows papilledema. Visual loss may occur due to OA. Usually there is no epileptic attack.

Investigations:
- *CT scan or MRI of brain*: Normal with no ventricular dilatation
- Lumbar puncture shows high CSF pressure (>30 cm CSF), but normal CSF constituents
- MR angiography or cerebral venography may be done to exclude cerebral venous sinus thrombosis.

Treatment: Weight reduction and avoid offending drugs. Loop diuretic or acetazolamide may be given. Occasionally, steroid may be used (reduces intracranial pressure).
- Repeated lumbar puncture may be done
- Surgical treatment (ventriculoperitoneal or lumboperitoneal shunt, especially if progressive vision loss. Optic nerve fenestration may be done).

BRAIN TUMORS

Primary brain tumors are rare, about 1% in adult, but higher in children. Metastatic tumors are common. Primary brain tumor does not metastasize to other parts due to absence of lymphatic drainage in brain.

Types:
- *Malignant*: Glioma (astrocytoma is common and glioblastoma multiforme is most aggressive). Others are oligodendroglioma, medulloblastoma, ependymoma and cerebral lymphoma
- *Benign*: Meningioma (common), neurofibroma, craniopharyngioma, pituitary adenoma, colloid cyst and pineal tumors.

Investigations:
- CT scan and MRI with contrast
- Chest X-ray and CT scan of chest
- USG of abdomen and pelvis—to see any primary lesion
- Bone scan
- Lumbar puncture and CSF study in some cases
- Biopsy.

Treatment: Surgery, chemotherapy and radiotherapy

WILSON'S DISEASE

It is an inborn error of copper metabolism, inherited as autosomal recessive, characterized by failure of biliary excretion of copper, excess deposition of copper in several organs with their damage. It is also called "hepatolenticular degeneration". The commonly affected organs are liver, basal ganglia of brain, cornea, kidney and skeleton. Ceruloplasmin production is less. Total body copper is increased.

Symptoms: Age 5–30 years. Hepatitis is common in children and neurological features in adult.

Features:
- *Liver*: Acute hepatitis may be recurrent, fulminating hepatic failure, chronic persistent hepatitis, chronic active hepatitis or cirrhosis
- *Neurological*: Extrapyramidal (parkinsonism, tremor, dysarthria, chorea, athetosis and dystonia), cerebellar syndrome and dementia. No sensory abnormality
- *Eye*: Kayser-Fleischer (KF) ring, common in 10–12 o'clock position (upper periphery), due to deposition of copper in Descemet's membrane of cornea. It is greenish brown pigmentation at the sclerocorneal junction. Rarely, sunflower cataract occurs due to deposition of copper in lens (does not impair vision)
- *Psychiatric problem*: Personality change, suicidal tendency and manic depressive psychosis
- *Other features*: Renal (renal tubular acidosis and nephrolithiasis), cholelithiasis, spontaneous abortion, amenorrhea, hemolytic anemia, aminoaciduria or Fanconi syndrome, and osteoporosis may occur.

Investigations:
- Serum ceruloplasmin (low)
- Serum free copper (high)
- *24-hour urinary copper*: High. 24-hour urinary copper after penicillamine therapy >25 mmol is a confirmatory test

- Liver biopsy with quantitative measurement of copper (high hepatic copper, usually not done).

Treatment:
- *Penicillamine*: 1–4 g (usually 1.5 g daily). Dose is reduced in remission, and continued lifelong, even in pregnancy
- *Trientine dihydrochloride*: 1.2–2.4 g daily and zinc acetate, 150 mg daily may be given as an alternative, helpful in maintenance therapy and in asymptomatic case
- Liver transplantation in fulminating hepatic failure or in advanced cirrhosis.

Prognosis: Excellent, if treatment is started before irreversible damage.

Follow-up: Regular measurement of urinary copper and CBC, LFT, and renal function test (RFT).

Some common definitions:
- *Paraplegia*: Complete paralysis of both lower limbs. It may be spastic or flaccid
- *Paraparesis*: Weakness of both lower limbs
- *Monoplegia*: Paralysis of one limb
- *Hemiplegia*: Paralysis of one-half of the body
- *Hemiparesis*: Weakness of one-half of the body
- *Quadriplegia*: Complete paralysis of all four limbs
- *Quadriparesis*: Weakness of four limbs.

SPASTIC PARAPLEGIA

It means paraplegia of UMN type.

Causes:
- Spinal cord compression due to any cause (see below)
- Demyelinating disease (multiple sclerosis and ADEM)
- Motor neuron disease (amyotrophic lateral sclerosis and primary lateral sclerosis)
- Friedreich's ataxia (early age)
- Hereditary spastic paraplegia
- Subacute combined degeneration
- Acute transverse myelitis
- Anterior spinal artery thrombosis or occlusion
- Tropical spastic paraplegia.

Note: The most common causes of spastic paraplegia—7 T's
- *T*rauma
- *T*uberculosis (Pott disease)
- *T*umor (meningioma, neurofibroma, lymphoma, leukemia, myeloma and glioma)
- *T*ransverse myelitis
- *T*abes dorsalis
- *T*welve (B12 deficiency)
- *T*hrombosis.

Symptoms:
- *Pain*: Localized over the spine or in a root distribution, aggravated by coughing, sneezing or straining

- *Sensory*: Paresthesia, numbness or cold sensations, especially in the lower limbs, which spread proximally to a level on the trunk
- *Motor*: Weakness, heaviness or stiffness of the limbs, most commonly the legs
- *Sphincter*: Retention followed by urinary incontinence.

Signs: UMN sign below the level of compression with LMN sign at the level of compression and segmental sensory loss (sensory loss up to a particular segmental level).

Investigations:
- X-ray, MRI of dorsolumbar spine
- Lumbar puncture and CSF study
- Other tests according to cause (tuberculosis and myeloma).

Treatment: Care of bowel, bladder, mouth and skin. Prevention of bed sore by changing of posture every 2–4 hours, using special bed (air cushion bed) and by physiotherapy. Specific treatment is given according to cause (anti-Koch's in Pott disease, surgical removal of tumor and drainage of abscess).

Causes of spastic paraplegia due to cerebral lesion:
- Parasagittal meningioma (usually falx meningioma)
- Thrombosis of superior longitudinal sinus
- Thrombosis of unpaired anterior cerebral artery
- Multiple cerebral infarctions
- Hydrocephalus
- Trauma
- In children, cerebral palsy (cerebral diplegia).

Noncompressive causes of spastic paraparesis or paraplegia:
- MND (amyotrophic lateral sclerosis)
- Subacute combined degeneration of spinal cord
- Transverse myelitis
- Multiple sclerosis
- Friedreich's ataxia
- Lathyrism
- Syringomyelia
- Vascular disease of spinal cord
- Hereditary spastic paraplegia
- Tropical spastic paraplegia
- Postvaccination
- Syphilitic amyotrophy
- Nonmetastatic manifestation of malignancy
- Radiation myelopathy
- Functional.

FLACCID PARAPLEGIA

It is the paraplegia of LMN type.

Causes:
- Guillain–Barré syndrome
- Motor neuropathy due to any cause
- Tabes dorsalis
- Friedreich's ataxia
- Progressive muscular atrophy (one type of MND)

- Acute inflammatory demyelinating polyradiculopathy (AIDP)
- Hysterical conversion reaction (HCR).

GUILLAIN–BARRÉ SYNDROME

It is a postinfective demyelinating neuropathy of unknown cause, characterized by demyelination of peripheral nerve or spinal root. It occurs 1–3 weeks after respiratory infection, postvaccination, surgery or diarrhea. Triggering factors are *Campylobacter jejuni*, *Cytomegalovirus*, *Mycoplasma*, herpes zoster virus, HIV and EBV infections. It may be immunologically mediated.

Symptoms:
- Weakness, usually starts in lower limbs, ascends rapidly and affects upper limbs (ascending paralysis), more marked proximally than distally. Facial and bulbar weakness, and respiratory weakness. Even respiratory failure may develop within hours
- Low back pain, distal paresthesia and pain may precede weakness.

Signs: Muscle tone and power are diminished, loss of all reflexes, sensory loss (minimum or absent), bilateral facial palsy (in 50% cases, unilateral in 25% cases), and sphincter involvement (rare).

Investigations:
- *Lumbar puncture and CSF study*: Typical finding is "albuminocytological dissociation" (albumin may be very high, >1,000 mg % and lymphocytes are slightly raised or normal, <20/mm^3)
- Repeated monitoring of respiratory function tests [forced vital capacity (FVC), forced expiratory volume in 1 second (FEV$_1$) and peak expiratory flow rate (PEFR)]
- Arterial blood gas analysis (respiratory failure may occur)
- Nerve conduction study (shows slow conduction or conduction block, demyelinating neuropathy, found after 1 week)
- Serum electrolytes.

Treatment: The patient should be treated in intensive care unit (ICU), respiratory function should be monitored regularly (vital capacity and arterial blood gases). It may require artificial ventilation.
- High-dose IV gamma globulin should be given to all patients, 400 mg/kg/day for 5 days, helpful if given within 14 days. Plasma exchange, if given within 14 days is equally effective
- Symptomatic treatment and physiotherapy.

Note: Steroid has no proven value (may worsen). Methylprednisolone with immunoglobulin has no proven benefit.

CHRONIC INFLAMMATORY DEMYELINATING POLYNEUROPATHY

It is an autoimmune demyelinating disease of peripheral nerves characterized by weakness and sensory loss in limbs, peripheral nerve enlargement and high CSF protein. It is common in young adult, males slightly more affected than female.

Symptoms: Onset is usually gradual, but sometimes subacute. Features are like GBS. Relapsing and remitting or progressive generalized neuropathy.

Sensory, motor or autonomic nerves can be involved, but signs are predominantly motor. Some patients may present with pure sensory ataxia.

Signs: Like GBS.

Difference between CIDP and GBS: CIDP is clinically similar to GBS except, it has a relapsing or steadily progressive course over months or years; autonomic dysfunction is generally less common. It is less common than GBS. CIDP responds to steroid, while GBS does not.

Investigations:
- CSF examination (high protein and acellular)
- *NCV of peripheral nerves*: GBS like feature
- MRI (plaques resembling multiple sclerosis are found in brain and spinal cord in some cases)
- Nerve biopsy (shows segmental demyelination).

Treatment: Depends on severity of disease—
- *Mild*: Follow-up only, spontaneous recovery may occur
- *Moderate*: Prednisolone 60–80 mg daily for 2–3 months, then taper slowly. IV immunoglobulin (0.4 g/kg/day for 5 days) with steroid. Plasma exchange (2–3 times per week for 6 weeks). If above treatment fails, azathioprine, methotrexate, ciclosporin and cyclophosphamide may be given
- *Severe disease and nonambulatory*: Plasma exchange 2–3 times/week for 6 weeks and prednisolone 60–80 mg/day.

SEIZURE AND EPILEPSY

Seizure: It means convulsion caused by abnormal, excessive or synchronous discharge of cerebral neurons.

Epilepsy: It is characterized by recurrent and paroxysmal attack of convulsion or seizure.

Causes of epilepsy:
- *Primary or idiopathic*: Common in early age, before 20 years
- *Secondary*:
  - Traumatic
  - Vascular: CVD and AVM
  - Infection: Meningitis, encephalitis, cerebral abscess, cerebral malaria, tuberculosis and HIV
  - Intracranial space occupying lesion: Tumor, secondaries, abscess, subdural hematoma
  - Inflammatory: SLE, vasculitis and sarcoidosis
  - Metabolic: Hypoglycemia, hepatic failure and renal failure
  - Cerebral anoxia: Asphyxia and carbon monoxide and nitrous oxide poisoning
  - Congenital: Tuberous sclerosis and cerebral palsy.

Classification:
- *Generalized*:
  - Generalized tonic–clonic seizure (grand mal)
  - Absence seizure (petit mal): Typical absence, atypical absence, absence with special features
  - Myoclonic seizure: Myoclonic atonic and myoclonic tonic
  - Tonic and atonic seizure.

- *Partial or focal*:
  - Simple partial: No impairment of consciousness (Jacksonian seizure)
  - Complex partial: Impairment of consciousness (psychomotor epilepsy)
  - Partial seizure evolving to secondary generalized seizure.
- *Unclassifiable seizure*: It does not fit to any category above.

Generalized seizures: There is diffuse involvement of both cerebral hemispheres, cellular, structural or biochemical abnormality. Consciousness is usually impaired and motor abnormalities are bilateral.

Grand mal or generalized tonic–clonic seizure (GTCS):
- *Prodromal symptoms or aura*: Nonspecific symptoms like change of mood, irritability, insomnia and hallucination may warn the patient that an attack is impending
- *Tonic phase*: Tonic spasm of all muscles and loss of consciousness. Typical epileptic cry due to spasm of respiratory and laryngeal muscles followed by clonic phase, lasts for 10–30 seconds
- *Clonic phase*: Spasm is followed by jerky movement of one or more limbs. There may be tongue bite, frothing around mouth, and incontinence of urine, which lasts for 1–3 minutes
- *Postictal phase*: The patient remains flaccid and unconscious, persists for some minutes, then gains consciousness, but is confused and disoriented for half an hour or more. After the seizure, patient feels severe headache and goes to sleep.

Typical absence seizure (Petit mal): Common in childhood below 14 years. There is transient loss of consciousness with or without falling, staring look or tilted up eyes. Attack may occur several times daily.

Myoclonic jerks: Simple twitching of single or multiple muscles or jerky movements mainly in arms.

Akinetic seizure: There is sudden fall on the ground without warning followed by gaining of consciousness immediately.

Partial seizures: Seizure activity is restricted to one part of cerebral cortex. There is structural abnormality of brain such as tumor and AVM.

Complex partial (psychomotor type or temporal lobe epilepsy): It usually arises from temporal lobe.
- Emotional state either with fear, horror or outrage
- Feeling of epigastric sensation
- Hallucinations of smell, taste, vision and hearing associated with disorientation and confusion
- *Disturbances of memory or perception*: Undue familiarity (déjà vu) or unreality (jamais vu)
- In a dreamy state, patient carries out purposeful action without subsequent memory.

Simple partial (Jacksonian epilepsy): There may be an irritative focus that starts at any part of cortex. Convulsion starts at a part of the body, and then spreads to whole body. After attack, there is paralysis of half of body called Todd's palsy.

Investigations:
- *Routine*: CBC, ESR, urea, creatinine, electrolytes, calcium, magnesium and blood sugar

- Chest X-ray
- CT scan or MRI of brain
- Video EEG.

Treatment: Explanation and reassurance.
- *Generalized seizures*: Drugs are sodium valproate 500–1,500 mg *or* carbamazepine 200–1,200 mg *or* phenytoin 200–400 mg. Others (lamotrigine, topiramate and vigabatrin)
- *Petit mal*: Ethosuximide 100–1,500 mg or sodium valproate
- *Psychomotor*: Carbamazepine and others (phenytoin and lamotrigine).

Advice to the patient: Must take the drug regularly, and should not work near fire and machine. Avoid swimming, cycling and driving. Precipitating factors should be avoided.

STATUS EPILEPTICUS

It is defined as persistent or prolonged seizure lasting for 30 minutes or longer or recurrent seizure with no recovery of consciousness in between.

Treatment: It is better to be treated in ICU. O_2 inhalation, airway should be kept clear. IV channel should be open.
- *Initially*: Injection diazepam, 10 mg IV over 5 minutes (or rectally). *Or* injection lorazepam 4 mg IV. Repeat after 15 minutes if attack recurs
- *If seizure continues after 30 minutes*: Injection phenytoin 15 mg/kg *plus* 10 mg/mL in saline at 50 mg/minutes *or* fosphenytoin 15 mg/kg with 10 mg/mL saline at 100 mg/min *or* phenobarbital 10 mg/kg with distilled water at 100 mg/min
- *If seizures persist over 90 minutes*: Intubation, ventilation, general anesthesia (injection thiopentone)
- *Once status is controlled*: Oral anticonvulsant should be continued.

DISEASE OF THE MUSCLES AND MYOPATHY

Some definitions:
- Myopathy means weakness of voluntary muscle
- Myositis means inflammation of muscle
- Muscular dystrophies are inherited disorders of muscle cells
- Myasthenia means fatigue or weakness, which worsens on exercise
- Myotonia is sustained contraction or slow relaxation after voluntary activity
- Channelopathies are ion channel disorders of muscles.

Symptoms: Weakness and difficulty in walking, combing, and raising upper limb above the head. Cramping, muscle pain and stiffness.

Signs: Depends on type.

Investigations:
- *CPK*: High, up to 40-fold in Duchenne type
- *EMG*: Short duration, and low-amplitude spiky polyphasic action potential
- ECG (cardiomyopathy and dysrhythmia), and echocardiography,
- *Muscle biopsy*: Shows variation of muscle fiber size, degenerative changes, regeneration and replacement by fat
- Blood sugar and lactic acid (to exclude mitochondrial myopathy)
- Molecular genetic testing.

Differences between neuropathy and myopathy:
- Myopathy usually involves proximal muscles (except myotonia dystrophica, which involves distal muscles)
- Neuropathy usually involves distal muscles (except diabetic amyotrophy, which involves proximal muscles).

Classification of muscular disease:
- *Genetic*: Muscular dystrophy and myotonic dystrophy
- *Acquired*:
    - Inflammatory: Polymyositis, dermatomyositis, viral, bacterial or parasitic, and sarcoidosis
    - Endocrine: Cushing's syndrome and thyroid disease
    - Myasthenic disease: Myasthenia gravis, Lambert–Eaton myasthenic myopathic syndrome
    - Metabolic: Myophosphorylase deficiency (McArdle's syndrome)
    - Channelopathy: Hypokalemic and hyperkalemic periodic paralysis
    - Drugs and alcohol.

MUSCULAR DYSTROPHY

It is a group of hereditary muscular disorder characterized by progressive degeneration of groups of muscles without involvement of nervous system.

Types:
- *Hereditary muscular dystrophy*:
    - Duchenne type (pseudohypertrophic)
    - Becker muscular dystrophy
    - Limb girdle myopathy
    - Facioscapulohumeral dystrophy.
- Myotonia dystrophica
    - Myotonia congenita
    - Others: Oculopharyngeal or ocular myopathy and congenital muscular dystrophy.
- *Congenital myopathy (rare)*: Central core, nemaline myopathy and myotubular myopathy.

Duchenne Muscular Dystrophy

It is inherited as X-linked recessive disorder (30% spontaneous mutation). It affects only males; age of onset is 3–4 years. The child presents with difficulty in walking or getting up from sitting or lying position. There is history of frequent fall and delayed motor activity (e.g. walking).

- *Gower's sign*: While the child gets up from lying position, he uses the hands to climb up
- Pseudohypertrophy in calf and deltoid muscles
- Waddling gait (duck like)
- *Other features*: Dilated cardiomyopathy, kyphoscoliosis, mental retardation and early respiratory involvement
- Prognosis is poor, chair bound by the age of 10 years and few survive up to 20 years
- *Causes of death*: Dilated cardiomyopathy and respiratory failure or inanition.

Becker Muscular Dystrophy

It is inherited as X-linked disorder, only males are affected and features are same as Duchenne type with the exception of:
- Onset is late (5-25 years). Less severe, less rapid progression and less cardiomyopathy
- Mental retardation and kyphoscoliosis are uncommon. Respiratory involvement is a late feature
- Chair bound at about 25 years after the onset. Survival up to fourth to fifth decade.

Limb Girdle Myopathy

It is inherited as autosomal dominant (type 1, 10%) and autosomal recessive (type 2, 90%), characterized by involvement of shoulder and pelvic girdle muscles. Age of onset is 10-30 years, male and female are equally affected. It may involve cardiac muscle (may cause conduction abnormality or heart failure). Intelligence is normal, face is normal, and muscle enzymes are normal or slightly elevated. Prognosis is poor, chair bound at 20-25 years of age (10-20 years after onset of disease).

Facioscapulohumeral Dystrophy

It is inherited as autosomal dominant, characterized by involvement of muscles of face and shoulder girdle. Onset is 10-40 years of age.
- Course is variable, but usually relatively benign
- There is wasting of muscles of face, neck and shoulder girdle (lower trapezei, pectoralis, biceps, triceps). Hypertrophy of the deltoid, winging of scapula (due to involvement of serratus anterior muscle). Pain in shoulder girdle is common. There may be distal lower limb weakness
- Face looks dull, expressionless, lips open and slack, inability to whistle, and puff the cheek
- *Eyes*: bilateral partial ptosis
- Intelligence is normal
- Muscle enzymes are usually normal or slightly elevated
- *Prognosis*: Normal life span, and slowly progressive.

Myotonia

It is the continued contraction of muscles after cessation of voluntary contraction.

Types: There are two types—(1) Myotonia dystrophica and (2) myotonia congenita (Thomsen's disease).

Myotonia Dystrophica

It is inherited as autosomal dominant. Males are affected more. Age of onset is usually 20-50 years.
- *In face*: Frontal baldness. Long, lean, triangular, sad and expressionless face. Wasting of temporalis and masseter
- *In eyes*: Partial ptosis (usually bilateral, may be unilateral) with smooth forehead. Cataract (stellate cataract). May be subcapsular fine deposit. Difficulty in opening the eyes after firm closure
- *In neck*: Wasting of sternomastoid and shoulder girdle muscles

- *In hands*: If the hands are closed tightly, it relaxes slowly if asked to open. Inability to relax hands after handshake. Percussion on thenar eminence shows depressions, which fill slowly
- *Other features*:
    - Percussion over the tongue shows depression
    - Wasting of distal muscles of arms and legs
    - Testicular atrophy and gynecomastia. Small pituitary fossa and hypogonadism may occur
    - In heart: Cardiomyopathy and conduction defect
    - Diabetes mellitus and impaired glucose tolerance (IGT) may occur
    - Intellect and personality: Mild deterioration
    - Low serum IgG levels
    - Tolerate anesthesia poorly.

Treatment: Only symptomatic. No specific treatment. May be treated by phenytoin. Procainamide or quinidine may be used, but may worsen cardiac conduction. Genetic counseling.

Myotonia congenita: It is inherited as autosomal dominant, characterized by failure to relax the muscle after forceful contraction. Present at birth with feeding difficulty, inability to open the eyes and a peculiar cry. It is mild disease, which improves with age. Procainamide, quinidine and mexiletine may be helpful. Life expectancy is normal.

ALZHEIMER'S DISEASE

It is a progressive and neurodegenerative disease characterized by memory loss, language deterioration, poor judgment, indifferent attitude and progressive dementia. However, motor function remains preserved. It appears first as memory decline and over several years, it disturbs cognition, personality, and person's ability to function. Confusion and restlessness may also occur.

Clinical features: It usually begins after the age 65 years. But it may occur as early as 40 years.
- Gradual decline in daily activities, ultimately profound disability, and dependent on others
- *Disturbance in memory*: Progressive loss of ability to learn, retain, and process new information and recall previously learnt information. Both short- and long-term memories are involved, commonly short term. Decline in language function, difficulty with names, word finding, and understanding what is being said
- *Apraxia*: Inability to perform skilled motor activity
- *Agnosia*: Failure to recognize objects, such as cloth, place and people
- *Frontal executive function*: Impairment of organizing, planning and sequencing
- Childish behavior, agitation, aggression, depression and paranoid delusion
- In early stage, patient may complain of any physical problem, but in later stage, usually he may be reluctant to seek medical attention (anosognosia).

Investigation:
- *Routine*: CBC, blood sugar, serum electrolytes, calcium, B12, thyroid function and chest X-ray
- CT scan or MRI of brain, EEG, and lumbar puncture and CSF study (also TPHA).

Treatment: Usually acetylcholinesterase inhibitor drugs (donepezil, galantamine and rivastigmine). Memantine (affects glutamine transmission) may be used. Antidepressant may be needed.

PARANEOPLASTIC SYNDROME

It is characterized by bizarre neurological presentation, multiple signs, and symptoms associated with malignancy unrelated to metastasis. Usually in elderly, most are associated with carcinoma of lung (small cell), ovary, breast, pancreas, prostate, nasopharynx and lymphoma.

Clinical Features: Varies with primary cause, and may precede clinical presentation of primary carcinoma in 50% cases.

Usual features are:
- *Neurological*: Neuropathy, cerebellar degeneration, motor neuron disease, myasthenic myopathic syndrome (Lambert–Eaton syndrome) and GBS
- *Musculoskeletal*: Polymyositis or dermatomyositis, clubbing and hypertrophic osteoarthropathy
- *Endocrine*: SIADH, ectopic ACTH syndrome and hypercalcemia
- Cachexia.

Investigations: X-ray of chest or other organ, USG of abdomen, CT scan or MRI, EMG, CPK and biopsy of muscle. Other investigations according to suspicion of cause.

Treatment: Primary cause should be treated.

NEUROFIBROMA

It is a benign tumor of peripheral nerves arising from neurilemmal sheath.

Neurofibromatosis: It is an autosomal dominant disease characterized by multiple neurofibroma with skin lesions like café au lait spots and axillary freckling.

Types: There are two types—
1. Type 1 or von Recklinghausen's disease or peripheral
2. Type 2 or central.

Features of type 1 neurofibromatosis: Multiple cutaneous neurofibroma, café au lait patches >6 (up to 5 may be found in normal person), axillary freckling, hamartoma of iris (Lisch nodules), optic glioma, and others (scoliosis, pseudoarthrosis and pulmonary stenosis).

Features of type 2 neurofibromatosis: Bilateral acoustic neuroma, glioma (cerebral or optic nerve), meningioma, spinal neurofibroma, schwannoma, and juvenile posterior subcapsular lenticular opacity.

Café au lait spot: These are round to ovoid, pale yellow or brown macules, and usually present on trunk. May be 1–15 cm. Up to 5 may be present in a normal person.

Lisch nodule: It is a melanocytic hamartoma of iris, clear to yellow or brown. It increases with age, present in patient older than 20 years.

Plexiform neurofibroma: In this type, entire nerve trunk and its branches are involved in diffuse neurofibromatosis with overgrowth of overhanging tissues, leading to gross deformities in temporal and frontal scalp. The most common sites are temporal region in relation to trigeminal nerve, upper eyelid and back of the neck.

Associated findings or complications of neurofibroma: Kyphoscoliosis, lung cyst (honeycomb lung), pseudoarthrosis and other orthopedic abnormalities, glioma, meningioma, medulloblastoma, pheochromocytoma (in MEN IIA), and posterior mediastinal tumor called dumb bell tumor, rarely sarcomatous change.

Phakomatosis: It is a group of diseases in which neurological abnormalities are associated with cutaneous disease. These are neurofibromatosis type 1, tuberous sclerosis, Von Hippel–Lindau syndrome and Sturge-Weber syndrome.

TUBEROUS SCLEROSIS

It is an autosomal dominant disease characterized by triad of mental retardation (or learning disability), epilepsy, and skin lesions. Family history, convulsion, and mental retardation are present.

Skin lesions: Papules on the face called adenoma sebaceum, subungual fibroma (nodule arising from the nail bed), shagreen patches (firm, flesh colored, patches of leathery thick skin over the lower back), ash leaf patches (hypopigmented areas of skin), and café au lait spots present in 30% cases.

Investigations: Skull X-ray shows tramline calcification at the basal ganglia. CT scan or MRI of brain.

Treatment: No specific treatment. Symptomatic treatment for seizure. Genetic counseling.

HYDROCEPHALUS

It is the excessive accumulation of CSF in brain caused either by increased CSF production, by reduced CSF absorption or by obstruction of circulation. As a result, there is ventricular dilatation.

Causes:
- Congenital malformations (infantile hydrocephalus). Head is enlarged in such case
- *Acquired causes (adult hydrocephalus)*:
  - *Mass lesions (mainly posterior fossa)*: Tumor, colloid cyst of 3rd ventricle, abscess and hematoma
  - Absorption blockages due to inflammation (meningitis and sarcoidosis), and subarachnoid hemorrhage
  - Idiopathic in many cases.

Symptoms: May be asymptomatic. Headache, cognitive impairment, features of raised intracranial pressure, and ataxia.

Treatment: Furosemide and acetazolamide may be given (decrease CSF production). Removal of tumor, if any. Serial lumbar puncture, ventriculoperitoneal shunt, and endoscopic 3rd ventriculostomy may be done.

Normal pressure hydrocephalus: It is a syndrome of enlarged ventricle with normal CSF pressure, characterized by triad of gait apraxia, dementia and urinary incontinence. Common in elderly. It is idiopathic in many cases, may be secondary to meningitis or subarachnoid hemorrhage. CT scan shows dilatation of ventricles but no cortical atrophy.

Treatment: Ventriculoperitoneal or less commonly ventriculoatrial shunt.

MULTI-INFARCT DEMENTIA

When dementia is due to multiple infarction of brain secondary to atherosclerosis, also called vascular dementia. It is common cause of dementia in elderly; occurs when a thrombus blocks small blood vessels in brain and destroys brain tissue. Overtime, as more small vessels are blocked, there is gradual mental decline. It typically begins in 60–75 years, more in men. In late stage, there is dementia, pseudobulbar palsy and shuffling gait (marche à petits pas), called atherosclerotic parkinsonism. Risk factors are advanced age, high BP, smoking, DM and dyslipidemia.

Symptoms: Often develop in a stepwise manner—
- Disturbance with recent memory, confusion, personality change, behavioral difficulty, aggressive, and wandering or getting lost in familiar places
- Loss of bladder or bowel control (incontinence)
- Emotional problems such as laughing or crying inappropriately
- Difficulty following instructions and problems handling money.

Investigation: MRI of brain shows multiple infarction of brain.

Treatment: No specific treatment. Only symptomatic and supportive, and control of risk factors (high BP, DM and dyslipidemia).

DIZZINESS AND VERTIGO

Dizziness: It means feeling of various types of sensations such as feeling of imbalance, light-headedness, faintness (a feeling of impending syncope), and giddiness.

Vertigo: It is a sensation of movement of body or surroundings, perceived as feeling of rotation. It is due to disturbance in vestibular system.

Both dizziness and vertigo may be accompanied by nausea and vomiting or difficulty with balance, gait or both. Vertigo can also present with nystagmus and blurring vision.

Causes of dizziness and vertigo: It may be central (brainstem or cerebellar lesion) or peripheral (labyrinthine or vestibular lesion)—
- *Central*: Brainstem or cerebellar hemorrhage or infarction, multiple sclerosis, acoustic neuroma, vertebral artery dissection, vertebrobasilar insufficiency, TIA, temporal lobe epilepsy and migraine
- *Peripheral*: Benign positional vertigo, Meniere's disease, vestibular neuronitis, labyrinthitis, otitis media, trauma (tympanic membrane rupture and temporal bone fracture), ototoxic drugs (aminoglycoside), and chronic motion sickness.

Investigations: CBC, ECG, echocardiography, chest X-ray, blood sugar, serum electrolytes, carotid Doppler study, MRI of brain and audiometry. Others according to suspicion of cause (pregnancy test).

Treatment: According to cause. Cinarizine, flunarizine and betahistine may be given.

SYNCOPE

It is defined as transient loss of consciousness due to inadequate blood supply to the brain.

Near syncope or presyncope: It is light-headedness and a sense of impending faint without loss of consciousness.

Causes:
- *Cardiac causes*: Arrhythmias (sick sinus syndrome, complete heart block, atrial fibrillation, ventricular tachycardia, ventricular fibrillation and asystole), aortic stenosis, tetralogy of Fallot, hypertrophic cardiomyopathy, left atrial myxoma, acute myocardial infarction and myocarditis
- *Vasovagal attack*: Prolong standing and strong emotion (pain and fear)
- *Orthostatic hypotension*: Drugs (nitrate, angiotensin-converting enzyme inhibitor and prazosin), and autonomic neuropathy
- *Cerebrovascular causes*: TIA, stroke and migraine
- *Other causes*: Cough syncope, micturition syncope and carotid sinus hypersensitivity syndrome.

Investigations: As in vertigo (see above).

Treatment: The patient should lie in horizontal position with legs elevated. If pulseless, CPR should be initiated. Synchronized DC shock may be needed. Treatment of cause.

Funny turn or blackout: It is characterized by altered consciousness, visual disturbance or falling. It is like dizziness. Causes are epilepsy, syncope due to any cause, nonepileptic attacks (pseudoseizure), panic attack, hypoglycemia, drop attacks, hydrocephalic attack, basilar migraine, severe vertigo, cataplexy, narcolepsy and sleep paralysis.

MÉNIÈRE'S DISEASE

It is a vestibular disorder of unknown origin characterized by recurrent attack of vertigo and progressive deafness. It is due to distension of endolymphatic system of inner ear (endolymphatic hydrops). Equal in both sexes, age 40–50 years.

Features: Recurrent attacks of severe vertigo, constant tinnitus increases during attack, feeling of fullness in the ear, severe nausea or vomiting, imbalance, and progressive hearing loss; recovers between attacks but later permanent and progressive.

Investigations: Audiometry, vestibular testing, and MRI to rule out other causes.

Treatment:
- Low-salt diet. Potassium sparing diuretic (spironolactone)
- *For vertigo, nausea and vomiting*: Prochlorperazine *or* cinnarizine *or* cyclizine can be given.
- Tablet diazepam 2–5 mg orally at 6 or 8 hours interval can also be given
- Betahistine to reduce the frequency and severity of attacks
- *For tinnitus*: Sound therapy and cognitive behavioral therapy

- Vestibular rehabilitation to cope with balance problems
- Surgery.

CENTRAL PONTINE MYELINOLYSIS

Rapid correction of hyponatremia by hypertonic saline (3%) results in central pontine myelinolysis, a dangerous complication. There may be various types of neurological deficits, from quadriparesis to coma and death. Rapid correction of hyponatremia by hypertonic saline should be avoided. Correction with IV normal saline and oral salt are sufficient. MRI of brain is the investigation of choice. No definitive treatment, only symptomatic and supportive.

NYSTAGMUS

It is the involuntary, rhythmical and oscillatory movement of one or both eyes, due to inability to maintain the posture of eyes, owing to the lack of balance of opposing ocular muscles. It is defined by the direction of fast phase and is exaggerated on gaze to that side. Nystagmus is significant, if sustained for more than few beats. It may be jerky or phasic, pendular or ataxic (internuclear ophthalmoplegia).

Types:
- *According to direction*: Horizontal, vertical and rotatory
- *According to site of lesion*: Cerebellar (toward the site of lesion), vestibular (away from the site of lesion), brainstem lesion (usually vertical, may be in other direction)
- *Others*: Positional nystagmus (associated with benign positional vertigo), ocular or fixation nystagmus (usually pendular type), optokinetic, and see-saw nystagmus.

Causes of horizontal nystagmus:
- Cerebellar and vestibular nystagmus
- Brainstem lesion
- *Others*: Ocular or fixation nystagmus (usually pendular type) and optokinetic. In normal person, in extreme lateral gaze.

Causes of vertical nystagmus: Brainstem lesion—upbeating (midbrain lesion) and downbeating (medulla associated with foramen magnum lesion). Rarely, ocular nystagmus.

Causes of vestibular nystagmus: Horizontal or rotatory, Not vertical. Two types—peripheral and central.
1. *Peripheral*: Lesion is in labyrinth or vestibular nerve. Fast component of nystagmus is contralateral to the site of lesion, and may be associated with cochlear lesion. Causes are—labyrinthitis (may be viral), Meniere's disease, acoustic neuroma, head injury, middle ear disease and vestibular neuronitis (presents with acute vertigo, tinnitus and deafness)
2. *Central*: Lesion is in vestibular nuclei. Causes are—cerebrovascular disease, multiple sclerosis, neoplasm, alcohol and anticonvulsant drugs.

Jerky or phasic nystagmus: It is characterized by eye movement faster in one direction than other. It is seen in horizontal direction, on lateral gaze in one or both directions. Causes are cerebellar lesion, vestibular lesion or lesions of their connection in the brainstem.

Pendular nystagmus: In this type, oscillations are equal in speed and amplitude in both directions of eye movement, seen in central gaze. Cause is poor visual acuity (in severe refractive error or macular disease), usually congenital and asymptomatic.

Ataxic nystagmus: In this type, on looking to one side, nystagmus is present in the abducting eye and there is failure of adduction of other eye. It is also called "dissociated nystagmus", present in internuclear ophthalmoplegia. Common cause is multiple sclerosis. However, on covering the abducting eye, adduction of other eye is normal. The lesion is in medial longitudinal bundle which connects 6th nerve nucleus on one side to the 3rd nerve nucleus on the opposite side of brainstem.

Optokinetic nystagmus: It occurs when the patient follows a rapidly moving scene (as during travelling in a train, eye remains fixed to a telegraph pole). It is a normal phenomenon.

See-saw nystagmus: In this condition, one eye raises and turns in and the other eye falls and turns out. It is due to parasellar tumor.

CHAPTER 13

Poisoning

INTRODUCTION

Common causes of poisoning: Paracetamol, salicylate (aspirin), tricyclic antidepressant (TCA), benzodiazepines, corrosives, organophosphorus, methanol, ethanol, ethylene glycol, kerosene, datura, cannabis and opioid.

General management (ABC):
- Airway should be kept clear (suction and airway tube)
- Breathing (O_2, ventilatory support, and endotracheal tube, if needed)
- Circulation [intravenous (IV) or central venous (CV) line, and IV fluid infusion]
- *Other treatments*: Gastric lavage except in corrosive poisoning, antidote if available, maintenance of water, electrolytes balance and nutrition.

PARACETAMOL POISONING

Lethal dose: Intake of 15 g of paracetamol is serious in most cases.

Mechanism: Toxic metabolite of paracetamol is N-acetyl-p-benzoquinone imine (NAPQI), which is normally conjugated with glutathione and excreted. In paracetamol poisoning, there is production of excess toxic metabolite and depletion of cellular glutathione. Toxic metabolite causes massive hepatic necrosis and hepatic failure (not by the drug itself). No liver damage until 18 hours. If blood level of paracetamol is >200 µg/mL in 4 hours, it indicates severe poisoning. Maximum liver damage occurs after 72–96 hours of ingestion.

Prothrombin time (PT) is prolonged with high serum glutamate-pyruvate transaminase (SGPT) and serum glutamic oxaloacetic transaminase (SGOT). May be hypo- and hyperglycemia, metabolic acidosis, arrhythmia, gastrointestinal tract (GIT) bleeding, cerebral edema, lactic acidosis and coma. Brainstem coning may occur after 96 hours.

Prognostic factors: Three important risk or prognostic markers for severe hepatic injury are—
1. Prothrombin time is >20 seconds in 24 hours
2. pH <7.3
3. Serum creatinine >300 µmol/L.

Without treatment, patient may develop fulminant hepatic failure. Renal failure may occur due to acute tubular necrosis in 25% cases.

Investigations: Serum paracetamol, blood glucose, SGPT, SGOT, PT, serum creatinine and electrolytes.

Treatment:
- Gastric lavage within 4 hours
- N-acetylcysteine (NAC) IV or methionine orally. More effective, if given within 10 hours. Protective effects decline rapidly and ineffective after 15–16 hours
- *If PT is prolonged*: Fresh frozen plasma
- Glucose may be given
- Dialysis, if renal failure. Forced diuresis has no role
- Liver transplantation should be considered in some cases of acute liver failure
- Monitor liver function test (LFT), electrolytes, glucose and creatinine.

Dose of NAC: Three consecutive doses are given in 21 hours.
1. *1st dose*: 150 mg/kg with 200 mL 5% dextrose over 1 hour, then
2. *2nd dose*: 50 mg/kg with 500 mL 5% dextrose over 4 hours, then
3. *3rd dose*: 100 mg/kg with 1,000 mL 5% dextrose over 16 hours.

Dose of oral methionine: If NAC is not available, methionine 2.5 g orally every 4 hours, total four doses can be given.

SALICYLATE (ASPIRIN)

Clinical features:
- Nausea, vomiting, epigastric pain, restlessness, sweating, tinnitus and deafness
- Direct stimulation of respiratory center causes hyperventilation
- *Neurological effects*: Agitation, confusion, tremor, delirium, stupor, convulsion and coma
- Petechiae and subconjunctival hemorrhages due to reduced platelet aggregation
- *If poisoning due to very high dose*: Respiratory paralysis and cardiovascular collapse.

Investigations:
- *Serum aspirin level*: In adults, >500 mg/L and 700 mg/L suggest serious and life-threatening poisoning, respectively
- Serum electrolytes, arterial blood gas (ABG) and pH (low PaCO$_2$ indicates respiratory alkalosis), and blood glucose
- Urine for ferric chloride test is positive.

Treatment:
- Gastric lavage up to 24 hours (better within 12 hours). Activated charcoal may be given
- Correction of water and electrolyte imbalance (IV fluid)
- *If severe metabolic acidosis*: IV sodium bicarbonate (8.4%)
- If serum salicylate >750 mg/L or 500 mg/L with severe acidosis, forced alkaline diuresis
- If no response or neurological feature with blood level >1,000 mg/L or 750 mg/L with renal failure or acidosis, then hemodialysis should be done.

TRICYCLIC ANTIDEPRESSANT

Clinical features:
- Drowsiness, confusion, delirium, hallucination, agitation, myoclonic fit, convulsion and coma
- *Pulse*: Tachycardia
- *Pupil*: Dilated and loss of accommodation. Divergent strabismus
- *Reflex*: Exaggerated, hypertonia or spasticity, and plantar extensor
- Retention of urine may occur
- *Electrocardiogram (ECG):* Sinus tachycardia, QRS is prolonged, P is small, and arrhythmia [supraventricular tachycardia (SVT) and ventricular tachycardia (VT)]
- Metabolic acidosis and cardiorespiratory failure in severe case
- Most patients recover in 48 hours. In some cases, may be persistent agitation, confusion, hallucination, and rapid jerky movement, which may persist for several days.

Investigations: Blood for TCA level, serum electrolytes and arterial blood gas analysis and ECG monitoring.

Treatment:
- Gastric lavage, if >250 mg tablet is taken. TCA causes delayed gastric emptying, so lavage can be given up to 12 hours. Activated charcoal may be given if the patient presents within 1 hour
- Protection of airway and oxygen, and IV fluid
- *Cardiac monitor*: If ECG shows prolong QRS (>0.16 s), arrhythmia may develop
- *If epileptic seizure*: IV lorazepam or diazepam should be given
- If acidosis, sodium bicarbonate (50 cc of 8.4%) should be given
- Supraventricular tachycardia and VT should be treated with sodium bicarbonate (50 cc of 8.4%) IV over 20 minutes (even without acidosis). If VT with low cardiac output, injection amiodarone 300 mg IV over 20–60 minutes
- Lipid emulsion therapy in severe intractable poisoning may be tried
- No role of forced diuresis or hemodialysis.

METHANOL (RECTIFIED SPIRIT)

Methanol or methyl alcohol is a component of varnishes, paint remover, windshield washer solution, and copy machine fluid. It is metabolized in liver (90%) by alcohol dehydrogenase to formaldehyde and formic acid. About 10% is excreted unchanged by lungs and kidneys.

Formic acid can cause retinal injury. There is reduced visual acuity, due to optic nerve damage by formic acid. Mydriasis, reduced visual reflexes to light, and hyperemia of optic disc are early features of methanol toxicity. If untreated, patient may develop blindness.

Clinical features:
- *Early manifestations (by methanol)*: Nausea, vomiting, abdominal pain, headache, vertigo, dizziness, ataxia, drowsiness, dysarthria, nystagmus, convulsion, confusion, stupor and coma
- *Later (by metabolite formic acid)*: Visual impairment, photophobia with optic disc and retinal edema, and impaired pupil reflexes. Retinal injury

may cause blindness. Ocular toxicity occurs 15–19 hours after ingestion. Pancreatitis and abnormal liver function may also occur
- *In severe cases*: Metabolic acidosis, bradycardia, myocardial depression and shock.

Investigations: Serum methanol level, serum electrolytes and creatinine, ABG, and plasma osmolality (high). Others—blood sugar, serum calcium and magnesium.

Treatment:
- Gastric lavage within first 4 hours. IV fluid and oxygen
- *Correction of acidosis*: Sodium bicarbonate in large dose (250 mL of 1.26% solution, repeated as necessary). Alkalinization enhances formic acid excretion
- *In early stage*: Antidote of methanol is ethanol or fomepizole. About 10 mL/kg of 10% ethanol IV or 1 mL/kg of 95% ethanol orally
- Thiamine (100 mg 6 hourly), pyridoxine (50 mg 6 hourly) and folate (50 mg 6 hourly)
- Folinic acid 30 mg IV every 6 hourly. It reduces ocular toxicity (accelerates metabolism of formic acid)
- *Dialysis*: Indicated, if ingestion of methanol >30 g or metabolic acidosis or blood methanol >500 mg/L.

ETHANOL OR ETHYL ALCOHOL

Ethanol is commonly ingested in beverages and deliberately with other substances in overdose. It is also present in many cosmetic and antiseptic preparations. Ethanol is a central nervous system (CNS) depressant. After absorption, it is oxidized to acetaldehyde and then to acetate.

Clinical features: Related to blood ethanol concentrations—
- *If 500–1,500 mg/L*: Emotional lability and mild impairment of coordination
- *If 1,500–3,000 mg/L*: Visual impairment, incoordination, slowed reaction time and slurred speech
- *If 3,000–5,000 mg/L*: Marked incoordination, blurred or double vision, and stupor. Occasionally, hypoglycemia, hypothermia and convulsion
- *If 3,000–5,000 mg/L*: Depressed reflexes, respiratory depression, hypotension, hypothermia and death (from respiratory or circulatory failure or aspiration).

Treatment: Gastric lavage, IV fluid and oxygen. Correction of acidosis by sodium bicarbonate in large dose (250 mL of 1.26% solution, repeated as necessary). Correction of hypoglycemia. Hemodialysis, if blood ethanol concentration exceeds 7,500 mg/L and if severe metabolic acidosis.

ETHYLENE GLYCOL

Ethylene glycol is a common constituent of antifreeze fluid used in car radiators, brake fluids and in lower concentrations, windscreen washes. It itself is nontoxic, but is metabolized to toxic products. Clinical features are same as methanol poisoning. Other toxic effects of ethylene glycol are:
- *Neurological*: Ophthalmoplegia, cranial nerve palsy, hyporeflexia and myoclonus

- Renal pain and acute tubular necrosis occur due to precipitation of calcium oxalate in kidneys
- Hypocalcemia, hypomagnesemia, and hyperkalemia are common.

Urinalysis under Wood's light in patient with ethylene glycol poisoning may reveal oxalate crystals in urine, but its absence does not exclude the diagnosis.

Treatment: Same like methanol. Correction of electrolytes (mainly hyperkalemia), hypoglycemia, hypocalcemia and hypomagnesemia.

ORGANOPHOSPHORUS COMPOUNDS

Organophosphorus insecticides (malathion and parathion) are irreversible inhibitors of acetylcholinesterase, resulting in accumulation of acetylcholine at muscarinic and nicotinic synapses. Due to acute cholinergic syndrome, features occur within minutes to hours.

Muscarinic effects:
- Constriction of pupil
- Increased salivation and lacrimation
- *Gastrointestinal tract*: Nausea, vomiting, abdominal pain, and urinary and fecal incontinence
- *Respiratory*: Breathlessness, wheezing, and excess bronchial secretion
- *In severe poisoning*: Bradycardia, hypotension, heart block, and pulmonary edema may occur.

Nicotinic effects: Muscle weakness, twitching or fasciculation of muscles.

Central nervous system effects: Headache, dizziness, confusion, drowsiness, fit and coma.

Investigations: Blood gas analysis, serum electrolytes, urea and creatinine, blood glucose, and ECG.

Treatment:
- Contaminated clothing should be removed. Airway should be cleared and high flow oxygen, if needed
- Gastric lavage may be done within an hour of intake, followed by oral activated charcoal
- If convulsion, IV diazepam
- Atropine 1.8–3 mg IV as bolus dose, then double the dose every 5 minutes until there are signs of atropinization (dry and hot skin, dry tongue, clear lung, tachycardia, and dilated pupil)
- Antidote like pralidoxime or obidoxime may be given
- Monitoring of ECG, blood gases, temperature, urea and electrolytes, amylase, and glucose.

Three types of illness may occur in organophosphorus compound poisoning:
1. Acute cholinergic phase (as described above)
2. Intermediate syndrome (IMS)
3. Organophosphate-induced delayed polyneuropathy (OPIDN).

Intermediate Syndrome

Begins 48 hours after poisoning, may be after 72–96 hours. Occurs after resolution of acute phase. Features are—
- Muscle weakness causing respiratory distress and failure

- Muscle weakness involves ocular, neck, and proximal limbs muscles, also respiratory muscles (intercostal muscles and diaphragm)
- Paralysis may continue for 2-18 days
- Usually, recovery occurs with adequate ventilatory care.

Treatment:
- Ventilator support
- Diazepam or midazolam may be used for sedation during ventilation
- Parenteral nutrition.

Organophosphate-induced Delayed Polyneuropathy

Occurs about 1-3 weeks after acute exposure.
- Cramping muscle pain in legs
- Acute weakness of muscles of upper and lower limbs causing shuffling gait, and foot and wrist drop. Muscle wasting and deformity causing claw hands
- Sensory loss is variable and is mild. Tendon reflexes are reduced or lost, absent ankle reflexes being a constant feature
- Recovery from OPIDN is incomplete. Although functional recovery after 1-2 years may occur in younger patients.

Treatment: No specific therapy. Regular physiotherapy.

BENZODIAZEPINE

It has low toxicity when taken alone in overdose, but can enhance CNS depression when taken with other sedative or alcohol.

Clinical features:
- Dizziness, drowsiness, confusion, hallucination and slurred speech
- Ataxia and reduced muscle tone
- Hypothermia
- Diplopia, strabismus, nystagmus, and normal pupil size
- *In severe poisoning*: Respiratory depression and hypotension may occur, even coma.

Investigations: Serum drug level, serum electrolytes and serum creatinine.

Treatment (ABC):
- Airway should be clear. If needed, oxygen inhalation
- Gastric lavage can be given, if >30 tablets are taken
- Activated charcoal may be given within 1 hour of ingestion of drugs
- Water and electrolytes balance
- Benzodiazepine antagonist flumazenil may be given (avoided in mixed TCA and benzodiazepine poisoning, also if history of epilepsy).

DATURA POISONING

Powder of datura seeds is used as a stupefying agent. Common places are railway station, launch or bus terminal and in hotels. Basic constituent of datura is atropine. Clinical features are due to excess anticholinergic activity.
- Patient is restless and confused with peculiar behavior
- There is pill-rolling movement of hands, incoherent talk and staggering gait

- Face is flushed, pupils widely dilated, and diplopia or photophobia may develop. Light reflex is lost
- Dryness of mouth, thirst and difficulty in speech
- Skin is hot and dry with rise of temperature
- Patient may progress to stupor and coma
- Death from respiratory failure.

Treatment (ABC):
- Clear the airway, ensure ventilation, maintain circulation, and maintain nutrition and hydration
- Stomach wash
- Antipyretic, if required, and tepid sponging for hyperpyrexia
- *Anticonvulsant*: Diazepam 10 mg intramuscular (IM)
- *Physostigmine*: 0.5 mg IV/IM at hourly interval
- *Pilocarpine*: 5 mg subcutaneously.

CANNABIS (MARIJUANA)

Cannabis is derived from dried leaves and flowers of *Cannabis sativa*. Usually, it is smoked but may be ingested as "cake", mixed with tea or injected intravenously.

Clinical features:
- Initially, there is euphoria, followed by perceptual alteration (distorted images, colors and sounds, and altered tactile sensation), and conjunctival congestion
- Visual and auditory hallucinations and acute psychosis, and confusion
- High dose can cause anxiety, depression, slurred speech and ataxia. Regular users are at risk of psychological dependence. Withdrawal symptoms are unusual
- Intravenous injection may cause watery diarrhea, tachycardia, hypotension and arthralgia
- Long-term use may cause schizophrenia in later life.

Treatment: Reassurance, psychotherapy. Sedation with IV diazepam 10–20 mg or chlorpromazine 50–100 mg IM in an adult is sometimes required. IV fluid for hypotension.

CORROSIVE POISONING

Common corrosives are acid, alkali, bleaching powder and household disinfectants (Harpic, Savlon and Dettol).

Clinical features: Burning and pain in mouth, throat and abdomen, nausea, and vomiting. Difficulty in swallowing. Cough may be due to chemical pneumonitis.

Treatment: Gastric lavage is contraindicated.
- Intravenous fluid to maintain water and electrolyte balance
- Parenteral nutrition if the patient is unable to take by mouth
- Intravenous antibiotic and analgesic (tramadol, morphine or pethidine).

Complications: Esophageal stricture, perforation of esophagus or stomach, and aspiration pneumonia.

OPIATE POISONING

Usually, morphine poisoning occurs if taken intravenously.

Clinical features:
- Difficulty in respiration, confusion, hallucination, slurred speech, stupor or even coma
- Ataxia and reduced muscle tone
- Pin point pupil, hypotension, relative bradycardia, and low respiratory rate
- *Abdomen*: Distended due to paralytic ileus
- Death due to respiratory depression.

Treatment: Maintenance of airway, breathing and circulation. Specific antidote is naloxone 0.8–2 mg IV, may be repeated if needed. Continuous monitoring of respiratory function.

KEROSENE POISONING

It is a common accidental poisoning in children. It is irritant to GIT and when absorbed, it depresses CNS. Aspiration in respiratory tract causes pneumonitis.

Clinical features:
- Smell of kerosene in breath and vomitus
- Pain and burning in throat, dry irritating cough and breathlessness
- Nausea, vomiting and abdominal pain
- Drowsiness, impaired consciousness and convulsion
- Death may occur due to respiratory failure or ventricular fibrillation.

Treatment:
- Gastric lavage and induced vomiting should be avoided
- Airway should be kept clear, maintenance of breathing and circulation. Oxygen inhalation, if needed
- Removal of contaminated clothing
- Liquid paraffin orally to delay absorption
- Antibiotic to prevent infection
- *Corticosteroid*: If chemical or aspiration pneumonia.

CHAPTER 14

Psychiatric Diseases

CLASSIFICATION OF PSYCHIATRIC DISEASES

There are two types—
1. *Major*: Schizophrenia, manic-depressive psychosis, major depression, dementia, and postpartum psychosis
2. *Minor*: Anxiety neurosis, obsessive–compulsive disorder (OCD), somatoform disorders, stress-related disorders, behavioral and personality disorders and eating disorders.

DELUSION

It is a false belief, which is not true, and the falsity cannot be corrected even after clear demonstration. Causes are schizophrenia, manic-depressive psychosis, dementia, alcohol, and drug abuse.

Types:
- *Delusions of control or influence*: Patient believes that his thoughts and actions are being controlled by outside force
- *Delusions of persecution*: Patient believes that attempts are being made to harm or poison him by their nearest relatives
- *Delusions of reference*: Patient believes that people refer to him in a special way, also believes that anyone is looking at him or talking about him
- *Delusion of broadcasting*: Patient believes that his thoughts are being broadcasted and everyone knows whatever he is thinking
- *Grandiose delusions*: It is the delusion of having power, wealth, knowledge or special relationship with important persons (e.g. prime minister and president)
- *Nihilistic*: Patient believes that he is dead or part or organ of his body is dead, the world and even time has been lost or destroyed. Found in severe depression
- *Delusion of infidelity*: Patient believes his wife to be unfaithful while in fact she is chaste

- *Hypochondriac*: Patient believes that something is wrong in his body and he has some serious disease, though he is actually healthy.

Illusion: It is the false interpretation of a real object. Patient imagines a rope to be a snake, voice of a bird to be voice of human. It has no significant diagnostic importance. It may be found in high fever, toxemia or anxiety.

HALLUCINATION

It is the false sense of perception without any real object.

Types:
- *Auditory hallucination*: Hearing of voice when nothing is present. Found in schizophrenia, severe depression, and bipolar disorder
- *Visual hallucination*: Seeing something while there is nothing. Found in dissociation and conversion disorder, organic mental conditions, substance abuse, and occasionally in schizophrenia and severe affective disorders
- *Tactile hallucination*: Sensation of being touched, and insects moving under the skin, while there is nothing. Found in cocaine abuse and occasionally in schizophrenia
- *Gustatory hallucination*: Abnormal taste sensation though there is nothing in mouth. Occurs in schizophrenia and severe depressive disorders
- *Olfactory hallucination*: Abnormal sense of smell while nothing is present. Occurs in schizophrenia and severe depressive disorders, but may be in temporal lobe epilepsy or irritation of olfactory bulb or pathways by tumor
- *Others*:
  - *Hypnagogic*: Vivid dream-like hallucination at the onset of sleep
  - *Hypnopompic*: Vivid dream-like hallucination on awakening
  - *Lilliputian hallucination*: Person thinks that people, animal or object seems to be smaller. May occur in substance use disorders.

Acute stress reaction: After a stressful situation like major accident, physical or sexual assault, serious illness like acquired immunodeficiency syndrome (AIDS) or cancer, there may be characteristic pattern of symptoms such as tension, anger, depression, increased activity or under activity, and withdrawal. These symptoms are transient, subsides within 3 days of their onset.

POST-TRAUMATIC STRESS DISORDER

It is defined as severe response to a stressful condition which is threatening or catastrophic in nature such as natural disaster, terrorist activity, serious accident, and witnessing violent death or even distressing medical treatment.

Symptoms: Recurrent thinking of the traumatic event, sleep disturbance, and nightmares from which the patient awakes in a state of anxiety, avoidance of situations, persons, activities or places similar to the traumatic event. Anxiety and depression.

Management: Reassurance and counseling. Antidepressant drug. A novel therapy called eye movement desensitization and reprocessing (EMDR) is effective.

ADJUSTMENT DISORDER

It is the psychological response to adapting new situations, which are distressing to the patient. It is less severe, but emotional reaction is more prolonged.

Situations such as change in work, school, living, migration, divorce and separation, death of close relative, onset of chronic or terminal illness, and long-term adjustment to sexual abuse.

These stresses can precipitate major depressive disorder, anxiety disorders, even schizophrenia. So, other psychiatric disorders must be excluded.

Symptoms: Develop within a month of the onset of stress, and features depend on the underlying condition. Improves with the removal of stressful condition. There may also be anger, aggressive behavior and excessive alcohol use, and depression or anxiety.

Management: Reassurance, explanation and advice. Does not require psychotropic medication. Sometimes benzodiazepines may be used. Psychotherapy. Usually resolves in time.

ANXIETY DISORDERS (ANXIETY NEUROSIS)

It is a disorder characterized by lack of concentration, loss of interest, and excessive worry, which are difficult to control and cause significant distress and impairment.

Types: There are three types—phobic, panic and generalized anxiety disorder.

Phobic disorder: It is an abnormal or excessive fear of an object or situation, which leads to avoidance of it, e.g. avoidance of journey by plane due to fear of crash. Types of phobia:

- *Simple phobia*: Fear of animal, height, closed or dark room, etc.
- *Social*: Fear of speech in a public gathering
- *Agoraphobia*: Fear of open space or street. Phobia outside home, so the patient remains homebound.

Panic disorder: It is a disorder in which there is sudden and unpredictable attack of severe anxiety associated with physical symptoms such as chest pain, palpitation, breathlessness, etc. Even when patient is well, he fears of another attack at any time. Symptoms are chest pain, palpitation, fear of suffering from serious illness such as heart attack or stroke, hyperventilation, difficulty in breathing, fear of losing control, going "crazy", passing out, fear of dying, anticipatory avoidance, and reluctant to go outside.

Generalized anxiety disorder: This is characterized by chronic uncontrollable worry, tension, and apprehension about everyday events and problems.

Symptoms:

- *Psychological*: Irritability, worry, fear, lack of concentration, and depersonalization
- *Somatic*: Palpitation, fatigue, tremor, dizziness, sweating, diarrhea, chest pain, insomnia and breathlessness.

Management of anxiety disorders:

- Explanation and reassurance, psychotherapy including relaxation and graded exposure (desensitization)

- *Drugs*: Benzodiazepines are useful. β-blocker such as propranolol for palpitation
- *For long-term treatment*: Selective serotonin reuptake inhibitor (SSRI) (escitalopram, fluoxetine, etc.).

OBSESSIVE COMPULSIVE DISORDER

It is characterized by unwanted thought, idea, impulse or image (obsession), which forces the person to do the act repeatedly to get rid of anxiety (compulsion). Example: Washing and rewashing of hands as if hands are not clear or contaminated.

Management:
- Explanation, reassurance, psychotherapy and behavioral therapy
- *Drugs*:
  - First-line: SSRI (sertraline and fluoxetine)
  - Second-line: Tricyclic antidepressant (TCA) (imipramine, clomipramine and amitriptyline)
  - Third-line: Combination of SSRI and TCA or antipsychotic.

DEPRESSION

It is defined as persistent mood disturbance such as loss of mood, interest, pleasure and retardation from physical and mental activities. Cardinal features are depressed mood, lack of enjoyment, negative thinking, reduced energy, and slowness of thought.

Types:
- *Primary*: No underlying cause
- *Secondary*: Due to some chronic illness and malignancy
- It may be unipolar or bipolar affective disorder.

Symptoms:
- *Psychological*: Lack of interest and concentration, guilty feeling, and unworthiness. Sometimes severe depressive psychosis is associated with restlessness, agitation and suicidal tendency
- *Somatic*: Anorexia, weight loss, headache, backache, amenorrhea, loss of libido, insomnia, early waking from sleep, and slowing of activity.

Management:
- *Supportive*: Psychotherapy and reassurance
- *Drugs*:
  - Selective serotonin reuptake inhibitor: Fluoxetine, paroxetine, citalopram, escitalopram and sertraline
  - Tricyclic antidepressant: Amitriptyline, nortriptyline and imipramine
  - For single episode, drug should be continued for at least 6–9 months and for multiple episodes, up to 2 years. Drug should not be discontinued abruptly.

MANIA AND HYPOMANIA

It is a disorder characterized by marked elevation of mood such as euphoria, overactivity, and disinhibition. Hypomania is the mild form of mania. It lasts a shorter time and is less severe with no psychotic features and less disability.

Clinical features of mania:
- *Mood*: Elevated or irritable, frequent swings from one mood to another, and flights of ideas
- *Talk*: Excessive, fast and pressurized
- *Energy*: Excessive
- Delusions of wealth, power, influence, religious significance and sometimes persecutory
- *Hallucinations*: Fleeting auditory
- *Behavior*: Disinhibition, excessive drinking, lost relationship (from promiscuity or irritability), social ostracism, and lost employment (from reckless or disinhibited behavior)
- Disturbance of memories. Insomnia, weight loss and increased libido
- Overspending of money leading to significant debts
- Mixed features of mania and depressive illness may be seen in the same episode.

Treatment: Explanation and reassurance, and psychotherapy.
- *Drugs*: Haloperidol 10–30 mg with procyclidine *or* chlorpromazine 200–600 mg *or* thioridazine 200–600 mg
- *To prevent relapse*: Lithium 400–1,200 mg single dose daily *or* carbamazepine *or* sodium valproate *or* clonazepam may be used.

BIPOLAR AFFECTIVE DISORDER (BIPOLAR MOOD DISORDER)

It is characterized by relapsing mood disturbance with periods of elevated mood known as mania and depressive mood. Depressive episode may not always be present. It was previously called "manic-depressive psychosis".

Clinical features:
- The patient may be cheerful, speaks fluently, and overtalkative
- Inappropriate behavior and social binding is completely lost
- *Delusion of grandiose type*: He may claim to have special powers or to be an important personality
- *Sleep*: Less, claiming to have many tasks
- *Idea*: Flights of ideas and rapid change of topics or shifting of ideas
- Overactivity
- *Insight*: Impaired, and hallucination may be present.

Treatment:
- Patient and family members should be educated about relapsing nature and measures to prevent further episode (adequate sleep and reduced stress)
- *Antipsychotics*: Dibenzodiazepines (olanzapine and quetiapine), phenothiazine (chlorpromazine and trifluoperazine) *or* butyrophenones (haloperidol) *or* thioxanthenes (flupentixol decanoate)
- *Prophylaxis to prevent recurrent episodes*: Lithium, carbamazepine, sodium valproate, lamotrigine and quetiapine may be used.

SCHIZOPHRENIA

It is a major psychiatric disorder characterized by disturbance of perception, thought, emotion, personality and social behavior.

Types:
- *Simple*: There is gradual loss of interest to surroundings, withdrawal from reality, lack of caring himself but not violent. Delusion and hallucination are uncommon
- *Hebephrenic*: Disorganized, disinhibited behavior, violent and irrelevant talk. Hallucination and delusion are present
- *Catatonic*: Patient maintains an odd posture for a prolong period, disturbance of behavior, there is homicidal and suicidal tendency
- *Paranoid*: Occurs at later age, persecutory delusions are main features. There is suspiciousness but personality is intact.

Clinical features:
- *Disturbance of thought*:
    - Speech may be uninformative and meaningless with irrelevant words
    - Thought insertion: Patient thinks that thoughts are being inserted in his mind
    - Thought withdrawal: Patient thinks that thoughts are being taken away from mind
    - Thought broadcasting: Patient thinks that everybody knows whatever he thinks
    - Delusion of control, grandiose, paranoid and hypochondriac are present.
- *Disorder of perception*: Hallucination, commonly auditory, may be visual
- *Disturbance of mood or emotion*:
    - Inappropriate emotional response (crying during laughing situation)
    - Blunt mood, rapid change of emotion, and perplexed mood (fearful without any reason).
- *Disturbance of behavior and activity*:
    - Violent, assaultive and destructive
    - Withdrawal of activity (does not take care of himself and does not eat)
    - Purposeless activity (continuous walking without any destination).
- Personality deterioration which affects family, work and personal relationship.

Features of acute schizophrenia:
- *A*: Auditory hallucination
- *B*: Broadcasting (insertion or withdrawal of thoughts)
- *C*: Controlled feelings, impulse or act ("passivity" phenomenon—patient thinks that somebody is controlling him)
- *D*: Delusional perception.

Above symptoms are often described as "*Schneider's first rank symptoms*".

Treatment: Acute schizophrenia may require hospital admission. Patient may be at risk of harming himself or others. Chronic schizophrenia can be treated at home.
- *General measures*: Explanation and reassurance. Environmental and social factors to be looked for. Counseling by nurses, doctors or social workers. After control of schizophrenic attack, social and occupational rehabilitation is required
- *Drug treatment*: Antipsychotic agents (called neuroleptics or major tranquillizers). Take 2-3 weeks for maximal effect. Once symptoms are controlled, drugs are continued to prevent relapse. Patient with first

episode of schizophrenia improves in 1–2 years. However, with multiple episodes, treatment may be required for many years
- *Antipsychotic drugs*:
  - Phenothiazine: Chlorpromazine 100–1,500 mg daily. *Or*, Fluphenazine 20–100 mg fortnightly. *Or*, butyrophenone (haloperidol, 5–30 mg daily). *Or*, thioxanthene (flupentixol, 40–200 mg fortnightly)
  - Newer drugs: Risperidone 2–16 mg daily, olanzapine 5–20 mg daily, quetiapine 150–400 mg daily, pimozide 4–30 mg daily, sulpiride 600–1,800 mg daily, and clozapine 25–900 mg daily.

Side effects of antipsychotic drugs:
- Weight gain due to increased appetite
- Metabolic (dyslipidemia and impaired glucose tolerance)
- Cardiac (QT prolongation)
- *Extrapyramidal*: Parkinsonism, akathisia (motor restlessness), acute dystonia, and tardive dyskinesia. More common in older (first generation) antipsychotics
- Sedation, postural hypotension, dry mouth, blurred vision, constipation, urinary retention, impotence and galactorrhea
- *Hypersensitivity reactions*: Cholestatic jaundice, photosensitive dermatitis, and blood dyscrasia (neutropenia with clozapine)
- *Ocular complications*: Corneal and lens opacities.

Eating disorders: It may be anorexia nervosa or bulimia nervosa.

Anorexia Nervosa

It is an eating disorder where body image is profoundly disturbed and despite emaciation, patient feels overweight and is afraid of weight gain. As a result, there is marked weight loss due to self-starvation. It is common in young teenage girls, rare after 30 years. More in higher social class, the girl is hard working, perfectionist and ambitious. Endocrine abnormality is present, which reverts to normal after improvement of the disease.

Diagnostic criteria:
- Weight loss, at least 15% of expected body weight
- Avoidance of high calorie diet
- Distortion of body image, patient regards herself fatty even she is thin or grossly underweight
- Amenorrhea for at least 3 months (in male, loss of sexual interest).

Clinical features:
- Patient may hide her emaciation by using loose-fitting clothes
- Physically overactive, performs excessive exercise, may use laxative or diuretic, and sometimes vomit after meal
- There may be downy, lanugo hair on trunk and limb. Hypotension, bradycardia, increased sensitivity to cold, constipation and peripheral cyanosis may be found
- Anxiety and depression are common. Psychosexual immaturity is present
- Osteoporosis may occur due to less estrogen. Bilateral parotid enlargement may be present.

Investigations:
- Low luteinizing hormone (LH), follicle-stimulating hormone (FSH), and estradiol. In male, low LH and testosterone

- Low T3, but normal T4 and thyroid-stimulating hormone (TSH)
- High cortisol and high growth hormone (GH). Dexamethasone suppression test may be abnormal. All revert to normal after therapy
- Glucose intolerance may occur due to starvation.

Physical effects of anorexia nervosa:
- *Cardiac*: ECG changes (T inversion, ST depression, and prolonged QT interval). Arrhythmia (sinus bradycardia and ventricular tachycardia)
- *Hematological*: Anemia, thrombocytopenia and leukopenia
- *Endocrine*: Delayed puberty or arrest, growth retardation, amenorrhea and sick euthyroid state
- *Metabolic*: Renal failure, renal stone and osteoporosis
- *Gastrointestinal*: Constipation and abnormal liver function test (LFT).

Treatment:
- *In mild case*: Treated in outdoor basis
- *Moderate-to-severe case*: Hospitalization. Controlled diet to increase weight, 1 kg weekly. Psychotherapy and behavioral therapy.

Prognosis: The 50% full recovery, 30% partial recovery, and 20% do not improve. 2–5% death from suicide or physical complication.

Bulimia Nervosa

It is an eating disorder characterized by uncontrolled, excessive eating (called binges), followed by self-induced vomiting. Patient's weight is usually normal or near normal.

Clinical features: Common in late adolescent female. Diagnostic criteria—
- Recurrent bouts of binge eating
- Lack of self-control and overeating during binges
- Self-induced vomiting, purgation or dieting after binges
- Weight maintained within normal limits.

Physical signs:
- Pitted teeth (from gastric acid due to repeated vomiting)
- Calluses on knuckles ("Russell's sign")
- Parotid gland enlargement.

Complications: Dental abnormality, esophageal tear due to excessive vomiting, electrolyte abnormalities, tetany due to hypokalemic alkalosis, cardiac arrhythmias, and renal problems.

Treatment:
- Cognitive behavioral therapy (CBT) achieves both short and long-term improvements
- Guided self-help and interpersonal psychotherapy may be helpful
- *Drugs*: SSRI (fluoxetine 60 mg daily).

Prognosis: Not associated with mortality like anorexia nervosa (AN). 10% remain unwell, 20% remain subclinical, and the remainder recover.

SOMATOFORM DISORDER

It is a group of disorders characterized by multiple somatic symptoms, without any demonstrable medical illness. Physical symptoms are due to psychological factors.

Types are
- *Somatization disorder (Briquet's syndrome)*: Multiple somatic symptoms, but no physical cause. Common in women. Usual complains are pain, vomiting, nausea, headache, dizziness, menstrual irregularity, and sexual dysfunction
- *Hypochondriasis*: Patient has a fear or belief that he or she has a serious, fatal disease that persists despite normal investigation
- *Body dysmorphic disorder*: There is feeling of disfigured appearance or body shape without reality. Patient even may request for cosmetic surgery
- *Somatoform autonomic dysfunction*: Related to autonomic nervous system. Complains are—
  - Cardiovascular (cardiac neurosis): Palpitation and chest pain
  - Respiratory: Hyperventilation and breathlessness
  - Gastrointestinal tract (GIT): Vomiting and irritable bowel syndrome.
- *Somatoform pain disorder*: There may be severe, persistent pain, which cannot be explained by a medical condition
- *Neurasthenia (chronic fatigue syndrome)*: Characterized by excessive fatigue after minimal physical or mental exertion. Also, poor concentration, dizziness, muscular aches, and sleep disturbance
- *Dissociative (conversion) disorder*: It is characterized by profound loss of awareness or cognitive ability without organic disease. The term dissociative (conversion) disorder has replaced "hysteria"
  - Conversion means unresolved conflict is converted into symbolic physical symptoms as a defense against it, e.g. paralysis, sensory loss, abnormal movements, aphonia, gait disturbance, and blindness
  - Dissociate means disintegration of different mental activity, e.g. amnesia, fugue and pseudoseizure
  - Sometimes, in dissociative disorder, there is rigidity, which increases more and more during more maneuvers.

General management of somatoform disorders:
- Reassurance, explanation, advice, psychotherapy and behavioral therapy
- Encourage to return to normal functioning
- *Drugs*: Antidepressant (sertraline, fluoxetine and escitalopram)
- Rehabilitation
- Shared care with general practitioner (GP).

Hysteria

It is a disorder in which patient develops symptoms of illness or mental symptoms for real or imagined gain without being fully aware of underlying motive. It is called conversion disorder.

Clinical features: It is common in young female and low socioeconomic group.
- *Neurological*: Gait disturbance, paraplegia, rigidity, aphonia, pseudoseizure, visual loss and sensory loss
- *Cardiovascular*: Palpitation and chest pain
- *Respiratory*: Breathlessness and hyperventilation
- *Gastrointestinal tract*: Nausea, vomiting, abdominal pain, feeling of lump in throat (globus hystericus), loss of appetite, and abstinence from food
- *Sexual*: Decreased libido or impotence
- Unexplained pain in different parts of the body.

Treatment: Explanation and reassurance. Removal of stress factor.
Drugs: SSRI, TCA and carbamazepine.

PUERPERAL DISORDERS

The three common psychiatric complications after childbirth.
1. *Postpartum blues*: Characterized by irritability, labile mood, and tearfulness. Symptoms begin soon after childbirth, peak on 4th day, and then resolve. Psychological and social supports are necessary. No drug is required
2. *Postpartum depression*: Occurs in 10–15% cases. Women with a previous history of depression are at risk. Explanation and reassurance are important. Psychotherapy and antidepressant may be given
3. *Puerperal psychosis*: Develops in the first 2 weeks after childbirth. Usually manic or depressive psychosis, although schizophrenia can occur.

Treatment: According to type of illness, e.g. depression and psychosis.

DEMENTIA

It is a disorder characterized by progressive deterioration of intellectual function, memory and personality due to progressive degeneration of brain. Consciousness is clear.

Causes:
- *Degenerative and hereditary*: Alzheimer's disease, Parkinson's disease, Pick's disease, Huntington's disease, and Wilson's disease
- *Vascular causes*: Multi-infarct dementia and diffuse white matter disease
- *Infections*: Human immunodeficiency virus (HIV), neurosyphilis, progressive multifocal leukoencephalopathy, Creutzfeldt–Jakob disease, and prion disease (kuru)
- *Inflammatory*: Multiple sclerosis and sarcoidosis
- *Connective tissue disease*: Systemic lupus erythematosus (SLE) and Sjögren's syndrome
- Drugs and toxins (sedative, heavy metal or carbon monoxide poisoning, and alcohol)
- *Trauma*: Head injury, chronic subdural hematoma, and punch drunk syndrome
- *Neoplastic*: Primary brain tumor and secondary metastasis
- *Endocrine causes*: Hypothyroidism, hypopituitarism, Addison's disease, Cushing's syndrome, and hypo- and hyperparathyroidism
- *Metabolic*: Renal failure, liver failure and respiratory failure
- *Vitamin deficiencies*: B1, B12 and B3 (nicotinic acid)
- *Others*: Normal pressure hydrocephalous.

Clinical features: Depends on cause.
- Common features are memory disturbance, disturbance of intellect (judgment and problem solving), and personality problem and disinhibition (not keeping clothes, exposing genitalia, etc.)
- Impairment of performance of activities of daily living, hallucination, agitation, insomnia, micturition and defecation at inappropriate place, and undue suspiciousness.

Investigations: According to suspicion of cause. Computed tomography (CT) or magnetic resonance imaging (MRI) of brain to identify brain atrophy and structural lesions.

Treatment: Treatment of underlying cause, if any.
- Usually symptomatic. Institutionalization may be required
- Explanation to family members and caregivers. Advise regarding exercise, structured activity, music therapy, bright light therapy, and environmental cues and instructions
- *Cholinesterase inhibitor drugs for memory disturbances*: Rivastigmine, donepezil, galantamine and tacrine
- *Symptomatic management of behavioral problems*: Haloperidol and thioridazine.

DELIRIUM

It is an acute, reversible mental disorder characterized by mental confusion, disorientation for time and place associated with emotional lability, illusion, auditory and visual hallucination, violent behavior.

Causes: Remember the formula—"*I WATCH DEATH*".
- *I*: Infection such as meningitis, encephalitis and septicemia
- *W*: Withdrawal of sedatives and alcohol
- *A*: Acute metabolic conditions such as electrolyte imbalance, hepatic and renal failure
- *T*: Trauma, head injury, and burn
- *C*: Central nervous system (CNS) lesion such as tumor, epilepsy and Wernicke's encephalopathy
- *H*: Hypoxia
- *D*: Deficiencies such as thiamine and B12
- *E*: Endocrine disorders such as hypothyroidism and adrenal insufficiency
- *A*: Acute vascular event such as transient ischemic attack (TIA), stroke, and shock
- *T*: Toxins and drugs
- *H*: Heavy metals such as lead and mercury.

Investigations:
- *Routine*: Complete blood count (CBC), erythrocyte sedimentation rate (ESR), serum urea, creatinine, electrolytes, calcium, magnesium, and glucose
- Renal, liver, and thyroid function tests. CT or MRI of brain
- *Others*: According to suspicion of cause.

Treatment:
- Treatment of underlying illness
- Maintenance of adequate hydration and nutrition, and correction of electrolyte imbalance
- *Psychotropic drugs*: For younger patients, haloperidol 5-10 mg orally every 12 hours, and for older patients, risperidone 2 mg orally olanzapine and thioridazine.

DELIRIUM TREMENS

It is a disorder due to sudden withdrawal of alcohol in a chronic alcoholic person, occurs 1-3 days after alcohol cessation. It is commonly seen a day or two after admission to hospital.

Clinical features:
- Disorientation, agitation, aggression and marked tremor
- Autonomic hyperactivity such as tachycardia, diaphoresis (excessive sweating), fever, anxiety, insomnia and hypertension
- Hallucinations, most frequently visual or tactile
- Features of dehydration.

Complications: Dehydration, secondary infection, hepatic disease, and Wernicke-Korsakoff syndrome.

Treatment:
- *General measures*: Hospitalization. Correction of electrolytes. Antibiotic, if infection
- *Benzodiazepines*: Lorazepam intravenously (IV) 0.1 mg/kg at 2.0 mg/min or diazepam 10–20 mg *or* chlordiazepoxide 30–60 mg orally
- Thiamine (vitamin B1) in high dose IV and other vitamin B complex
- Phenytoin or carbamazepine, if previous history of withdrawal fits.

SUBSTANCE ABUSE

It is the dependence on and misuse of both illegal and prescribed drugs. In addition to alcohol and nicotine, many psychotropic drugs that are taken for prolonged period, resulting in dependency, affect mood and mental function, and even occupational disturbance. Also, causes withdrawal symptoms on abrupt cessation.

Common drugs and substances which are misused:
- *Sedatives*: Benzodiazepines and barbiturates
- *Narcotics*: Morphine, heroin and pethidine
- *Stimulants*: Cocaine, amphetamine and ecstasy [3,4-methylenedioxy-methamphetamine (MDMA)]
- *Hallucinogens*: Cannabis, solvents and lysergic acid diethylamide (LSD).

Clinical features: Vary according to the drug taken.

Treatment: Explanation, reassurance and patient's cooperation and will are the vital parts. Gradual reduction of dose. Substitute or antagonist should be considered. Preventive measure to stop selling of the drugs by the chemist.

Factitious disorder: There is repeated and deliberate production of signs or symptoms of a disease to get medical care. Common in young women. Example: Deliberate intake of thyroxine to reduce weight, which can cause factitious thyrotoxicosis.

Münchausen's syndrome: This is a severe form of factitious disorder in which the patient makes signs and symptoms of disease for hospital admission repeatedly, sometimes visiting several hospitals in 1 day.

Advice: Reassurance and psychotherapy.

CHAPTER 15

Vitamins

INTRODUCTION

Vitamins are organic substances required in small quantities for a variety of biochemical functions, which are usually not synthesized in the body and supplied in the diet. Vitamins are of two types:
1. *Fat-soluble vitamins*: A, D, E and K
2. *Water-soluble vitamins*: B complex and vitamin C.

VITAMIN A (RETINOL)

Source: Milk, egg, butter, cheese, egg yolk, fish liver oil. Also green leafy vegetables, carrot and mango (beta-carotene).

Functions: It is essential for normal retinal function, cell growth and differentiation, mainly in epithelial cells. It is necessary for normal wound healing.

Deficiency may cause:
- Night blindness
- Xerosis of conjunctiva (dryness)
- Xerophthalmia
- Bitot's spots
- Keratomalacia
- Blindness
- Dryness of skin (Toad's skin).

Treatment: Vitamin A 30,000–50,000 IU orally daily for 5 days.

Prevention: Intake of food rich in vitamin A. Single prophylactic oral dose of 60 mg retinyl palmitate (providing 200,000 IU retinol) to all preschool children. Pregnant women and lactating mothers should eat dark green, leafy vegetables, and yellow fruits. Vitamin A 20,000 IU every week.

Toxicity: Prolonged use may cause toxicity called hypervitaminosis A. It may cause liver and bone damage, hair loss, double vision, vomiting, headaches, and other abnormalities. Retinol is teratogenic.

VITAMIN D (CHOLECALCIFEROL)

Source: Sunlight, fish oil, egg yolk, milk, margarine, and fortified cereals. Natural form of vitamin D is cholecalciferol or vitamin D3, formed by action of UV light on 7-dehydrocholesterol in skin. Vitamin D is converted in liver to 25-hydroxycholecalciferol, which is further hydroxylated in kidney to 1,25-dihydroxycholecalciferol, which is the active form of vitamin D.

Functions: Absorption of calcium from gut and mineralization of bone.

Causes of deficiency: Lack of exposure to sunlight, malabsorption, and less intake in food.

Deficiency may cause: Rickets in child and osteomalacia in adult.

Rickets

It is a disease of children due to deficiency of vitamin D.

Clinical features:
- Irritability, restlessness, sweating in forehead, and muscle hypotonia
- Delayed development
- Swelling of costochondral junctions of ribs called "rickety rosary"
- Craniotabes (small unossified areas in membranous bones of skull that yield to finger pressure with a cracking feeling). Bossing of frontal and parietal bones. Delayed anterior fontanelle closure
- Enlargement of epiphyses at the lower end of radius
- Harrison's sulcus—depression of lower ribs along the attachment of diaphragm
- *When the child begins to walk*: May be knock-knee or bowing legs
- Kyphosis, lordosis, and pelvic deformity may occur. Delayed dentition
- Abdominal distention due to weak abdominal muscle called potbelly
- Prone to respiratory infection
- X-ray of knee or wrist joints will show typical finding.

Treatment: Oral vitamin D3, 300,000–600,000 IU single dose or 2,000–5,000 IU daily for 4–6 weeks. Then, maintenance dose of 400–600 IU daily. Calcium supplement, 350–1,000 mg daily.

Osteomalacia

It is the disease in adult due to vitamin D deficiency. There is softening of bone due to defective mineralization. Causes are lack of exposure to sunlight, less intake in diet, malabsorption, obstructive jaundice, and chronic kidney diseases.

Clinical features: May be asymptomatic.
- Muscle and bone pain. Increased bone fragility and fracture
- Proximal muscle weakness and waddling gait
- X-ray shows pseudofracture called Looser's zone.

Treatment:
- Vitamin D 10,000–25,000 IU daily for 2–4 weeks
- *Maintenance*: 800–1,600 IU daily for few months
- Diet rich in vitamin D. Oral calcium 1,000–1,200 mg daily may be given.

Toxicity: Prolonged and excessive use of vitamin D may cause hypervitaminosis D, characterized by nausea, vomiting, polyuria, and other features of hypercalcemia.

Prevention: Regular intake of food rich in calcium, e.g. milk. Adequate sunlight exposure.

VITAMIN E (TOCOPHEROL)

Source: Vegetable and seeds oil, soya oil, sunflower and nuts.
Function: It is an important antioxidant, which protect cells and membranes from free radicals.
Deficiency may cause: Mild hemolytic anemia, ataxia, areflexia, visual scotoma and infertility.
Treatment: Vitamin E 100–400 mg orally daily.

VITAMIN K

Source:
- *Vitamin K1 (phylloquinone)*: Green vegetables, dairy product, liver and soybean oil.
- *Vitamin K2 (menaquinone)*: Intestinal bacterial flora.

Vitamin K-dependent clotting factors: II, VII, IX, and X, which are produced in the liver.
Functions: It acts as a cofactor in production of gamma-carboxyglutamic acid, which helps in the production of these coagulation factors.
Causes of deficiency: Less intake in food, obstructive jaundice, malabsorption syndrome, and prolonged use of antibiotic, which destroys bacterial flora.
Deficiency: Delayed coagulation and bleeding tendencies.
Treatment: Vitamin K 10 mg IV for 3–5 days.

THIAMINE (VITAMIN B1)

Source: Cereals, beans, peas, grains, yeast, pork, beef and liver.
Function: It is an essential coenzyme for decarboxylation of pyruvate to acetyl coenzyme A.
Causes of deficiency: Dietary deficiency, chronic alcoholism, and prolonged use of polished rice (causes beriberi).
Disease caused by deficiency: Beriberi and Wernicke's encephalopathy.
Beriberi: It is a disease caused by deficiency of vitamin B1.
Types: Two types in adults—
1. *Dry (or neurological) beriberi*: Features are peripheral neuropathy, tingling, numbness, wasting of muscles, loss of reflexes, and wrist and foot drop. Wernicke's encephalopathy. Korsakoff's psychosis
2. *Wet (or cardiac) beriberi*: Features are generalized edema. There may be biventricular heart failure and pulmonary edema.

Treatment: Injection B1 intravenous (IV) 50–100 mg for 3–5 days, then oral therapy. Diet rich in vitamin B1 should be given.

Wernicke's Encephalopathy

It is the acute cerebral manifestation of vitamin B1 deficiency, common in chronic heavy drinking of alcohol and inadequate diet. It may also occur after repeated vomiting, prolonged starvation or diarrhea. Lesion may be in brainstem (causing ophthalmoplegia, nystagmus and ataxia), superior vermis of cerebellum (causing ataxia), dorsomedial nucleus of thalamus, and adjacent area of gray matter (causing amnesia).

Clinical features:
- *Cognitive changes*: Acute confusion, disorientation, drowsiness or altered consciousness
- *Eye changes*: Bilateral symmetrical ophthalmoplegia, bilateral or unilateral paralysis of lateral conjugate gaze, horizontal or vertical nystagmus, and abnormal pupillary reflex. Rarely, ptosis, miosis, and unreactive pupil
- *Gait ataxia*: Broad-based gait, cerebellar signs, and vestibular paralysis
- When associated with memory disturbance and confabulation, it is called Korsakoff's psychosis. Loss of recent memory is common, but past memory may be normal. Confabulation means falsification of memory with clear consciousness. The patient makes new stories unrelated to truth.

Investigations: Diagnosis is clinical. Computed tomography (CT) scan is normal and cerebrospinal fluid (CSF) is also normal, but slight rise of protein may occur.

Treatment: Injection B1, 500 mg IV over 30 minutes tds 2 days, then 500 mg IV or IM daily for 5 days. Then, oral B1 100 mg tds and other B complex vitamins. If promptly treated, it is reversible. If not treated promptly, lesion may be irreversible.

RIBOFLAVIN (VITAMIN B2)

Source: Milk, cheese, eggs, liver, kidney, cereal and bread.

Deficiency: Vitamin B2 deficiency affect lips and tongue. It may cause glossitis, angular stomatitis, cheilosis, and seborrheic dermatitis. Genitals and skin areas rich in sebaceous glands may be affected.

Treatment: Riboflavin 10 mg daily orally.

NIACIN (VITAMIN B3)

Source: Meat, cereals, liver, kidney and fish.

Deficiency: It causes pellagra, characterized by dermatitis, diarrhea and dementia (3 D's).
- *Dermatitis*: It occurs on the sun-exposed areas, mainly limbs and neck (necklace area), but not on face. Skin lesions are erythema, vesiculation, cracking and pigmentation
- *Diarrhea*: It is associated with anorexia, nausea, glossitis and dysphagia
- *Dementia*.

Treatment: Nicotinic acid 100 mg 8 hourly daily orally or parenterally.

Toxicity: Reversible hepatotoxicity. Dose above 200 mg daily causes vasodilatory symptoms (flushing and hypotension).

PYRIDOXINE (VITAMIN B6)

Source: Milk, egg, meat, wheat, corn and cabbage.

Causes of deficiency: Pyridoxine-inactivating drugs (e.g. isoniazid), protein-energy malnutrition (PEM), malabsorption, and alcoholism or excessive loss.

Deficiency may cause: Peripheral neuropathy, mouth sores and glossitis. Isonicotinylhydrazide (INH) and penicillamine may antagonize the action of pyridoxine and mimic pyridoxine deficiency.

Treatment: Oral pyridoxine 10–20 mg daily (very high doses of vitamin B6 taken for several months may cause sensory polyneuropathy).

BIOTIN (VITAMIN B7)

Deficiency: It may occur due to intake of large quantities of raw eggs. It may cause scaly dermatitis, alopecia and paresthesia.

Treatment: Biotin 10 mg daily.

VITAMIN B12 (CYANOCOBALAMIN)

Source: Foods of animal origin such as liver, meat, fish and egg. No plant source

Functions: It acts as coenzyme for methionine synthesis and L-methylmalonyl CoA mutase

Causes of deficiency: Inadequate dietary intake (strict vegetarians), pernicious anemia, partial or total gastrectomy (intrinsic factor deficiency), and ileal disease (resection and Crohn's disease)

Deficiency may cause: Macrocytic or megaloblastic anemia, glossitis, subacute combined degeneration of spinal cord, peripheral neuropathy, dementia, and optic atrophy

Treatment: Injection hydroxycobalamin 1,000 μg IM for 5 days 2–3 days apart. Then maintenance dose 1,000 μg every 3 months for lifelong.

FOLATE

Source: Green vegetables, potato, peas, beans, meat, liver and kidney.

Function: It acts as a coenzyme for one carbon transfer in nucleic acid and amino acid metabolism.

Causes of deficiency: Less vegetable intake, malabsorption, more demand (such as pregnancy), and drug (methotrexate).

Deficiency may cause: Macrocytic or megaloblastic anemia. Neural tube defects such as spina bifida, anencephaly and encephalocele.

Treatment: Folic acid 5 mg daily for 3 weeks, then 5 mg weekly as maintenance dose. In pregnancy, folic acid is given to prevent megaloblastic anemia and fetal neural tube defect.

VITAMIN C (ASCORBIC ACID)

Source: Fresh citrus fruits and vegetables.

Functions: It is a powerful reducing agent and is involved in the hydroxylation of proline to hydroxyproline, which is necessary for the formation of collagen.

Causes of deficiency: Less intake of fresh fruits and vegetables.

Scurvy

It is disease due to vitamin C deficiency. It is of two types—infantile and adult scurvy.

Features:
- Swollen and spongy gums (particularly the papilla between teeth is called scurvy bud), which bleed easily. Teeth become loose and fall easily
- *Cutaneous bleeding*: Perifollicular hemorrhage, bruise and ecchymoses. Bleeding into joints (hemarthrosis), and gastrointestinal bleeding
- Anemia and poor wound healing
- *In infants*: Subperiosteal hemorrhage leads to painful limbs, occurs at the end of long bones, usually seen after 2 weeks of onset of clinical symptoms. There may be enlargement of costochondral junction (scorbutic rosary). Infants become very irritable and even do not allow to touch.

Treatment:
- *Vitamin C 250 mg*: 3-4 times daily orally
- *Diet*: Fresh fruits (orange, mango, pineapple, guava, etc.) and liver extract
- Bottle-fed infants should be given fruit juice. Nursing mother should take sufficient vitamin C, which is secreted in breast milk.

Toxicity: Daily intake of more than 1 g/day may cause diarrhea and formation of renal oxalate stones.

ZINC

Source: Red meat, seafood, meat, dairy products, and wholemeal bread.

Deficiency may cause:
- Growth retardation (dwarfism, hypogonadism, constipation and diarrhea)
- Acrodermatitis enteropathica (characterized by growth retardation, hair loss and diarrhea)
- In starvation, zinc deficiency causes thymic atrophy.

Treatment: Zinc supplementation should be given.

PROTEIN-ENERGY MALNUTRITION

It is a syndrome due to deficiency of protein, energy or both.

Types: There are three types of PEM—
- Marasmus: Deficiency in calorie intake
- *Kwashiorkor*: Protein malnutrition is predominant
- *Marasmic kwashiorkor*: Marked protein and calorie deficiency, most severe form of malnutrition.

Marasmus

It is defined as a malnutrition where both protein and energy deficiency occurs.

Clinical features:
- *Emaciation*: There is obvious muscle wasting and loss of body fat resulting in wrinkling and loosening of skin. Weight loss. Muscles are flabby with hypotonia

- Peculiar old man-like facies (monkey facies)
- Milestone of child development are delayed (standing, sitting, crawling and walking)
- Hair is thin and dry. Eyes are sunken and anterior fontanelle is depressed
- Diarrhea. Signs of infection may be present. No edema.

Treatment: Diet should contain protein, fat and carbohydrate. Minerals and vitamins should be added. Infection should be controlled and underlying cause should be treated.

Kwashiorkor

It is a malnutrition where there is severe deficiency of proteins in infants and young children soon after weaning. It is often precipitated by infections such as measles, malaria, and diarrheal illnesses.

Clinical features:
- Child is apathetic and lethargic with severe anorexia
- Generalized edema
- *Skin*: Erythematous, pigmentated, thick and shiny, and occasionally desquamation
- Muscles are flabby. Hair is dry, sparse lusterless, and may be reddish or yellow in color
- Abdomen is distended due to hepatomegaly and/or ascites.

Treatment: Diet should contain milk, milk proteins, fish, egg and fruits. Vitamins and minerals should be added.

Complications: Hypoglycemia, shock, hypothermia, and severe infection.

Investigations:
- *Complete blood count*: Anemia due to folate, iron, and copper deficiency
- Serum electrolytes
- Serum total protein and albumin to globulin (A:G) ratio
- Stool Routine microscopic examination (to see parasite)
- Chest X-ray (to exclude tuberculosis).

CHAPTER 16

Electrolyte and Acid-base Imbalance

INTRODUCTION

Normal range of serum electrolytes:
- *Sodium*: 135–145 mmol/L
- *Potassium*: 3.5–5.2 mmol/L
- *Chloride*: 95–107 mmol/L
- *Bicarbonate*: 21–28 mmol/L.

HYPERNATREMIA

When serum sodium level is above upper normal limit.

Causes:
- *Pure or predominant water depletion due to*: Less intake, fever and hot environment
- Hyperosmolar nonketotic diabetic coma (HONC) or hyperosmolar hyperglycemic state (HHS)
- Diabetes insipidus
- Excessive normal saline infusion.

Clinical features: May be asymptomatic. Altered mental status (confusion, stupor and coma).

Treatment: Water by mouth or nasogastric tube or dextrose in aqua or half strength normal saline IV. Treatment of underlying disorder.

HYPONATREMIA

When sodium is below the lower normal limit.

Causes:
- *True hyponatremia (hypovolemic)*: There is real loss of sodium
  - *GIT cause*: Vomiting, diarrhea and pancreatitis
  - *Renal cause*: Diuretic phase of acute renal failure (ARF), chronic kidney disease (CKD), tubulointerstitial disorder and salt-losing nephropathy
  - *Endocrine cause*: Addison's disease
  - *Drugs*: Diuretic.

- *Hypervolemic or dilutional*: No sodium loss and water volume is relatively high. Causes are—
  - Congestive cardiac failure (CCF)
  - Nephrotic syndrome
  - Cirrhosis of liver.
- *Euvolemic*:
  - SIADH (syndrome of inappropriate antidiuretic hormone secretion)
  - Psychogenic polydipsia
  - Postoperative hyponatremia
  - *Iatrogenic*: Dextrose in aqua infusion.
- *Pseudohyponatremia*: Body sodium is normal, but serum sodium is low due to interference of laboratory tests by the following conditions:
  - Hyperglycemia
  - Paraproteinemia
  - Hyperlipidemia.

Clinical features: May be asymptomatic, weakness, lassitude, tiredness, muscle cramp, dizziness, giddiness, confusion, stupor or even coma.

Treatment: According to type and cause—
- *True hyponatremia*: Sodium should be corrected. In mild case—oral salt is sufficient. If serum sodium is <125 mmol/L, intravenous (IV) normal saline
- *Hypervolemic or dilutional*: Water restriction, 600–1,000 mL/day, diuretic, and treatment of underlying cause
- *Euvolemic*: Water restriction and treatment of cause, e.g. SIADH.

Note: About 3% saline should not be given in most cases, may be required in selected cases. It should be used with caution, as rapid correction may cause central pontine myelinolysis (CPM).

HYPERKALEMIA

When serum potassium is high above the normal limit.

Causes:
- High potassium intake (oral or IV fluid with potassium, food or drugs containing potassium)
- *Renal diseases*: Acute and chronic renal failure. Impaired tubular secretion of serum potassium (renal lupus, amyloidosis and transplanted kidney)
- *Endocrine diseases*: Addison's disease, diabetic ketoacidosis and primary hypoaldosteronism
- *Drugs*: Potassium sparing diuretics (spironolactone, amiloride and triamterene), angiotensin-converting enzyme (ACE) inhibitor, nonsteroidal anti-inflammatory drug (NSAID) and cyclosporine
- *Miscellaneous*: Metabolic acidosis, rhabdomyolysis, tumor lysis syndrome, digoxin poisoning, vigorous exercise, hyperkalemic periodic paralysis, hyporeninemic hypoaldosteronism [type IV renal tubular acidosis (RTA)], and transfusion of stored blood
- *Pseudohyperkalemia*: Due to abnormal release of serum potassium from abnormal or damaged cells, also called spurious hyperkalemia
  - If blood is kept at room temperature for long time before analysis
  - Acute leukemia [due to very high white blood cell (WBC)]
  - Hemolysis

- Thrombocytosis
- Infectious mononucleosis.

Electrocardiogram (ECG) changes in hyperkalemia: T is tall, peaked and tented (in chest leads). Later, P is wide, small, and ultimately absent. PR interval is prolonged and QRS is wide, slurred and bizarre.

Clinical features: May be asymptomatic.
- Muscular weakness, may be severe causing flaccid paralysis, and tingling around lip or finger
- Loss of tendon jerk and paralytic ileus (abdomen is distended)
- Sudden death due to cardiac arrest or arrhythmia.

Treatment:
- Withdrawal of potassium, and potassium containing food and drug
- Injection 10% calcium gluconate, 10–20 cc IV slowly over 10 minutes. May be repeated (it protects the myocardium, also reduces the risk of cardiac arrest)
- Injection 50 mL of 50% glucose IV plus injection insulin 10 units. It can be repeated
- Correction of acidosis by IV sodium bicarbonate (1.26%), 500 mL 6–8 hourly (until serum HCO_3 is normal)
- Injection furosemide may be given
- Treatment of primary cause
- In some cases, exchange resins (calcium resonium 15–30 g orally)
- Nebulized salbutamol. It causes potassium entry into the cell
- If all fail, hemodialysis or peritoneal dialysis.

Note: Hyperkalemia is dangerous, if serum potassium is >7 mmol/L. May cause cardiac arrest in systole.

HYPOKALEMIA

When serum potassium is below normal physiological limit.

Causes:
- *Diuretic (thiazide, furosemide)*: The most common cause
- *Gastrointestinal (GI) loss*: Diarrhea, vomiting, purgative abuse, villous adenoma and ileostomy
- *Renal loss*: Renal tubular acidosis type I and II, renal tubular necrosis (diuretic phase), diuretic phase of ARF, relief of urinary tract obstruction, Bartter syndrome, Liddle's syndrome and Gitelman syndrome
- *Endocrine cause*: Cushing's syndrome and Conn's syndrome (primary hyperaldosteronism)
- *Others*: Heart failure, liver failure, nephrotic syndrome, drug (salbutamol and fenoterol), insulin therapy (in diabetic ketoacidosis), alkalosis, hypokalemic periodic paralysis, and interstitial renal disease
- *Intracellular shift*: Metabolic alkalosis and insulin therapy.

Clinical features:
- May be asymptomatic (if serum potassium >2.5 mmol/L)
- If severe hypokalemia (serum potassium <2.5 mmol/L)
  - Muscular weakness, paralysis and loss of tendon reflex
  - Abdominal distension with sluggish or absent bowel sound due to paralytic ileus and constipation
  - Arrhythmia and increased digoxin toxicity.

Treatment:
- If serum potassium is >2.5 mmol/L—oral potassium therapy
- If severe or serum potassium is <2.5 mmol/L—potassium is given in infusion (with normal saline)
- Treatment of primary cause.

Note: Potassium should never be given directly IV. Failure to correct hypokalemia may be due to concurrent hypomagnesemia. So, it should be measured and corrected.

Electrocardiogram changes in hypokalemia: U wave is prominent in chest leads (common). Others are ST depression, T is small or inverted, and prolonged PR interval.

HYPOMAGNESEMIA

Normal value: 0.5–1 mmol/L.

Causes:
- *Less intake*: Starvation, malnutrition, chronic alcoholism, and prolong parenteral nutrition
- *Gastrointestinal tract loss*: Prolong vomiting, chronic diarrhea, laxative abuse, nasogastric suction, small bowel bypass surgery and GI fistula
- *Renal loss*: Diuretic, recovery phase of acute tubular necrosis, drugs (gentamicin and cisplatin), primary hyperaldosteronism, diabetic ketoacidosis, and others (Bartter syndrome and Gitelman syndrome)
- *Miscellaneous*: Acute pancreatitis.

Clinical features: Usually associated with hypocalcemia. Features of tetany, cardiac arrhythmia (mainly torsades de pointes), and central nervous system (CNS) abnormality (irritability, dizziness, giddiness and seizure).

Treatment: IV magnesium chloride, 0.5 mL/kg in first 24 hours. Treatment of primary cause.

METABOLIC ACIDOSIS

It is a disorder characterized by reduction in plasma bicarbonate and rise in hydrogen ion concentration (low pH).

Causes: Acute and chronic renal failure, diabetic ketoacidosis, lactic acidosis, diarrhea, poisoning with methanol and ethanol, aspirin poisoning, and starvation.

Clinical features: Confusion, drowsiness, Kussmaul breathing (deep sighing respiration) and arrhythmia

Treatment: Treatment of primary cause. Injection sodium bicarbonate (1.26%). Correction of dehydration and other electrolyte imbalance.

METABOLIC ALKALOSIS

It is a disorder characterized by rise in plasma bicarbonate and fall in hydrogen ion concentration (increased pH).

Causes: Vomiting, aspiration of gastric contents, ingestion of alkali or overuse of antacid, diuretic, IV bicarbonate, acetate or citrate, hyperaldosteronism, Cushing's syndrome or excess use of steroid.

Clinical features: May be asymptomatic. Confusion, stupor or even coma. May cause tetany.

Treatment: IV fluid, usually normal saline. Treatment of primary cause. Correction of potassium.

RESPIRATORY ACIDOSIS

It is a disorder characterized by increased pCO_2 and low pH due to inadequate ventilation.

Causes:
- *Respiratory center depression*: Head injury, cardiovascular disease (CVD), encephalitis, and overdose of morphine, pethidine and sedative
- *Lung disease*: Collapse, extensive fibrosis, massive pleural effusion, and large pneumothorax
- *Neuromuscular*: Poliomyelitis and myopathy
- *Miscellaneous*: Kyphoscoliosis, Pickwickian syndrome and morbid obesity.

Treatment: Treatment of primary cause. Nebulized bronchodilator. O_2 inhalation. In severe case, ventilatory support.

RESPIRATORY ALKALOSIS

It is a disorder characterized by low pCO_2 and high pH secondary to hyperventilation.

Causes:
- Hysterical hyperventilation and anxiety
- Pregnancy
- *Respiratory*: Pulmonary embolism and pneumonia
- *Central nervous system*: Meningitis and encephalitis
- *Others*: Salicylate poisoning, metabolic acidosis, and vigorous assisted ventilation.

Treatment: Correction of cause and rebreathing in a closed bag.

CHAPTER 17

Pediatrics

INTRODUCTION

Common disease in children like measles, mumps, whooping cough, rheumatic fever, infectious disease, cardiac, respiratory, protein energy malnutrition (kwashiorkor and marasmus), etc. are described in the respective chapters. Only few are described here.

CEREBRAL PALSY

It is a disorder of posture and movement resulting from permanent, nonprogressive insult to the developing fetal and infant brain. Predominantly involves motor systems but may be disturbance of sensation, perception, cognition, communication, behavior, epilepsy and secondary musculoskeletal problem.

Causes: Intrauterine hypoxia, perinatal asphyxia and hypoxic ischemic encephalopathy, birth trauma, intrauterine maternal infection, infection (meningitis and encephalitis), intracerebral hemorrhage, neonatal sepsis, low birth weight (LBW), kernicterus, hypoglycemia or other metabolic abnormalities and congenital brain malformation.

Types:
- *Spastic (75%)*: Hemiplegic, diplegic (lower limbs more affected), quadriplegic and monoplegic (rare)
- Ataxic (15%)
- Dyskinetic (choreoathetosis, tremor, rigidity and dystonia)
- Hypotonic (1%)
- Mixed type.

Symptoms: Not achieving or delay of milestones of development (neck control, sitting, standing, crawling, walking and holding things) and involuntary movements (choreoathetosis). Other symptoms (seizure, mental retardation, speech disturbance and visual disturbance such as squint, refractive error, defect in choroid or retina and blindness, defect in hearing and interaction).

Signs: Due to involvement of pyramidal, extrapyramidal and cerebellum. Usual findings are—
- Spasticity (scissoring and tight tight Achilles tendon), exaggerated reflex and ataxia
- Involuntary movements, occasionally hypotonia
- *Other findings*: Microcephaly, squint, persistence of primitive reflexes (palmer reflex, Moro reflex).

Investigations: Diagnosis is clinical. Computed tomography (CT) scan or magnetic resonance imaging (MRI) of brain may be done to exclude other neurological disorders.

Management: Counseling of parents.
- *Symptomatic treatment*: For seizures, anticonvulsants (phenytoin and phenobarbitone). For spasticity, baclofen, diazepam, clonazepam and tizanidine. In some cases, botulinum toxin to reduce spasticity
- *Others*: Physiotherapy, speech therapy, psychotherapy, social and rehabilitation, educational therapy and orthopedic measures
- Follow-up, to assess improvement of the disabilities.

FEBRILE CONVULSION OR FEBRILE SEIZURE

It is defined as seizure during fever between 6 months to 5 years of age in the absence of intracranial infection. It is the common seizure disorder of children less than 5 years, more common in male. Occurs among developmentally normal children following viral infection (90%), pneumonia, otitis media, tonsillitis, dysentery and urinary tract infection (UTI).

Diagnostic criteria:
- *Age*: 6 months to 5 years with a peak age of 14–18 months
- Temperature >38.8° C or 101.8° F
- *Seizures*: Mostly generalized, tonic clonic, usually once within 24 hours, last from few seconds to few minutes, but not exceeding 15 minutes. Usually one seizure attack in one episode, rarely two
- Absence of signs of meningitis (e.g. bulging fontanelle, stiff neck, stupor and irritability)
- No residual neurological deficit.

Investigations: Complete blood count (CBC), blood culture/sensitivity (C/S), throat swab C/S, urine routine examination and C/S, lumbar puncture and cerebrospinal fluid (CSF) study, and X-ray of chest. Others—blood sugar, serum electrolytes and calcium.

Note: Electroencephalogram (EEG) and neuroimaging are not required in simple febrile seizure.

Treatment: For acute episode—
- Explanation and reassurance to the parents
- Maintaining airway, breathing and circulation
- *For fever*: Tepid sponging, fanning and paracetamol. Excess clothing is removed (ice cold water should be avoided)
- *Control of convulsion*: Diazepam per rectally (0.5 mg/kg) or intravenously (0.2–0.3 mg/kg)
- *For infection*: Antibiotic (e.g. amoxicillin and ceftriaxone).

Prevention of recurrence:
- *Intermittent prophylaxis*: Oral diazepam (1 mg/kg/day 8 hourly) with paracetamol should be given at the onset of fever, usually for 2–3 days
- *Continuous prophylaxis*: Not recommended, but may be considered if occurrence of seizure after 6 years of age, despite intermittent prophylaxis.

Counseling to parents: About the natural history, treatment and prognosis.

Prognosis: Generally good. Benign condition and recurrence is high in one-third of cases—50% in under 1 year of age, and 30% in other situation. Frequency decreases after 5 year of age. In about 2% cases, may turn to epilepsy in later childhood.

Atypical febrile convulsion: If convulsion associated with fever persists >15 minutes, occurs more than once in 24 hours, focal or unilateral in nature, followed by Todd's paralysis, but no significant other cause or central nervous system (CNS) infection, it is called atypical febrile convulsion. EEG may be abnormal for 2 weeks or more following the attack.

Treatment: Continuous prophylaxis therapy may be given, sodium valproate 30–60 mg/kg/day in two divided dose. Continued for at least 2 years fit free or until the child is 6 years old whichever comes earlier.

NEONATAL PNEUMONIA

It is the infection and inflammation of lung parenchyma.

Causes:
- *Early onset neonatal pneumonia, in first 7 days*: Escherichia coli, group B *Streptococcus*, *Klebsiella*, *Staphylococcus aureus*, *Streptococcus pneumoniae* and *Pseudomonas*
- *Late onset neonatal pneumonia, after 3 weeks*: S. pneumoniae, S. aureus, Klebsiella, Streptococcus and Pseudomonas.

Symptoms: Fever (moderate-to-high), cough, respiratory distress, not able to drink or stop feeding, convulsion and stridor.

Signs: Wheeze, cyanosis, fast breathing and chest indrawing. In chest, bronchial breath sounds, rhonchi and few crepitations.

Investigations: CBC, C-reactive protein (CRP), X-ray of chest posteroanterior (PA) view, arterial blood gas analysis, nasopharyngeal or tracheal aspirate for C/S.

Treatment: Counseling to parents and breastfeeding to be continued.
- Airway should be kept clear, O_2 inhalation and bronchodilator
- *Antibiotic*: Injection ampicillin 50–100 mg/kg/day in four divided dose *plus* injection gentamycin 2.5 mg/kg/day, 8–12 hourly or cefotaxime 150 mg/kg/day or injection ceftriaxone 75 mg/kg/day. Antibiotic can be changed according to C/S.

BRONCHIOLITIS

It is an acute viral infection of bronchioles resulting in inflammatory obstruction.

Causes: Respiratory syncytial virus (common). Other organisms—Influenzae, parainfluenza viruses, adenovirus, metapneumovirus, rhinovirus and sometimes mycoplasma.

Risk factors: Prematurity, low socioeconomic status, nonbreastfeeding, crowded environment, passive smoking and indoor air pollution.

Symptoms: Common in children <2 years of age, peak 2-6 months. It occurs in epidemics, particularly during winter and rainy season. Runny nose, fever, usually low grade, cough, respiratory distress, loss of appetite, irritability and crying.

Signs: Tachypnea, flaring alae nasi, movement of accessory muscles of respiration, suprasternal, intercostal and subcostal recession, cyanosis, multiple rhonchi and crepitations. Liver and spleen are palpable due to downward pushing of diaphragm by hyperinflated lung.

Investigations:
- *X-ray of chest*: Shows hypertranslucency and hyperinflation, and interstitial shadow
- *Complete blood count*: Normal
- *Blood gas analysis*: Shows low oxygen
- Virus isolation from nasopharyngeal secretion by polymerase chain reaction (PCR) or culture.

Treatment: Counseling the parents about the diseases.
- *Mild case*: May be treated at home—normal feeding, cleaning nose with normal saline drop, and bathing with lukewarm water
- *Severe case*: Hospitalization if central cyanosis, unable to take food, restlessness, severe respiratory distress or chest indrawing, and grunting
  - Propped up position and oxygen inhalation
  - Correction of dehydration, if needed intravenous (IV) fluid
  - Nebulized salbutamol, 0.03 mL/kg/dose
  - For fever: Tepid sponging and paracetamol
  - Antiviral: Nebulized ribavirin, especially in cyanotic congenital heart disease, bronchopulmonary dysplasia and immunodeficiency
  - Steroid: Short course prednisolone, mainly if family history of atopy.

Prognosis: Good, most case recover in 5-7 days. 30-50% may develop bronchial asthma, especially if family history of asthma.

MENINGITIS

It is the inflammation of leptomeninges (pia and arachnoid mater) by invasion of micro-organism.

Causes: It may be bacterial, viral, tuberculous (TB), and others (parasitic and fungal).

Bacterial (or pyogenic) meningitis: Causative organisms are—
- *Neonatal period (under 2 months)*: E. coli, Pseudomonas, group B *Streptococcus* and proteus
- 2 months to 6 years: *Haemophilus influenzae*, S. pneumoniae and *Neisseria meningitidis*
- Above 6 years: S. pneumoniae and N. meningitidis.

Symptoms:
- *In children*: High fever, nausea, vomiting, headache, photophobia, impaired consciousness and recurrent convulsion
- *In neonates*: Presentations are nonspecific. Reluctant to feed, high-pitched cry, vacant look, hypo or hyperthermia, jitteriness, convulsion, respiratory distress and features of sepsis.

Signs:
- Altered sensorium or altered consciousness or stupor. Bulging of anterior fontanelle (in neonates and infants)
- *Signs of meningeal irritation*: Neck rigidity and Kernig's sign (may not be present in children <18 months)
- *In meningococcal septicemia*: Typical skin rash in different parts of body, and even features of shock.

Investigations:
- *Complete blood count*: Shows polymorphonuclear leukocytosis
- Blood C/S (may reveal the organism in 80% cases)
- *Lumbar puncture and CSF study*: High pressure, cloudy or purulent color, cytology (300–2,000 cell/mm^3 and high neutrophil), biochemistry (high protein, low glucose and corresponding blood sugar should be done). Gram staining may show the organism
- *Bacterial antigens*: May be detected by latex agglutination test or PCR for DNA (deoxyribonucleic acid) of causative agent
- Culture and sensitivity.

Treatment:
- *General*: Maintenance of nutrition, IV fluid, and 10% dextrose (if hypoglycemia). For fever, tepid sponging and paracetamol. For convulsion—diazepam, phenytoin and phenobarbitone
- *Specific*:
  - Ampicillin 400 mg/kg/day *plus* chloramphenicol 100 mg/kg/day 6 hourly or ceftriaxone (100 mg/kg/day) once daily
  - Vancomycin, if pneumococcus is suspected. Antibiotic may be changed according to C/S
  - Injection dexamethasone IV 0.15/kg/dose 6 hourly for 2 days.

Duration of treatment: 7 days (if meningococcus), 10 days (if *H. influenzae*), and 14 days (if pneumococcus).

Complications:
- *Acute complications*: Hydrocephalus, subdural effusion, empyema, ventriculitis, cerebral abscess, cerebral infarction and cranial nerve palsy
- *Long-term complications*: Cerebral palsy (CP), deafness, mental retardation, epilepsy, visual impairment, and learning and language disability.

VIRAL MENINGITIS

Causes:
- *Enterovirus (the most common)*: Coxsackievirus, echovirus, poliovirus and human enterovirus
- *Other viruses*: Herpes simplex virus (HSV), varicella zoster, cytomegalovirus (CMV), measles, Epstein–Barr virus (EBV).

Clinical features: Same as bacterial meningitis.

Investigations:
- *Complete blood count*: Normal, may be leukopenia with lymphocytosis
- *Lumbar puncture and CSF study*: Clear fluid, cytology (lymphocytosis), and biochemistry (normal protein and glucose)
- *Others*: Blood glucose, electrolytes and creatinine.

Treatment: General measures are as in bacterial meningitis. In HSV, aciclovir 10 mg/kg 8 hourly for 14–21 days.

TUBERCULOUS MENINGITIS

Caused by *Mycobacterium tuberculosis*.

Clinical features:
- History of contact with TB patient
- History of fever, loss of weight, night sweating, nausea, vomiting, headache and irritability
- Convulsion, drowsiness, dizziness or impaired consciousness
- Signs of meningeal irritation (neck rigidity and Kernig's sign)
- Cranial nerve palsy (3rd and 6th nerve).

Investigations:
- *Complete blood count*: High erythrocyte sedimentation rate (ESR)
- *Cerebrospinal fluid study*: High pressure, straw color, high lymphocyte, high protein, low sugar, high adenosine deaminase (ADA), acid-fast bacillus (AFB) may be positive, and PCR
- *Mantoux test (MT)*: May be positive
- *X-ray of chest*: May show primary focus
- CT or MRI of brain.

Complications: Hydrocephalus, cranial nerve palsy, deafness, blindness, hemiplegia or paraplegia, and mental retardation.

Treatment: Anti TB [rifampicin, isonicotinylhydrazide (INH), and pyrazinamide] for 2 months, then INH and rifampicin for 10 months. Prednisolone 1–2 mg/kg/day for 4–6 weeks, then taper over 2–4 weeks. Pyridoxine to prevent peripheral neuropathy.

Note: Ethambutol is avoided in children, as they cannot complain of the features of optic neuritis (may become blind).

DIARRHEA

It means frequent passage of loose stools.

Causes:
- *Virus*: Rotavirus and Enterovirus
- *Bacteria*: E. coli, Shigella, Salmonella, Campylobacter, and Vibrio cholerae
- *Parasitic*: Giardia lamblia and Entamoeba histolytica.

Pathological consequence: During diarrhea, three important clinical consequences occur:
1. Loss of water and electrolytes (sodium, chloride, potassium and bicarbonate)
2. Loss of zinc, which delays recovery of patients and make the child vulnerable to suffer afterward
3. Weight loss due to less intake of food, less absorption, and increased nutrient requirements.

Acute watery diarrhea: When diarrhea persists <14 days.

Symptoms: Patient passes loose watery stool several times (>3 times) daily that do not contain blood. Sometimes may have associated vomiting and low-grade fever.

Signs: Signs of dehydration, abdominal distension and sign of severe malnutrition.

Signs of dehydration: Lethargy, absent tears, sunken eyes, pinched face, dry tongue, unable to drink or drink poorly, and skin pinch goes back very slowly.

Assessment of patient with diarrhea:
- Frequency of diarrhea and presence of blood
- History of vomiting, attacks of crying with pallor and urine output
- History about foods and feeding
- Local reports of cholera outbreaks.

Investigations:
- Stool for routine microscopic examination and C/S
- Complete blood count and peripheral blood film (PBF), serum urea, creatinine and electrolytes, and blood sugar
- *Others*: Plain X-ray of abdomen and ultrasonography (USG).

Treatment: Rehydration therapy, zinc supplement, continued feeding, and antibiotic in specific cases.

Rehydration
- *No signs of dehydration*: Plan "A" (treatment at home)—advice to the mother about the following:
  - Child is given more fluid to prevent dehydration until diarrhea stops
  - More food to prevent under nutrition
  - If no improvement or baby drinks poorly or unable to drink or breastfeed or becomes more sick or develops fever or blood appears in stool, child should be transferred to the hospital or health center.
- Rehydration at home with oral rehydration solution (ORS) or home-based fluids after each loose stool as follows:
  - *Less than 2 years*: 50–100 mL
  - *2–10 years*: 100–200 mL
  - *10 years and above*: As much as possible.
- *Some dehydration*: Plan "B"
  - *Rehydration with ORS solution*: 75 mL/kg given in 4 hours at OPD and the child is monitored
  - Encourage mother for breastfeeding
  - After 4 hours of oral rehydration, the child's hydration status should be reassessed. If no signs of dehydration, treatment is like plan A. If signs of severe dehydration, treatment is like plan C.
- *Rehydrate as follows (4 hourly)*:
  - *Up to 4 months*: 200–400 mL
  - *4–12 months*: 400–700 mL
  - *12 months to 2 years*: 700–900 mL
  - *2 years up to 5 years*: 900–1,400 mL.
- *Severe dehydration*: Plan "C"

Rapid IV rehydration 100 mL/kg, best IV fluid is Ringer's lactate solution (also called Hartmann's solution) or cholera fluid. If not available, then 5% dextrose in normal saline can be used
  - *Infant under 12 months*: 30 mL/kg in 1 hour, then 70 mL/kg in 5 hour
  - *Older children*: 30 mL/kg in 30 minutes, then 70 mL/kg in two-and-a half hour.

- *Monitoring*: Reassess the child every 15–30 minutes until a strong radial pulse is present. When full amount of IV fluid has been given, reassess the child's hydration status
  - *If sign of severe dehydration still present*: Repeat IV fluid
  - *If signs of some dehydration*: Discontinue IV fluid and treat as plan B
  - *If no signs of dehydration*: Discontinue IV fluid and treat as plan A.

Zinc supplementation
- *<6 months*: 10 mg/day for 10–14 days
- *>6 months*: 20 mg/day for 10–14 days.

Continued feeding
- *<6 months*: Breastfeeding
- *>6 months*: Breastfeeding plus freshly prepared high energy complementary foods like mashed rice, mashed banana and fresh fruit juice.

Antimicrobials for specific disease
- *Cholera*: Tetracycline (>8 years), doxycycline and co-trimoxazole
- *Amoebiasis*: Metronidazole, tinidazole and nitazoxanide
- *Giardiasis*: Metronidazole and tinidazole
- *Shigella*: Ciprofloxacin, pivmecillinam and nalidixic acid.

NEONATAL JAUNDICE

It is the yellow coloration of skin and mucous membrane of newborn baby. In adult, jaundice is seen when serum bilirubin is >3 mg/dL, but in newborn, jaundice is seen when serum bilirubin is >5 mg/dL.

Causes: According to age—
- *Early jaundice (jaundice within 10 days of age)*:
  - Within first 2 days: Hemolytic disease of newborn [Rh incompatibility, ABO incompatibility, and glucose-6 phosphate dehydrogenase (G6PD) deficiency], congenital spherocytosis, congenital TORCH infection (toxoplasmosis, rubella, cytomegalovirus and herpes)
  - Within 3–10 days: Physiological jaundice, prematurity, hypoglycemia, sepsis, congenital hemolytic anemia, congenital nonhemolytic hyperbilirubinemia (Gilbert's syndrome, Dubin–Johnson syndrome, Crigler–Najjar syndrome and Rotor syndrome).
- *Prolonged jaundice (jaundice >10 days)*:
  - Prolonged unconjugated hyperbilirubinemia: Breast milk jaundice, sepsis, hypothyroidism, galactosemia, RH-incompatibility, G6PD deficiency and congenital hemolytic anemia
  - Prolonged conjugated hyperbilirubinemia: Intrahepatic cholestasis (septicemia, UTI, hepatitis, galactosemia, alpha-1 antitrypsin deficiency, hypothyroidism and idiopathic neonatal hepatitis), and extrahepatic cholestasis (biliary atresia and choledochal cyst).

Investigations:
- *Complete blood count with PBF*: It shows leukocytosis in sepsis, PBF shows fragmented or nucleated red blood cell (RBC) in hemolytic disease, serum bilirubin (high), serum glutamic oxaloacetic transaminase (SGOT), serum glutamic pyruvic transaminase (SGPT), and alkaline phosphatase (all may be high)
- Blood grouping ABO (to see ABO incompatibility) and Rh typing of mother and baby (negative mother and positive baby if Rh incompatibility)

- *Coomb test*: Positive (if Rh incompatibility)
- *Reticulocyte count*: High in hemolytic disease
- *Others*: Enzyme assay, TORCH screening, USG of hepatobiliary system, chest X-ray and blood C/S.

Treatment: Counseling to parents and breastfeeding to be continued. IV fluid may be needed. Spontaneous recovery in physiological jaundice. In other cases, to reduce bilirubin:
- *Sunlight exposure*: In early morning for 10-20 minutes every day.
- *Phototherapy*:
  - If serum bilirubin >15 mg/dL for term baby
  - If serum bilirubin 10-12 mg/dL for preterm baby.
- Exchange transfusion when bilirubin >20 mg/dL with anemia in Rh incompatibility and ABO incompatibility
- Intravenous immunoglobulin may be helpful
- Treatment of underlying cause.

ABO Incompatibility: If mother has O group and baby has A or B group, it causes hemolysis of RBC of the baby.

Rh incompatibility: Here, baby is Rh positive and mother is Rh negative. Rh antibody enters into fetal bloodstream resulting in destruction of fetal RBC.

KERNICTERUS

It is a neurological syndrome that occurs as a result of excess bilirubin in blood and its deposition within the brain, mainly in basal ganglia. Also involves hippocampus, subthalamic nuclei and thalamus. Cerebral cortex is spared.

Causes: Prematurity, hemolytic disease of newborn, congenital familial nonhemolytic jaundice, neonatal hepatitis and congenital spherocytosis.

Clinical features: Usually occur if bilirubin is >20 mg/dL.
- *Early signs*: Lethargy, poor feeding and loss of Moro reflex
- *Acute bilirubin encephalopathy, three phases*:
  - Phase I (hypotonia, lethargy, poor suck and depressed sensorium)
  - Phase II (hypertonia progressing to opisthotonus, rigidity and oculogyric crisis)
  - Phase III (high pitched cry, convulsion, hypotonia and death).
- *Chronic bilirubin encephalopathy*:
  - In the first year of life: Opisthotonus, extrapyramidal rigidity, irregular movements and convulsion
  - Later, in older children: Mental retardation, deafness, athetosis, poor formation and green discoloration of teeth.

Treatment: Kernicterus is irreversible, and management is only symptomatic and supportive.

LOW BIRTH WEIGHT

It means baby with birth weight <2.5 kg irrespective of gestational age, includes preterm or prematurity and small for date or small for gestational age, also called intrauterine growth retardation (IUGR).
- *Preterm*: When baby is born before 37 weeks of gestation
- *Term*: When baby is born at 37-42 weeks of gestation

- *Post-term*: When baby is born after 42 weeks of gestation
- *Very LBW baby*: When birth weight is <1,500 g, but >1,000 g
- *Extremely LBW baby*: When birth weight is <1,000 g or less
- *Incredible LBW baby*: When birth weight is <750 g or less
- *Small for date or gestational age*: Gestation is full-term, but baby is malnourished.

Causes of prematurity:
- *Fetal*: Fetal distress, multiple gestations and erythroblastosis fetalis
- *Placental*: Placental dysfunction, placenta previa and abruptio placentae
- *Uterine*: Bicornuate uterus and incompetent cervix
- *Maternal*: Teenage mother, pre-eclampsia, chronic medical illness (cyanotic heart disease and renal disease), infections (UTI and chorioamnionitis, listeria, bacterial vaginosis and group B streptococcus)
- *Others*: Diabetes mellitus, Rh incompatibility, premature rupture of membrane and polyhydramnios.

Causes of IUGR:
- *Fetal*: Chromosomal disorder (trisomy), congenital rubella, syphilis, radiation and multiple gestations
- *Placental*: Decreased placental weight or cellularity or both, villous placentitis, tumor (chorioangioma and hydatidiform mole), placental separation or infarction, and twin-twin transfusion syndrome
- *Maternal*: Toxemia of pregnancy, hypertension, renal disease, hypoxemia (high altitude and cyanotic heart or lung disease), malnutrition, chronic illness, sickle cell anemia and drugs (narcotics and alcohol).

Complications of preterm baby:
- *Respiratory*: Respiratory distress syndrome or hyaline membrane disease, pneumothorax and apnea
- *Cardiovascular system (CVS)*: Patent ductus arteriosus (PDA) and bradycardia with apnea
- *Gastrointestinal tract (GIT) and hepatic*: Necrotizing enterocolitis, poor motility and hyperbilirubinemia
- *Hematologic*: Early anemia and disseminated intravascular coagulation (DIC)
- *Neurological*: Intraventricular hemorrhage, hypotonia, seizure and retinopathy of prematurity
- *Electrolyte imbalance*: Hyponatremia, hypernatremia and hyperkalemia
- *Metabolic*: Hypothermia, hypocalcemia, hypoglycemia and hyperglycemia
- *Others*: Infection, neonatal death, stillbirth, CP and seizure.

Complications of IUGR: Meconium aspiration syndrome and transient hypo- or hyperglycemic episode.

NEONATAL CONVULSION

It is defined as paroxysmal alteration in neurological function such as behavior, motor, autonomic function, either one or all three within 28 days of birth.

Causes:
- Hypoxic ischemic encephalopathy (the most common)
- Birth trauma (especially during forceps delivery), intraventricular, subdural or subarachnoid hemorrhage, and congenital anomaly of brain

- *Infection*: Meningitis, viral encephalitis and TORCH syndrome
- *Metabolic*: Hypoglycemia, hypocalcemia, hypomagnesemia, hyponatremia, hypernatremia and inborn errors of metabolism
- Kernicterus, pyridoxine dependency or deficiency, and maternal narcotic addiction.

Investigations:
- Complete blood count with ESR, blood sugar, serum electrolytes, serum calcium and serum magnesium
- Arterial blood gas analysis
- *If indicated*: Lumbar puncture and CSF study
- Ultrasonography of head.

Treatment:
- Maintenance of airway and circulation. Mouth gag between jaws to prevent tongue bite
- Reduction of body temperature by tepid sponging
- Intravenous 10% dextrose, 2 mL/kg over 2-5 minutes
- Intravenous 10% calcium gluconate, 1 mL/kg mixed with distilled water with cardiac monitoring
- Injection pyridoxine 50-100 mg single dose
- *For convulsion*: Lorazepam 0.05 mg/kg or diazepam 0.3 mg/kg IV or phenobarbitone 10-20 mg/kg IV, may be repeated 5-10 mg/kg. For maintenance dose 3-6 mg/kg in two separate doses. *Or* phenytoin 20 mg/kg IV may be given
- If the baby is neurologically normal, drug may be discontinued. If neurologically abnormal, drug should be continued.

PERINATAL MORTALITY

Perinatal period is 28 weeks of gestation to 7 days after birth. Perinatal mortality is the number of stillbirths and deaths in the first week of life (early neonatal mortality).

Causes:
- *Fetal*: Placental insufficiency, intrauterine infection, severe congenital anomalies, abruptio placentae and hydrops fetalis
- *Preterm*: Respiratory distress syndrome, intraventricular hemorrhage, infection, necrotizing enterocolitis and bronchopulmonary dysplasia
- *Full-term*: Congenital anomalies, birth asphyxia, trauma, infection, meconium aspiration pneumonia, and ABO and Rh incompatibility

CHAPTER 18

Genetics

AUTOSOMAL DOMINANT DISEASE

It has the following characters:
- Consecutive generations are affected
- Half of the offspring are affected
- Both male and female are equally affected
- Unaffected individual cannot transmit the disease
- Age of onset of the disease is variable. Affected person may remain symptom free up to adult life.

Some autosomal dominant diseases: Neurofibromatosis, tuberous sclerosis, Huntington's disease, adult polycystic kidney disease, Marfan syndrome, familial adenomatous polyposis coli, pseudoxanthoma elasticum and Peutz–Jeghers syndrome.

AUTOSOMAL RECESSIVE DISEASES

It has the following characters:
- Half of the children of unaffected carriers will be carriers
- It affects both male and female
- If both parents are carriers, one in four of children of heterozygous parents will be affected and half will be carrier
- Usually only one generation is affected
- Consanguinity increases the risk of autosomal recessive disorders.

Some autosomal recessive diseases: Hereditary hemochromatosis, cystic fibrosis, Wilson's disease, albinism, xeroderma pigmentosum, ataxia-telangiectasia, phenylketonuria and alkaptonuria.

X-LINKED RECESSIVE DISORDERS

It has the following characters:
- Only males are affected and females are carrier
- Unaffected female carriers transmit the disease

- A female carrier will transmit the disease to half of her sons and half of her daughters will be the carrier
- Affected males cannot transmit the disease to their sons, but all the daughters will be carrier.

Some X-linked recessive disorders: Hemophilia A and B, glucose-6 phosphate dehydrogenase deficiency, Duchenne muscular dystrophy, Alport syndrome and fragile X syndrome.

X-Linked Dominant

It has the following characters:
- X-linked diseases are rarely dominant
- Females who are heterozygous for the mutant gene and males who have only one copy of the mutant gene on their single X chromosome will manifest the disease
- Half of the male or female offspring of an affected mother will have the disease
- All the female offspring of an affected man will have the disease
- Affected man will always have affected daughter, but never son
- Women are more affected than men, M:F = 1:2
- Affected males tend to have the disease more severely than the heterozygous female.

Some of the X-linked dominant diseases: Vitamin D-resistant rickets or familial hypophosphatemic rickets, and oro-facio-genital syndrome.

Nongerm line cytoplasmic inheritance (e.g. gene on mitochondrial DNA): It has the following characters
- Males and females are affected
- No males transmit the disease
- Variable proportion of offspring from female are affected.

DOWN SYNDROME

It is a chromosomal abnormality, trisomy 21 (47, XX/XY, +21), caused by the presence of all or part of an extra 21 chromosome.

Types:
- *Trisomy 21 (47, XX/XY, +21)*: The most common (95%)
- Mosaic variant
- Translocation variant.

Clinical features:
- *Face*: Flat with flat nasal bridge and low set small ears
- *Mouth*: Appears small and tends to remain open with high-arched palate
- *Tongue*: Appears protruding with large and horizontal fissure
- *Eyes*: Epicanthic folds and slanting eyes, Brushfield spots on iris (yellow speckles), and conjunctivitis
- *Neck*: Short and wide
- *Hands*: Single palmar crease (simian) and short stubby finger. Hand looks small and round (short and broad hands) and has clinodactyly (short inward curving of little finger)
- *Foot*: Gap between first and second toe
- *Cardiac*: Ventricular septal defect (VSD) is common, also atrial septal defect (ASD), patent ductus arteriosus (PDA), tetralogy of Fallot, and mitral regurgitation due to endocardial cushion defect

- *Others*: Short stature, hypotonia, joint hyperextensibility, straight pubic hair and low IQ (from mild-to-severe)
- The child is fond of music.

Note: Down syndrome is related to maternal age during pregnancy (incidence is high with more maternal age).

Investigations: Karyotyping. Regular follow-up to see complications.

Complications:
- High incidence of leukemia (in neonates, acute myeloid leukemia and in older children, acute lymphoid leukemia)
- Duodenal atresia
- Presenile dementia of Alzheimer's type
- Autoimmune hypothyroidism may occur
- Mental retardation (mild-to-severe)
- Lenticular opacity.

Prenatal screening:
- *First trimester*: Nuchal translucency, human chorionic gonadotropin (hCG) and pregnancy-associated plasma protein-A (PAPP-A)
- *At 13–20 weeks*: Maternal serum for alpha-fetoprotein, hCG, unconjugated estriol (uE3), fetal ultrasonography (USG) and amniocentesis.

Turner Syndrome: For details, see in the chapter 'Endocrinology'.

NOONAN SYNDROME

It is also called male Turner. It may affect both male and female equally.
- Female patients have Turner's phenotype, but with normal 46, XX. They have normal ovarian function and normal fertility
- In male, there is 46, XY. Cardiac lesion is present, more on right side (e.g. pulmonary stenosis). In Turner syndrome, left-sided cardiac lesion is more.

Clinical features:
- Short stature
- Mental retardation (common)
- Downward slanting and wide-spaced eyes
- Low set ear
- Webbing of the neck
- Low posterior hairline
- Pulmonary stenosis.

KLINEFELTER SYNDROME

It is a chromosomal abnormality in which there is an extra X chromosome associated with hypogonadism (due to small testis). Common karyotype abnormality is usually 47, XXY which results from nondisjunction during meiosis in one of the parents, may be 46, XY or 47, XXY mosaic.

Clinical features:
- Tall stature (arm span greater than height and leg is more long, lower extremity is greater than upper extremity). Tallness is due to androgen deficiency with lack of epiphyseal closure in puberty
- Obesity
- Gynecomastia (carcinoma of breast may develop in 20% cases)

- *Eunuchoid body proportion*:
  - *Absence or rudimentary external genitalia*: Small penis and testis (volume <5 mL)
  - Absence of secondary sexual characters (axillary, pubic hair and beard).
- In mosaic, there may be normal puberty. Diagnosis is done during routine investigation for infertility.

Usual presentations of Klinefelter syndrome: Poor sexual development, infertility, gynecomastia, and small or undescended testis.

Associations in Klinefelter syndrome: Type 2 diabetes mellitus, low T4, bronchial asthma, carcinoma of breast in male is more in Klinefelter syndrome.

Investigations:
- Serum testosterone (low) and gonadotropic hormones [increased follicle-stimulating hormone (FSH) and luteinizing hormone (LH)]
- Serum estrogen (increased)
- Azoospermia is universal
- Chromosomal analysis (two or more X-chromosome, one or more Y-chromosome).

Treatment: No specific treatment. Androgen (testosterone may be used in oral, injection, patch, gel and pellet). Plastic surgery for gynecomastia. Lifespan is usually normal.

Abnormality of testis in Klinefelter syndrome: Both testes are small and firm. These show seminiferous tubules dysgenesis. Hyalinization and fibrosis are present within the seminiferous tubules. Leydig cell function is impaired, resulting in hypogonadism. Also, there is azoospermia and high gonadotropin.

Features of eunuchoid body proportion: Features are apparent from childhood.
- Tall stature with long leg
- Hairless face (also sparse body hair)
- High-pitched voice
- Small and poorly-developed external genitalia
- Immature personality.

CHAPTER 19

Miscellaneous

SNAKE BITE

Features are due to different toxins by different snakes like hematotoxin, cardiotoxin, neurotoxin, myotoxin, nephrotoxin and allergic toxin.

Clinical features:
- *Local features*: There may be fang marks, pain, numbness, tingling, local edema, redness, warmth, bleeding from site, blister and necrosis
- *General*: Nausea, vomiting, headache, dizziness, fever and urticaria
- *Neurological*: Cranial nerve palsy, ptosis, squint, facial weakness and respiratory paralysis
- *Muscular*: Weakness and paralysis
- *Cardiac*: Tachycardia, hypotension, shock, cardiac failure and arrhythmias
- *Renal*: Oliguria, anuria or even renal failure
- *Hematological*: Bleeding, thrombosis, deep vein thrombosis (DVT), and disseminated intravascular coagulation (DIC)
- Cobra and krait cause constitutional symptoms more than local symptoms. Neurotoxicity is more
- Russell and scaled vipers cause severe local symptoms and hemorrhagic tendency.

Treatment:
- *General*: Maintenance of airway, breathing, and circulation. Immobilization and pressure bandage above the bite, and local care of wound. Intravenous (IV) fluid and maintenance of nutrition. Antibiotic and analgesic, if needed. Antihistamine in some cases. Corticosteroid in severe shock and allergic reactions. Management of complication, if any
- *Specific*: Antidote (polyvalent anti-snake venom IV).

SHOCK

Shock is a clinical syndrome characterized by inappropriate and inadequate tissue perfusion resulting in widespread reduction of oxygen and metabolic requirements of the tissues, leading to tissue damage or organ failure and death. There are four types:

1. *Hypovolemic shock*: There is reduction of blood volume, so less stroke volume and cardiac output
2. *Cardiogenic shock*: It is due to failure of heart to maintain effective pump
3. *Obstructive shock*: There is compression of heart, so impairment of forward flow of blood
4. *Distributive shock*: There is severe impairment of peripheral circulation. Cardiac output may be normal or even high, but still inadequate tissue perfusion.

Clinical features of different shock: Some features are common in any shock and some are due to the cause.

Hypovolemic Shock

There is reduction of blood volume, so less cardiac output and low blood pressure (BP). If not properly treated, there is severe hypotension, tissue hypoxia, and damage to vital organs.

Causes:
- *Blood loss*: Bleeding due to any cause (hematemesis, melena and multiple injury)
- *Fluid and electrolytes loss*: Vomiting, diarrhea, heat stroke, aspiration of fluid, and excessive sweating
- *Plasma loss*: Burn and exfoliative dermatitis.

Signs: Pinched face, sunken eyes, cold and clammy extremities, low BP (systolic BP <100 mm Hg and narrow pulse pressure), tachycardia, low volume pulse, rapid and shallow respiration, and oliguria (urinary output <30 mL/h). Drowsiness, dizziness, irritability, confusion, stupor and coma. If persists for long time, multiple organ failure and death may occur.

Treatment (ABC):
- *A*: Airway should be kept clear
- *B*: Breathing should be maintained and oxygen inhalation
- *C*: Circulation, IV channel or central venous (CV) line
- *Position*: Supine or leg raised
- Replacement with blood, plasma or IV fluid (crystalloids such as normal saline, Ringer's lactate or colloids such as albumin, dextran, and haemaccel)
- Treatment of primary cause (bleeding, diarrhea, etc.).

Cardiogenic Shock

There is impairment of cardiac function due to myocardial damage. Its causes are acute myocardial infarction (MI), acute myocarditis, cardiac arrest, prolonged cardiac bypass surgery, dilated cardiomyopathy, dissecting aneurysm of ascending aorta, arrhythmia, acute valvular dysfunction [acute mitral regurgitation (MR) or aortic regurgitation (AR) and severe aortic stenosis (AS) or mitral stenosis (MS)], rupture of ventricular septum or wall, and ventricular aneurysm.

Signs: Features of primary disease (e.g. MI), raised jugular venous pressure (JVP), pulsus alternans, gallop rhythm [in left ventricular failure (LVF)], and bilateral basal crepitations (in pulmonary edema). Central venous pressure (CVP) and pulmonary artery occlusion pressure (PAOP) are increased.

Treatment: Treatment of primary cause and general measures of shock (as above).
- Ionotropic drugs (dopamine, dobutamine, dopexamine and enoximone)
- *Other therapy*: Diuretic. Vasodilator therapy to reduce afterload (captopril and enalapril). Mechanical support of myocardium (intra-aortic balloon counter pulsation).

Obstructive Shock

Heart is unable to contract due to mechanical obstruction compressing the heart. Its causes are cardiac tamponade, massive pulmonary embolism, and tension pneumothorax.

Signs: Features of primary disease (e.g. cardiac tamponade and tension pneumothorax) and raised JVP. Pulsus paradoxus, soft heart sounds (in cardiac tamponade), and Kussmaul's sign.

Treatment: General measures as above and treatment of primary cause (e.g. aspiration in cardiac tamponade).

Distributive Shock

There is severe peripheral vasodilation and increased capillary permeability, cardiac output may be normal or even high, but still inadequate perfusion.

Causes: Septic shock, anaphylactic shock, neurogenic shock, vasodilator drug toxicity, and endocrine (Addisonian crisis, thyrotoxic crisis, myxedema coma, and hypopituitarism).

Treatment: General measures of shock and treatment of primary cause.

Septic Shock

It is characterized by development of shock due to septicemia or endotoxin produced by different microorganisms. It may be associated with diabetes mellitus (DM), malignancy, immunosuppressive therapy, hepatobiliary, gastrointestinal tract (GIT), and gynecological and urinary abnormalities.

Causative organisms: Gram-negative (*Escherichia coli*, *Klebsiella*, *Proteus*, *Pseudomonas* and *Serratia*). Also, gram-positive organisms and *Bacteroides*.

Features: High fever with chill and rigor, warm periphery, high volume, bounding pulse, signs of DIC, and multiple organ failure. Other features of shock (as in hypovolemic shock).

Treatment: General management (ABC, see above)
- *Antibiotic*: Broad spectrum *plus* metronidazole
- *Other therapy*:
  - Blood transfusion if anemia, correction of electrolytes, calcium, magnesium and albumin
  - Respiratory support (if needed, mechanical ventilation)
  - Methylprednisolone 1 g with 200 cc 5% DA IV daily for 5 days.

Anaphylactic Shock

Anaphylaxis is a serious allergic reaction due to acute immunoglobulin E (IgE)-mediated immune reaction involving antigen, mast cell, and basophil.

Causes: Drugs (penicillin, cephalosporins, vancomycin, insulin, anti-snake venoms, and radiographic contrast media), blood transfusion, foods (fish, egg, milk, peanut, strawberry and soya product), insect bite (bee, wasp sting), and serum and vaccines (ATS and anti-rabies vaccine).

Clinical features:
- *General*: Local tingling, itching, urticaria, angioedema, flushing, warm periphery, edema of face, pharynx, and larynx
- *Respiratory*: Bronchospasm, dyspnea, wheeze and stridor due to laryngeal edema
- *Abdominal*: Nausea, vomiting, abdominal pain, and diarrhea
- *Cardiovascular*: Tachycardia, hypotension, arrhythmia, MI, collapse, and death.

Treatment: ABC as above. Position (supine or leg raised).
- *Intravenous fluid*: Normal saline or 5% DNS (dextrose normal saline)
- Intravenous hydrocortisone 100–200 mg and IV antihistamine (chlorphenamine 10–20 mg). Intramuscular (IM) adrenaline 0.5 mg may be given
- Intubation may be necessary, if hypoxia or hypotension is severe.

Prevention: Avoidance of allergen (food and drugs). Patient's education regarding use of adrenaline, hydrocortisone during emergency, maintains a *"Medic alert bracelet"* naming the culprit allergen. Desensitization in some case, where allergen is unavoidable.

Neurogenic Shock

It is caused by major brain or spinal cord injury, which disrupt brainstem and neurogenic vasomotor control. There is arteriolar and venous dilatation which causes pooling of blood in the venous system, decreased venous return and cardiac output, resulting in shock.

Clinical features: Same like other shock. Extremities are warm.

Treatment: General measures as in other shock. IV fluid to maintain normal circulation. Norepinephrine may be necessary to maintain increase vascular resistance. Treatment of primary cause.

PROXIMAL MYOPATHY

It means weakness of upper arm and thigh muscles. Patient complains of difficulty in raising the arm above the head, combing and standing from sitting.

Causes:
- Dermatomyositis or polymyositis
- Myasthenia gravis and myasthenic myopathic syndrome (Eaton–Lambert syndrome)
- Myopathy (limb girdle, facioscapulohumeral and mitochondrial) except myotonic dystrophy
- Cushing's syndrome, diabetic amyotrophy, thyrotoxicosis, hypothyroidism and hyperparathyroidism
- Polymyalgia rheumatica and osteomalacia
- Familial periodic paralysis
- Alcohol and drugs [steroid, chloroquine, amiodarone, lithium, and zidovudine (ZDV)]
- McArdle's syndrome (myophosphorylase deficiency, there is stiffness and cramps of muscle after exercise, which is hard and painful on movement).

WEGENER'S GRANULOMATOSIS (GRANULOMATOSIS WITH POLYANGIITIS)

It is a disorder of unknown etiology characterized by necrotizing granulomatous vasculitis of upper and lower respiratory tract with glomerulonephritis (focal, segmental and necrotizing).

Clinical features: Affects both male and female.
- *Nasal*: Discharge, epistaxis, nasal obstruction, nasal crust, rhinitis and sinusitis. If untreated, destruction of nasal bone and cartilage causes depressed nose and deafness due to inner ear involvement
- *Respiratory*: Cough, hemoptysis, chest pain and breathlessness
- *Eye*: Conjunctivitis, episcleritis, iritis, proptosis, diplopia and loss of vision
- *Renal*: Features of glomerulonephritis or renal failure.

Investigations:
- Complete blood count (CBC), erythrocyte sedimentation rate (ESR) (leukocytosis with very high ESR), and C-reactive protein (CRP) (high)
- Urine routine microscopic examination (RME)
- Serum urea, creatinine and electrolytes. Serum complement (normal or slightly high)
- Chest X-ray (shows single or multiple nodules and migrating lung lesion in 50% cases)
- Magnetic resonance imaging (MRI) of chest may be done
- Biopsy from nasal lesions and kidney (shows necrotizing vasculitis with granuloma formation)
- Cytoplasmic antineutrophil cytoplasmic antibodies (c-ANCA): Positive (helpful for diagnosis and to see the relapse).

Treatment:
- Intravenous methylprednisolone 0.5–1 g for 3 days, then oral prednisolone (0.5 mg/kg) and IV cyclophosphamide (0.5–1 g every 2 weeks for 3 months). Once remission occurs (takes 3–6 months), maintenance therapy with low dose prednisolone and azathioprine, methotrexate (MTX) or mycophenolate mofetil
- Or, oral cyclophosphamide (2 mg/kg) *plus* prednisolone (1 mg/kg)
- Rituximab in combination with high dose steroid is equally effective
- Plasmapheresis should be considered for fulminant lung disease
- Oral co-trimoxazole (960 mg, three times weekly) is given to prevent pneumocystis pneumonia
- Regular follow-up should be done to check for recurrence. Measurements of ESR, CRP and c-ANCA should be done.

TAKAYASU'S DISEASE

It is a chronic, inflammatory, granulomatous panarteritis of unknown cause involving the elastic arteries commonly aorta and its major branches, carotid, ulnar, brachial, radial and axillary. Occasionally, may involve pulmonary artery, rarely abdominal aorta, and renal artery. It is also called pulseless disease or aortic arch syndrome. There are four types:
1. *Type 1*: Involves aortic arch and its major branches
2. *Type 2*: Involves descending aorta and abdominal aorta
3. *Type 3*: Involves both type 1 and type 2. This may be complicated by AR
4. *Type 4*: Involves the pulmonary arteries.

Clinical features: Common in young female, 25–30 years (F:M ratio is 8:1), more in Asians.
- *In acute stage*: May present with fever, malaise, weight loss, arthralgia, myalgia and high ESR
- *In chronic case*: Dizziness, giddiness, headache, blurring of vision, syncope, and claudication in the upper limb
- May be features of AR, renal artery stenosis or anginal pain, and hypertension.

Signs: All pulses of upper limbs are absent, but present in lower limbs (called reverse coarctation syndrome). BP is undetectable in upper limb and normal or high in lower limb. Carotid bruit may be present, also renal bruit. Signs of AR may be present. There may be less development of upper part of the body. Fundoscopy shows wreath-like anastomosis around the optic disk.

Investigations:
- Complete blood count (high ESR and normocytic normochromic anemia) and CRP (high)
- Chest X-ray shows cardiomegaly and widening of aorta
- *Magnetic resonance imaging*: Helpful to detect inflammatory thickening of the affected vessel walls
- *Computed tomography (CT) angiography*: Helpful to detect stenosis, occlusion, and condition of arteries
- Aortography of aortic arch and its branches (shows narrowing, coarctation, and aneurysmal dilatation)
- *Serum immunoglobulin*: High.

Treatment:
- Prednisolone 40–60 mg daily or 1–2 mg/kg
- *If difficult to taper steroid, or in refractory case*: MTX 25 mg per week may be given with prednisolone. *Or*, MTX, mycophenolate mofetil or azathioprine may be added with prednisolone, which is more effective than prednisolone alone
- Cyclophosphamide may be used in resistant case
- Anti-TNF (tumor necrosis factor) agents such as etanercept and infliximab may be given in relapse
- Reconstructive vascular surgery in selected case
- Angioplasty and stenting or bypass surgery may be done, if vascular complication
- Treatment of hypertension.

Complications: Heart failure, stroke, seizure, organ failure, retinopathy and renovascular hypertension.

GIANT CELL ARTERITIS OR TEMPORAL ARTERITIS

It is an inflammatory granulomatous arteritis of unknown cause involving large arteries, predominantly affecting temporal and ophthalmic artery. Common in female (F:M = 4:1), 60–75 years of age. It may be associated with polymyalgia rheumatica.

Clinical features:
- Headache, mostly on temporal and occipital region with local tenderness. Pain in face, jaw and mouth
- Temporal artery is thick, hard, tortuous and tender. Jaw claudication and worse on eating

- Sudden painless temporary or permanent loss of vision in one eye. Rarely transient ischemic attack (TIA), brainstem infarct, and hemiparesis may occur
- Systemic features such as severe malaise, tiredness, weakness, weight loss, arthralgia, myalgia and fever. Pyrexia of unknown origin (PUO) may be the only feature and common in elderly
- Fundoscopy shows optic disc is pale and swollen with hemorrhage.

Investigations:
- Complete blood count, ESR (normocytic normochromic anemia, very high ESR), and CRP (high)
- *Antinuclear antibodies (ANA) and ANCA*: Negative
- Temporal artery biopsy should be done
- Ultrasound of the temporal arteries and ^{19}fluorodeoxyglucose positron emission tomography (PET) scan may be done.

Treatment:
- Prednisolone 60–100 mg/day for 1–2 months, then taper slowly, continued for long time
- Low dose aspirin
- Monitoring ESR and CRP (markers of disease activity)
- If relapse, MTX or azathioprine may be added.

Polymyalgia Rheumatica

It is characterized by severe pain and stiffness of the muscles of shoulders, neck, hips, lower back and thigh, in limb girdle pattern, occurs alone or with giant cell arteritis (GCA).

Clinical features: Common in middle age above the age of 50 years, more in women.
- Pain and stiffness, worse in the morning, lasting from 30 minutes to several hours. The patient complains of difficulty in combing the hair and raising from sitting. General features like tiredness, fever, weight loss, depression and occasionally nocturnal sweating
- On examination, stiffness and painful restriction of active shoulder movement, but passive movements are preserved. Muscles may be tender, but weakness and muscle wasting are absent.

Investigations: Diagnosis is clinical.
- *Complete blood count and ESR*: Shows anemia (mild normochromic and normocytic). High ESR and CRP are the hallmark
- Serum alkaline phosphatase and gamma-GT may be high in acute inflammation
- Temporal artery biopsy shows GCA in 10–30%.

Treatment: Prednisolone, 15–30 mg/day. Dose should be tapered when symptoms improve, 10–15 mg for 8 weeks. Then maintenance of 5–7.5 mg daily and continued for 12–24 months. MTX or azathioprine may be given. Prophylaxis against osteoporosis should be given in patients with low bone mineral density (BMD).

POLYARTERITIS NODOSA

It is a multisystem necrotizing vasculitis involving medium and small vessels accompanied by severe systemic manifestations. Occasionally, associated with hepatitis B antigenemia. Usually in middle age, 40–50 years, more in male, and the M:F is 2:1.

Clinical features:
- *General features*: Fever, malaise, weakness, weight loss, headache and myalgia
- *Neurological*: Peripheral neuropathy, mononeuritis multiplex, cardiovascular disease (CVD), and seizure may occur
- *Gastrointestinal tract*: Abdominal pain, nausea, vomiting, cholecystitis, pancreatitis or appendicitis, gastrointestinal (GI) bleeding
- *Renal*: Severe hypertension and renal impairment. May be hematuria and proteinuria
- *Cardiac*: Coronary arteritis causes MI and heart failure. Pericarditis also occurs
- *Skin*: Rash, palpable purpura, nodule, ulceration, infarction, livedo reticularis, subcutaneous hemorrhage, and gangrene
- Raynaud's phenomenon may be present
- *Musculoskeletal*: Arthritis, arthralgia and myalgia
- *Lung*: Involvement is rare.

Investigations:
- Complete blood count and ESR (shows anemia, neutrophilic leukocytosis, and high ESR)
- *Hepatitis B surface antigen (HBsAg)*: Positive in 10–30% cases
- Biopsy of muscle or sural nerve or from an affected organ (shows features of vasculitis)
- Angiography (to see microaneurysms in hepatic, intestinal or renal vessels, if necessary)
- *Others*: Electrocardiogram (ECG) and abdominal ultrasound, if needed.

Treatment: Prednisolone 1 mg/kg body weight with cyclophosphamide 2 mg/kg for 6–12 months. Maintenance with azathioprine or MTX.

MICROSCOPIC POLYANGIITIS

It is characterized by necrotizing vasculitis with few or no immune complex affecting small vessels such as capillaries, arterioles and venules. It is common in elderly, above the age of 57 years, more in female.

Clinical features: General features such as fever, weight loss, arthralgia and myalgia.
- *Renal*: Rapidly progressive glomerulonephritis (RPGN) causing renal failure
- *Pulmonary*: Hemoptysis, cough, breathlessness and pleural effusions (15%)
- *Cutaneous*: Palpable purpura, skin rash, nodule and ulceration
- *Gastrointestinal*: Abdominal pain, nausea, vomiting and diarrhea
- *Neurological*: Peripheral neuropathy and mononeuritis multiplex.

Investigations:
- Complete blood count, ESR (shows high ESR, anemia, leukocytosis and thrombocytosis)
- Perinuclear antineutrophil cytoplasmic antibodies (p-ANCA) (positive in 75%)
- *Chest X-ray*: May be normal and infiltration due to hemorrhage
- *Kidney biopsy*: Shows necrotizing arteritis.

Treatment: Prednisolone 1 mg/kg *plus* cyclophosphamide 2 mg/kg for 3–6 months, then maintenance with azathioprine or MTX.

CHURG–STRAUSS SYNDROME (ALLERGIC ANGIITIS OR GRANULOMATOSIS)

It is a small and medium vessel necrotizing granulomatous vasculitis characterized by cutaneous vasculitic lesions, respiratory involvement, and asthmatic symptoms with eosinophilia [which are less in polyarteritis nodosa (PAN)]. It is common in males, in fourth decade. Triad of asthma, eosinophilia and positive p-ANCA strongly suggest Churg–Strauss syndrome.

Clinical features:
- Nasal polyp, allergic rhinitis, and adult onset asthma usually occur before vasculitis by many years. Pulmonary infiltrate and eosinophilia are the main features
- Fever, arthralgia, myalgia and weight loss. Skin rash and tender nodules
- Mononeuritis or polyneuropathy
- Gastrointestinal and cardiac involvement and hypertension may occur
- Glomerulonephritis (rare).

Investigations:
- Complete blood count with ESR (eosinophilia is common)
- Chest X-ray (shows transient patchy pneumonia like shadow)
- Perinuclear antineutrophil cytoplasmic antibodies (usually positive) and c-ANCA (negative, done to exclude Wegener's granulomatosis)
- Kidney biopsy, lung or calf muscle biopsy may be done
- Antinuclear antibodies and anti-double-stranded deoxyribonucleic acid (anti-dsDNA) [to exclude systemic lupus erythematosus (SLE)].

Treatment: High dose prednisolone and cyclophosphamide. Then maintenance therapy with low dose prednisolone and azathioprine, MTX and mycophenolate mofetil. Major life-threatening organ involvement may require treatment with pulse IV methylprednisolone.

BEHÇET'S SYNDROME

It is a vasculitis of unknown cause, characterized by recurrent oral, genital ulcer, ocular and skin lesion. It may be joint and neurological lesion. It mainly involves small arteries and venules. Common in male.

Clinical features: Oral and genital ulcers are present in most patients.
- Recurrent oral ulceration, deep and multiple, and genital ulcers
- *Skin*: Erythema nodosum, diffuse pustular rash, and erythema multiforme
- *Ocular*: Recurrent uveitis, iridocyclitis, retinal vascular lesions, optic atrophy, and can cause loss of vision in 50%
- Recurrent thrombophlebitis may occur, leading to venous thrombosis. Less often, superior or inferior vena cava thrombosis, abdominal pain, and bloody diarrhea may occur
- Seronegative arthritis, involving knees, ankles and wrists
- Asymptomatic proteinuria is a recognized feature, but rarely may cause renal amyloidosis
- Neurological complications occur in 5% cases. Organic confusional state, meningoencephalitis, transient or persistent brainstem syndromes.

Investigations: No specific investigations. Pathergy test is a useful diagnostic sign. It is demonstrated by pricking the skin by needle, there is pustule formation at venipuncture site within 24–48 hours.

Criteria for diagnosis: It is a clinical diagnosis. No specific test is required.
- Recurrent oral ulcers, at least three times in 12 months
- *Plus two of the following*:
  - Recurrent genital ulceration
  - Eye lesion
  - Skin lesion
  - Positive pathergy test.

Treatment:
- *For oral ulcer and genital ulcer*: Topical steroid. Thalidomide 100–300 mg/day for 28 days is effective in resistant oral and genital ulcer
- Colchicine is effective in erythema nodosum and arthralgia
- Systemic steroid, immunosuppressive agent or cyclosporine are used for uveitis and neurological disease
- Anti-TNF agent can be used in severe uveitis, neurological, and gastrointestinal manifestations.

GOODPASTURE SYNDROME

It is a clinical syndrome of glomerulonephritis and pulmonary hemorrhage mediated by anti-GBM (glomerular basement membrane) antibody, usually IgG type which binds with glomerular or alveolar basement membrane. More in males, 20–40 years, exclusively in smokers. Females are affected more after the age of 60 years.

Clinical features:
- Initially upper respiratory tract infection (cough, recurrent hemoptysis, and dyspnea)
- Then renal involvement (proteinuria and hematuria) due to progressive, proliferative glomerulonephritis or features of renal failure
- In one-third cases, no lung injury and only glomerulonephritis is present
- Systemic features like fever, malaise, arthritis, headache and weight loss are not common, but may occur. Hypertension is usually not a feature. Chest pain and pleurisy are also rare.

Investigations:
- Complete blood count
- Chest X-ray (shows blotchy opacities due to lung hemorrhage)
- Ultrasonography (USG) of abdomen to see KUB (kidney, ureter and bladder)
- Anti-GBM antibody is positive (usually IgG) and p-ANCA (positive in 30% cases)
- Antinuclear antibodies (negative) and complements (normal)
- Lung function test. Restrictive lung disease may occur in advanced stage
- In sputum (hemosiderin-laden macrophage may be present)
- Kidney biopsy (shows proliferative or crescentic glomerulonephritis).

Treatment:
- *Plasmapheresis*: To remove circulating antibodies
- Methylprednisolone IV, 1–2 g/day for 3 days
- Cyclophosphamide 2–3 mg/kg/day may be given

- Occasionally, kidney transplantation may be done. Recurrence may occur in transplanted kidney.

RESTLESS LEG SYNDROME (ALSO CALLED EKBOM SYNDROME)

It is a neuromuscular abnormality, characterized by discomfort or abnormal sensation in the calf or feet requiring irresistible and frequent movement of affected limb. When associated with iron deficiency anemia and chronic kidney disease (CKD), it is called secondary restless leg syndrome (RLS). It is common in normal population (1–5%), in middle age. But frequency increases up to 20–30% after 60 years. It may be familial in one-third cases, multiple members in family may be affected, occasionally inherited as autosomal dominant.

Clinical features: It is worse in the evening or at the onset of sleep at night, interfering with sleep. It commonly involves lower limbs, may also involve upper limbs. It is exaggerated by pregnancy, inactivity, caffeine and sleep disturbance.

Treatment: Clonazepam (0.5–2 mg), levodopa (100–200 mg), and dopamine agonist (pramipexole or ropinirole). Narcotics, benzodiazepine and anticonvulsant may be helpful. Treatment of primary cause such as CKD.

HELLP SYNDROME (OR HELP SYNDROME)

It occurs in a patient with pre-eclampsia. It stands for:
- *H*—hemolysis
- *EL*—elevated liver enzymes
- *LP*—low platelet

The HELLP syndrome is a variant of pre-eclampsia, affects 1 in 1,000 pregnancies, common in multiparous women, in last trimester of pregnancy or within the first week of delivery. Perinatal mortality is 10–60% and maternal mortality is 1.5–5%. In 15% cases, BP may be normal and proteinuria may be absent (liver disease is associated with hypertension, proteinuria and fluid retention. Serum transaminases are high. Hepatic infarction and rupture may occur).

Investigations:
- *Complete blood count*: Low platelet, increased reticulocyte count
- *Liver function test (LFT)* [serum glutamate-pyruvate transaminase (SGPT) and serum glutamic-oxaloacetic transaminase (SGOT)]: High
- *Urine RME*: Proteinuria
- Ultrasonography of hepatobiliary system
- *Others*: Blood sugar, electrolytes, calcium, magnesium and prothrombin time (PT).

Treatment: Prompt delivery is indicated in pregnancy ≥34 weeks of gestation or maternal disease (multiorgan dysfunction, DIC, liver infarction or hemorrhage, renal failure, and abruptio placentae).

In <34 weeks, IV dexamethasone may be given. Other therapies:
- Control of hypertension
- Platelet and blood transfusion may be necessary
- *If convulsion*: Magnesium sulfate intravenously
- *In severe renal failure*: Dialysis may be necessary.

Complications:
- *Maternal*: DIC, abruptio placentae, acute renal failure, pulmonary edema, subcapsular liver hematoma, and retinal detachment
- *Fetus/neonate*: Prematurity, intrauterine growth retardation, sequelae of abruptio placentae, and perinatal mortality.

HEREDITARY HEMORRHAGIC TELANGIECTASIA (OSLER–WEBER–RENDU DISEASE)

It is inherited as an autosomal dominant, characterized by multiple telangiectasia in skin and mucous membrane in different parts of the body.

Symptoms:
- Epistaxis (common), usually recurrent and sometimes the only feature
- Gastrointestinal tract bleeding (hematemesis and melena) and bleeding from other sites
- Pulmonary arteriovenous fistula may develop causing hemoptysis, cyanosis, and clubbing
- Anemia (due to chronic blood loss, especially from GIT)
- Paradoxical embolism, stroke and cerebral abscess may occur.

Signs: Telangiectasia (localized collection of multiple noncontractile capillaries, found in lip, face, under the surface of tongue, buccal mucosa, nasal mucosa, nail bed, palm, feet and GIT).

Treatment: Continuous iron therapy. If frequent epistaxis, estrogen therapy is used. Antifibrinolytic agent, aminocaproic acid, may be given. Laser therapy may be used for cutaneous and mucosal lesions.

DROWNING

It is defined as death due to asphyxia following immersion in water. In some cases, no water enters into the lungs and death occurs due to severe laryngospasm, which is called "dry drowning".

"Near drowning" is defined as survival for longer than 24 hours after suffocation by immersion.

After drowning, the victim becomes unconscious and does not breathe unless there is rescue.

Pathogenesis: After drowning, there is rapid ventilation-perfusion imbalance with hypoxemia and development of severe pulmonary edema. As fresh water is hypotonic, it is rapidly absorbed across the alveolar membrane, impairs surfactant function that leads to alveolar collapse. Absorption of large amount of hypotonic fluid results in hemolysis. In saltwater drowning, there is alveolar edema, as salt water is hypertonic.

Clinical features: Hypoxemia, metabolic acidosis, lung injury, and acute respiratory distress syndrome (ARDS).

Complications: Dehydration, hypotension, hemoptysis, rhabdomyolysis, renal failure, arrhythmia and death.

Management:
- *Prehospital management*: Person should be taken out from water. Mouth should be cleaned, mouth-to-mouth breathing. If not breathing, CPR should be started (two breaths followed by 30 chest compressions).

This cycle is continued until the person starts breathing or emergency help arrives
- *Hospital management*: Oxygen inhalation, maintenance of water and electrolyte balance, adequate nutrition, and hydration. If no spontaneous breathing, endotracheal intubation should be done. Antibiotic, if infection.

HEAT-RELATED ILLNESS

Exposure to excessive heat may cause heat cramps, heat syncope, heat exhaustion, and heat stroke.

Heat Stroke

It occurs when body temperature is >40°C on exposure to high atmospheric temperature. There is failure of thermoregulation.

Clinical features: High body temperature with no sweating and red, hot and dry skin. Nausea, vomiting and throbbing headache. Rapid and shallow breathing. Muscle weakness or cramps, tachycardia, dizziness, confusion, disorientation, seizure and unconsciousness.

Complications: Hypovolemic shock, lactic acidosis, DIC, rhabdomyolysis, hepatic and renal failure, pulmonary edema, and cerebral edema.

Investigations: Diagnosis is clinical. Investigations are done to see the effect: CBC, blood sugar, serum electrolytes, liver and renal function tests, creatine phosphokinase (CPK) (high), coagulation screening (for DIC), and chest X-ray.

Treatment: The patient is transferred to cool environment and clothing is removed, and O_2 inhalation.
- Body should be cooled by spraying cold water, fanning, if possible, with air cooler or conditioner. Ice packs in axilla, neck and groin may be used
- Intravenous infusion to correct hypotension and dehydration
- Benzodiazepine to prevent shivering
- If patient is unconscious, immediately transfer to hospital.

ALCOHOLISM

Alcohol becomes harmful when taken more than 21 units in men and 14 units in women weekly. There may be social, psychological and physical problems with excessive use of alcohol.

Features of acute alcohol intoxication: Emotional and behavioral disturbance, hypoglycemia, aspiration of vomitus, respiratory depression, accidents, and injuries.

Complications of chronic alcohol misuse:
- *Social problems*: Disturbance of work, unemployment, marital disharmony, child abuse, financial difficulties, violence and traffic offences
- *Psychological*: Depression, anxiety, attempted and completed suicide, and auditory hallucination. Alcohol withdrawal symptoms appear 1–3 days after the last drink and may cause seizures. Delirium tremens (associated with severe alcohol withdrawal)

- *Physical*: Involves multiple systems of the body.
  - Neurological: Peripheral neuropathy, cerebellar degeneration, cerebral hemorrhage, and dementia
  - Hepatic: Fatty liver, alcoholic hepatitis, cirrhosis and liver cancer
  - Gastrointestinal tract: Esophagitis, gastritis, pancreatitis, esophageal cancer, and Mallory–Weiss syndrome
  - Respiratory: Pulmonary tuberculosis (TB), pneumonia and other chest infections
  - Skin: Spider naevi, palmar erythema, Dupuytren's contracture, and telangiectasia
  - Cardiac: Cardiomyopathy, arrhythmia and hypertension
  - Hematological: Macrocytosis
  - Musculoskeletal: Myopathy, osteopenia and fracture
  - Endocrine and metabolic: Pseudo-Cushing's syndrome, hypoglycemia and gout
  - Reproductive: Hypogonadism, fetal alcohol syndrome, and infertility
  - Wernicke's encephalopathy: Nystagmus, ophthalmoplegia, ataxia and confusion
  - Korsakoff syndrome: Short-term memory deficit and confabulation.

Clinical features of alcohol withdrawal:
- Restlessness, anxiety and panic attack
- Tachycardia, sweating and pupil dilatation
- Nausea and vomiting. Delusion, convulsion and delirium tremens (agitation, hallucinations and illusions).

Treatment of chronic alcoholism:
- Counseling regarding the harmful effects and safe level of alcohol consumption, and psychotherapy
- Maintenance of balanced diet with vitamins, especially thiamine
- Disulfiram may be used.

DELIRIUM TREMENS

It is a severe alcohol withdrawal syndrome characterized by restlessness, agitation, insomnia, hallucination, illusion, delusion and tremor. Its signs are sweating, tachycardia, tachypnea and pyrexia. It has a significant mortality and morbidity. Its features usually occur 1–3 days after withdrawal.

Treatment: Hospitalization of patient.
- Correction of electrolyte abnormalities and dehydration and control of infection, if any
- Parenteral thiamine slowly (250 mg daily for 3–5 days). If Wernicke–Korsakoff encephalopathy, thiamine slowly (500 mg daily for 3–5 days)
- Prophylactic phenytoin or carbamazepine, if there is a previous history of withdrawal fits.

Specific drug treatment: Diazepam 10–20 mg or chlordiazepoxide 30–60 mg. Repeat 1 hour after the last dose, depending on response.

Then, fixed-schedule regimens:
- Diazepam 10 mg every 6 hours for four doses, then 5 mg 6-hourly for eight doses
- Chlordiazepoxide 30 mg every 6 hours for four doses, then 15 mg 6-hourly for eight doses

- Additional benzodiazepine when symptoms and signs are not controlled.

WERNICKE ENCEPHALOPATHY

It is the acute cerebral manifestation of vitamin B1 deficiency, commonly in heavy drinking of alcohol for long time and inadequate diet. It occurs after repeated vomiting, alcoholism, prolonged starvation or diarrhea.

Site of lesion: In brainstem (causing ophthalmoplegia, nystagmus and ataxia), superior vermis of cerebellum (causing ataxia) and dorsomedial nucleus in thalamus and adjacent area of gray matter (causing amnesia).

Clinical features:
- *Cognitive changes*: Acute confusion, disorientation, drowsiness or altered consciousness
- *Eye changes*: Bilateral symmetrical ophthalmoplegia, bilateral or unilateral paralysis of lateral conjugate gaze, horizontal or vertical nystagmus, and abnormal pupillary reflex. Rarely ptosis, meiosis and unreactive pupil
- *Gait ataxia*: Broad-based gait, cerebellar sign, and vestibular paralysis
- When associated with memory disturbance and confabulation, it is called Korsakoff's psychosis. Loss of recent memory is common, but past memory may be normal.

Note: Following points are important—
- Confabulation means falsification of memory with clear consciousness. The patient makes several new stories unrelated to the truth
- *In alcoholic*: If repeated vomiting is associated with confusion, drowsiness with eye abnormality, Wernicke encephalopathy should be suspected.

Diagnosis: Mainly clinical. CT scan (normal). Cerebrospinal fluid (CSF) is also normal, but slight rise of protein may occur.

Treatment: Injection vitamin B1, 500 mg IV over 30 minutes 8 hourly for 2 days, then 500 mg IV or IM daily for 5 days. Then oral B1 100 mg 8 hourly and other B complex vitamins. If promptly treated, it is reversible. Correction of dehydration and electrolyte imbalance.

ADULT STILL'S DISEASE

It is a disease of unknown cause, characterized by high fever, seronegative arthritis, skin rash, and polyserositis. It is usually diagnosed by exclusion of other diseases.

Clinical features: Common in young adult, 16–35 years of age, rare after 60 years.

Diagnostic criteria of Adult Still's disease: Five or more criteria including two or more majors with exclusion criteria.

Major criteria:
- Quotidian fever >39°C, lasting 1 week or longer
- Arthralgia or arthritis, lasting 2 weeks or longer (knee, wrist and ankle)
- Typical rash (evanescent macular, maculopapular, salmon-colored, non-pruritic, common in chest, and abdomen)
- Leukocytosis >10,000/mm^3 with >80% neutrophil (leukocytosis may be very high, >40,000).

Minor criteria:
- Sore throat
- Recent development of significant lymphadenopathy (usually cervical, may be generalized)
- Hepatomegaly or splenomegaly
- Abnormal LFTs
- Antinuclear antibodies and rheumatoid arthritis (RA) are negative.

Exclusion criteria: Infection, malignancy and other rheumatic disease.

Investigation:
- *Complete blood count and ESR*: Leukocytosis (may be very high) and high ESR
- *Serum ferritin*: Very high
- Liver function test (may be high SGPT and SGOT)
- X-ray of chest (may be pleural effusion and cardiomegaly due to pericardial effusion)
- Ultrasonography of whole abdomen (may be ascites, hepatosplenomegaly and lymphadenopathy).

Treatment:
- *For pain and fever*: Nonsteroidal anti-inflammatory drug (NSAID) (high dose aspirin 1 g 8-hourly). Other NSAID, indomethacin and ibuprofen, may be helpful
- *If no response*: High dose prednisolone (60–100 mg/day). When fever subsides, dose is tapered slowly
- *Other drugs*: Chloroquine, hydroxychloroquine, MTX, sulfasalazine, azathioprine and cyclophosphamide
- *In chronic or resistant case*: TNF antagonists such as etanercept or interleukin-1 receptor antagonist such as anakinra or interleukin-6 receptor antagonist such as tocilizumab may be given.

RHABDOMYOLYSIS

It is defined as acute muscle destruction associated with high myoglobinemia and myoglobinuria.

Causes: Trauma (crush injury), vigorous exercise, convulsion or epilepsy, electrocution, hypothermia, heat stroke, alcoholism, polymyositis, neuroleptic malignant syndrome, burn, septicemia, infection (influenzae and Legionnaire's disease), and ecstasy or amphetamine abuse.

Rhabdomyolysis is associated with high aspartate transaminase (AST), CPK, creatinine, potassium, phosphate and uric acid. Calcium is low, because free calcium is bound by myoglobin.

Rhabdomyolysis and Renal Failure

Muscle injury due to any cause followed by acute renal failure is highly suggestive of rhabdomyolysis. Myoglobin is highly toxic to renal tubules and precipitates renal failure. Urine is red, but no red blood cells (RBCs).

Investigations: Urine for ammonium sulfate test and spectroscopic examination of urine to detect myoglobin.

Treatment: Adequate hydration and alkalinization of urine to reduce precipitation of myoglobin in renal tubules. Dialysis, if renal failure.

Loop diuretic should be avoided, as it may cause acidic urinary pH and aggravating renal failure.

TOXIC SHOCK SYNDROME

It is characterized by high fever, hypotension, diffuse macular rash, and desquamation of palms and soles with widespread multiorgan involvement caused by toxic shock syndrome toxin 1 by *Staphylococcus aureus* or enterotoxin secreted by *Streptococcus pyogens*.

Cause: Toxic shock syndrome toxin-1 in menstruating women and enterotoxin in nonmenstruating.

Source of infection: In *S. aureus* infection, usually from tampons used during menstruation, also infection in nasopharynx, rectum, wound and abscess. In *Streptococcus* β hemolyticus, due to soft tissue infection such as necrotizing fasciitis, myositis or cellulitis or secondary to pneumonia, osteomyelitis or peritonitis.

Clinical feature: In menstruating women, onset begins 2–3 days after menstruation.
- High fever >39°C. Hypotension (systolic BP <90 mm Hg or postural diastolic drop)
- Widespread erythematous macular skin rash
- *Multiple organ involvement*:
    - Gastrointestinal tract: Vomiting or diarrhea, and abdominal pain
    - Mucosal involvement: Oropharyngeal, vaginal and conjunctival
    - Muscular: Myalgia (high CPK)
    - Central nervous system (CNS): Drowsiness, confusion, disorientation, alteration in consciousness, and no focal neurological sign
    - Skin: Desquamation of palms and soles during recovery
    - Hepatic: High bilirubin, SGPT and low albumin
    - Hematological: Thrombocytopenia <100,000/mm^3 and DIC
    - Renal: High urea and creatinine.

Investigations:
- *Complete blood count and ESR*: Shows leukocytosis with thrombocytopenia
- *Blood for culture/sensitivity (C/S)*: Usually negative
- High endocervical swab for C/S
- *Disseminated intravascular coagulation screening*: PT, activated partial thromboplastin time (APTT), D-dimer, fibrin degradation products (FDP)
- *Liver function test*: High bilirubin, SGPT, SGOT and albumin (low)
- *Renal*: Urea and creatinine (high)
- *Others*: Serum electrolytes, blood sugar, chest X-ray, and USG of whole abdomen.

Treatment:
- Intravenous fluid, correction of water and electrolyte balance, and nutritional support. Inotropic support, if needed. Surgical debridement, if needed
- Broad-spectrum antibiotic (for *S. aureus*, flucloxacillin or vancomycin *plus* clindamycin. Linezolid may be given. For *S. pyogenes*, Penicillin G 2–4 g IV 4-hourly *plus* clindamycin 600–900 mg IV 8-hourly *plus* Ig 2 g/kg single dose).

PICKWICKIAN SYNDROME

It is also called obesity hypoventilation syndrome, characterized by gross obesity associated with failure to breathe properly enough resulting in hypoxemia and hypercapnia. Most patients suffer from obstructive sleep apnea syndrome.

Clinical features: Gross obesity. Sleep disturbance or sleep apnea, daytime sleepiness, and snoring. Airway obstruction may be present. Features of polycythemia. Respiratory failure (reduced respiratory drive. Usually $PaCO_2$ is normal, but may be high). Serum leptin (high).

Treatment: Weight reduction. Smoking should be stopped. Respiratory stimulants such as theophylline, acetazolamide and medroxyprogesterone may be given. Continuous positive airway pressure (CPAP) or bilevel positive airway pressure (BiPAP) may be used for sleep apnea.

Complications: Pulmonary hypertension, cor pulmonale, sleep apnea syndrome, secondary polycythemia, and type II respiratory failure due to alveolar hypoventilation.

HEREDITARY ANGIOEDEMA

It is inherited as autosomal dominant, due to deficiency or inactivity of C1 esterase inhibitor (C1-INH), a component of complement system. As a result, there is uncontrolled activation of C1 with increased local bradykinin concentration giving rise to pain and swelling. Common in late childhood or early adolescence.

Clinical features: Angioedema in face, extremities, GIT and upper airways. Recurrent acute abdomen and laryngeal obstruction. No urticaria, no allergy, and no itching.

Attack may be spontaneous or triggered by trauma, infection, dental procedures or emotional stress. Usually, family history is present. Patient can present with combination of cutaneous angioedema, abdominal pain or acute airway obstruction.

Investigations:
- *During acute attack*: Serum C4 is low
- Confirmed by measurement of serum C1-INH.

Treatment:
- *During acute attack*: Purified C1-INH infusion. Bradykinin receptor antagonist (icatibant) or plasma kallikrein inhibitor (ecallantide) may be used. Fresh frozen plasma may be used. Steroid and adrenaline are ineffective
- *For prevention*: Danazol or stanozolol may be given, which increase C1-INH, C2 and C4 by hepatic synthesis. However, these should be avoided in children. Screening of the family members.

FAMILIAL PERIODIC PARALYSIS

It is inherited as autosomal dominant, characterized by episodic extreme weakness which progresses from proximal to distal due to low potassium. Cranial and respiratory muscles are spared. There are three types:
1. *Hypokalemic*: Lasts for days. It is the common type, called hypokalemic periodic paralysis

2. *Hyperkalemic*: Lasts for hours (myotonia of tongue, eye may occur, common in <10 years of age)
3. *Normokalemic*: Rare.

Cause: Unknown, there is shift of potassium from extracellular fluid to intracellular fluid. It may be confused with thyrotoxic periodic paralysis (TPP).

Clinical features: Patient feels weakness with activity, which usually occurs periodically after some precipitating factors. Usually occurs during rest after prolonged exercise, and also while the patient is asleep.

Precipitating factors: High carbohydrate meal, cold, rest after exercise, alcohol, anxiety or tension.

Treatment:
- *During acute attack*: Potassium with normal saline infusion (potassium is never given directly intravenously)
- Long-term treatment with potassium supplement. Potassium sparing diuretic (spironolactone) is given. Acetazolamide may be helpful to prevent attack.

HYPERKALEMIC PERIODIC PARALYSIS

It is inherited as autosomal dominant characterized by severe weakness, usually after exercise. It starts in childhood and remits after the age of 20 years. Attack persists for 30–120 minutes. Myotonia of tongue and eye may occur.

Treatment: The IV calcium gluconate during acute attack. Acetazolamide or thiazide diuretic may be helpful.

THYROTOXIC PERIODIC PARALYSIS

If a thyrotoxic patient develops sudden or periodic weakness, it is called thyrotoxic periodic paralysis. It is due to hypokalemia (caused by entry of potassium into the cell), common in Asians. It may occur following excess carbohydrate or glucose or heavy exercise. It persists up to 7–72 hours. Treatment of thyrotoxicosis improves the condition.

CARCINOID SYNDROME

It is characterized by systemic symptoms that occur when secretory products released from carcinoid tumor enter into systemic circulation. Secretory products are serotonin or 5-hydroxytryptamine (5-HT), bradykinin, histamine, tachykinin and prostaglandin.

Sites: Carcinoid tumor is derived from enterochromaffin cells, 90% found in GIT (common in ileum, also appendix and rectum) and 10% in lung. In appendix, it is usually benign and presents as appendicitis (10%).

Clinical features: Asymptomatic, until metastasis. Only 5% develop carcinoid syndrome, when metastasis to the liver. Features are:
- Recurrent attack of bluish red flushing mainly on the face and neck, and wheezing. Flushing is the hallmark
- Abdominal pain, recurrent diarrhea, and vomiting. Pellagra and photosensitive dermatitis may occur
- There may be hypotension, bradycardia and facial edema

- Cardiac abnormalities are found in 50% cases, usually right sided. Tricuspid regurgitation and pulmonary stenosis. Left-sided cardiac valves are not affected, but bronchial carcinoid causes left-sided valvular lesion
- Hepatomegaly, which is firm and irregular due to metastasis.

Investigations:
- The 24 hours urine for 5-HIAA (5-hydroxyindoleacetic acid)
- Ultrasonography of abdomen (to see hepatic metastasis). CT scan may be done
- Color Doppler echocardiography to see cardiac lesion
- *Serum chromogranin A*: High.

Treatment:
- Surgery or embolization for solitary liver metastasis or bronchial carcinoid
- Octreotide or lanreotide improves the syndrome in 90%. Long-acting octreotide sometimes inhibits tumor growth
- Interferon and chemotherapy may be used which reduces tumor growth, but does not prolong survival
- Nicotinamide is helpful for pellagra
- Survival is 5–10 years.

PSEUDOMEMBRANOUS COLITIS

It is an inflammatory colitis characterized by bloody diarrhea due to *Clostridium difficile* that occurs after antibiotic therapy, commonly clindamycin, cephalosporin, ampicillin and amoxicillin. About 5% healthy adults and 20% elderly are healthy carriers of this organism.

Pathogenesis: Two types of toxins—A (enterotoxin) and B (cytotoxin) are responsible. Colonic mucosa may be ulcerated, occasionally covered by creamy white membrane-like material, so it is called pseudomembranous colitis. It is confused with ulcerative colitis.

Clinical features: It is common in first few days of using antibiotic, even up to 6 weeks after stopping drug. Usually there is bloody diarrhea, abdominal pain, and cramps.

Investigations: Stool for enzyme-linked immunosorbent assay (ELISA) (detecting A or B toxin). Stool for routine examination (RE) and C/S (positive in 90% cases). Colonoscopy (shows erythema, wide area of plaque, and adherent pseudomembrane) and biopsy should be taken.

Treatment: Offending drug should be stopped, correction of dehydration by IV infusion. Metronidazole 400 mg 8 hourly or vancomycin 125 mg qds for 7–10 days. In severe case, IV Ig may be given.

Complications: Toxic dilatation, perforation and ileus may occur.

KALLMANN SYNDROME

It is due to isolated gonadotropin-releasing hormone (GnRH) deficiency, characterized by hypogonadotropic hypogonadism with anosmia. GnRH deficiency leads to failure of luteinizing hormone (LH), follicle-stimulating hormone (FSH), and testosterone production. It is often familial, may be inherited as X-linked, autosomal dominant or autosomal recessive.

Clinical features: It is common in male and less in female (male to female ratio 4:1).
- Features are short stature, absence of secondary sexual characters (sparse body hair, under developed penis, and small testis), and anosmia
- Associated with cleft lip and palate, high-arched palate, nystagmus and sensorineural deafness. Renal agenesis may occur. May be cryptorchidism, cerebellar dysfunction, cerebral abnormality, and color blindness.

Investigation: Measurement of GnRH. MRI of brain to exclude other abnormalities.

Treatment: The GnRH hormone therapy restores pituitary function. In female, cyclic estrogen and progesterone therapy should be given. Fertility is possible.

TUMOR LYSIS SYNDROME

It is characterized by hyperuricemia, hyperkalemia, hyperphosphatemia and hypocalcemia, caused by destruction of large number of neoplastic cells during or shortly (1–5 days) after chemotherapy. Acidosis and acute renal failure may occur.

Investigations:
- *Serum uric acid, phosphate and lactate dehydrogenase (LDH)*: High
- Serum calcium (low), serum potassium (high), serum urea, and creatinine (high, if renal failure).

Treatment: Identification of risk and prevention are most important.
- *Preventive measures*: Allopurinol, urinary alkalinization, and plenty of fluid
- Symptomatic hypocalcemia should be corrected
- *If renal failure*: Dialysis and hemodialysis is preferred.

KIKUCHI DISEASE

It is a rare and benign disorder of unknown etiology, characterized by lymphadenopathy with or without systemic features. It is also known as histiocytic necrotizing lymphadenitis.

Clinical features: Common in female.
- Lymphadenopathy (common), usually localized, involving cervical lymph nodes (80%), mainly posterior chain. May be generalized affecting axillary, inguinal and mesenteric nodes
- Fever, headache, nausea, vomiting, malaise, arthralgia, myalgia, night sweat, rash, abdominal or thoracic pain, and weight loss
- There may be maculopapular or morbilliform rash, nodules, urticaria and malar rash
- Hepatosplenomegaly
- *Neurological manifestation*: Aseptic meningitis, acute cerebellar ataxia, and encephalitis.

Investigations:
- *Complete blood count*: Shows mild granulocytopenia or atypical lymphocytes. ESR and CRP may be high
- Lactate dehydrogenase may be high, if liver is involved
- Antinuclear antibodies and anti-dsDNA may be done to exclude SLE

- *Fine-needle aspiration cytology (FNAC) or biopsy of lymph node shows*: Necrotizing lymphadenitis
- *Others*: Chest X-ray and USG of whole abdomen.

Treatment: Usually supportive. Reassurance.
- Fever and pain may be treated with NSAID
- Steroid is indicated in severe extranodal disease, involvement of liver (elevated LDH) or nervous system, severe lupus-like syndrome or generalized Kikuchi disease. Prednisolone 50–60 mg daily orally with tapering as symptoms resolve
- Immunosuppressive drugs are used with steroid in severe and life-threatening cases
- Some patients respond to minocycline, ciprofloxacin, chloroquine and hydroxychloroquine.

Prognosis: Kikuchi disease is generally benign and self-limiting with a good prognosis. It usually resolves over several weeks to 6 months. Recurrence is unusual (3%) and fatalities are rare.

CAVERNOUS SINUS THROMBOSIS

In any patient with infection in upper lip followed by headache, fever and proptosis, is highly suggestive of cavernous sinus thrombosis.

Mechanism: Facial veins drain into sinus. The most common source of infection is due to squeezing of nasal furuncle without antibiotic cover. Other sources of infection are otitis media, sinusitis and dental infection. The most common organism is *S. aureus*.

Causes or predisposing factors:
- Infections of the face, nose, ear, teeth and sinuses
- Thromboembolism due to inherited thrombophilic disease (deficiency of antithrombin III and protein S and C), hyperviscosity syndrome, immobilization, pregnancy, puerperium, oral contraceptive pill, and Behçet's syndrome.

Clinical features:
- Severe periorbital headache and bilateral proptosis with ophthalmoplegia. Fundoscopy shows papilledema
- Fever and periorbital edema usually develop later.

Investigations: High resolution CT scan or MRI of orbit.

Treatment: IV flucloxacillin 500 mg 6 hourly and heparin. Steroid may be used.

Complications: Ocular swelling, chemosis, and ophthalmoplegia due to compression of 3rd, 4th and 6th cranial nerves and drowsiness.

FLUID RETENTION SYNDROME (IDIOPATHIC EDEMA)

This syndrome is characterized by periodic episodes of edema frequently accompanied by abdominal distension without any detectable cause. It exclusively occurs in women.

Clinical features:
- Edema is intermittent and often worse in the premenstrual phase
- The patient complains of swelling of the face, hands, breasts, thighs and feeling of being bloated

- Also, there may be headache, blurring of vision, abdominal pain, and diarrhea
- Sodium retention during the day causes increase in body weight, followed by increased sodium excretion during recumbency which causes reduction of weight (usually at night). Diurnal variation of weight >1.5 kg over 12 hours.

Investigations: Done to exclude other diseases.

Treatment: Restriction of salt intake, wearing of elastic stockings, rest in supine position for several hours in each day, and regular exercise. Diuretic may help initially, but later lose their efficacy. Angiotensin-converting enzyme (ACE) inhibitors may be given. Progesterone and bromocriptine may be used.

HICCOUGH

It is a disorder due to sudden spasmodic involuntary contraction of the diaphragm with the glottis remaining closed. It is caused by irritation of diaphragm or phrenic nerve.

Causes below the diaphragm:
- *Stomach*: Gastric distension (due to air swallowing, overeating and hasty ingestion food and fluids) and neoplasm
- *Esophagus*: Obstruction and reflux esophagitis
- Intestinal distension
- *Hepatobiliary*: Hepatomegaly, hepatitis, hepatic failure, and cholecystitis
- *Pancreatic*: Pancreatitis and malignancy
- Subphrenic abscess, peritonitis and CKD.

Causes above the diaphragm:
- *Respiratory*: Pneumonia, empyema, neoplasm and respiratory failure
- *Cardiac*: Myocardial infarction, pericarditis and aneurysm.

Other causes:
- *Central nervous system*: Neoplasm, infection (encephalitis), CVD and trauma
- *Metabolic*: Hypocapnia (hyperventilation), diabetic ketoacidosis, and electrolyte imbalance
- Alcohol ingestion and mechanical ventilation
- *Surgery*: General anesthesia and postoperative
- *Psychogenic*: Emotional excitement, stress and laughing
- Idiopathic.

Investigations: According to history and suspicion of causes.
- Complete blood count and liver and renal function test (serum urea, creatinine, and electrolytes)
- Chest X-ray, USG of abdomen, upper GI endoscopy, and echocardiography
- Bronchoscopy and chest fluoroscopy
- Computed tomography of the head, chest and abdomen.

Treatment: Breathing and rebreathing into a paper bag. Breath holding and drinking cold water. Valsalva maneuver, sneezing and gasping (fright stimulus). Stimulation of vagus by carotid sinus massage. Relief of gastric distension by belching or antacid or insertion of nasogastric tube. Treatment of primary cause.

Drugs:
- Chlorpromazine 25–50 mg or haloperidol 5 mg tds
- Domperidone 10 mg tds or metoclopramide 10 mg tds
- Benzodiazepines (lorazepam and diazepam) and anticonvulsants (phenytoin and carbamazepine)
- Baclofen or gabapentin. Occasionally general anesthesia.

CYSTIC FIBROSIS

Cystic fibrosis (CF) is an autosomal recessive disease characterized by abnormal transport of chloride and sodium ions across the epithelium, causing thick and viscous secretions, leading to bronchopulmonary infection and pancreatic insufficiency.

Clinical features: In neonate—failure to thrive, meconium ileus, and rectal prolapse.

In children and young adult:
- *Respiratory*: Recurrent infection (by *S. aureus* and *Pseudomonas aeruginosa*) and features of bronchiectasis (cough with profuse expectoration, wheeze and hemoptysis). May be pneumothorax, lung collapse, respiratory failure, cor pulmonale, asthma, otitis media, sinusitis and nasal polyps
- *Abdominal*: Pancreatic insufficiency causing steatorrhea, malabsorption, cholesterol gallstone, secondary biliary cirrhosis, portal hypertension, distal intestinal obstruction syndrome (meconium ileus equivalent syndrome). Also increased incidence of peptic ulceration and GI malignancy
- *Others*: CF-related diabetes, infertility, delayed puberty and skeletal maturity, arthritis, osteoporosis, cutaneous vasculitis, and clubbing with hypertrophic osteoarthropathy.

Investigations:
Routine—
- Complete blood count, blood sugar, LFTs, serum creatinine, and electrolytes
- Throat swab and sputum culture
- The X-ray of chest (shows hyperinflation and bronchiectasis) and spirometry (to see obstructive defect)
- Ultrasonography of whole abdomen (fatty liver, cirrhosis and chronic pancreatitis).

Specific: Sweat test (high sweat chloride >60 mmol/L).

Treatment:
- *General measures*: Nutritional support and fat-soluble vitamin supplement (A, D, E and K). Strict glucose control and smoking must be stopped. Vaccination for influenza and pneumococcus
- *For respiratory problems*:
  - Regular chest physiotherapy, mucolytic, inhaled bronchodilator, and steroid
  - Antibiotic, if infection. Also, prophylactic antibiotic (oral ciprofloxacin or nebulized colomycin, and levofloxacin). Azithromycin 500 mg orally three times weekly

- o Recombinant human deoxyribonuclease (rhDNase) from early childhood (regardless of disease status)
- o Ivacaftor, an oral drug, is a potentiator of cystic fibrosis transmembrane conductance regulator (CFTR) channel
- o *For advanced lung disease*: Oxygen, diuretics (for cor pulmonale), noninvasive ventilation, and lung or heart–lung transplantation.
- *For abdominal problems*: Pancreatic enzyme and vitamin supplement, and ursodeoxycholic acid for impaired liver function. Liver transplantation may be needed in cirrhosis
- Gene therapy is a possibility in future. Genetic counseling.

OXYGEN THERAPY

To treat hypoxemia and to ensure adequate arterial oxygen saturation (pO_2 >90%).

Methods: nasal cannulae, face mask or venturi mask, CPAP (useful in obstructive sleep apnea syndrome), and BiPAP [useful in neuromuscular disease, chronic obstructive pulmonary disease (COPD), and postoperative respiratory insufficiency].

Indications:
- *In chronic condition*: Low-flow oxygen in COPD (high flow should be avoided. Because, in such case, respiratory center is insensitive to high CO_2 retention and hypoxia is the only stimulant to respiratory center. So total correction of hypoxia may aggravate respiratory failure)
- *In acute conditions*: Acute severe asthma, major trauma, MI, left ventricular failure (acute pulmonary edema), ARDS, massive hemorrhage, anaphylaxis and shock, during resuscitation.

Complications:
- In COPD or chronic bronchitis, it aggravates respiratory failure
- *In lung*: Pulmonary edema, ARDS and progressive decrease in lung compliance
- *In premature infants and neonates*: Retrolental fibroplasia, blindness and bronchopulmonary dysplasia.

PAGET'S DISEASE

It is characterized by excessive and disorganized resorption and formation of bone, resulting in deformity and fracture. The commonly involved bones are pelvis, femur, tibia, lumbar spines, skull and scapula. It is common above 55 years, rare below 40 years. It is more in temperate climate. Its cause is unknown. There is increased osteoclastic bone resorption and increased osteoblastic activity, followed by abnormal bone formation. Bone formation exceeds resorption, the new bone is bigger, but weaker and filled with new blood vessels.

Clinical features: It is common in female, M:F = 2:3. It may be asymptomatic.
- Bone pain, joint pain, stiffness, bowing of legs, deformities (in weight-bearing bones such as femur, tibia), pathological fracture, enlarged head, and other bony swelling
- *Neurological features*: Deafness, cranial nerve defect, nerve root pain, spinal cord compression, and spinal stenosis may occur due to enlargement of affected bone

- Warm skin over affected bone and high-output cardiac failure due to hyperdynamic circulation.

Investigations:
- *Bone X-ray*: Shows enlargement of bone with typical lytic and sclerotic lesion
- Serum alkaline phosphatase (high) and urinary hydroxyproline (high)
- Isotope bone scan, CT scan or MRI of bone may be done
- Rarely bone biopsy
- *Calcium and phosphate*: Normal (calcium may be high in prolonged immobilization or fracture).

Treatment:
- *For pain*: NSAIDs
- *To prevent further bone breakdown*:
  - *Bisphosphonates*: Pamidronate, zoledronate, risedronate, etidronate and tiludronate. Hypocalcemia may occur, so calcium and vitamin D should be given
  - *Calcitonin*: Subcutaneously 100–200 IU, three times weekly, for 2–3 months.
- *Surgery*: Joint replacement or osteotomy. Neurosurgery in spinal cord compression.

Complications: Bone fractures, deformities, deafness, high-output heart failure, secondary osteoarthrosis, optic atrophy, spinal cord compression, spinal stenosis, and osteosarcoma (rare but serious).

CHARCOT–MARIE–TOOTH DISEASE

It is a group of heterogeneous motor and sensory neuropathy. It may be inherited as autosomal dominant or recessive or X-linked.

Clinical features:
- Usually presents with foot deformities or gait disturbance in early childhood or early adult life. Bilateral pes cavus and clawing of toes are present. Distal weakness and wasting that begins in leg, progress slowly, involves both lower limbs up to middle of legs, giving rise to inverted champagne bottle (stork or spindle legs) appearance
- Dorsiflexion (weak in both feet), ankle jerk (absent bilaterally), and plantar response (equivocal)
- *Sensory*: Mild impairment of superficial and deep sensation up to mid-thigh (marked sensory loss with trophic ulcer may be found)
- *Gait*: Steppage gait with foot drop
- Later wasting and weakness in upper limbs may occur.

Investigation: Nerve conduction study.

Treatment: Symptomatic and supportive. Physiotherapy and orthopedic measure may be given.

HUMAN IMMUNODEFICIENCY VIRUS INFECTION (ACQUIRED IMMUNODEFICIENCY SYNDROME)

Human immunodeficiency virus (HIV): It is a single-stranded RNA virus, belongs to lentivirus group of retrovirus family. There are two types: HIV-1 and HIV-2.

Human immunodeficiency virus disease: Spectrum of disorders are—
- Primary infection with or without acute HIV syndrome
- Asymptomatic infected state, even in advanced disease
- Acquired immunodeficiency syndrome (AIDS).

Acquired immunodeficiency syndrome: HIV-infected individual with CD4 T cell count <200 cells/mm^3 regardless of the presence of symptoms *or* HIV-infected individual with AIDS-defining conditions (category C) regardless of CD4 count is called acquired immunodeficiency syndrome.

Modes of transmission of HIV: Sexual contact (more in homosexuals, multiple sexual partners, and uncircumcised persons), transplacental, perinatal and breastfeeding, parenteral exposure to infected body fluid, sharing of needles, IV drug abuser, blood and blood product transfusion, occupational transmission, and organ transplantation including cornea.

Routes not involved in transmission of HIV: Close personal contact (sleeping, shaking hands and kissing), social contact (at school, swimming pool, and shopping mall), sharing toilet, staying in a common ward in hospital, sharing utensils, insect or animal bite. Also, respiratory droplets, sputum, through health workers like doctors and nurses.

Natural history of HIV or AIDS:
- *Primary infection*: It is symptomatic in 70–80% cases, usually occurs 2–6 weeks after exposure. Features are fever with rash, pharyngitis with cervical lymphadenopathy, myalgia, arthralgia, headache and mucosal ulceration
- *Asymptomatic infection*: Patient remains asymptomatic but potentially infectious to others, may persist for 5–10 years. There may be anemia, leukopenia, lymphopenia and reduced CD4 count. Also, there is cutaneous anergy
- *Mildly symptomatic disease (HIV symptomatic or indicator diseases, category B)*: Constitutional (low-grade fever, night sweat and weight loss), oral hairy leukoplakia, recurrent oropharyngeal candidiasis and vaginal candidiasis, herpes zoster (in more than one dermatome), immune thrombocytopenic purpura (ITP), chronic diarrhea, peripheral neuropathy, cervical dysplasia, and severe pelvic inflammatory disease.

Acquired immunodeficiency syndrome: AIDS-defining diseases are (category C)—
- Esophageal candidiasis and chronic cryptosporidial diarrhea
- Cryptococcal meningitis, cerebral toxoplasmosis, and progressive multifocal leukoencephalopathy
- Cytomegalovirus (CMV) retinitis or colitis
- Chronic mucocutaneous herpes simplex and Kaposi's sarcoma
- Invasive cervical cancer, non-Hodgkin's lymphoma (including Burkitt's lymphoma), and primary cerebral lymphoma
- Disseminated *Mycobacterium avium* intracellulare, pulmonary or extrapulmonary TB, and *Pneumocystis jirovecii pneumonia (PCP)*
- Recurrent non-typhi salmonella septicemia, HIV-associated wasting, and HIV-associated dementia
- Extrapulmonary coccidioidomycosis and extrapulmonary histoplasmosis.

Common infections in AIDS: *P. jirovecii*, *Candida albicans*, *Cryptococcus neoformans*, *Toxoplasma gondii*, *Mycobacterium* (typical and atypical), CMV, amoebiasis and *Cryptosporidium*.

Human immunodeficiency virus-related cancer: AIDS-defining cancers (Kaposi's sarcoma and non-Hodgkin's lymphoma) and non-AIDS defining malignancies (anal cancer and Hodgkin's disease).

Cutaneous manifestations of HIV:
- Early (Herpes simplex, varicella-zoster, and human papillomavirus)
- Late (Kaposi's sarcoma, molluscum contagiosum, and chronic mucocutaneous herpes simplex).

Findings in mouth cavity in HIV patient: Hairy leukoplakia, oropharyngeal candidiasis, aphthous ulcer, herpes simplex, and periodontal disease.

Causes of diarrhea or enteropathy in HIV patient: CMV, *Cryptosporidium*, *Microsporidium*, *M. avium intracellulare*, and other (*Isospora*, *Giardia*, *Entamoeba histolytica*, *Salmonella*, adenovirus and bacterial overgrowth). The patient presents with dysphagia, retrosternal pain, watery diarrhea accompanied by blood, colicky abdominal pain, weight loss, and fever.

Major causes of pulmonary disease in HIV: Pneumonia (*P. jirovecii* and bacterial), TB, fungus (*Histoplasma* and *Cryptococcus*), and malignancy (non-Hodgkin's lymphoma and Kaposi's sarcoma).

Neurological manifestations in AIDS patient:
- *Acute meningitis*: May be aseptic meningitis, multiple cranial nerve palsy
- *Encephalitis*: Herpes simplex, varicella zoster virus, and *T. gondii*
- Primary CNS lymphoma (5%)
- Acquired immunodeficiency syndrome dementia complex and progressive multifocal leukoencephalopathy
- Retinitis (CMV and toxoplasmosis)
- Autonomic neuropathy
- *Spinal cord, root and peripheral nerve disease includes*: Peripheral neuropathy, HIV myelopathy, Guillain-Barré syndrome (GBS), transverse myelitis, brachial neuritis, and polyradiculitis.

Ocular diseases in AIDS: CMV retinitis and *T. gondii* retinitis.

Renal: Acute renal failure, CKD, HIV immune complex kidney diseases, and thrombotic microangiopathy.

Cardiac: Dilated cardiomyopathy, ZDV-induced cardiomyopathy, and coronary artery disease.

Endocrine: Hypoadrenalism, hypogonadism and hypopituitarism.

Hematological: Anemia, leukopenia, thrombocytopenia, lymphoma and pancytopenia.

Investigations for newly diagnosed (asymptomatic) HIV-infected patient:
- *Routine tests*: CBC, peripheral blood film (PBF), LFT, renal function test, lipid profile, blood glucose, urinalysis and chest X-ray
- *Specific*: HIV antibody (confirmatory), HIV rapid antibody test (should be confirmed with ELISA and Western blot), CD4 count, viral load and HIV genotype.

Diagnosis of HIV or AIDS: Screening by ELISA (positive 3–12 weeks after infection), confirmation by Western blot.

Pretest and post-test counseling for suspected HIV or AIDS patient:
- *Pretest counseling*: Purpose of test should be discussed, assessment of risk factors, explanation of natural history, mode of transmission and reduction of risk of HIV, coping strategy, explanation of test procedure, and informed consent.
- *Post-test counseling*:
  - If the test is negative: Discussion regarding behavior modification including safer sex and needle exchange. A second test should be carried out 3 months after last exposure
  - If the test is positive: Explanation of significance and implications of result, urgent medical follow-up, strategy regarding fear of disclosure and social rejection, verbal and written information, and emotional and practical support by providing phone number and name.

Aims of treatment: To reduce viral load to undetectable level, to improve CD4 count to >200 cells/mL, to improve quantity and quality of life and to reduce transmission.

Treatment of AIDS:
- *General management*: Advice on diet, nutrition, smoking, alcohol, drug misuse, and exercise. Proper advice on reducing the risk of HIV transmission including sexual practice, psychological support for patient, family, friends and care givers, and information about childbearing
- *Drug treatment*: Depends on clinical assessment, laboratory investigations including viral load and CD4 counts, and also individual circumstances.

Drugs used in HIV-infected patients:
- *Reverse transcriptase inhibitors (RTIs)*: ZDV, didanosine, lamivudine, abacavir, nevirapine, efavirenz and etravirine
- *Protease inhibitors*: Indinavir, ritonavir, lopinavir, atazanavir and fosamprenavir
- *Entry inhibitors*: Enfuvirtide, maraviroc and raltegravir
- *Treatment of CMV retinitis in HIV*: Ganciclovir.

Prevention of HIV infection: Safe sexual practice, effective treatment of sexually transmitted infection (STI), screening of blood and blood products, use of clean needles and syringes, and anti-retroviral drugs to reduce mother-to-child transmission.

Treatment of a person exposed to HIV infection: When risk is significant, in both occupational and nonoccupational settings, lopinavir, tenofovir and emtricitabine are given. First dose is given as soon as possible, preferably within 6–8 hours, and 4 weeks of therapy is recommended. Protection is not absolute and seroconversion may occur.

Treatment of HIV positive pregnant woman:
- *Antepartum*: Lopinavir with ZDV and lamivudine from 20 weeks to all mothers or oral ZDV for those with viral loads <10,000 copies/mL and wild type virus who are willing to have cesarean section.
- *During delivery*:
  - Zidovudine IV infusion at the onset of labor given to those on ZDV alone or those on highly active antiretroviral therapy (HAART) but with detectable virus, and undergoing normal vaginal delivery
  - Delivery by caesarean section reduces the risk of transmission.

- *After delivery*: Neonate should get oral ZDV for 6 weeks and breastfeeding should be avoided.

PNEUMOCYSTIS JIROVECII PNEUMONIA

Pneumocystis jirovecii (previously called *Pneumocystis carinii* or PCP) is an opportunistic fungus that causes pneumonia in HIV or AIDS patient, when CD4 is <200/mm^3. PCP may also occur in immunosuppressed due to cancer, corticosteroid or other immunosuppressive drugs, organ or bone marrow transplantation.

Clinical features: Develop slowly over weeks, may take months.
- Shortness of breath on exertion and cough (usually dry)
- Fever, malaise, weight loss, and night sweat
- Tachypnea, tachycardia and cyanosis. Fine crepitations may be present.

Investigations:
- *Chest X-ray*: Shows bilateral perihilar interstitial infiltrates
- *High-resolution computed tomography (HRCT) of chest*: Shows ground-glass appearance
- *Sputum for cytology or polymerase chain reaction (PCR)*: Organism may be found in 50–90% cases (by silver or Giemsa staining or immunofluorescent technique. Organism cannot be cultured)
- Bronchoscopy and bronchoalveolar lavage (shows organisms in 90–95% cases)
- Blood gas analysis (pO$_2$ is low and <90% on exercise)
- Polymerase chain reaction amplification of fungal DNA in blood
- Lung function tests (restrictive pattern with reduced diffusion capacity) and lung biopsy
- Lactate dehydrogenase (high).

Treatment:
- Intravenous co-trimoxazole (120 mg/kg daily in divided doses for 21 days) is the first-line treatment
- *If allergic to co-trimoxazole*: IV pentamidine (4 mg/kg/day) or dapsone and trimethoprim are given for same duration
- Atovaquone or combination of clindamycin and primaquine may be given
- *Prednisolone*: 40 mg bid for 5 days, then 40 mg daily for 5 days and 20 mg daily for 11 days
- Systemic corticosteroid may be used in severe cases
- Continuous positive airway pressure or mechanical ventilation (if patient remains severely hypoxic or becomes too tired).

CHAPTER 20

Diseases of the Eye

RED EYE

In this condition, the eye appears red due to any disease which affects the eyelids and its hair follicles (adnexal cause), conjunctiva (bulbar and tarsal), cornea, etc.

Causes:
- *Lid diseases*: Stye, chalazion, blepharitis and allergy
- *Conjunctival diseases*: Conjunctivitis (viral or bacterial), vernal (allergic or seasonal) conjunctivitis and subconjunctival hemorrhage
- *Corneal diseases*: Keratitis, corneal ulcer (bacterial and fungal), foreign body, trauma, abrasion, herpes zoster ophthalmicus and dry eye
- *Scleral inflammation*: Episcleritis, scleritis and postoperative
- *Uveal or iris inflammation*: Anterior uveitis (iritis and iridocyclitis), posterior uveitis (choroiditis and choroidoretinitis), and intermediate uveitis
- *Other causes*: Acute glaucoma, postoperative endophthalmitis, disease of orbit (such as malignant exomphalos, tumor and orbital cellulitis), and idiopathic orbital inflammatory disease.

Red flags for red eye (following symptoms require urgent referral):
- Severe pain in eye and watering of eye
- Photophobia
- Reduced vision, particularly if sudden
- Colored halos around a point of light in patient's vision
- Proptosis, double vision and reduced or absent eye movement
- Smaller pupil in affected eye (mid dilated and fixed pupil)
- History of trauma or foreign body.

Plus on medical assessment:
- High intraocular pressure (IOP)
- Corneal epithelial disruption
- Shallow anterior chamber
- Ciliary flush
- Absent or sluggish pupillary response.

DISEASE OF EYE LIDS

- Misdirected or ingrowing lashes (trichiasis)
- Loss of eyelashes (madarosis)
- Depigmentation of eyelashes (poliosis)
- Entropion (inward folding of eyelid)
- Ectropion (outward folding of eyelid)
- Ptosis (drooping of upper eyelid)
- Blepharitis (inflammation of lid margin)
- Xanthelasma
- *Causes of localized eyelid swelling*: Stye, chalazion, papilloma, sebaceous cyst, marginal cyst of Zeis, basal cell cancer (BCC) (rodent ulcer), and lacrimal gland and lacrimal sac disorders.

Blepharitis

It is the inflammation of the eyelid margin.

Causes:
- Irritation due to dust, smoke and cosmetics
- Uncorrected refractive error
- Dandruff or seborrhea of scalp
- Chronic conjunctivitis
- Dry eye.

Types:
- *Anterior*: Inflammation of anterior lid margin (staphylococcal and seborrheic or mixed)
- *Posterior*: Inflammation of posterior lid margin (meibomian seborrhea and meibomianitis)
- Mixed anterior and posterior.

Clinical features: Redness, itching and crusting of lid margins, ulcer at lid margins, and burning sensation of eye. In posterior blepharitis, oily secretion is produced from meibomian glands if pressure is applied over tarsal plate, frothy discharge is secreted with capped meibomian gland.

Treatment:
- *Maintenance of lid hygiene*: Cleaning of lid margin with moistened cotton (with clean boiled water). Lid scrub with baby shampoo.
- *Specific treatment*:
  - Combination of antibiotic-steroid ointment three times daily for 2–4 weeks
  - Chloramphenicol eye drop or ciprofloxacin eye drop, one drop 6 hourly for 7 days
  - Artificial tear, one drop three times daily for 2–4 weeks
  - In posterior blepharitis: Tetracycline 250 mg 6 hourly for 1 week, then 12 hourly for 12 weeks. *Or*, doxycycline 100 mg 12 hourly for 1 week then daily for 12 weeks.
- General hygiene to be improved and treatment of scalp dandruff if any
- Refer to ophthalmologist to check for refractive error.

Stye (External Hordeolum)

It is the acute suppurative inflammation of the follicle of eyelash and Zeis glands due to *Staphylococcus*.

Causes: Low general resistance, diabetes mellitus (DM), and uncontrolled refractive error.

Clinical features: Acute pain and localized, hard, red, tender swelling of lid margins and discharge. In advanced stage, a pus point is visible at the lid margin.

Treatment:
- Removal of affected eyelashes. Hot compression with clean boiled water and cotton pad 3-4 times (10 minutes each) daily for 7 days
- Antibiotics eye drop or ointment (chloramphenicol or ciprofloxacin eye drop—one drop 4-6 hourly in the affected eye for 10 days)
- Sometimes systemic antibiotics (flucloxacillin) may be needed
- Surgical drainage may be necessary in some cases.

Internal Stye (Hordeolum Internum)

It is the abscess of meibomian gland. It often causes less swelling than external stye. It may occur as primary staphylococcal infection of the meibomian gland or due to secondary infection in a chalazion (infected chalazion). Symptoms are similar to stye, except that pain is more intense. Treatment is similar to hordeolum externum.

Chalazion

It is the chronic inflammation of meibomian gland, also called a tarsal or meibomian cyst.

Causes: Poor general condition, DM and refractive error.

Clinical features: Swelling of the eyelid which is nontender, firm and tense nodular.

Treatment: If it is small, it may resolve spontaneously. In moderate to large chalazion—incision and curettage under local anesthesia.

Entropion

Inward turning of eyelids margin is called entropion. It is due to degenerative changes or secondary to scarring. It commonly affects the lower lid, but can affect both.

Clinical features: Increase with age (rare <40 years). Eyelashes rub on cornea and causes irritation, watering, pain, corneal vascularization, ulceration and infection.

Treatment: Taping the lower lid to cheek can give temporary relief. Refer for rapid surgical correction. Artificial tear and antibiotic, when needed.

Ectropion

Turning outward or outrolling of eyelid margin is called ectropion. It is common in elderly patient or patient with facial nerve palsy. It causes dry eye, watering, discomfort, exposure keratitis and conjunctivitis. Refer for surgery.

DACRYOCYSTITIS

It is the infection of lacrimal sac, secondary to obstruction of nasolacrimal duct at the junction of lacrimal sac. It may be congenital or may be in adult. Adult dacryocystitis are due to *Staphylococcus, Streptococcus,* and pneumococcus. It may be acute and chronic.

Acute dacryocystitis: Symptoms are pain, redness, and swelling over the lacrimal area and watering and discharge from the eye. In severe case, there is cellulitis of surrounding area. Signs are red, tense swelling, and tenderness over lacrimal sac area, and mucoid or purulent discharge. Regurgitation test is usually positive.

Treatment:
- *Systemic antibiotic*: Flucloxacillin 500 mg or cephradine 500 mg 6 hourly for 2 weeks
- *Topical antibiotic*: Ciprofloxacin eye drop four times daily for 2 weeks
- Analgesics and warm compression for pain
- *Surgery*: Dacryocystorhinostomy (DCR) 6–8 weeks after the acute attack. Dacryocystectomy (DCT) in older patient.

Chronic dacryocystitis: Features are constant epiphora, mild conjunctivitis, and mild discharge, which occur regularly. It is common in female, middle-aged, and elderly with poor personal hygiene and low socioeconomical group. The eye does not look inflamed.

Treatment: DCR operation. DCT in elderly if tear film deficiency.

Ingrowing Lashes (Trichiasis)

It is the misdirection of eyelashes causing trauma to cornea and conjunctiva.

Features: Irritation, foreign body sensation, pain, lacrimation, congestion, and with or without recurrent infection. In severe cases, ingrowing lashes may damage the cornea.

Treatment: Epilation (removal of eye lash by epilation forceps).

Loss of Eyelashes (Madarosis)

It means decrease in number or complete loss of eyelashes. It is usually due to blepharitis. Other causes are picking or rubbing, alopecia areata, discoid lupus erythematosus, and also idiopathic. Treatment of cause if possible.

Depigmentation of the Eyelashes (Poliosis)

Depigmentation or whitening of the eyelashes is called poliosis. Vitiligo can affect the eyelids. There is usually a family history. It may be associated with other autoimmune disease (e.g. thyroid disease) and Vogt–Koyanagi–Harada syndrome. Treatment of primary cause.

CONJUNCTIVITIS

It is the inflammation of conjunctiva due to any cause. It may be acute, subacute and chronic.

Causes:
- *Infection*: Bacterial (*Staphylococcus, Streptococcus* and pneumococcus), viral (adenovirus, herpes simplex virus, and enterovirus), trachoma, tuberculosis (TB), and parasitic
- *Allergic*: Dust, pollen, animal dander and cold
- *Others*: Chemical or toxic, contact lens and idiopathic.

Clinical features: Redness (conjunctival congestion), discharge (watery or purulent or mucoid), itchy eyes, stickiness of eye lids, foreign body sensation, irritation, and chemosis (edema). It may be preauricular lymphadenopathy (in viral and chlamydial conjunctivitis), subconjunctival hemorrhage and swollen lids.

Treatment:
- Isolation of patient, maintenance of personal hygiene, cleaning of eyelashes, dark glass and cold compression
- *In bacterial conjunctivitis*:
  - Chloramphenicol or ciprofloxacin or moxifloxacin eye drop 1 hourly in severe case. Otherwise, 6 hourly for 7–14 days
  - Antibiotic eye ointment at bed time (tetracycline or chloramphenicol)
  - *In gonococcal conjunctivitis*: Gentamicin or tobramycin eye drop.
- In viral conjunctivitis: General measures (as above). Artificial tear and antibiotic eye drop to prevent secondary infection.
- *In allergic conjunctivitis*:
  - Avoidance of allergen
  - Topical anti-allergic eye drop: Sodium cromoglycate, ketotifen, olopatadine or fluorometholone
  - Topical steroid: In severe case for short duration
  - Systemic anti-allergic drug (antihistamine such as fexofenadine and cetirizine).

Ophthalmia Neonatorum

Acute purulent conjunctivitis in the 1st month of life is called ophthalmia neonatorum.

Causes: *Neisseria gonorrhoeae*, *Staphylococcus*, *Streptococcus*, chemicals, herpes simplex virus (HSV) type-2, and chlamydia.

Clinical features: Eyelids are severely edematous and tender, profused purulent discharge, severe conjunctival congestion, severe chemosis, pseudomembrane formation, fever, lymphadenopathy, keratitis, etc.

Treatment: General measure and depends on cause—
- If *N. gonorrhoeae* is suspected, intravenous (IV) ceftriaxone with gentamicin drop and ointment should be given
- If bacterial, tobramycin eye drops and gentamicin ointment
- If viral, acyclovir eye ointment
- In chlamydia, tetracycline eye ointment and oral erythromycin.

Pterygium

It is a degenerative condition of subconjunctival tissue, presenting as a triangular fold of conjunctival tissue involving up to the cornea. Apex is toward the cornea, more common on the nasal side, and less on temporal side. Types are progressive pterygium and atrophic pterygium.

Causes: Ultraviolet irradiation, prolonged exposure to hot, sandy or dusty weather and chronic dryness of eye.

Clinical features: Usually no symptoms in early stages. A dirty white or fleshy mass is seen growing on to cornea from nasal side. May be slight irritation or foreign body sensation. Diminution of vision may occur due to astigmatism produced by traction on the cornea. Gross diminution of vision occurs when it encroaches upon the pupillary area.

Treatment: Surgical excision with autograft.

Subconjunctival Hemorrhage

It is the bleeding under the conjunctiva.

Causes: Trauma, conjunctivitis, postoperative, whooping cough, repeated vomiting, hypertension (HTN), DM, any bleeding disorder or antiplatelet, and anticoagulant therapy.

Treatment: Avoid dust, fume, and cold. Use of dark glass and lubricant tear drop. Treatment of primary cause (e.g. DM and HTN). Cold compression, rest, and fluorometholone eye drop if needed. Resolves in 3 weeks.

CORNEAL ULCER

Loss of corneal epithelium with stromal inflammation with or without hypopyon.

Causes: It may be infective and noninfective.
- *Infective*: Bacterial (staphylococcal, streptococcal, pneumococcal, *N. gonorrhoeae*), viral (herpes simplex virus and herpes zoster virus), fungal (*Aspergillus fumigatus* and *Aspergillus niger*), and protozoal
- *Noninfective*: Trauma, foreign body, chemical, allergic, neurotropic and neuroparalytic.

Symptoms: Pain with irritation and redness of affected eye, photophobia, watering and discharge from eye, and decreased vision.

Signs: Decreased vision and edematous lid. Pupil constricted with irregular margin and posterior synechiae. Iris may be grey. Cornea stains positive with fluorescein dye. Satellite lesion is seen in fungal type of corneal ulcer. Hypopyon in anterior chamber.

Investigations: Corneal scraping for staining with Gram stain and KOH, C/S. Sac patency test and blood sugar.

Treatment: Patient should be referred for immediate consultation with an ophthalmologist.
- *Bacterial corneal ulcer*:
  - Topical antibiotic eye drop: Moxifloxacin alone or with gentamicin/tobramycin, one drop 2 hourly in affected eye. Frequency of dose will depend on severity
  - Atropine eye drop: One drop 8 hourly
  - Systemic antibiotic: Ciprofloxacin 500 mg 12 hourly may be given, if hypopyon
  - Systemic analgesic if pain.
- *Fungal corneal ulcer*:
  - Natamycin (5%) eye drop: One drop half to 1 hourly initially and then tapered accordingly
  - Atropine (1%) eye drop: One drop 8 hourly
  - Systemic analgesics, if pain.
- *Other treatment*:
  - Steroid is contraindicated. Avoid application of water to eye
  - Oral vitamin C, multivitamins and vitamin B complex
  - Control of DM.

KERATITIS

Keratitis means inflammation of the cornea. Keratoconjunctivitis means inflammation of cornea and conjunctiva. It may be due to:
- Trauma and dry eye
- *Viral*: Herpes simplex virus type 1 or 2 and adenovirus
- *Foreign body*: Contact lens and blepharitis
- *Autoimmune disease*: Rheumatoid arthritis, systemic lupus erythematosus (SLE), and Sjögren's syndrome.

Clinical features: Painful red eye, blurring of vision, photophobia, watering, and reduction of visual acuity.

Treatment: Usually symptomatic.
- Artificial tears have soothing effect
- Chloramphenicol or moxifloxacin eye drop to prevent secondary bacterial infection
- Specific treatment of cause should be given whenever possible
- If stain negative or signs of uveitis or stromal opacity, steroid eye drop may be given.

Viral Keratitis

It may occur due to infection with herpes simplex virus type 1 or 2, adenovirus.

Symptoms: Redness, watering, discomfort, photophobia and foreign body sensation.

Signs: Lid may be edematous, circumciliary congestion, and corneal sensation may be reduced. Fluorescein stain may show erosions with lateral branches and knobbed ends. "Dendritic pattern" is the pathognomonic sign.

Treatment: Avoid application of water to eye.
- Topical antiviral eye drop, also acyclovir (3%) ointment five times daily for 14 days, then three times daily for 14 days
- Artificial tear
- Atropine or homatropine eye drop, 1–2 drops three times daily if severe pain
- *If recurrent*: Above plus oral acyclovir tablet twice daily for 6 months.

UVEITIS

It is the inflammation of the uveal tract (iris, ciliary body and choroid).

Causes:
- Idiopathic
- *Endogenous cause*: Immune complex mediated and microorganism
- *Secondary to systemic diseases*: Seronegative arthritis, TB, syphilis, leprosy, sarcoidosis, herpes simplex virus and sympathetic ophthalmitis, etc.
- *Exogenous cause*: Trauma.

Types: Four types—
1. Anterior uveitis is inflammation of the anterior part of uveal tract. It includes iris (iritis), or both iris and ciliary body (iridocyclitis). Common type

2. Intermediate uveitis is inflammation of the middle part of uveal tract
3. Posterior uveitis is inflammation of the posterior part of eye that affects choroid, optic nerve, head and retina. It includes choroiditis, chorioretinitis, retinitis and neuroretinitis
4. Panuveitis is inflammation affecting the whole uveal tract.

Symptoms: Pain, red eye, photophobia, watering, blurring or dimness of vision, and floaters. May be unilateral or bilateral.

Signs: By slit lamp examination, keratic precipitate, pupil (normal or synechiae), and intraocular pressure (may be normal or raised). May be hypopyon (inflammatory exudates in anterior chamber) and hyphema (blood in the anterior chamber, if trauma).

Investigations:
- *Routine*: Complete blood count (CBC), erythrocyte sedimentation rate (ESR), chest X-ray (posteroanterior), MT, and random blood sugar (RBS)
- *Other*: According to suspicious of cause—antinuclear antibodies (ANA), and serological tests for syphilis, toxoplasma and human immunodeficiency virus (HIV).

Treatment:
- *Topical steroid*: Dexamethasone or prednisolone acetate eye drop, frequent instillation, and then tapered accordingly (total 6 weeks treatment)
- Atropine (1%) or homatropine eye drop, one drop three times daily for 14 days
- *Systemic steroid*: If topical drops fail to control the inflammation
- In severe case, immunosuppressive agents may be used (e.g. cyclophosphamide, chlorambucil, azathioprine and methotrexate)
- Treatment of specific disease
- Systemic steroid or immunomodulators needed in chronic or systemic disease
- Subconjunctival mydricaine injection may be given by ophthalmologist in severe case.

EPISCLERITIS

It is the inflammation of thin layer of vascular tissue overlying sclera. The patient presents with diffuse inflammation of eye with minimal tenderness, discomfort, mild watering and localized redness.

Treatment: For pain, NSAID (ibuprofen 400 mg 8 hourly or ketorolac 0.5% eye drops 6 hourly). Steroid (fluorometholone) eye drop, 4–6 hourly may be given.

SCLERITIS

Inflammation of sclera due to any cause. Can be unilateral or bilateral. It may be anterior uveitis (98%) or/and posterior uveitis. May be diffuse, nodular, or necrotizing.

Causes:
- Trauma, surgery
- *Autoimmune collagen disorders*: Especially rheumatoid arthritis. Others are Wegener's granulomatosis, polyarteritis nodosa, SLE and ankylosing spondylitis

- *Metabolic disorders*: Gout and thyrotoxicosis
- *Some infections*: Particularly herpes zoster ophthalmicus, chronic staphylococcal and streptococcal infections have also been known to cause scleritis
- *Granulomatous diseases*: Tuberculosis, syphilis, sarcoidosis and leprosy can also cause scleritis
- *Miscellaneous*: Irradiation, chemical burns, Vogt-Koyanagi-Harada syndrome, and Behcet's disease.

Symptoms: The patient presents with painful and red eye. Vision may be blurred and visual acuity decreases. Eye is tender. There may be scleral nodules, uveitis and keratitis.

Treatment: Topical steroid and systemic NSAID for pain. If severe, systemic steroid may be given. Sometimes intraocular steroid injection. Treatment of primary cause.

Complications: Cataract, glaucoma, retinal detachment and staphyloma due to scleral thinning.

FOREIGN BODY IN EYE (SUPERFICIAL)

Symptoms: The patient has definitive complains of something falling and feeling in eye, watering from affected eye, and photophobia.

Signs: Foreign body in eye and conjunctival congestion.

Treatment: Removal of foreign body by slit lamp (examined under topical anesthesia). Broad-spectrum antibiotic eye drop (ciprofloxacin). Artificial tear—frequent drops are applied. No pad and bandage. Eye ointment at bed time. Avoid application of water in eye. Oral vitamin C.

CHEMICAL INJURIES

Injury by any chemicals such as detergents, cleansing agents, acid or alkali. Common alkalis are liquid ammonia, caustic soda, and potash lime. Common acids are sulfuric acid (in battery), hydrochloric acid, nitric acid, and acetic acid.

Features: Redness, watering, and pain in affected eye. Critical signs are epithelial defect, corneal hemorrhage, corneal edema and limbal ischemia.

Treatment: Irrigation with water or normal saline (by lid eversion or double lid eversion) to remove offending agent. Topical steroid—dexamethasone eye drop, one drop 1 hourly for 7–10 days. Topical antibiotic eye drop—ciprofloxacin or moxifloxacin. Topical antiglaucoma drops—timolol maleate 12 hourly. Artificial tears and antibiotics. Surgical treatment. If severe, immediate hospitalization.

CATARACT

Opacity of lens or its capsule causing gradual dimness of vision is called cataract.

Causes:
- *Congenital*: Maternal infection [TORCH (toxoplasmosis, other agents, rubella, cytomegalovirus and herpes simplex) syndrome] and familial.

- *Acquired*:
  - Age: Elderly
  - Metabolic: Diabetes mellitus, galactosemia, hypocalcemia and Wilson's disease
  - Drug-induced: Corticosteroids, phenothiazines and amiodarone
  - Traumatic: Direct intraocular injury to the lens and post-intraocular surgery
  - Inflammatory: Uveitis
  - Hereditary: Down syndrome, dystrophia myotonica and Lowe syndrome.

Clinical features: Painless gradual dimness of vision, halos around light and diplopia.

Investigations:
- Preoperative evaluation of visual acuity, papillary reaction, fundus evaluation, intraocular pressure, and lacrimal sac assessment
- Blood sugar, electrocardiography (ECG) and conjunctival swab for C/S.

Treatment:
- Extracapsular cataract extraction (ECCE)
- Small-incision cataract surgery (SICS) with PCIOL
- *Phacoemulsification (PHACO) and PCIOL*: The surgery may be done as day care
- Femtosecond laser-assisted cataract surgery.

GLAUCOMA

It is a disease characterized by increased intraocular pressure within the eyeball that leads to damage to the optic disc with gradual loss of vision.

Types:
- *Congenital*: May be primary and secondary
- *Acquired*:
  - Open-angle glaucoma: Primary open-angle glaucoma (POAG), secondary open-angle glaucoma, normal tension glaucoma, juvenile open angle glaucoma and ocular HTN
  - Angle-closure glaucoma: Primary angle-closure glaucoma (PACG) and secondary angle-closure glaucoma and (SACG)
  - Primary angle-closure glaucoma is most dangerous as it may present as an acute attack.

Primary Open-angle Glaucoma

Primary open-angle glaucoma is the common type of glaucoma. HOP result from reduced outflow of aqueous humor through the trabecular meshwork.

Common risk factors: After 40 years, race (more in black), positive family history, HTN and retinal disease (central retinal vein occlusion and retinitis pigmentosa). Common in high myopic eye.

Clinical features: Usually asymptomatic. There is gradual loss of peripheral visual field and loss of vision, identified during a routine ophthalmic examination. There is raised IOP and optic disc shows enlarged cup with thin neuroretinal rim and visual field defect.

Treatment: Aims to reduce the IOP, either by reducing aqueous production or by increasing aqueous drainage.

- *Medical*: Timolol one drop 12 hourly, dorzolamide one drop 8 hourly, and brimonidine
- *Surgical*: Trabeculectomy and selective laser trabeculoplasty (SLT).

Acute Angle-closure Glaucoma

Acute angle-closure glaucoma (AACG) is an ophthalmic emergency. There is sudden rise in intraocular pressure over 50 mm Hg. This occurs due to reduced aqueous drainage due to narrow angle, when the ageing lens pushes the iris forward against trabecular meshwork.

People mostly at risk are those with shallow anterior chambers such as hypermetropes and women. The attack is more likely to occur under reduced light conditions when the pupil is dilated.

Clinical features: Sudden severe painful red eye, blurring of vision, nausea, vomiting and severe headache, photophobia and lacrimation.

On examination:
- Eye lid edematous
- *Conjunctiva*: Ciliary congestion and chemosis
- Cornea is hazy, edematous and insensitive
- Pupil is semidilated and nonreactive to light and accommodation
- Shallow anterior chamber
- Intraocular pressure very high, 50–100 mm Hg.

Treatment:
- Immediate hospitalization
- Tablet acetazolamide 500 mg stat, then one tablet four times daily
- Topical pilocarpine, two drops to both eye 8 hourly
- Dexamethasone eye drop one drop 6 hourly
- *Antiglaucoma eye drop*: Timolol/dorzolamide/brimonidine, one drop 12 hourly
- Systemic analgesics and antiemetics may be given
- *After 1 hour*: Pilocarpine continued 6 hourly until pupil constricted
- *If no response, usually after 48 hours, surgical management*:
  ○ Laser peripheral iridotomy in both eyes
  ○ If synechia is more than 50%, or IOP >35 mm Hg, then trabeculectomy under IV mannitol coverage.

Primary Angle-closure Glaucoma

Elevation of IOP occurs as a result of obstruction of aqueous outflow by partial or complete closure of the angle by the peripheral iris. Risk factors are—age above 60 years, more in females, and positive family history. Also it is precipitated by working in dark place, prolong close work, watching cinema and TV in dark room.

Treatment: Medical treatment (as for POAG) and surgical (consider lens extraction and/or trabeculectomy). Laser peripheral iridotomy to prevent attack until surgery.

CHAPTER 21

Diseases of the Ear, Nose and Throat

OTALGIA (EARACHE)

It means pain in the ear, which can be due to local cause in the ear or referred cause from other sites.

Causes:
- *External ear*: Furuncle, impacted wax, otitis externa, otomycosis, myringitis bullosa, herpes zoster and malignant neoplasms
- *Middle ear*: Acute otitis media, eustachian tube obstruction, mastoiditis, extradural abscess, aero-otitis media, and carcinoma of middle ear.

Referred causes:
- *Tooth*: Caries tooth, apical tooth abscess, impacted molar teeth, malocclusion, gingivitis and ill-fitting denture
- *Tongue or oral cavity*: Ulcer, glossitis, malignancy and tuberculosis (TB)
- *Temporomandibular joint disorders*: Osteoarthritis, recurrent dislocation and rheumatoid arthritis
- *Tonsil*: Acute tonsillitis, peritonsillar abscess, benign or malignant ulcers of soft palate, and tonsil and its pillars
- *Throat*:
  - Pharynx: Pharyngeal abscess (parapharyngeal and retropharyngeal), ulcer, foreign body (FB), and malignancy
  - Larynx: Epiglottitis, laryngeal edema, TB laryngitis, and malignancy.
- *Others*: Acute maxillary sinusitis, nasal and maxillary malignant growth, elongated styloid process, cervical spondylosis, and injuries of cervical spine.

Note: Remember the formula: "*5T-O*" (*T*ooth, *T*ongue or oral cavity, *T*emporomandibular joint disorders, *T*onsil, *T*hroat and *O*thers).

EAR WAX

It is the mixture of secretion of ceruminous and pilosebaceous glands in which desquamated keratin debris, dust, and broken hair are added. It is usually asymptomatic or there may be blockage feeling, itching, irritation, deafness (when wax blocks external auditory canal), earache, tinnitus and vertigo.

Treatment: Removal of wax. If hard and impacted, first softening with solvent (liquid paraffin, wax soap, and olive oil), then removal by aural syringing with sterile water. If not possible, it can be removed by ring probe or Hartmann aural forceps or wax hook for dry wax.

FOREIGN BODY IN EAR

It may be nonliving or living FB.
- *Nonliving FB*: It is common in children. Piece of paper, grain (rice and wheat), and metallic parts. In adults, broken matchsticks or cotton bar. FB should be removed with forceps, in some case, syringing and suction may be needed. Rounded FB should be removed with hook
- *Living FB*: Flies, mosquito, ant and cockroach. First the insect should be killed, then removed. For killing of living object, oily solution is better
- In some cases, maggots (larva of flies) may be found in the ear. Before removal, these should be killed by chloroform, turpin oil, and water instillation, and then removed by forceps.

TEAR OR TRAUMATIC RUPTURE OF TYMPANIC MEMBRANE

Injury to the tympanic membrane may be due to:
- Pricking the ear by match sticks, hair pin, pencil and cotton bar (common cause)
- Trauma during removal of FB
- Slapping, blast injury, and head injury
- Rapid descent in a nonpressurized aircraft
- Forceful inflation of eustachian tube.

Features: Acute pain at the time of rupture, conductive type of deafness (mild to moderate), tinnitus (may be persistent in cochlear damage), and rarely vertigo. On examination, tear in the tympanic membrane or bleeding from ear may be visible (blood clot may be found in the meatus).

Treatment: Avoid cleaning of the ear, syringing, ear drops, swimming or bathing in ponds. Most cases heal rapidly. Nasal decongestant and antibiotic may be needed. If fails to heal, myringoplasty may be needed.

OTITIS EXTERNA

It is the acute or chronic infection of skin of external ear. It may be localized (furuncle) or generalized or diffused. It may spread to pinna and epidermal layer of tympanic membrane.

Causes:
- *Trauma to the ear canal*: Scratching with cotton bar, hair pins or match sticks, instrument to remove FBs, and cleaning of ear canal
- *Invasion by organism such as*: Bacteria (*Staphylococcus aureus*, *Pseudomonas pyocyaneus*, *Bacillus proteus*, and *Escherichia coli*), fungus (otomycosis), and viral (herpes zoster, herpes simplex, and bullous myringitis)
- *Reactive otitis externa*: Eczematous or seborrheic otitis externa, and keratosis obturans.

Note: Diabetics and immunosuppressed patients can develop severe necrotizing otitis externa.

Clinical features:
- *Acute otitis externa (<6 weeks duration)*: Ear pain often severe, discharge which may be offensive, and hearing loss. Pre or postauricular lymphadenopathy may be present. Ear canal looks red, swollen and inflamed. Moving pinna may be painful
- *Chronic otitis externa (>3 months duration)*: Persistent discharge from the ear, hearing loss, and canal stenosis may occur.

Investigation: Swab for culture and sensitivity (C/S) if any discharge. Complete blood count (CBC), erythrocyte sedimentation rate (ESR), and blood sugar.

Treatment:
- *Analgesics*: Paracetamol, ibuprofen *or* other nonsteroidal anti-inflammatory drug (NSAID), if pain
- *Topical antibiotics and/or steroid drops*: Dexamethasone 0.05%, framycetin sulfate 0.5%, gramicidin 0.005%, hydrocortisone acetate 1% *or* gentamicin 0.3%
- *Broad-spectrum systemic antibiotics*: For cellulitis and acute tender lymphadenitis
- Ear toileting. If needed, careful removal of exudates and debris.

FURUNCULOSIS

It means boil in the ear canal, usually by *Staphylococcus*. Pain in the ear, more by movement of the pinna, pressure on tragus, jaw movements, and chewing. Mild deafness due to meatal occlusion.

Treatment: If no surrounding cellulitis, analgesic, hot compression, and topical antibiotics. Ear wick with glycerine-soaked pack. If surrounding cellulitis, flucloxacillin 250–500 mg 6 hourly for 7 days. If abscess, incision and drainage.

OTOMYCOSIS

It is the fungal infection of external auditory canal due to *Aspergillus niger*, *Aspergillus fumigatus* or *Candida albicans*. It is found in hot and humid climate, may be caused by use of topical antibiotics.

Features: Itching, pain, watery and purulent discharge with musty odor, blockage of ear, and deafness. Fungal mass looks greyish-white or black like filter paper.

Diagnosis: Microscopic examination of ear swab is confirmatory.

Treatment: Removal of fungal mass. Ear toileting, local antifungal nystatin, clotrimazole, povidone iodine, and 2% salicylic acid in alcohol, may be given. If bacterial infection, topical antibiotic, amphotericin B, with steroid may be used. Perchloride of mercury in alcohol 1:4,000 (adult) and 1:8,000 for child is another best option.

ACUTE SUPPURATIVE OTITIS MEDIA

It is the acute inflammation of middle ear by pyogenic organisms. It is common in children <10 years of age, mostly in lower socio-economic group, bath in unhygienic and contaminated water.

Predisposing factors: Recurrent common cold, upper respiratory tract infection (URTI), nasal allergy, enlarged adenoid, tonsillitis, sinusitis, measles, diphtheria, whooping cough, rhinitis, tumors or polyp of nasopharynx, and cleft palate.

Common organisms: *Streptococcus pneumoniae, Haemophilus influenzae,* and *Moraxella catarrhalis.* Other are *Streptococcus pyogenes, S. aureus,* and *Pseudomonas aeruginosa.*

Stages with features: There are five stages.
1. *Stage of tubal occlusion*: Due to edema and hyperemia of nasopharyngeal end of eustachian tube. There may be mild deafness and earache, but no fever. Tympanic membrane is retracted, lusterless, and there may be some effusion. Tuning fork test shows conductive deafness
2. *Stage of presuppuration or exudation*: Inflammatory exudate in middle ear and tympanic membrane is congested. Severe throbbing earache, deafness, and tinnitus may be present. High fever and restlessness in children. Tympanic membrane is uniformly red. Tuning fork tests shows conductive deafness
3. *Stage of suppuration*: Formation of pus in middle ear, also in mastoid air cells. There is severe earache and deafness. In children, high fever, vomiting, and convulsion. Tympanic membrane is red and bulged with loss of landmarks. There is tenderness over mastoid antrum. A yellow spot may be seen on tympanic membrane when rupture is imminent. X-ray of mastoid will show clouding of air cells due to exudate. With rupture of tympanic membrane, symptoms subsides, and pain diminishes with release of pus
4. *Stage of resolution*: If proper treatment is started early or if mild infection, resolution may start even without rupture of tympanic membrane. External auditory canal may contain blood-stained discharge. Tympanic membrane color becomes normal. If perforation, discharge subsides and it may heal up. Sometimes, dry perforation may persist
5. *Stage of complication*: If failure of resolution, there may be acute mastoiditis, subperiosteal abscess, facial paralysis, labyrinthitis, petrositis, extradural abscess, meningitis, brain abscess or lateral sinus thrombophlebitis.

Treatment:
- *For pain*: Paracetamol *or* NSAID
- *Antibiotic*: Amoxicillin *or* ampicillin for 10 days. Cefuroxime, cefixime *or* erythromycin may be used
- *Decongestant nasal drops*: Oxymetazoline *or* xylometazoline
- *Oral nasal decongestant*: Pseudoephedrine alone *or* with antihistamine
- *Others*: Dry local heat, ear toilet, and helps to relieve pain
- *Surgery*: Myringotomy (incision of the drum to remove pus).

CHRONIC SUPPURATIVE OTITIS MEDIA

It is the long-standing infection of a part or whole of the middle ear cleft, characterized by ear discharge, permanent perforation, and conductive hearing loss.

Organisms: *P. aeruginosa, Proteus, E. coli, S. aureus, Bacteroides fragilis* and anaerobic streptococci.

Causes: It may be due to sequelae of acute otitis media, inadequate or inappropriate antibiotic therapy, upper airway sepsis, malnutrition, anemia, immunosuppression, measles and cholesteatoma.

Types: Clinically, it is divided into two types—
1. *Tubotympanic (central perforation)*: Also called *safe* or *benign* type. It involves anteroinferior part of middle ear cleft. No risk of serious complications
2. *Atticoantral or tympanomastoid (attic or marginal perforation)*: Also called *unsafe* or *dangerous* type. It involves posterosuperior part of cleft, associated with attic or marginal perforation. Risk of complications are more, may be associated with cholesteatoma, granulation or osteitis.

Clinical features:
- *Ear discharge*: In tubotympanic, profuse, nonoffensive, mucoid or mucopurulent. In atticoantral, scanty, purulent and foul smelling
- *Hearing loss*: Conductive type. It may be mixed in atticoantral
- *Perforation*: Central in tubotympanic, attic or marginal in atticoantral
- Cholesteatoma present in atticoantral variety.

Investigations: The C/S of ear discharge, audiogram, mastoid X-ray, and computed tomography (CT) scan of temporal bone.

Treatment:
- Thorough and regular aural toileting with antiseptic solution. If not available, then with hydrogen peroxide
- *Ear drop*: Antibiotic ear drop such as neomycin, gentamicin, polymyxin and chloromycetin with steroid drop
- Systemic antibiotic, if needed
- *Decongestant nasal drops*: Oxymetazoline or xylometazoline
- *Surgery*: It is the mainstay of treatment in atticoantral variety. Atticotomy and modified radical mastoidectomy may be done
- After primary treatment, hearing can be restored by reconstructive surgery (tympanoplasty or myringoplasty) in both types.

Complications:
- *Extracranial*: Acute mastoiditis, subperiosteal abscess, facial nerve paralysis, labyrinthitis, petrositis, osteomyelitis of temporal bone, septicemia, pyemia and otogenic tetanus
- *Intracranial*: Extradural or subdural abscess, meningitis, perisinus abscess, brain abscess, sigmoid sinus thrombosis, otitic hydrocephalus, and encephalitis.

ACUTE MASTOIDITIS

It is the inflammation of mucosal lining of air cell (both antrum and mastoid), invariably accompanied with acute suppurative otitis media (ASOM), common in children, caused by *Streptococcus* beta-hemolytic.

Symptoms: Pain behind the ear, creamy and profuse ear discharge, fever, and increasing deafness.

Signs: Tenderness and swelling over mastoid. Tympanic membrane is red, bulged or may be perforated. If tympanic membrane is normal, the patient does not have acute mastoiditis.

Investigation: CBC (high neutrophil). CT scan shows opacity and air cell coalescence.

Treatment:
- Hospital admission immediately after diagnosis
- *Broad-spectrum antibiotic*: Start amoxicillin or ampicillin. According to C/S. Metronidazole orally and chloramphenicol ear drop is added
- *Surgery*: Myringotomy to drain pus. Cortical mastoidectomy, if subperiosteal abscess or no rapid response or if leading to complication.

OTOSCLEROSIS

It is the abnormal bone remodeling of middle ear, in which new bony deposits occur within the stapes footplate and cochlea, causing ankylosis or fixation. Usually bilateral, starts unilaterally, may be hereditary, more in female, common in second and third decade, and worse during pregnancy.

Features: Progressive deafness, which is usually bilateral. May be tinnitus, paracusis, and giddiness. Stapedotomy or stapedectomy may be done with replacement by prosthesis. Hearing aid is an alternative.

PRESBYCUSIS

It is a degenerative disorder of cochlea, also called senile deafness. It is the common cause of sensorineural deafness in elderly (>60 years). It may be due to loss of outer hair cells (sensory), loss of ganglion cells (neural) or strial atrophy (metabolic), or mixed.

Audiometry: Bilateral symmetrical high frequency sensorineural hearing loss (SNHL) is the diagnostic criteria.

There is gradual deafness and higher frequencies are affected most. Patient cannot tolerate high-pitched sound and speech. Treatment is high-frequency specific hearing aid.

CHOLESTEATOMA

It means presence of keratinizing squamous epithelium within the middle ear or mastoid. May present with foul-smelling otorrhea. Examination shows defect in tympanic membrane, with white and cheesy material. It can erode local structures such as ossicles or facial nerve, may extend intracranially to cause meningitis or intracranial abscess. Treatment is mastoid surgery to remove the sac of squamous debris and reconstruction of ossicle and tympanic grafting.

DEAFNESS

It means impairment of hearing. It is mainly of three types—conductive, sensorineural and mixed.

Conductive deafness: It means deafness due to any disease process which interferes with conduction of sound to reach cochlea.

Causes:
- *Congenital*: Atresia or microtia of external ear, Treacher-Collins syndrome, ossicular chain deformity, fused ossicles, and congenital otosclerosis
- *Acquired*: Impacted wax or FB, otitis externa, bullous myringitis, traumatic rupture of tympanic membrane, trauma to middle ear,

ossicular dislocation, ASOM, chronic suppurative otitis media (CSOM), secretory otitis media, otosclerosis, TB or syphilitic otitis media, neoplasm, eustachian tube obstruction, dysfunction, barotrauma, enlarged adenoid, and growth in nasopharynx.

Sensorineural: It results from lesions of cochlea, vestibulocochlear nerve or central auditory pathways. It may be congenital or acquired.
- *Congenital*: Pendred syndrome, Waardenburg syndrome, Klippel–Feil syndrome, congenital rubella, congenital syphilis, prolonged labor, perinatal hypoxia, premature birth, and phenylketonuria
- *Acquired*: Infections of labyrinth, trauma to labyrinth or 8th nerve, noise-induced hearing loss, ototoxic drugs, presbycusis, Ménière's disease, acoustic neuroma, sudden hearing loss, familial progressive SNHL, and systemic disorders [diabetes mellitus (DM), hypothyroidism, kidney disease, autoimmune disorders, multiple sclerosis, and blood dyscrasias].

Mixed: Where both conductive and sensorineural deafness occurs. It may be due to blast injury, CSOM, otosclerosis and presbycusis.

Others: Psychological deafness [hysterical conversion reaction (HCR) and malingering].

Investigation:
- *Rinne test*: In conductive deafness, bone conduction is more than air conduction (BC > AC), but in sensorineural, AC is more than BC (AC > BC)
- *Weber test*: Lateralized to diseased ear in conductive and lateralized to better ear in sensorineural deafness
- Audiometry
- X-ray of temporal or mastoid bone, CT scan or magnetic resonance imaging (MRI)
- *Audiological basic investigations*: Pure tone audiometry (PTA), impedance and speech recognition threshold (SRT)
- *Others*: Blood sugar, thyroid function, Venereal Disease Research Laboratory (VDRL), and *Treponema pallidum* hemagglutination assay (TPHA), according to cause.

NOSE

Foreign Body in the Nose

It is common in children. Pieces of paper, chalk, button, pebbles and seeds are common. Unilateral nasal discharge which is often foul smelling and occasionally bloodstained. Pieces of paper or cotton swabs can be easily removed with forceps. In babies and uncooperative children, general anesthesia may be needed, if impacted. Its complications are nasal infection, sinusitis, rhinolith formation, and inhalation into the tracheobronchial tree.

Sinusitis

It is an infection of paranasal sinuses due to bacterial (*S. pneumoniae* and *H. influenzae*) or occasionally fungal. It is commonly associated with URTI and bronchial asthma. There are four types:
1. *Acute sinusitis*: 1 week to 1 month
2. *Recurrent acute sinusitis*: >4 episodes of acute sinusitis per year

3. *Subacute sinusitis*: 1–3 months
4. *Chronic sinusitis*: >3 months.

Acute Sinusitis

Acute inflammation of mucosa of paranasal sinus is called acute sinusitis. It is common in maxillary, ethmoid, frontal and sphenoid sinus.

Causes: Most cases of acute sinusitis are secondary to—
- Nasal infections, common cold, influenza, measles and whooping cough
- *Nasal obstructions*: Deviated nasal septum (DNS), nasal polyp, hypertrophied turbinates, nasal packing, FB and enlarged adenoid
- *Dental*: Apical abscess, periodontal abscess, and dental extraction
- *Trauma or injury to sinus*: Fracture and gunshot wound
- *Predisposing factors*: Cold and wet environment by smoke, dust fume, overcrowding and occasionally by swimming and diving in water.

Symptoms:
- History of URTI, dental infection or recent extraction
- Pain over the sinus, often referred to supraorbital region. Pain is usually throbbing and is aggravated by bending, coughing or walking
- Adults usually present with nasal blockage or congestion with discharge, headache, dental or facial pain or pressure, reduction or loss of sense of smell or altered smell
- Children often present with nonspecific symptoms like URTI, nasal blockage or congestion, discolored nasal discharge, and cough during day or night.

Signs:
- Tenderness over the sinuses and on percussion of upper teeth
- Mucopus in nose or nasopharynx. Nasal mucosa is congested
- X-ray shows opacity or a fluid level in the antrum. CT scan shows fluid level or opacity, or mucosal thickening within the sinus.

Treatment: Most cases resolve spontaneously in 7–10 days.
- Steam inhalation
- *Antibiotics*: Co-amoxiclav *or* cephalexin, ampicillin, amoxicillin, azithromycin and moxifloxacin
- *Analgesic*: Paracetamol, ibuprofen *or* other NSAID
- *Nasal decongestant*: 1% ephedrine *or* 0.05% oxymetazoline
- *Steroid nasal sprays*: Fluticasone propionate *or* beclomethasone two puffs each nostril 12 hourly
- If not relieved, sinus is punctured under local anesthesia and drained out.

Chronic Sinusitis

Sinusitis lasting for months or years is called chronic sinusitis.

Causes:
- Repeated attack of acute sinusitis, and upper and lower respiratory tract infection
- *Nasal obstructions*: DNS, nasal polyp, hypertrophy turbinates, nasal packing, FB, and enlarged adenoid
- *Others*: Allergic rhinitis, chronic dental sepsis, poor nutrition, air pollution, and damp environment.

Common organisms are *H. influenzae, S. aureus,* gram-negative *Proteus, E. coli, Klebsiella, P. aeruginosa,* and fungal.

Features: Nasal obstruction, headache, dull ache over the sinus, foul-smelling discharge, and epistaxis.

Investigation: X-ray of paranasal sinus (PNS) and CT scan is more diagnostic.

Treatment: Conservative, as in acute sinusitis. If fails, surgery should be done.

Epistaxis

Bleeding from nose is called epistaxis. Little's area is a frequent site of epistaxis for children.

Causes:
- *Local*: Trauma (foreign bodies, nose-picking, and nasal fractures), iatrogenic (surgery and intranasal steroids), DNS, neoplasm (nasal, paranasal sinus, nasopharyngeal), and idiopathic
- *General*: Severe hypertension, anticoagulants or antiplatelet agents, coagulation disorders (hemophilia and Christmas disease), and Osler–Weber–Rendu syndrome (familial hemorrhagic telangiectasia)
- Spontaneous epistaxis is common in children and young adults. It arises from Little's area, may be precipitated by infection or minor trauma, easy to stop, and tends to recur.

Treatment:
- *Immediate first aid measures*: External digital compression of anterior lower portion of external nose, ice packs, and leaning forward. The patient should avoid swallowing of blood, as this causes nausea
- Anterior or posterior nasal pack. If not improved, simple local anesthetic cautery with silver nitrate stick
- *If bleeding continues*: Resuscitation with intravenous (IV) fluid *or* blood transfusion and oxygen inhalation
- Treatment of cause, if any (control of hypertension, stop antiplatelet *or* anticoagulant)
- If the above treatments fail, endoscopic cauterization, endoscopic sphenopalatine artery ligation *or* interventional arterial embolization can be done.

Rhinitis

It is defined as sneezing, nasal discharge or nasal blockage. It may be seasonal (only certain times of the year), perennial (all year), intermittent (<4 days/week or <4 weeks at a time) or persistent.

Causes:
- *Allergic*: Allergen such as pollen, animal dander, fungi or molds, and occupational allergens (flour, latex)
- *Nonallergic*: Vasomotor, triggered by physical or chemical agents such as cold air, tobacco, perfume, and drug-induced.

Symptoms: Nasal discharge, itching, sneezing with or without nasal blockage or congestion. It may be tiredness, fever, malaise, sore nose, and pharynx.

Investigation: CBC shows high eosinophil, serum immunoglobulin E (IgE) (raised), and skin prick test may detect allergen. X-ray of PNS or CT scan.

Treatment:
- Avoid allergen exposure
- Saline nose drops and steam inhalation
- *Antihistamine*: Effective against sneezing and itching of eyes and palate
- *Decongestants*: Xylometazoline and oxymetazoline nasal drops or sprays
- *Anti-inflammatory drugs*: Topical corticosteroid, e.g. beclometasone, fluticasone propionate, fluticasone furoate or mometasone furoate spray
- *Leukotriene antagonists*: Montelukast 10 mg daily in the evening
- *Immunotherapy*: Patients with seasonal allergic rhinitis not responding to standard drugs can be given oral and injectable vaccines
- *Surgery*: In some cases, reduction of nasal turbinate, submucosal diathermy, and surface electrocautery may be done.

Nasal Polyps

It means non-neoplastic masses of edematous nasal or sinus mucosa. There are two types:
1. Ethmoidal polyp
2. Antrochoanal polyp.

Causes: Chronic rhinosinusitis, bronchial asthma, aspirin intolerance, cystic fibrosis, allergic fungal sinusitis, Kartagener's syndrome, Young syndrome, Churg–Strauss syndrome, nasal mastocytosis, and neoplasm.

Features: Nasal blockage or nasal stuffiness, loss of sense of smell (partial or total), sneezing and watery nasal discharge due to allergy, epistaxis and headache due to sinusitis. Change in voice. Reddish mass may be seen protruding from nostril.

Management:
- *Topical steroid*: Nasal drops (fluticasone) until polyps shrink (maximum 1 month), then steroid nasal spray to prevent recurrence
- *Antibiotics*: If purulent nasal discharge
- *Surgical*: Polypectomy, if medical treatment fails. May be simple polypectomy or FESS (functional endoscopic sinus surgery).

Anosmia and Hyposmia

Anosmia is the complete loss of sense of smell and hyposmia means partial loss of sense of smell.

Causes: Nasal obstruction due to upper respiratory infection and nasal polyps.

Others: Sinonasal disease, old age, drug therapy, head injury, trauma and idiopathic. Hyposmia is common in elderly, postmenopausal and smokers.

Treatment: According to cause.

Deviated Nasal Septum

It may be due to trauma or developmental anomaly. It may be associated with external deformity. It occurs at any age and any sex, but more in males and adults. It is usually asymptomatic. It may cause unilateral nasal blockage, anosmia, nasal obstruction, sinusitis, epistaxis and headache.

Treatment: If asymptomatic, no treatment. If troublesome symptoms, surgery may be necessary (submucosal resection or septoplasty).

Septal Perforation

It can cause bleeding, crusting and discomfort. Its causes are trauma, nose picking, cocaine use, postoperative and delayed drainage of septal abscess. Rarely in syphilis, malignancy and systemic lupus erythematosus (SLE).

Treatment: No treatment if asymptomatic, otherwise treat symptomatically (e.g. Vaseline or Naseptin nasal cream for crusting). Surgical closure is often not successful. Refer to ENT specialist, if suspicion of malignancy.

Snoring

It is an undesirable disturbing nasal sound that occurs during sleep.

Causes:
- *In children*: DNS and adenotonsillar hypertrophy
- *In elderly*: No obvious cause. It may be due to DNS, hypertrophied turbinate, sleep apnea, obesity and abnormal faciomaxillary bone development, and short neck.

Treatment: If any, treatment of primary cause. Surgical correction (in children, removal of enlarged adenoid and correction of DNS). Sometimes uvulopalatopharyngoplasty may be done. In sleep apnea, continuous positive airway pressure (CPAP) or bilevel positive airway pressure (BiPAP) machine may be used for adult.

THROAT

Tonsillitis

Acute tonsillitis: Acute inflammation of palatine tonsil. Children and young adults are prone to infection. It may be acute parenchymous and acute follicular type.

Causes:
- *Bacterial*: Streptococcus beta-hemolyticus, *S. aureus*, *Haemophilus* and *Pneumococcus*
- *Viral*: Influenza, parainfluenza, adenovirus and rhinovirus.

Symptoms: Sore throat, difficulty in swallowing, high fever, headache and earache.

Signs: Tonsils are enlarged and congested. Fetid breath (foul-smelling breath due to pus). Enlarged, tender jugulodigastric or tonsillar lymph node. Pseudomembrane may be found in streptococcal tonsillitis (yellowish, thin and can be removed easily with swab).

Investigation: CBC with ESR and throat swab for C/S.

Treatment:
- *General treatment*: Bed rest, soft diet, fluid intake, and warm saline gurgling
- *Specific treatment*: Systemic antibiotic. Penicillin is the drug of choice. Oral penicillin-V 250 mg 6 hourly for 5–7 days. In severe case, broad-spectrum antibiotic, amoxicillin, cephalexin, erythromycin and roxithromycin
- *Analgesics and antipyretics*: Paracetamol, ibuprofen or other NSAID.

Chronic tonsillitis: Chronic inflammation of palatine tonsil in which inflammation and repair occurs simultaneously.

Types: There are two types—Chronic parenchymatous (common in children and adolescents) and chronic fibrotic (common in elderly).

Features: Repeated sore throat, difficulty in swallowing, irritating cough, and earache. Tonsils are enlarged and fibrotic, nontender bilateral enlarged jugulodigastric lymph node, and inspissated pus may come out on pressing the anterior pillar.

Investigations: CBC with ESR, throat swab for C/S.

Treatment: Tonsillectomy under general anesthesia (GA), if conservative treatment fails and proper indication is there. Bronchial asthma and severe allergic rhinitis, and it is better to avoid operative treatment.

Peritonsillar Abscess

It means collection of pus in peritonsillar space which lies between the capsule of tonsil and superior constrictor muscle. It usually follows acute tonsillitis, may be caused by *S. pyogenes*, *S. aureus* or anaerobic organisms. Features are high fever with chills and rigor, severe throat pain, pain during swallowing, foul-smelling breath, ipsilateral ear pain, trismus, malaise, body ache, headache and nausea. The tonsil, pillars and soft palate on the involved side are congested and swollen. Uvula is swollen and edematous and cervical lymphadenopathy is common.

Treatment: Hospitalization, IV fluids, and broad-spectrum IV antibiotic. NSAID, and sometimes pethidine may be required. Oral hygiene should be maintained.

Tumor of Tonsil

Commonly squamous cell carcinoma. May be adenocarcinoma, lymphoma, and sarcoma.

Features: It is common in elderly, present with sore throat or FB sensation in throat, dysphagia, earache and speech abnormality. Unilateral enlargement of tonsil or ugly ulcer over one tonsil.
Diagnosis by fine-needle aspiration cytology (FNAC) and biopsy.

Treatment: Early stage and tonsillectomy. In advanced stage, tonsillectomy with block dissection of cervical node, followed by radio and chemotherapy.

Enlarged Adenoid

It is a nasopharyngeal mass of lymphoid tissue, situated in posterosuperior wall. It is common in children.

Features: Nasal obstruction, mouth breathing, nasal voice, snoring, earache, may be otitis media, mouth breathing, drooling of saliva, may be chronic pharyngitis, and laryngitis. Mouth is always open. General features are pinched nose, loss of nasolabial furrow, and dribbling of saliva. Soft tissue X-ray of nasopharynx shows the enlarged adenoid. Adenoidectomy is the treatment of choice.

Hoarseness (Dysphonia)

It means change in quality of voice affecting pitch, volume or resonance. It occurs when vocal cord function is affected by local, neurological or muscular problems.

Causes:
- *Local*: URTI (common), excessive use of voice (singers, teachers and politicians), laryngitis, epiglottitis, acute laryngotracheobronchitis, trauma (shouting, coughing, vomiting and instrumentation), and carcinoma
- *Systemic disease*: Hypothyroidism and acromegaly
- *Neurological*: Laryngeal nerve palsy, motor neuron disease, myasthenia gravis, and multiple sclerosis
- *Muscular*: Muscular dystrophy
- *Functional*: HCR.

Acute Pharyngitis

It means acute inflammation of pharynx.

Causes:
- *Infection*: Viral (rhinovirus, influenza, parainfluenza, measles, chickenpox, coxsackie, herpes simplex, infectious mononucleosis, and cytomegalovirus), bacterial (Group A beta-hemolytic *Streptococcus*, diphtheria, *Gonococcus* and *Chlamydia*), and fungal (*Candida*)
- *Others*: Vincent's angina (due to gram-negative fusiform bacilli and spirochaetes) and hematological (agranulocytosis, acute leukemia, and aplastic anemia).

Investigation: Throat swab for C/S, CBC and ESR.

Treatment: Complete bed rest, antibiotic, analgesic for fever and pain, and maintenance of oral hygiene.

Chronic Pharyngitis

Causes:
- Mouth breathing
- Recurrent acute pharyngitis, after tonsillectomy, and allergy
- Chronic rhinitis, sinusitis, chronic tonsillitis, and dental sepsis
- Chronic irritants. Excessive smoking, chewing of tobacco and betel nut, heavy drinking or highly spiced food
- *Environmental pollution*: Smoke, dust or irritant industrial fumes

Treatment: Antiseptic or warm saline gurgling, and treatment of primary cause.

Acute Laryngitis

It is the acute superficial and catarrhal inflammation of laryngeal mucosa.

Causes:
- *Infectious*: Upper respiratory infection such as viral (influenza, measles and chickenpox) and bacterial (*S. pneumoniae*, *H. influenzae*, beta-hemolytic *Streptococcus*, *S. aureus* and whooping cough)
- *Noninfectious*: Excessive use of voice, smoking, allergy, inhalation of fume or gas, laryngeal trauma, and endotracheal intubation.

Features: Hoarseness or complete loss of voice, discomfort or pain in throat, dry cough worse at night, dryness of throat, malaise and fever. Vocal cords are red and swollen. It is diagnosed by indirect and fiber-optic laryngoscopy.

Treatment: Vocal rest, steam inhalations (also menthol or tincture benzene), avoidance of smoking, and alcohol. Cough suppressant, antihistamine and nasal decongestant may be used. Antibiotic, if secondary infection. Sometimes steroids may be given following thermal and chemical burn.

Chronic Laryngitis

It is a chronic diffuse symmetrical or localized inflammation of larynx.

Causes:
- Excessive or faulty use of voice (actors, singers and teachers)
- Chronic exposure to dust and fumes, smoking or alcohol
- *Sequelae* of acute laryngitis or recurrent laryngitis
- Chronic infection in paranasal sinuses, teeth, tonsils, lungs and laryngeal TB.

Features: Hoarseness, dry cough, and discomfort in throat. Vocal cords are red, swollen and may be nodular. It is diagnosed by indirect and fiber-optic laryngoscopy.

Treatment: Voice rest, speech therapy, and steam inhalation with menthol should be started. Avoid smoking, alcohol, dust and fumes. Treatment of primary cause. Stripping of vocal cords, and removal of hyperplastic and edematous mucosa may be done.

Acute Epiglottitis

It is the acute inflammation of supraglottic structures such as epiglottis, aryepiglottic folds, and arytenoid cartilage. It is common in children of 2–7 years of age, but can also affect adults. *H. influenzae* is common organism.

Features: Pain on swallowing, dyspnea, which is rapidly progressive, stridor and high fever. Epiglottis is red and swollen, may be edema and congestion of supraglottic structure. X-ray of neck lateral view may show swollen epiglottis (thumb sign).

Treatment: Immediate hospitalization. Death may occur if delayed treatment. Antibiotics (IV ampicillin or ceftriaxone) should be started immediately. IV hydrocortisone or dexamethasone to relieve edema. Intubation or tracheostomy, if respiratory obstruction. Steam inhalation, voice rest, and IV infusion.

Acute Laryngotracheobronchitis

It is an acute inflammation of larynx and tracheobronchial tree. It is common in children between 6 months and 3 years of age, mostly viral (parainfluenza type I and II), and also bacterial (*Streptococcus* and *H. influenzae*).

Features are croupy cough, hoarseness, high fever, difficulty in breathing, may be cyanosis, and collapse. Indirect laryngoscopy shows congested and edematous larynx, and dry crust over glottis and subglottis. Swab C/S from larynx may be done.

Treatment: Broad-spectrum parenteral antibiotic. Steroid may be given. If respiratory distress, tracheostomy should be done.

Carcinoma Larynx

Common in male, fifth to sixth decade. Causes are smoking, alcohol, previous radiation to neck, genetic factors, occupational exposure to asbestos, mustard gas or other chemical and petroleum products.

Anatomically, there are three types—supraglottic, glottic (common), subglottic (or infraglottic), and transglottic. Histologically, 90-95% are squamous cell carcinoma. 5-10% are verrucous carcinoma, spindle cell carcinoma, and sarcomas.

Symptoms:
- *Supraglottic*: Usually asymptomatic. There may be throat pain, dysphagia, and cervical lymphadenopathy. Hoarseness, weight loss, respiratory obstruction, and halitosis are late features
- *Glottic*: Hoarseness of voice, stridor and laryngeal obstruction
- *Subglottic*: Hemoptysis is common, may be stridor, and laryngeal obstruction. Hoarseness is a late feature.

Signs: Raised nodule, may be ulcerative, and vocal cords may be fixed.

Investigation:
- Flexible fiber-optic or rigid laryngoscopy or video laryngoscopy or direct laryngoscopy
- X-ray of chest, X-ray of neck lateral view, CT scan, and MRI
- Biopsy and histopathology.

Treatment: Radiotherapy or surgery or both or surgery followed by radiotherapy and chemotherapy.

CHAPTER 22

Gynecology

AMENORRHEA

It means absence of menstruation. It is of two types:
1. *Primary amenorrhea*: Patient has never menstruated
2. *Secondary amenorrhea*: Previously, there was menstruation, but cessation or no menstruation later for 6 months or more, e.g. during pregnancy (the most common), lactation and after menopause. It may be due to other diseases (severe anemia and Sheehan's syndrome).

Amenorrhea may also be:
- *True amenorrhea*: In which menstruation is absent or suppressed due to physiological or pathological cause
- *Concealed amenorrhea (cryptomenorrhea)*: Menstruation has occurred but patient is unaware of it as menstrual blood fails to come out due to obstruction in genital tract.

Primary Amenorrhea

It means absence of menstruation by 16 years of age in presence of normal secondary sex characters or by 14 years of age if secondary sex characters have not developed.

Causes:
- *Physiological*: Before puberty, pregnancy, lactation and after menopause
- *Pathological*: Disease of uterus, ovary, hypothalamo-pituitary axis, thyroid and adrenal gland.
  - Disease of uterus: Congenital absence or gross hypoplasia of uterus, hysterectomy, disease of endometrium, tubercular endometritis, postradiation and synechiae
  - Disease of ovary: Absence or rudimentary ovary, oophorectomy, polycystic ovarian syndrome (PCOS), premature ovarian failure, resistant ovarian syndrome (Savage's syndrome), irradiation and ovarian neoplasm
  - Disease of hypothalamo-pituitary axis: Hypopituitarism due to any cause, e.g. encephalitis, meningitis, traumatic fracture of base

of skull, infiltrative disease like sarcoidosis, hypophysectomy, pituitary disorder (prolactinoma), Sheehan's Syndrome and craniopharyngioma
- Endocrine: Hyperthyroidism, Addison's disease and diabetes mellitus (DM)
- Chromosomal abnormality: Abnormal chromosomal pattern (Turner syndrome)
- Any acute and chronic illness: DM, tuberculosis (TB), environmental factors and anorexia nervosa.

Diagnosis:
- Details history (age, history of pregnancy, family history and any history of primary disease)
- Physical examination and pelvic examination.

Investigation:
- *Routine*: Complete blood count (CBC), fasting blood sugar (FBS), serum creatinine, urine routine microscopic examination (RME), chest X-ray (CXR) and ultrasonography (USG) of whole abdomen
- *Special*: Pregnancy test, radiology and imaging [computed tomography (CT) scan and magnetic resonance imaging (MRI)], hormone assay [luteinizing hormone (LH), follicle-stimulating hormone (FSH), testosterone, prolactin and thyroid functions], karyotype, biopsy (endometrial and gonadal), USG or transvaginal sonography (TVS), hysteroscopy, laparoscopy and hysterosalpingography.

Treatment:
- *Treatment of cause*: If no cause is found and treatment is delayed up to 18 years of age. Spontaneous menstruation may occur due to late menarche
- *Treatment of pathological amenorrhea*: Reassurance, psychotherapy and maintenance of nutrition
- *Surgical treatment*:
  - Imperforate hymen or transverse vaginal septum: Cruciate incision of membrane and drainage of blood under general anesthesia
  - Vaginal agenesis: Vaginal reconstruction surgery and bilateral wedge resection of polycystic ovaries.
- *Hormone therapy*: For pituitary and thyroid disease.

Secondary Amenorrhea

Causes:
- *Uterine factors*: Tubercular endometritis, postradiation, synechiae and surgical removal
- *Ovarian factors*: PCOS, premature ovarian failure, resistant ovarian syndrome (Savage's syndrome), hyperestrogenic state (persistent follicles in metropathia and feminizing tumor of ovary-like granulosa cell tumor), masculinizing tumor of ovary (Sertoli–Leydig cell tumor), and hypoestrogenic state (ablation of ovaries and pelvic radiation)
- *Pituitary factors*: Adenoma (prolactinoma), Cushing's disease, acromegaly, Sheehan's syndrome and Simmonds disease (unrelated to pregnancy)
- *Hypothalamic factors*: Psychogenic shock, stress, anorexia nervosa, strenuous exercise, pseudocyesis, congenital malformation, trauma

(accident and surgery), radiotherapy, infection (tubercular or sarcoid granulomas), and tumors (craniopharyngioma and meningioma)
- *Adrenal factors*: Adrenal tumor or hyperplasia and Cushing's syndrome
- *Thyroid factors*: Hypothyroid state
- *General disease*: Malnutrition, TB, chronic nephritis, and diabetes
- *Iatrogenic*: Contraceptive pills (post-pill amenorrhea), psychotropic phenothiazine derivative drugs, and antihypertensive drugs.

Investigation: According to history and physiological examinations as primary amenorrhea.

Treatment: According to cause.

OLIGOMENORRHEA

It means menstruation cycle occurring more than 35 days apart, may be both infrequent and irregular, or may be regularly infrequent.

Causes:
- *Constitutional and physiological*: Familial, following menarche and preceding the menopause
- *Hormonal*: Ovarian dysfunction and ovarian estrogen-producing tumor
- *Uterine cause*: Infection, traumatic curettage, myomectomy and uterine hypoplasia
- Any cause like primary amenorrhea
- Systemic disease.

Investigation and treatment are same as those for amenorrhea. No need to treat in majority of cases (constitutional and unassociated with infertility). Induction of ovulation or to increase the frequency of ovulation (if associated with infertility).

MENORRHAGIA (HYPERMENORRHEA)

It means menstrual bleeding which is excess in amount or duration or both at normal regular menstruation cycle.

Causes:
- *Uterine cause*: Fibroid, adenomyosis, retroversion of uterus, endometriosis, endometrial carcinoma and foreign body [intrauterine contraceptive device (IUCD)]
- Dysfunctional uterine bleeding (DUB)
- *Systemic disorder*: Blood dyscrasias (leukemia and aplastic anemia), immune thrombocytopenic purpura (ITP), and coagulation disorder.

Investigations: According to history and physiological examinations—
- *Routine*: CBC, FBS, serum creatinine, urine RME, CXR and USG of whole abdomen
- Coagulation screening [prothrombin time (PT), activated partial thromboplastin time (APTT), fibrin degradation product (FDP) and D-dimer]
- Thyroid function tests
- Hysteroscopy.

Treatment: According to cause. Correction of anemia, anti-fibrinolytic agent (tranexamic acid), and progestogen therapy. Surgical (myomectomy, polypectomy). If all fail, then hysterectomy.

POLYMENORRHAGIA (EPIMENORRHAGIA)

Polymenorrhagia is cyclical bleeding which is both excessive and too frequent (in less than 21 days). Causes and treatment are like menorrhagia.

METRORRHAGIA (METROSTAXIS)

Metrorrhagia is bleeding of any amount which is acyclical and which occurs irregularly or continuously. Causes are cervical carcinoma, endometrial polyp, endometrial carcinoma, abnormal pregnancy (abortion, ectopic pregnancy), and exogenous estrogen administration.

DYSMENORRHEA

It means painful menstruation, which interferes with day-to-day activities.

Types:
- *True (primary or spasmodic)*: It means where there is no identifiable pelvic pathology. It is common in young girls. Pain occurs few hours before or after the onset of menstruation, colicky in nature, radiates to inner thigh. It may be associated with nausea, vomiting, sweating, diarrhea and frequency of micturition.

Treatment: Reassurance, regular physical exercise, analgesic [nonsteroidal anti-inflammatory drug (NSAID), ibuprofen, naproxen and mefenamic acid], antispasmodic (hyoscine), start 2 days before expected date. If no response, oral contraceptive pill (OCP) may be given, started from day 5 to day 25 of menstrual cycle, with a break of 7 days, and continue for 6 months.

- *Congestive dysmenorrhea (secondary dysmenorrhea)*: Painful menstruation associated with pelvic pathology (not uterine).

Treatment: According to cause.

DYSFUNCTIONAL UTERINE BLEEDING

It means abnormal uterine bleeding without any detectable pelvic pathology, tumor, inflammation or pregnancy.

Types:
- *Primary*:
  - Ovular type: DUB with ovulation in which there is normal or heavy menstruation bleeding. May be due to irregular ripening or shedding of endometrium
  - Anovular: DUB in absence of ovulation. It may be metropathia hemorrhagica (short period of amenorrhea followed by prolonged and heavy menstrual bleeding), threshold bleeding of puberty menorrhagia and premenopausal.
- *Secondary*: Due to systemic disease (hypothyroidism and blood dyscrasia). No detectable disease in genital tract
- *Iatrogenic*: Due to administration of contraceptives (oral, injectable and IUCD), and sex hormones.

Diagnosis: Detailed history and physical examination should be done. CBC, erythrocyte sedimentation rate (ESR), Mantoux test (MT), bleeding and coagulation profile [bleeding time (BT), clotting time (CT), PT and APTT], USG of whole abdomen, CXR, hysteroscopy, and diagnostic endometrial curettage.

Treatment:
- *General treatment*: Explanation and reassurance, correction of anemia (blood transfusion, hematinics and vitamin), sedative and NSAID
- *Hormone therapy*: To stop bleeding, tablet norethisterone 5 mg 1 tablet 8 hourly for 10 days. Then 5 mg, from 5th day to 25th day of cycle, for 9–12 months. Combined oral contraceptive may be given, from 5th day of withdrawal bleeding to 25th day for 3–6 cycles
- *Surgical measures*: Dilatation and curettage (D&C) and endometrial ablation. If all fails, hysterectomy.

MENOPAUSE

It means permanent cessation of menstruation for at least 1 year at the end of reproductive life. Age of menopause—48–55 years or average 51 years. Menopausal symptoms are (also called climacteric symptoms):
- *Vasomotor symptoms*: Hot flushes, night sweating and insomnia
- *Cardiovascular system*: Palpitation, hypertension and ischemic heart disease
- *Psychological*: Depression, anxiety, insomnia and lethargy
- *Neurological*: Headache, dizziness, irritability and vertigo
- *Urogenital*: Incontinence, nocturia, urgency, dysuria, dyspareunia, vaginal dryness and atrophy and loss of libido
- *Musculoskeletal*: Osteoporosis, bony pain and fracture
- *General features*: Obesity, loss of appetite, constipation, weakness, skin pigmentation and atrophy of breast and uterus.

Treatment: Explanations and reassurance. Calcium, vitamin D, calcitriol, calcitonin and physical exercise. Drug therapies are:
- *Hormone therapy*: Effective in 80–90% of women
  - Estrogen (better in hysterectomized patient)
  - Combined estrogen and progesterone (given in those with intact uterus), for 21 days then stopped for 1 week
  - Mixed estrogen and androgen preparations
  - SERM (selective estrogen receptor modulator): Raloxifene, given one tablet daily
  - Tibolone: One tablet daily.
- For severe hot flushes, antidepressant, vitamin E or gabapentin may be given.

HORMONE REPLACEMENT THERAPY

Short-term hormone replacement therapy (HRT) is used for relief of symptoms of peri- and postmenopausal estrogen deficiency. Carefully balance risk against benefits for each individual.

Indications:
- Relief of symptoms of menopause
- Asymptomatic women with risk factors (premature menopause, gonadal dysgenesis and oophorectomy)
- Hysterectomy before menopause even if ovaries are conserved.

Contraindications:
- Uncontrolled HTN
- History of endometrial or breast cancer

- Unexplained vaginal bleeding
- Cardiovascular disease and liver disease
- Porphyria
- History of hormone-dependent cancer (breast and endometrium)
- Thromboembolic disease.

Complications of hormone replacement therapy:
- Endometrial carcinoma
- Breast cancer
- Gall bladder disease (cholelithiasis)
- *Others*: Precipitation of myocardial infarction (MI), HTN, changes in liver function and thromboembolism.

Choice of preparation: Start with low dose for 3 months. Tablets, patches, gels and implants are available:
- *Women without uterus*: Estrogen alone. If history of endometriosis, add a progestogen (endometrial foci may remain despite hysterectomy)
- *Women with an intact uterus*: Progestogen is needed for the last 12–14 days of cycle or intrauterine system (IUS) to prevent endometrial proliferation.

Benefits of hormone replacement therapy:
- Relief of symptoms (hot flush, night sweat, etc.)
- Relief of urogenital symptoms (urgency, frequency, dysuria and dyspareunia)
- Prevents postmenopausal osteoporosis
- Prevents recurrent urinary tract infection (UTI)
- Prevents coronary heart disease [estrogen reduces serum cholesterol, low-density lipoprotein (LDL) and increases high-density lipoprotein (HDL)]
- Improvement of psychological symptoms.

POSTMENOPAUSAL BLEEDING

Bleeding per vagina after menopause is called postmenopausal bleeding (usually after 6–12 months of amenorrhea).

Causes:
- *Injuries*: Direct trauma, decubitus ulcer and foreign body
- *Infections*: Vaginitis, endometritis, pyometra and hematometra
- *Vagina*: Atrophic vaginitis, trichomoniasis and moniliasis
- *Cervix*: Chronic cervicitis and cervical erosion
- *Endometrium*: Senile endometritis
- Carcinoma of the cervix, endometrium, vagina, vulva, fallopian tubes and ovary
- Indiscriminate use of estrogen for climacteric syndrome
- *Dysfunctional uterine bleeding*: Metropathia hemorrhagica and threshold bleeding
- Blood dyscrasias.

Investigations: Detailed history (age, history of pregnancy, family history, and any history of primary disease) and physical examination should be done:
- *Routine*: CBC, FBS, serum creatinine, urine RME, CXR and USG of whole abdomen

- *Specific*:
  - Ultrasonography of uterus and adnexa
  - Diagnostic curettage
  - Cervical smear and biopsy
  - Endocervical aspiration cytology (to exclude endometrial malignancy)
  - Fractional curettage (if cervical cytology is negative)
  - Hysteroscopic evaluation and biopsy
  - Laparoscopy (ovarian or adnexal mass)
  - Cystoscopy and sigmoidoscopy (if needed).

Treatment: According to cause—
- If no cause is detected, follow-up
- *Recurrent or continuous bleeding*: Hysterectomy with bilateral salpingo-oophorectomy.

ECTOPIC PREGNANCY

In ectopic pregnancy, fertilized ovum is implanted in a site other than uterine cavity. There are two types:
1. Acute ectopic or acute tubal or ruptured ectopic pregnancy (40%)
2. Subacute or chronic ectopic pregnancy (60%).

Sites: Fallopian tube (the most common, 95%), ovary, cervix, rudimentary horn of bicornuate uterus, abdominal cavity and broad ligaments.

Causes: Pelvic inflammatory disease (PID), tubercular salpingitis, congenital anomalies of fallopian tube, pelvic tumor, tubal surgery, transmigration of ovum and assisted reproductive technique.

Features: In acute attack—
- Amenorrhea and symptoms of early pregnancy
- Severe abdominal pain, vaginal spotting or bleeding and features of shock (hypotension, tachycardia, cold clammy extremities and pallor)
- On examination, extreme tenderness in abdominal and pelvic region on affected side. In delayed case, whole abdomen becomes distended.

Investigation: USG and serum β-hCG.

Treatment:
- Resuscitation [intravenous (IV) fluid and blood transfusion]
- *Surgical management*: Laparoscopic removal. *Or*, salpingotomy, salpingectomy and salpingo-oophorectomy
- *Medical management*: Methotrexate 50 mg/m^2 IM, when patient is hemodynamically stable.

FIBROID UTERUS (MYOMA)

It is a benign tumor arising from myometrium, composed of smooth muscle and fibrous connective tissue (also called fibromyoma or leiomyoma). There are three types:
1. Subserous
2. Interstitial or intramural
3. Submucous.

Clinical features: Common in 35–45 years, rarely before 20 years of age. It may be asymptomatic.

- *Menstrual disturbances*: Menorrhagia, dysmenorrhea, metrorrhagia and continuous and irregular bleeding
- *General*: Anemia, palpitation, lassitude and loss of weight
- *Pressure symptoms*:
  - Urinary bladder: Frequency of micturition and retention of urine
  - Gastrointestinal tract (GIT): Constipation
  - Presence of tumor-like sensation of weight in pelvis
  - Edema and varicosities of legs
  - Low back pain.
- *Physical sign*: Mass is hard, rounded or lobulated. On per vaginal examination, mass is felt attached to uterus.

Differential diagnosis:
- Ovarian tumor
- Pregnancy
- Adenomyosis.

Treatment:
- No treatment for small symptomless tumor
- Correction of anemia
- *Surgical treatment needed if*: Larger than 12–14 week's size, if growing rapidly, if subserous or pedunculated, doubt about nature, and persistent menorrhagia causing significant anemia.

Options of surgical operation: Total abdominal hysterectomy and myomectomy.

Indication of myomectomy: Younger age (<40 years), desires pregnancy or desires conservation of reproductive function, unexplained infertility and repeated pregnancy loss.

Complications of fibroid:
- Degeneration
- Torsion
- *Hemorrhage*: Rupture of large vein on the surface intraperitoneal hemorrhage
- *Pseudo Meigs syndrome*: Subserous pedunculated type by mechanical irritation
- Infection
- Malignant change.

ABORTION

It is the expulsion of product of conception before the age of viability [usually 28 weeks or <1,000 g in weight. According to World Health Organization (WHO), it is 500 g or less]. Miscarriage means spontaneous abortion, not induced. Types are: it may be spontaneous and induced.
- Spontaneous abortion, which may be—
  - Threatened abortion
  - Inevitable abortion
  - Incomplete abortion
  - Complete abortion
  - Missed abortion
  - Septic abortion
  - Habitual abortion.

- Induced abortion, which may be—
  - Legal or therapeutic abortion
  - Criminal abortion.

Threatened Abortion

It means abortion has started but may be arrested, pregnancy may continue.

Features:
- History of amenorrhea and suggestive of pregnancy
- Bleeding per vagina, which is slight, may stop spontaneously
- Usually no pain, may be low backache or dull lower abdominal pain
- *PV examination*: Cervical os is closed
- Uterine size corresponds to the duration of gestation.

Investigation: USG (1st). Others—CBC, ESR, blood grouping, and Rh typing. Serial serum β-hCG levels (helpful to assess fetal well-being).

Treatment:
- Complete bed rest at least 1 week after bleeding stops. Sedatives may be used
- *Hormonal treatment*: Progestogen may be given if deficiency or defective placentation (such as allylestrenol tablet 5 mg 8 hourly. *Or* dydrogesterone tablet, 10 mg 8 hourly. *Or* injection hCG 1,500 unit twice a week. *Or* injection 17- α hydroxyprogesterone, 250 mg IM twice a week)
- *General measures*: Control of any medical problem (DM, HTN and anemia).

Advice to the patient:
- The patient is advised to preserve the vulval pads and anything expelled out per vagina, for inspection. Also to report if bleeding and/or pain becomes aggravated. Routine checkup of pulse, temperature and vaginal bleeding
- Rest and limit activities for at least 2 weeks and avoid heavy work. Coitus is avoided. Reexamine after 1 month.

Inevitable Abortion

It means abortion has started and process is irreversible.

Features:
- History of amenorrhea and suggestive of pregnancy
- Vaginal bleeding, initially scanty, later excessive and may be accompanied with clots
- Pain in lower abdomen, may be severe and may radiate to the back
- Internal os of cervix is dilated and products of conception may be felt through it
- Ultrasonography may be done.

Treatment:
- *Resuscitation*: IV infusion, blood is sent for grouping and cross matching. Blood transfusion may be needed
- If bleeding is continued, IV oxytocin or ergometrine 0.5 mg, IM or IV
- *Evacuation of uterus*:
  - If pregnancy is <12 weeks: Suction and curettage under general anesthesia
  - If pregnancy is >12 weeks: IV oxytocin drip to expel uterine contents. If placenta is retained, it is removed under general anesthesia.

Incomplete Abortion

It means, some part of products of conception are expelled, some part is left inside of the uterus.

Features:
- History of amenorrhea and suggestive of pregnancy. There is history of expulsion of part of conception product per vagina
- Pain in lower abdominal and colicky in nature. Persistence of vaginal bleeding
- *PV examination reveals*: Uterus smaller than duration of gestation or amenorrhea, cervical os is open and part of product of conception is found (incomplete).

Investigation: USG shows retained contents.

Treatment: Conservative followed by evacuation. Avoid pregnancy for at least 3 months.

Complete Abortion

It means all the products of conception are expelled. Features are history of amenorrhea and expulsion of product of conception per vagina. Pain is subsided after expulsion. Vaginal bleeding becomes trace or absent. USG shows empty cavity of uterus.

Treatment: Only supportive. Rest and limit activities for few days.

Missed Abortion

In this type of abortion, embryo or fetus is dead and retained or it does not develop within the uterus for 4 weeks or more.

Features:
- History of amenorrhea but regression of pregnancy symptoms such as nausea and vomiting
- Repeated vaginal bleeding or brownish vaginal discharge
- Uterus does not increase and may even decrease in size, cervix is not dilated and tightly closed.

Investigation: USG is done to confirm diagnosis.

Treatment: Evacuation is done by suction and curettage under general anesthesia, if—
- Spontaneous expulsion does not occur within 4 weeks
- When there is excessive bleeding or infection or disseminated intravascular coagulation (DIC)
- Patient is anxious to evacuate the products of conception.

Complications: Hypofibrinogenemia and severe bleeding. In such case, blood transfusion, platelet transfusion, cryoprecipitate, fibrinogen infusion and aminocaproic acid may be given. If intractable bleeding despite all measures, hysterectomy should be done.

Habitual Abortion (Recurrent Miscarriage)

It is defined as three or more consecutive spontaneous abortion before 20 weeks. Multiple factors are responsible for habitual abortion:
- Genetic or chromosomal abnormalities
- Anatomical defect or malformation of uterus (congenital anomalies such as double uterus, septate or bicornuate uterus, hypoplastic uterus

and cervical incompetence). Acquired abnormalities such as cervical incompetence, fibroid uterus, etc
- *Endocrine and metabolic*: Uncontrolled diabetes, hypertension, thyroid disorder, luteal phase defect, excess secretion of LH, Rh incompatibility and progesterone deficiency
- Infection of genital tract
- Inherited thrombophilia
- Immunological cause
- *Antiphospholipid antibodies (APA)*: Lupus anticoagulant and anticardiolipin antibodies
- Cervical incompetence.

Investigations:
- *Blood*: CBC, ESR, blood grouping and Rh typing (both husband and wife), and blood glucose
- Karyotyping of both husband and wife
- Antinuclear antibody (ANA) and antiphospholipid antibody
- TORCH screening
- Serological test for syphilis both in wife and husband
- Thyroid, liver and renal function test
- Ultrasonography
- Hysteroscopy, laparoscopy and hysterosalpingography in some cases
- Hormone assay.

Treatment:
- *General*: Bed rest, good nutrition, avoid coitus and physical activity, weight lifting, and psychological support
- *Specific treatment*:
  - For cervical incompetence: Shirodkar sutures
  - Retroversion: Correction with pessary
  - Aspirin or heparin for antiphospholipid syndrome
  - Folic acid
  - Hormone therapy (progesterone as indicated)
  - Treatment of cause (such as thyroid, DM, HTN and antiphospholipid syndrome).

Septic Abortion

When abortion is complicated by infection of uterus or its contents or genital tract is called septic abortion. Infection is common in induced abortion than spontaneous. Organisms are—*Escherichia coli*, *Bacteroides*, anaerobic streptococci, clostridia, streptococci and staphylococci.

Features:
- History of pregnancy followed by passage of products of conception per vagina. Usually illegal termination by an unauthorized person (usually concealed)
- High fever with chills and rigors, lower abdominal pain, tachycardia, headache, body ache, anorexia, nausea and vomiting. Offensive vaginal discharge. Patient looks toxic
- Examination reveals offensive purulent vaginal discharge, tender uterus and cervix feels soft with tender fornices.

Investigations:
- Complete blood count, ESR, blood grouping and Rh typing (both husband and wife), blood sugar, and blood culture/sensitivity (C/S)

- High vaginal and endocervical swab for C/S
- Urine RME and C/S
- Ultrasonography
- Coagulations screens (serum fibrinogen, BT, CT, PT, APTT, FDP, D-dimer).

Complications:
- *Immediate complications*: Hemorrhage, injury to uterus, endotoxic shock, thrombophlebitis, generalized peritonitis, acute renal failure and DIC
- *Remote complication*: Chronic debility, chronic pelvic pain, dyspareunia, ectopic pregnancy, secondary infertility and emotional depression.

Treatment:
- Patient should be hospitalized, IV fluids, antipyretic and sedatives. Oxytocin infusion may be given to control bleeding
- *Broad-spectrum antibiotics*: Ampicillin, flucloxacillin, ceftriaxone *plus* gentamycin *plus* metronidazole
- Evacuation of uterus after 12–24 hours of antibiotics therapy
- Treatment of complications.

Therapeutic Abortion

It means induction of abortion on medical ground. Indications are:
- *Disease of mother*: Heart disease, severe hypertension, renal disease, malignancy, severe hyperemesis gravidarum, any severe psychiatric problem of mother and infection of mother (like rubella)
- Unwanted pregnancy or pregnancy due to rape
- Fetal disease or malformation like anencephaly, Down syndrome and neural tube defect.

ENDOMETRIOSIS

It means presence of functioning endometrial tissue other than uterine endometrium.

Sites:
- *Common site*: Ovary (the most common, 65%), Pouch of Douglas, pelvic peritoneum, uterosacral ligaments, rectovaginal septum, sigmoid colon, appendix, pelvic lymph nodes and fallopian tubes
- *Other site*: Outer coat of uterus, myometrium (adenomyosis), round ligament of ovary, intestine, bladder, ureter, vagina, vulva, abdominal scar, lungs and pleura.

Clinical features: May be asymptomatic. There may be—
- Dysmenorrhea (common), menorrhagia, dyspareunia and infertility
- *Others*: Chronic pelvic pain, abdominal pain and unexplained fever. Other features according to site of involvement.

Investigations: USG, CT scan, MRI and CA-125 may be done. Laparoscopy is gold standard. Laparotomy in some case.

Treatment:
- *In asymptomatic case*: Follow-up. Analgesic, if pain. Married women are encouraged for pregnancy
- *Hormonal treatment*: Estrogen, progesterone, combined estrogen and progesterone, danazol and gonadotropin-releasing hormone (GnRH) analogues

- *Surgery*: In ovarian endometriosis—
  - Small endometrioma (<3 cm): Aspirated laparoscopically
  - Large endometrioma (>4 cm): Ovarian cystectomy and adhesiolysis
  - If advanced stage and if >40 years with complete family: Hysterectomy with bilateral salpingo-oophorectomy should be done
  - In other sites: Surgical excision in endometriosis of abdominal scar, umbilicus, bladder, gut, cervix, vagina, lung and pleura. Removal of ovaries may help in regression of the lesions.

CHOCOLATE CYST

Chocolate cysts are noncancerous, old blood-filled cysts within the ovaries. It looks brown, tar-like, melted chocolate. It is also called ovarian endometriomas.

Features: Irregular painful periods, pelvic pain not related to menstrual cycle, pain during coitus and infertility in some women.

Investigations: USG of lower abdomen.

Treatment: In asymptomatic case, follow-up. Ovarian cystectomy, laparoscopy may be needed. Medical treatment like endometriosis.

ADENOMYOSIS

It may be defined as the growth of endometrial tissue into the myometrium.

Features: Usually above 40 years, may be asymptomatic. Menorrhagia (common), dysmenorrhea, dyspareunia, frequency of urination and lower abdominal pain. Abdominal examination may reveal enlarged uterus (size does not exceed 12–14 weeks gestation). Per vaginal examination reveals uniformly enlarged uterus.

Investigations: Ultrasound and color Doppler TVS and MRI.

Treatment: Hormone therapy not beneficial. Surgery is done. Most patients are usually aged and parous. So, total abdominal hysterectomy with or without salpingo-oophorectomy is the treatment of choice.

PELVIC INFLAMMATORY DISEASE

It means infection and inflammation of upper genital tract involving uterus (endometrium), fallopian tubes, ovaries, pelvic peritoneum and surrounding structures, not associated with pregnancy or surgery.

Causative organisms are: *Neisseria gonorrhoeae* and chlamydia trachomatis. Other causes are *Gardnerella vaginalis, Peptostreptococcus, Streptococci, Haemophilus influenzae* and *Pneumococci*.

Risk factors: Sexual activity, multiple partners, frequent vaginal douching, IUCD, previous PID, low socio-economic status, malnutrition and multiparity.

Clinical features: May be asymptomatic.
- Lower abdominal and pelvic pain
- Irregular and excessive vaginal bleeding, painful coitus and abnormal purulent vaginal discharge. May be associated menorrhagia, metrorrhagia and urinary symptoms
- Fever, lassitude, headache, backache, nausea and vomiting.

Sequelae: Long-term sequelae are chronic pelvic pain, ectopic pregnancy and infertility.

Investigations:
- Complete blood count, ESR, urine RME and blood sugar
- High vaginal swab, discharge from urethra or Bartholin's gland and cervical canal for C/S
- Ultrasonography of lower abdomen
- Laparoscopy (gold standard).

Treatment: Bed rest and analgesics in severe case.
- *Outpatient antibiotics regimen*:
  - Levofloxacin 500 mg (or, ofloxacin 400 mg) orally daily with or without metronidazole 500 mg 12 hourly for 14 days
  - Ceftriaxone 250 mg IM single dose *plus* doxycycline 100 mg orally 12 hourly with or without metronidazole 500 mg 12 hourly for 14 days.
- *Inpatient antibiotics regimen*:
  - Cefoxitin 2 g IV 6 hourly for 2–4 days *plus* doxycycline 100 mg orally 12 hourly for 14 days
  - If *pelvic abscess*: Clindamycin 900 mg IV 8 hourly *plus* gentamicin 2 mg/kg IV (loading dose), followed by 1.5 mg/kg IV (maintenance dose) 8 hourly.
- Treating sexual partners may be necessary in some case
- Laparoscopy or laparotomy may be needed. Surgery may be required in some cases, even hysterectomy with or without salpingo-oophorectomy.

OVARIAN TUMOR

It may be benign or malignant.
- *Benign*: Serous cystadenoma, mucinous cystadenoma, teratoma, dermoid cyst, androblastoma, fibroma, thecoma, granuloma cell tumors, and Sertoli–Leydig cell tumors
- *Malignant*: Serous cystadenocarcinoma, mucinous cystadenocarcinoma, teratoma, dysgerminoma and yolk sac tumors.

Features: May be asymptomatic, detected on routine examination.
- Abdominal swelling or lump in lower abdomen
- Dull abdominal pain and discomfort
- Local symptoms related to gastrointestinal or urinary due to pressure effects.

Investigation: USG, CT scan of abdomen and CA-125.

Complications: Torsion or rupture of cyst, hemorrhage, infections and malignant changes.

Management: If small and benign, follow-up. If large, surgery.

Malignant Ovarian Tumor

Causes: Unknown, multiple factors may be responsible, such as—hereditary, nulliparity, infertility, early menarche and late menopause and streak gonad in Turner syndrome.

Features:
- Rapidly growing mass in lower abdomen
- Loss of weight, malaise and weakness

- Edema of feet and vulva
- Menstrual abnormality is conspicuously absent except in functioning tumor
- *Features of metastases*: According to organ involvement (respiratory distress, ascites and pleural effusion).

Investigation: As above.

Management: In early stage, surgery (hysterectomy with bilateral salpingo-oophorectomy with omentectomy). In advanced cases—Chemotherapy, radiotherapy or combination.

CARCINOMA CERVIX

Types: Squamous cell carcinoma (90%), adenocarcinoma (5%) and mixed (5%).

Risk factors:
- *Age*: Perimenopausal women, early marriage and early sexual intercourse
- Women with high risk human papillomavirus (HPV) infection
- *Parity*: Multiparous, early age of first pregnancy and frequent childbirth
- Low socio-economic status and poor maintenance of local hygiene
- No circumcision of male partner
- *Others*: OCP, smoking and genital infection (chlamydia, HIV and HSV-2).

Features: Common in middle age and elderly. In early stage, usually asymptomatic, discovered incidentally during routine examination.
- Irregular uterine bleeding or discharge or both, usually after coitus or any trauma to cervix. Later, there may be severe bleeding
- Offensive vaginal discharge, initially creamy white but later dirty brown
- *Features of advanced cancer*: Frequency of micturition, dysuria, urinary incontinence, rectal pain, deep pelvic pain, low backache, sciatica, ureteric colic, edema of legs, loss of weight, anorexia and malaise
- *Features of metastases*: According to involvement of organ
- PV examination shows hard, friable, fixed cervix and bleeding on examination.

Investigations:
- *For diagnosis*: Pap smear, cervical biopsy, colposcopy and colpomicroscopy
- *For staging*: Hysteroscopy, cystoscopy and endocervical curettage
- *To see metastases*: Chest and skeletal X-ray, intravenous urogram (IVU), USG, proctoscopy or sigmoidoscopy and barium enema. If needed, CT scan or MRI
- *Routine*: CBC, ESR, serum creatinine, electrolytes, blood sugar, urine RME and USG of abdomen

Management: Treatment depends on staging.
- Surgery (Wertheim's hysterectomy) for early cervical cancer (Stage I and IIA)
- *In advanced cases*: Radiotherapy with or without chemotherapy and surgery is also sometimes used
- Radiotherapy (in all stages) for invasive carcinoma
- If metastasis, palliative radio or chemotherapy
- *General*: Maintenance of nutrition, correction of anemia, NSAID (if pain), control of bleeding and infection.

Preventive: Identifying "high-risk" factors, prophylactic HPV vaccine and secondary prevention by cervical screening.

Complication: Hemorrhage, ureteric pain, pyometra, vesicovaginal fistula, rectovaginal fistula, and death due to uremia, hemorrhage, and sepsis.

ENDOMETRIAL CARCINOMA

Types: Adenocarcinoma (common), adenocarcinoma with squamous elements, papillary serous carcinoma, mucinous adenocarcinoma, clear cell adenocarcinoma, secretory carcinoma, squamous cell carcinoma and mixed carcinoma.

Risk factors:
- *Age*: Postmenopausal, 55–60 years, also in late menopause
- *Parity*: Common in nulliparous (also in virginity)
- *Estrogen*: Persistent stimulation of endometrium with estrogen
- *Corpus cancer syndrome*: Encompasses obesity, hypertension and diabetes mellitus
- Unopposed estrogen stimulation in ovarian or PCOS
- Tamoxifen used for breast cancer
- Family history or personal history of colon, ovarian or breast cancer
- Fibroid, endometrial hyperplasia and atrophic endometritis
- Past history of pelvic radiation.

Clinical features:
- Postmenopausal bleeding (75%), usually slight, irregular or continuous and sometimes excessive
- In premenopausal women, there may be irregular and excessive bleeding
- Watery, offensive discharge due to pyometra and colicky pain due to uterine contractions
- Few patients remain asymptomatic.

PV examination: In early stage, uterus is atrophic, normal or enlarged. In advanced stage, irregular, enlarged and fixed. Blood or purulent offensive discharge.

Investigation: USG of lower abdomen or TVS, hysteroscopy, endometrial biopsy and fractional curettage.

To check for metastases: CT scan, MRI and positron emission tomography (PET) scan.

Management: Surgery, radiotherapy, chemotherapy and combination therapy. Depends on stage:
- *In Stage I and II*: Total abdominal hysterectomy with bilateral salpingo-oophorectomy with resection of draining lymph node
- *In stage III and IV*: Radiotherapy followed by surgery, if possible. Chemotherapy may be necessary.

Prevention: Weight control, reduce estrogen use in postmenopausal women and secondary prevention by screening.

CHAPTER 23

Obstetrics

HYPEREMESIS GRAVIDARUM

Hyperemesis gravidarum is a complication in pregnancy characterized by severe nausea, vomiting, weight loss and possibly dehydration, electrolytes and acid-base imbalances, and nutritional deficiencies. It usually occurs in 4th to 6th weeks of pregnancy and it may be worse around 9–13 weeks. Vomiting is so severe that interferes with daily physical activities of pregnant woman. Symptoms usually improve by 20th week.

Risk factors: First pregnancy, multiple pregnancy, hydatidiform mole and family history of hyperemesis gravidarum.

Features: Repeated vomiting, oliguria, epigastric pain and constipation may occur. Weakness, sleep disturbance, depression, anxiety, irritability, mood changes and decreased concentration may occur.

Differential diagnosis: Acute hepatitis, gastroenteritis, peptic ulcer disease, cholecystitis and appendicitis.

Treatment: Reassurance. Hospitalization in severe case.
- Increased oral or intravenous (IV) fluid intake
- Advice to take dry toast or biscuit and avoidance of fatty and spicy foods
- *Antiemetics*: Prochlorperazine, metoclopramide, promethazine, vitamin B_6 or trifluoperazine
- *Nutritional supplementation*: Vitamin B1, vitamin B6, vitamin C and vitamin B12.

Complications:
- Dehydration, ketoacidosis and acute renal failure
- *Neurologic complications*: Wernicke's encephalopathy, beriberi due to thiamine deficiency, pontine myelinolysis, peripheral neuritis, Korsakoff psychosis, convulsions and coma
- Retinal hemorrhage
- Jaundice, hepatic failure, stress ulcer in stomach and esophageal tear (Mallory-Weiss syndrome)
- Hypokalemic hypochloremic alkalosis
- Hypoprothrombinemia due to vitamin K deficiency.

ANTEPARTUM HEMORRHAGE

It is defined as bleeding from or into genital tract, occurring from 24th week of pregnancy and before birth of the baby.

Causes:
- *Placental bleeding (70%)*: Placenta previa (35%), abruptio placentae (35%), and vasa previa
- Unexplained (25%)
- *Extraplacental cause (5%)*: Cervicitis, cervical polyp, trauma, carcinoma cervix, varicose vein and local trauma.

Management: Hospitalization and complete bed rest. Correction of anemia, if needed blood transfusion, and oxygen inhalation. Follow-up and checkup. If needed, caesarean section.

Placenta Previa

When the placenta is implanted partially or completely over the lower uterine segment, it is called placenta previa.

It is of four types:
- Type-I (low lying)
- Type-II (marginal)
- Type-III (incomplete or partial central)
- Type-IV (central or total).

Another classification:
- Mild degree (Type I and II anterior)
- Major degree (Type II posterior, III and IV).

Symptoms: History of amenorrhea and sudden onset of painless, recurrent and fresh vaginal bleeding.

Risk factors: Age more than 35 years, multiparous, twins, preterm delivery, previous caesarean section, previous placenta previa, smoking, endometrial damage and placental abnormality.

Investigations:
- Ultrasonography (USG)
- Complete blood count (CBC), erythrocyte sedimentation rate (ESR), blood grouping and rhesus (Rh) typing
- Urine routine microscopic examination (R/M/E)
- *Others*: Blood sugar, serum creatinine and electrocardiogram (ECG).

Treatment: Hospitalization and complete bed rest. Correction of anemia, if needed blood transfusion. The aim is to continue pregnancy for fetal maturity without compromising maternal health.
- It depends on amount of blood loss, gestational age, and fetal maturity. If <36 weeks pregnancy with small bleeding—bed rest, correction of anemia, avoid sexual intercourse, and frequent follow-up. Dexamethasone injection is given to speed up fetal maturity
- If >36 weeks or with significant bleeding, cesarean section should be done.

Complications:
- *Maternal complications*:
  - During pregnancy: Antepartum hemorrhage (APH), malpresentation and premature labor

- During labor: Early rupture of membrane, cord prolapse, slow dilatation of cervix, intrapartum hemorrhage and postpartum hemorrhage (PPH)
- During puerperium: Puerperal sepsis, subinvolution, and embolism.
- *Fetal complications*: Low birth weight, asphyxia, intrauterine death, birth injuries and congenital malformation.

ABRUPTIO PLACENTA

It is a type of APH in which bleeding occurs due to premature separation of normally situated placenta.

It is of three types:
1. *Revealed*: Blood comes out of the cervical canal to be visible externally (most common)
2. *Concealed*: Blood does not come out of cervical canal and is not visible outside (rare)
3. *Mixed*: Some part of blood remains inside and some is expelled out.

Symptoms: History of amenorrhea and painful vaginal bleeding.

Signs: Uterus is hard and tender. Fetal heart sound may be absent or there may be fetal distress.

Risk factors: Multigravida, trauma to cervix, hypertension, preeclampsia, sudden decompression like artificial rupture of membrane, external cephalic version and folic acid deficiency.

Treatment: Resuscitation followed by termination of pregnancy. Induction of labor is done by low rupture of membranes and oxytocin drip may be added. In some cases, caesarean section.

POSTPARTUM HEMORRHAGE

Bleeding from or into the genital tract after delivery of the baby up to the end of puerperium.

Causes:
- *Uterine causes (atonic uterus, 80%)*:
  - Grand multipara, multiple pregnancy, hydramnios and big baby (>4 kg)
  - Placenta previa and abruption, and adherent placenta (accreta, increta and percreta)
  - Prolonged labor (>12 hours) and mismanaged third stage of labor
  - Malnutrition, anemia and anesthesia
  - Septate or bicornuate uterus and uterine fibroid
  - Others: Obesity, previous PPH, age >40 years, tocolytic drugs (ritodrine), $MgSO_4$, and nifedipine.
- Traumatic (20%)
- *Retained tissues*: Part of placenta and blood clots cause PPH due to imperfect uterine retraction
- Blood coagulation disorders.

Types of PPH: It may be primary and secondary.
- *Primary*: If bleeding occurs within 24 hours after birth of baby. It is of two types—

- Third stage hemorrhage: Bleeding occurs before expulsion of placenta.
- True PPH: Bleeding occurs after expulsion of placenta (majority).
- *Secondary*: Excessive vaginal bleeding after 24 hours of delivery. Usually during 5th to 12th day after delivery. Causes are postpartum infection with retained placental tissue or clot.

Management:
- *General measures*: IV line, blood for grouping and crossmatching, IV infusion with normal saline or haemaccel till blood is available, and blood transfusion when available
- *If uterus is hard and contracted*: Exploration of trauma and hemostatic sutures if tear.
- *If uterus is atonic*:
  - Uterine massage, IV methergine and injection oxytocin drip. If the uterus fails to contract, then
  - Uterus exploration under general anesthesia. Injection 15-methyl prostaglandin (PG) F2α or misoprostol (PGE1). When uterine atony is due to tocolytic drugs, calcium gluconate is given
  - Uterine massage and bimanual compression
  - Uterine tamponade: Tight intrauterine packing and balloon tamponade
  - Surgery: If all fails, hysterectomy may be needed.

Prevention of Postpartum Hemorrhage:
- *Antenatal care*:
  - Correction of anemia and hemoglobin should be >10 g/dL
  - Screening and regular follow-up of high-risk patients. Delivery should be done in a well-equipped hospital
  - Blood grouping should be done for all women so that no time is wasted during emergency.
- *Intranatal*:
  - Slow delivery of the baby is done
  - During caesarean section, spontaneous separation and delivery of placenta reduce blood loss
  - Active management of third stage
  - Routine examination of placenta and membranes should be done to see if there is any missing part
  - If induced or accelerated labor by oxytocin, infusion should be continued for at least 1 hour after delivery
  - Exploration of uterovaginal canal after difficult labor or instrumental delivery
  - Observe the patient for 2 hours after delivery. Patient is sent to ward if uterus is hard and contracted.

Retained Placenta

It means a placenta that is not expelled out even 30 minutes after the birth of the baby (WHO 15 minutes).

Risk factors:
- *Placental abnormalities*: Placenta accreta, increta and percreta and previous retained placenta
- Grand multipara, preterm delivery and induced labor

- Previous injury or surgery of uterus and uterine abnormality
- Constriction ring.

Complications: Uterine inversion, shock, PPH, puerperal sepsis, subinvolution and recurrence in next pregnancy.

Management: IV cannula and blood is sent for grouping. CBC with ESR.
- Oxytocin drip
- Transfer patient to theater for manual removal of placenta
- Broad-spectrum antibiotic with metronidazole.

PREECLAMPSIA

It is characterized by hypertension, >140/90 mm Hg with proteinuria after 20th week in a previously normotensive and nonproteinuric woman.

Risk factors are:
- Primigravida
- Family history of hypertension and preeclampsia
- Placental abnormality, molar pregnancy and multiple pregnancy
- Obesity and insulin resistance
- Preexisting vascular disease
- *Thrombophilias*: Antiphospholipid syndrome, protein C and S deficiency and factor V Leiden.

Clinically, it is of two types:
1. *Mild*: When blood pressure (BP) is 140–160/90–110 mm Hg
2. *Severe*: When BP is >160/110 mm Hg

Features: Common in primigravida (70%).
- Hypertension
- *Proteinuria 2+ in urine*: In the absence of urinary tract infection, it is considered significant
- *Edema*: Pitting edema over the ankles after 12 hours bed rest may be generalized
- *Other features*: Headache, sleep disturbance, diminished urinary output, epigastric pain and eye symptoms (blurring, scotomata, dimness of vision and complete blindness).

Investigations:
- Urine shows proteinuria—24-hours urine for protein measurement (high). May be hyaline casts, epithelial cells or red cells
- *Fundoscopy*: In severe cases, it may show retinal edema, constriction of arterioles, nicking of veins and hemorrhage
- Serum uric acid level (high). May be thrombocytopenia and abnormal coagulation profile. Hepatic enzyme may be high
- Complete blood count, blood sugar, coagulation profile and liver function test.

Management: Preeclampsia usually regresses within 48 hours of delivery.
- Hospitalization and rest. Antihypertensive (methyldopa, labetalol, nifedipine and hydralazine)
- Frequent follow-up of mother and fetus
- If the mother's and baby's condition is stable, delivery can be done at 37–38 weeks of pregnancy
- If condition is severe or fetal distress is present, delivery can be done earlier.

Complications:
- *Maternal*: Eclampsia, hemorrhage, oliguria and anuria, dimness of vision, blindness, preterm labor, HELLP (hemolysis, elevated liver enzymes, and low platelet count) syndrome, cerebral hemorrhage, acute respiratory distress syndrome (ARDS), PPH, shock, sepsis and abruptio placentae
- *Fetal*: Intrauterine death, intrauterine growth restriction (IUGR), asphyxia and prematurity.

ECLAMPSIA

Preeclampsia when complicated with grand mal seizures (generalized tonic-clonic convulsions) and/or coma is called eclampsia. The UK Eclampsia Trial definition consisted of—*seizures* occurring in pregnancy or within 10 days of delivery and with at least two of the following features documented within 24 hours of seizure:

- *Hypertension*: Diastolic blood pressure (DBP) at least 90 mm Hg (if DBP is less than 90 mm Hg on booking visit) or DBP increment of 25 mm Hg above booking level
- Proteinuria one "*plus*" or at least 0.3 g/24 hours
- Thrombocytopenia less than 100,000/dL
- Raised aspartate aminotransferase (AST) greater than 42 IU/L.

Complications:
- *Injuries*: Tongue bite, injuries due to fall from bed and bed sore
- *Pulmonary*: Edema, aspiration pneumonia, adult respiratory distress syndrome and embolism
- Hyperpyrexia
- *Cardiac*: Acute left ventricular failure and cardiomyopathy
- Renal failure
- *Hepatic*: Necrosis and subcapsular hematoma
- *Cerebral*: Edema, hemorrhage and neurological deficits
- Retinal detachment
- *Hematological*: Thrombocytopenia and disseminated intravascular coagulation (DIC)
- *Postpartum*: Shock, sepsis and psychosis.

Management:
- Hospitalization
- ABC (airway, breathing and circulation) and oxygen 8–10 L/min
- Control BP
- *Control of convulsions*:
  - $MgSO_4$, 4 g (20% solution) IV over 3–5 minute followed by 10 g (50%), deep intramuscular (IM) (5 g in each buttock). Maintenance dose is 5 g (50%) IM 4 hourly in alternate buttock
  - Diazepam and phenytoin may be used. Diazepam or diazemuls 5–10 mg, or lorazepam 2–4 mg given as a slow IV bolus
  - Delivery should be done as early as possible.

PUERPERAL PYREXIA

Fever reaching 100.4°F (38°C) or more (measured orally) on two separate occasions at 24 hours apart (excluding 1st 24 hours) within first 10 days after delivery is called puerperal pyrexia.

Causes:
- Puerperal sepsis
- Urinary tract infections (such as cystitis and pyelonephritis)
- Mastitis and breast abscess
- Wound infections [in culture/sensitivity (C/S) or episiotomy]
- Pulmonary infections (such as pneumonia)
- Pelvic thrombophlebitis
- *Others*: Malaria, pharyngitis and gastroenteritis.

Investigations: CBC with ESR, blood sugar, USG (whole abdomen mainly pelvis), chest X-ray, urine R/M/E, blood C/S, computed tomography (CT) scan or magnetic resonance imaging (MRI) of lower abdomen, and high vaginal or endocervical swab for C/S. Others—blood urea, creatinine and electrolytes.

Treatment:
- *General measures*: Antipyretics, IV fluids, maintenance of nutrition and care of wound if any
- Broad-spectrum IV antibiotics (e.g. ceftriaxone, amikacin and metronidazole).

Puerperal Sepsis

Infection of genital tract that occurs after delivery during puerperal period.

Predisposing factors:
- Preterm labor, premature rupture of membranes and rupture of membrane for more than 18 hours
- Retained placental tissue or membranes
- Prolonged labor, obstructed labor, cesarean delivery
- Traumatic vaginal delivery and repeated vaginal examination
- Hemorrhage (antepartum or postpartum)
- Systemic disease [malnutrition, anemia, immunocompromised and diabetes mellitus (DM)].

Organisms: *Escherichia coli*, *Streptococcus pyogenes*, *Staphylococcus aureus*, *Klebsiella*, *Pseudomonas*, *Proteus*, chlamydia, *Peptococcus*, *Bacteroides* and *Clostridia*.

Clinical features:
- Fever, may be high with chill and rigor, malaise, headache, tachycardia, breathlessness, cough, abdominal pain and dysuria
- Local vaginal discharge, which may be offensive and copious. Uterus is tender and soft, and may be associated wound infection of perineum, vagina or cervix
- *Spreading infections (extrauterine)*: Pelvic peritonitis, parametritis, pelvic abscess, thrombophlebitis, septicemia and endotoxic or septic shock.

Investigations: As in puerperal pyrexia.

Treatment:
- Hospitalization. Complete bed rest, IV fluid infusion and correction of anemia
- *Antibiotics*: C/S should be sent. Then empirical broad-spectrum antibiotics should be started. Gentamicin *plus* clindamycin *plus* metronidazole should be continued until the infection is controlled for at least 7–10 days (antibiotics may be changed according to C/S report).

- *If severe sepsis*: Combination of piperacillin-tazobactam or carbapenem *plus* clindamycin. If methicillin-resistant *Staphylococcus aureus* (MRSA) infection, it should be treated with vancomycin
- *Care of wound*: Cleaning and debridement of wound
- If retained placenta, it should be removed. Ruptured tubo-ovarian abscess should be removed
- Laparotomy and hysterectomy are indicated if rupture or perforation, multiple abscesses, and gangrenous uterus or gas gangrene infection is confirmed.

PUERPERAL PSYCHIATRIC DISORDERS

- *Maternity blues (postpartum blue)*: It is characterized by brief episodes of emotional lability, irritability and tearfulness, and it occurs in 50% of women after delivery. Symptoms begin soon after childbirth, typically on 4th day. Only reassurance is given and it resolves spontaneously within few days to weeks
- *Postpartum psychosis*: Onset is usually within first 2 weeks of delivery but can occur several weeks later. There is a strong association with a personal or familial history of bipolar disorder. Classical features of affective psychosis, disorientation, confusion, suspiciousness, concealment and impulsivity are common. Severely depressed patient may have delusional ideas that the child is deformed, evil or affected in some way, which may lead to attempt to kill the child or suicide. Priority is to ensure the safety of both mother and baby. The response to antipsychotic with antidepressants is generally good. Recurrence rate in subsequent puerperium is 20–30%, but some will progress to psychotic episodes not associated with childbirth, usually bipolar disorder
- *Postpartum depression*: It occurs during first postpartum year in 10% of mothers, usually in first 3 months, with a higher prevalence in developing countries. Risk factors are first pregnancy, poor relationship with partner, ambivalence about pregnancy, emotional personality traits, previous history of depression or postpartum depression, and antenatal depression and antenatal anxiety. Depressive illness after childbirth is clinically similar to other depressive illnesses, but lack of emotional bonding with the baby is common. Explanation and reassurance are important. Antidepressant drugs may be needed.

ANEMIA IN PREGNANCY

It is quite common.

Complications are:
- *During pregnancy*: Preeclampsia, intercurrent infection, heart failure and preterm labor
- *During labor*: Postpartum hemorrhage, cardiac failure and shock
- *Puerperium*: Puerperal sepsis, subinvolution, poor lactation, venous thrombosis and pulmonary embolism.

Treatment:
- *If severe anemia*: Blood transfusion
- *If iron deficiency anemia*: Oral or IV iron therapy
- *If megaloblastic anemia*: Oral folic acid and IM vitamin B_{12}.

HYPERTENSION IN PREGNANCY

- It may be preexisting or pregnancy induced
- *In mild cases with blood pressure less than 160/100 mm Hg*: Adequate rest (physical and mental) and low salt. If no response, antihypertensive should be given
- *In severe cases or in cases of superimposed preeclampsia*: The patient should be hospitalized and treated as preeclampsia.

Antihypertensive drugs: Methyldopa, labetalol, nifedipine or hydralazine may be used if BP is high [avoid beta-blocker and angiotensin-converting enzyme (ACE) inhibitor].

Obstetric management:
- *In mild cases*: Continue the pregnancy up to the term and spontaneous labor is awaited
- *In severe or complicated cases*: The aim is to try to continue the pregnancy for at least 34 weeks, may be up to 37th week for fetal maturity and then to terminate the pregnancy.

DIABETES MELLITUS AND PREGNANCY

It may be preexisting diabetes mellitus or gestational diabetes mellitus.

Complications:
Fetal:
- Teratogenicity (if DM is present in early pregnancy, in first 6 weeks). May be cardiac, renal and skeletal malformations (caudal regression syndrome and neural tube defect)
- Fetal macrosomia (if DM is present in later pregnancy)
- Neonatal hypoglycemia
- Increased risk of polycythemia, hyperbilirubinemia and hypocalcemia
- Hyaline membrane disease
- Intrauterine fetal death (IUFD) and stillbirth.

Maternal:
- Polyhydramnios
- Preeclampsia
- Recurrence of gestational diabetes mellitus (GDM) in subsequent pregnancies is about 50%
- Also APH, PPH, puerperal pyrexia and puerperal sepsis.

Management:
 Restriction of diet: Calorie intake 200–2,500 for normal and 1,200–1,800 for obese.
- Regular exercise
- If needed, insulin
- Metformin or glibenclamide may be given in GDM
- With good glycemic control and patients who do not require insulin may wait for spontaneous onset of labor. Elective delivery (induction or caesarean section) is considered in patients requiring insulin or with complications (macrosomia) at around 38 weeks.

Gestational Diabetes Mellitus

It is defined as any degree of glucose intolerance with the onset or first recognition during pregnancy. Approximately 7% of all pregnancies are complicated by GDM. More than 50% women ultimately develop diabetes in the next 20 years and this is linked with obesity. Mostly they develop type-2 diabetes mellitus (T2DM).

Screening for GDM: Oral glucose tolerance test (OGTT) with 75 g of glucose is used between 24 weeks and 28 weeks of gestation. Blood glucose is measured at fasting, and 1 and 2 hours after glucose load. GDM is diagnosed if blood glucose is—fasting ≥5.1 mmol/L, or after 1 hour ≥10 mmol/L, or after 2 hours ≥8.5 mmol/L.

All woman with high risk should have OGTT. Measurement of hemoglobin A1c (HbA1c) and/or blood glucose should be done at booking visit.

Risk factors for gestational diabetes:
- Older women (40 years or over)
- Obesity
- Family history of T2DM or first-degree relative (mother or sister) who had GDM
- *Family origin*: South-Asian, black Caribbean and Middle-east
- Gestational diabetes mellitus during previous pregnancies
- History of previously macrosomia or large-weight baby (>4.5kg)
- Gestational diabetes mellitus may occur with no risk factors.

Complications: As above in DM but congenital malformation is less in GDM.

Management of GDM:
- Dietary modification. Reduction of refined carbohydrate
- *Monitoring of blood glucose regularly*: Preprandial glucose should be <5.5 mmol/L, 1 hour postprandial should be <7.8 mmol/L and 2 hours postprandial should be <6.4 mmol/L
- *If drug is necessary*: Metformin or glibenclamide is safe (does not cross placenta). Insulin may be required (other oral therapy or injectable incretin base therapy should not be used)
- After delivery, glucose usually becomes normal. Follow-up is necessary. All women with GDM should have fasting glucose measure 6 weeks postpartum and HbA1c measured annually
- There is risk of T2DM, 15–50% in 5 years. So, dietary and life style advices are necessary.

BRONCHIAL ASTHMA IN PREGNANCY

- *Uncontrolled asthma is associated with*:
  - Maternal complications: Hyperemesis gravidarum, hypertension, preeclampsia, hemorrhage and complicated labor
  - Fetal complications: IUGR, low birth weight, preterm baby, increased perinatal mortality and neonatal hypoxia.
- *Management of asthma in pregnancy*:
  - All inhalers are safe and effective
  - β_2-agonist (both short and long acting), inhaled steroids, theophylline, oral prednisolone and chromone are safe
  - If the patient was getting leukotriene receptor blockers, it can be continued (e.g. montelukast)
- *Management during labor*: Treatment should be continued. If patient on prednisolone >7.5 mg/day for >2 weeks prior to delivery, it should be changed to IV hydrocortisone, 100 mg 6–8 hourly during labor

- Breastfeeding should be continued. Very little drug is excreted in breast milk (<1% of maternal theophylline is excreted in milk)
- Acute attack during delivery is rare, probably due to endogenous steroid production. PG should be avoided, as it may induce bronchospasm.

POSTPARTUM CARDIOMYOPATHY

If any patient develops cardiac failure in the last trimester of pregnancy or within 6 months after delivery in the absence of previous heart disease, it is called postpartum or peripartum cardiomyopathy. It is a type of dilated cardiomyopathy and the cause is unknown. Immune and viral causes are postulated. Other factors are advanced age, multiple pregnancy, multiparity, and hypertension in pregnancy. It commonly occurs immediately after or in the month before delivery (peripartum).

Symptoms: It occurs usually in multipara and age above 30 years. The patient usually presents with respiratory distress, orthopnea, features of heart failure (weakness, pain in abdomen and swelling in legs), and cough with frothy sputum due to pulmonary edema.

Signs: Signs of heart failure. Atrial fibrillation or other arrhythmia may occur.

Diagnostic criteria (four criteria):
1. Presentation in the last month of pregnancy or within 6 months of delivery
2. Absence of an obvious cause for heart failure
3. Previously normal cardiac status
4. Echocardiographic evidence of systolic left ventricular dysfunction.

Treatment:
- Symptomatic for heart failure (diuretics, ACE inhibitor and digoxin)
- Beta-blocker may be helpful in some cases
- Inotropic agent may be given
- The patient should avoid subsequent pregnancy due to risk of relapse. However, if the heart size is normal in the first episode following heart failure, subsequent pregnancy is tolerated in some cases. If the heart size remains enlarged, further pregnancy causes refractory chronic heart failure.

Bibliography

1. ABM Abdullah. Case History and Data Interpretation in Medical Practice, 3rd edn. Jaypee Brothers Medical Publishers (P) Ltd, 2015.
2. ABM Abdullah. Long Cases in Clinical Medicine, 6th edn. Jaypee Brothers Medical Publishers (P) Ltd, 2019.
3. ABM Abdullah. Practical Manual in Clinical Medicine, 1st edn. Jaypee Brothers Medical Publishers (P) Ltd, 2015.
4. ABM Abdullah. Short Cases in Clinical Medicine, 7th edn. Elsevier India, 2018.
5. AK Khurana. Comprehensive Ophthalmology, 7th edn. Jaypee Brothers Medical Publishers (P) Ltd.
6. Bhuiyan SN. Clinical Guide to Obstetrics And Gynaecology, 7th edn. Publisher: Muhammad Asheek Bhuiyan.
7. DA, Cox TM, John D. Oxford Textbook of Medicine, 5th edn. Oxford: Oxford University Press, 2012.
8. Dhingra PL, Dhingra S. Diseases of Ear, Nose and Throat, 7th edn. Elsevier India.
9. Dooley JS, Lok A, Burroughs A, Heathcote J. Sherlock's Diseases of the Liver and Biliary System (Sherlock Diseases of the Liver), 12th edn. Blackwell Scientific Publications, Oxford, 2011.
10. Douglas G, Nicol F, Robertson C. Macleod's Clinical Examination, 13th ed. Churchill Livingstone Elsevier, 2013.
11. Firkin F, Chesterman C, Rush B, Penington D. de Gruchy's Clinical Haematology in Medical Practice, 6th edn. Oxford: Blackwell Scientific, 2012.
12. Glynn & Drake. Hutchison's Clinical Methods, 24th edn. WB Saunders, 2017.
13. Haque MS. Basic Ophthalmology, 2nd edn. Capital Book Center, Bangladesh.
14. James WD, Berger T, Elston D. Andrew's Diseases of the Skin Clinical Dermatology, 11th edn. Philadelphia: WB Saunder, 2011.
15. Konar H. DC Dutta's Textbook of Gynecology, 9th edn. Jaypee Brothers Medical Publishers (P) Ltd.
16. Konar H. DC Dutta's Textbook of Obstetrics, 9th edn. Jaypee Brothers Medical Publishers (P) Ltd.
17. Kumar P, Clark M. Kumar & Clark's Clinical Medicine, 9th edn. London: Elsevier, 2017.
18. Longo DL, Fauci AS, Kasper DL, et al. Harrison's Principles of Internal Medicine, 19th edn. New York: McGraw Hill, 2015.
19. Papadakis MA, McPhee SJ, Rabow MW. Current Medical Diagnosis and Treatment. New York: Mc Graw Hill, 2019.
20. Raiston SH, Penman ID, Strachan MWJ, Hobson RP. Davidson's Principles and Practice of Medicine, 23rd edn. Elsevier, 2018.
21. Ryder REJ, Mir MA, Freeman EA. An Aid to the MRCP PACES, 3rd edn. Oxford: Blackwell Publishing, 2003.

22. SK De. Fundamentals of Ear Nose and Throat and Head Neck Surgery. 11th Edition.
23. SN Chugh. Bedside Medicine Without Tears, 2nd edn. Jaypee Brothers Medical Publishers (P) Ltd, 2011.
24. SN Chugh. Clinical Methods in Medicine, 1st edn. Jaypee Brothers Medical Publishers (P) Ltd, 2008.
25. Talley NJ, O'Connor S. Clinical Examination: A Systematic Guide to Physical Examination, 6th edn. Elsevier Australia, 2009.
26. Wilkinson IB, Raine T, Wiles K, et al. Oxford handbook of clinical medicine, 10th edn. Oxford: Oxford University Press, 2017.

Index

A

Abdomen 7
   ultrasonography of 134, 161
   X-ray of 134, 192
ABO incompatibility 338
Abortion 404, 408
   complete 408, 410
   criminal 409
   habitual 408, 410
   incomplete 408, 410
   induced 409
   inevitable 408, 409
   legal 409
   missed 408, 410
   septic 408, 411
   spontaneous 408
   therapeutic 409, 412
   threatened 408, 409
Abruptio placenta 115, 419
Acanthosis nigricans 73, 237
Acetoacetate 196
Acetone 196
   breath 155
Achalasia cardia 65, 67
Acid-base imbalance 325
Acid-fast bacillus 83, 125, 243, 259
Acidosis
   correction of 301
   metabolic 300, 328
   respiratory 329
   severe metabolic 299
Acne vulgaris 242
Acquired immunodeficiency syndrome 307, 370, 371
   diagnosis of 372
   natural history of 371
   treatment of 373
Acromegaly 149
Actinomyces israelii 44
Activated partial thromboplastin time 191, 361, 403
Acute exacerbation 40
   treatment of 47
Acute respiratory distress syndrome 45, 48, 74, 356, 422
Acyanotic Fallot 15

Addison's disease 86, 143, 145, 250, 315, 325
Addisonian crisis 84, 86, 146
Adenocarcinoma 43, 415, 416
Adenoma 142
   adrenal 147
Adenomyosis 408, 413
Adenosine deaminase 83, 125, 259
Adjustment disorder 308
Adrenal cortex, diseases of 143
Adrenal medulla, diseases of 143
Adult polycystic kidney disease 204
Adult Still's disease 359
Aedes aegypti 166
Agnosia 291
Agoraphobia 308
Air embolism 115
Akinetic seizure 287
Albendazole 183-185
Albinism 341
Alcohol 84, 117, 121, 264
   intoxication, acute 357
   withdrawal, clinical features of 358
Alcoholism 357
Alemtuzumab 107
Alkaline phosphatase 118
Alkalosis 142
   metabolic 328
   respiratory 329
Alkaptonuria 341
Allergens 39
Allergic alveolitis, extrinsic 57
Allergic angiitis 353
Allergic reaction 115
Allergies 200
Allopurinol 199, 205
Alopecia 250
   areata 250
   totalis 250
   causes of 250
   universalis 250
Alpha-glucosidase inhibitors 156
Alpha-thalassemia 95, 96
Alport syndrome 200, 342
Aluminum-containing antacids 85
Alzheimer's disease 291, 315
Amblyopia, nutritional 264

Amenorrhea 160, 401
  concealed 401
  history of 409
  primary 160, 401
  secondary 160, 401, 402
  true 401
Amiodarone 267
Amitriptyline 309
Amniotic fluid embolism 115
Amoebiasis 86, 173
Amphotericin B
  conventional 182
  deoxycholate 183
Amyloidosis 108
Amyotrophy
  diabetic 348
  syphilitic 284
Analgesic 388
  nephropathy 210, 213
Ancylostoma duodenale 184
Ancylostomiasis 184
Androgen 146
Anemia 73, 90, 92, 101, 208, 424
  aplastic 99, 101, 403
  autoimmune hemolytic 96
  correction of 95
  dimorphic 91
  dyshemopoietic 90
  features of 101
  hemorrhagic 90
  investigations of 91
  pernicious 93, 250
  severe 401
  sideroblastic 90, 92
  specific cause of 91
  triad of 95
Aneurysm, ventricular 20
Angina 11
  pectoris 17
Angioedema, hereditary 362
Angiotensin-converting enzyme
    inhibitor 7, 153, 198, 238, 326
Angle-closure glaucoma, acute 385
Angular cheilitis 93
Ankylosing spondylitis 5, 222
Anorectum 252
Anorexia 68, 73, 88, 164
  nervosa 84, 85, 312, 313
    physical effects of 313
Anosmia 395
Anterior spinal artery thrombosis 283
Anthrax 186
  cutaneous 186
  gastrointestinal 187
  inhalational 187
Antianginal drugs 17

Antibiotic 133, 212, 393, 395, 423
  therapy 83
  topical 378, 388
Antibody 88
  antinuclear 108, 200, 225, 244, 351
  antiphospholipid 411
  test 225
Anticholinergic 85
  drug 40
Anticoagulant 62, 65
  therapy 108
Antiepileptics 185
Antifibrotic therapy 57
Antigen
  bacterial 334
  detection of 181
  serum prostate-specific 218
Anti-hepatitis
  A virus 118
  E virus 118
Antihistamine 116, 395
Antihypertensive drugs 425
Anti-inflammatory drugs 395
Anti-Koch's
  disease 284
  therapy 211, 233
Anti-mitochondrial antibody 124
Antiplatelet 226
  prolonged use of 65
  therapy 17
Antipsychotic drugs 312
  side effects of 312
Antistreptolysin O titer 242
Antitubercular drugs 59
  first-line 59
  second-line 59
Anti-tuberculosis 117
Antral biopsy 69
Anuria 198
  causes of 198
Anxiety 39, 85
  disorders 308
    management of 308
  neurosis 306, 308
Aorta, coarctation of 16, 161
Aplastic crisis 98
Appendicitis, acute 76, 84
Appendicular lump, treatment of 76
Apraxia 291
  constructional 128
Arnold-Chiari lesion 280
Arrhythmia 27
Arsenic 264
  toxicity, chronic 245
Arsenicosis 244
Artemether plus lumefantrine 180

Arterial blood gas 154, 155
   analysis 56, 191
Arteriovenous malformation 277
Arteritis, temporal 350
Arthralgia 47, 221
Arthritis 12, 221, 235
   hemophilic 222, 234
   inflammatory 221
   juvenile idiopathic 221, 235
   mechanical 221
   noninflammatory 221
   psoriatic 229
   seronegative 221, 229
   seropositive 221
   treatment of 229
   types of 238
Arthrocentesis 235
Arthropathy 151
   neuropathic 222
Arthroscopy 232
Artificial tear 225
Asbestosis 62
Asboe-Hansen signs 240
Ascariasis 184
Ascaris lumbricoides 184
Ascites 124
Ascitic fluid 83
   aspiration of 125
   color 125
Ascorbic acid 322
Aspergillus
   flavus 131
   fumigatus 388
   niger 388
Aspiration 45, 123, 125, 193
   pneumonia, recurrent 67
Aspirin 65, 299
   intolerance 395
Asthenia 73
Asthma 39, 41, 42
   acute severe 40
   chronic 40
   drugs-induced 41
   episodic 40
   exercise-induced 41
   intermittent 40
   management of 41, 426
   nocturnal 39
   occupational 41
   uncontrolled 426
Ataxia 266
   telangiectasia 341
Atherosclerosis 136, 214
Athetosis 274
Atresia, duodenal 343
Atrial ectopics 31
Atrial fibrillation 29

Atrial flutter 31
Atrial pacing 36
Atrial septal defect 13, 161, 342
Atrioventricular block 32
Attack, acute 17
Audiometry 391
Auditory hallucination 307
Auspitz's sign 238
Autoimmune collagen disorders 382
Autonomic dysfunction 176, 207
Autonomic failure, primary 270
Autosomal dominant disease 341
Autosomal recessive diseases 341
Azithromycin 170, 253

B

Bacillary dysentery 172
Bacillus anthracis 186
Bacillus calmette-guérin 241
Bacillus cereus 85
Back pain, low 408
Bacteria 335
   gram-negative 211
Bacteriuria, asymptomatic 211, 212
Bacteroides fragilis 389
Bardet–Biedl syndrome 160
Bariatric surgery 86
Barium
   enema 78, 79
   meal 87
Barrett's esophagus 66, 68
Bartter syndrome 327
Basal ganglia 271
Becker muscular dystrophy 289, 290
Behavioral disorders 306
Behçet's disease 257, 277
Behçet's syndrome 64, 242, 353
Bell's palsy 262, 263
Bence–Jones protein 114
Benzodiazepine 303, 317
Beriberi 417
   dry 320
   neurological 320
   wet 320
Berry aneurysm 277
Beta-blocker, contraindications of 10
Beta-hydroxybutyric acid 196
Betamethasone 251
Beta-thalassemia 95
Bicarbonate 325
Biguanides 156
Bile
   acid malabsorption 87
   salt 196
Bilevel positive airway pressure 362, 396

Biliary atresia, extrahepatic 117
Bilirubin 100, 196
   excess production of 117
   reduced hepatic uptake of 117
Biochemistry 83
Biological therapy 224
Biopsy 68, 216, 232
Biotin 322
Bipolar affective disorder 310
Bipolar mood disorder 310
Birth weight, low 338
Bisphosphonate 65, 229
Bitot's spots 318
Biventricular failure, causes of 8
Black urine, causes of 197
Bladder
   emptying, incomplete 211
   involvement 270
   neck obstruction 205
   stone 215
   tumor, invasive 217
Blalock-Taussig shun 15
Bleeding 129
   continuous 407
   cutaneous 323
   disorder 65
   gastrointestinal 127
   manifestations 101
   per vagina 409
   placental 418
   postmenopausal 406
   primary prevention of 130
   recurrent 407
   spots 101
   time 100, 108
Blepharitis 376
Blindness 318
Bloating 88
Blood 196
   dyscrasias 403
   gas analysis 333
   glucose 155
      monitoring of 152
   loss 90, 205, 346
   pressure 5, 136
      diastolic 422
      low 190
   sugar 200
   tests 70
   transfusion 115
Blumer's shelf 73
Body dysmorphic disorder 314
Body mass index 158
Bone 68, 78
   age 160
   disease 178, 207
   marrow 95, 99, 101, 103, 104, 108
      examination 92
      secondary deposit of 107
      study 105, 111
      transplantation 101, 102
   mineral density 145, 351
   X-ray of 229
Borderline lepromatous leprosy 187
Borderline leprosy 187
Borderline tuberculoid 187
Bordetella pertussis 175
Bortezomib 114
Bouchard's node 228
Bowen's disease 245
Bradycardia, causes of 28
Brain 68
   abscess 260
   magnetic resonance imaging of 259, 266, 281, 316
   tumor 282
      primary 315
Breast abscess 423
Breastfeeding 427
Breathlessness 49
Briquet's syndrome 314
Broad-spectrum antibiotic 74, 127, 260, 391, 412
Bronchial asthma 39, 395, 426
   drugs used in 40
   management of 40
   types of 40
Bronchial carcinoma 43, 53, 267
   types of 43
Bronchiectasis 42, 67
   dry 42
   sicca 42
Bronchiolitis 332
Bronchitis
   acute 48
   chronic 47, 102
Bronchodilator 47, 57
Bronchopneumonia 46
Bronze diabetes 130
Brucella agglutination test 178
Brucellosis 177
Brugia malayi 183
Brushfield spots 342
Budd-Chiari syndrome 99
Bulbar palsy 65
   progressive 275
Bulbar poliomyelitis 190
Bulimia nervosa 313
Bull's eye lesion 241
Bullous diseases 239
Bullous pemphigoid 240
Bumetanide 201
Bundle branch block 32
Burr-hole aspiration 261
Butyrophenone 273

C

Café au lait spot 292
Calcinosis 226
Calcium 85, 87, 208
Campylobacter jejuni 195, 285
Cancer
  colon 86
  colorectal 80
Candida 23
  albicans 64, 253, 257, 372, 388
Candidiasis 64, 65
Cannabis 304
Carbimazole 138
Carbohydrate malabsorption 87
Carbon monoxide poisoning 315
Carcinoembryonic antigen 73
Carcinoid syndrome 363
Carcinoma 64, 217
  anaplastic 141
  breast 343
  cervix 415
  colon 80, 82
  endometrial 416
  esophagus 65, 67
  follicular 141
  gallbladder 134
  hepatocellular 130
  large cell 43
  larynx 399
  pancreas 75, 117
  papillary 140
  periampullary 117
  pharynx 65
  primary 132
  prostate 197
  secondary 132
  stomach 72, 84, 86
  undifferentiated 141
Cardiac failure, congenital 1, 7, 136, 199, 326
Cardiomyopathy 25
  dilated 26
  hypertrophic 25
  postpartum 27, 427
  restrictive 26
Cardiovascular disease 103, 352
Cardiovascular system 1, 149, 339, 405
Carditis, signs of 11
Carfilzomib 115
Carpal tunnel syndrome 268
Casts 196
Cataract 383
Catarrhal phase 164
Cat-scratch disease 242
Cavernous sinus thrombosis 366
Cefixime 170, 253
Cefotaxime 127
Ceftriaxone 170, 253
  plus amoxyclav 127
Ceiling test 279
Celiac disease 64, 86, 88
Cells, epithelial 196
Central nervous system 55, 84, 104, 207, 258, 302, 316, 328, 329, 361
  infection of 257
Central retinal vein occlusion 264
Cerebellar
  hemangioblastoma 102
  lesions 280
  signs 281
  syndrome 280
Cerebral
  circulation 151
  edema 277
    features of 129
  embolism 278
  hemorrhage 277, 278, 422
  infarction 277, 278
    multiple 284
  lesion 284
  malaria 180
  palsy 330
  tumor 271
  vasodilator 277
  venography 281
Cerebrospinal fluid 60, 255, 258, 321, 331
  study 335
Cerebrovascular accident 204, 276
Cerebrovascular disease 85
  types of 278
Ceruloplasmin production 282
Cervix 406
Chagas disease 65
Chalazion 377
Chancroid 254
Channelopathy 289
Charcot's joint 151, 222
Charcot-Marie-Tooth disease 267, 370
Chemical injuries 383
Chemotherapy 73, 76, 112, 132, 217
  intravesical 217
  perioperative 73
Chest
  high-resolution computed tomography of 374
  physiotherapy 56
  X-ray of 1, 39, 333, 335
Chicken pox 177
Chlamydia psittaci 44
Chlamydia trachomatis 253, 413
Chloasma 247
Chlorambucil 107
Chlorhexidine 64
Chloride 325

Chloroquine 179, 224, 264
Chlorpromazine 117, 270
Chocolate cyst 413
Cholangiocarcinoma 117
Cholangitis, sclerosing 117
Cholecalciferol 319
Cholecystectomy 81
Cholecystitis
   acute 84, 133
   chronic 134
Choledocholithiasis 117, 121
Cholera 173
Cholestasis, transient intrahepatic 117
Cholesteatoma 391
Cholesterol, total 157
Cholestyramine 87
Chorea 273
   benign familial 273
   gravidarum 273
Choriomeningitis, lymphocytic 259
Christmas disease 108, 111, 197
Chromones 40
Chromosome analysis 104
Chronic alcoholism 126
   treatment of 358
Chronic cold agglutinin disease 97
Chronic kidney disease 10, 69, 84, 90, 141, 199, 206, 227, 267, 325, 355
   causes of 206
   stages of 207
Chronic myeloid leukemia 102, 105
   treatment of 106
   types of 105
Chronic obstructive pulmonary disease 55, 69, 102, 369
Churg-Strauss syndrome 56, 353, 395
Chyle 196
Cincent's angina 64
Ciprofloxacin 170, 199, 205, 253
Cirrhosis 119
   causes of 131
   decompensated 126
   primary biliary 117, 121, 123
Cisplatin 267
Clarithromycin 47
Claudication 151
Clindamycin 174
Clobetasol propionate 251
Clomipramine 309
Clonazepam 355
Clopidogrel 65
Clostridium difficile 85
Clostridium tetani 175
Coagulation
   defect 108
   disorder 403
   screen 100, 108
Coagulopathy 129

Coal worker's pneumoconiosis 62
Coartemether 180
Coccidioides 257
Coccidioidomycosis 242
Cognitive behavioral therapy 313
Cold
   agglutinin disease 97
   antibodies 94
   clammy skin 166
   hemagglutinin disease 97
Colitis
   ischemic 86
   pseudomembranous 364
Collagen disease 108, 124, 199, 243, 267
Collagen vascular disease 231, 279
Colon cancer, hereditary nonpolyposis 75, 81
Coma 100
   hyperosmolar nonketotic diabetic 151, 155
Common bile duct 117
Community-acquired pneumonia 45
   causes of 44
Complement fixation test 181
Complete blood count 2, 40, 47, 68, 76, 88, 91, 98-101, 119, 122, 165, 166, 205, 223, 226, 231, 232, 238, 242, 258, 324, 331, 333, 334, 335, 337, 349, 351, 355, 361, 388
Computed tomography 2, 316
   angiography 350
   scan 118
Condylomata lata 255
Conjugation, impaired 117
Conjunctiva, xerosis of 318
Conjunctival diseases 375
Conjunctivitis 253, 378
   allergic 379
   bacterial 379
   gonococcal 379
Conn's syndrome 143, 147, 327
Connective tissue
   disease 315
   disorders 37
Constipation 84, 89
Contact dermatitis 248
   acute irritant 248
   allergic 248
   chronic irritant 249
   irritant 248
   occupational 249
   treatment of 249
Continuous positive airway pressure 362, 396
Conversion disorder 314
Convulsion
   control of 331
   neonatal 339

Coomb test 46, 338
Corneal diseases 375
Corneal ulcer
  bacterial 380
  fungal 380
Corona virus 85
Coronary artery
  bypass surgery 18
  disease 16
Coronary circulation 151
Corpus cancer syndrome 416
Corrosive poisoning 304
Corticospinal tract sign lesion 281
Corticosteroid 40, 305
  inhaled 47
Corticotropin-releasing hormone test 144
Cortisol, low 146
Corynebacterium diphtheriae 174
Cotrimoxazole 170
Cough
  variant asthma 41
  whooping 107, 175, 330
Coxiella burnetii 44, 171
Coxsackievirus 259
C-reactive protein 78, 114, 231
Cretinism 135, 137
Creutzfeldt-Jakob disease 280, 315
Crigler-Najjar syndrome 117
Crohn's disease 64, 77-80, 87, 93, 242
Cryoglobulinemia 243
Cryptococcus neoformans 51, 257, 372
Cryptomenorrhea 401
Cryptosporidium parvum 85
Cullen's sign 74
Cushing's disease 114, 144, 145, 402
Cushing's syndrome 108, 143, 144, 160, 228, 289, 315, 327, 348
Cyanide poisoning 264
Cyanocobalamin 322
Cyanosis 175
  central 14
Cyclophosphamide 114, 350
Cyclosporine 117, 199, 205
Cyst 192
  features of 192
  renal 102, 213
Cystic fibrosis 341, 368, 395
Cysticercosis 185, 257
Cystinuria 215
Cystitis 211
Cytology 83
Cytomegalovirus 44, 115, 117, 209, 285, 371, 383
Cytotoxic drugs 64, 84, 87

D

Dacryocystitis 377
  acute 378
  chronic 378
Dapsone 267
Dark-ground illumination 255
Datura poisoning 303
De Quervain's thyroiditis 135, 138
Deafness 264, 391
Dehydration 215, 336, 417
  features of 195
  severe 336
  signs of 85, 336
Delirium 316
  tremens 316, 358
Delusion 306
Dementia 94, 271, 306, 315, 321
Demyelinating disease 264, 283
Dendritic pattern 381
Dengue 108, 117
  fever 166
  hemorrhagic fever 65, 166
  shock syndrome 166
  viral infection, manifestations of 166
Dental procedure 25
Deoxyribonucleic acid, anti-double-stranded 230
Depression 85, 309
  postpartum 315, 424
  respiratory center 329
Dermatitis 243, 321
  exfoliative 239
Dermatomyositis 73, 231, 237, 289
  causes of 231
  childhood 231
  primary idiopathic 231
Dermatophyte infection 246
Dermis 236
Descemet's membrane 282
Desmopressin 111
Dexamethasone 114, 277
Diabetes insipidus 150, 264, 325
  cranial 150
Diabetes mellitus 10, 41, 65, 81, 119, 130, 144, 151-153, 191, 200, 206, 213, 236, 263, 264, 267, 402, 425
  complications of 151
  diagnosis of 151
  etiological classification of 152
  gestational 152, 425, 426
  insulin-dependent 198
  management of 153, 155
  noninsulin-dependent 198
Diaphragm 367

Diarrhea 47, 85, 87-89, 99, 321, 335, 336
  acute 85
  bloody 86
  chronic 85, 86
  factitious 86
  watery 335
Diethylcarbamazine 183
Diffuse goiter, diffuse 139
Digoxin 84
Dimercaprol 245
Dimercaptosuccinic acid 245
Diphenyl hydantoin 247
Diphtheria 174, 267
  antitoxin 174
  pertussis and tetanus 175
Diphyllobothrium latum 86, 93
Direct agglutination test 181
Diseases modifying anti-rheumatic drugs 224
Disseminated infection 253
Disseminated intravascular coagulation 98, 115, 361
Dissociative disorder 314
Distal tubular acidosis 215, 219
Distension 88
Diverticular diseases 89
Diverticulitis 86, 89
Diverticulosis 89
Dizziness 294
  causes of 294
Domperidone 68, 84
Down syndrome 342, 343
Doxycycline 47, 171, 172, 183
Drowning 356
Drugs 84, 121, 228, 264, 267, 270, 315, 326
  therapy 40, 56, 129, 231, 271
  treatment 311
Dubin-Johnson syndrome 117
Duchenne muscular dystrophy 289, 342
Duodenal ulcer, chronic 65
Dwarfism 160
Dysarthria 275
Dysentery, amoebic 173
Dysfunctional uterine bleeding 404, 406
Dyskinesia 274
Dyslipidemia 11, 208
Dysmenorrhea 404
  congestive 404
  secondary 404
Dyspepsia, nonulcer 71
Dysphagia 65, 67, 226, 275
Dysphonia 275, 397
Dystonia 274
Dystrophy, facioscapulohumeral 289, 290
Dysuria 198

E

Ear
  discharge 390
  diseases of 386
  drop 390
  external 386
  foreign body in 387
  low set 343
  middle 386
  wax 386
Earache 164, 386
Eating disorder 83, 306, 312
Eaton-Lambert syndrome 348
Ebstein's anomaly 3, 4, 12
Echinococcus granulosus 192
Echovirus 257, 259
Eclampsia 422
Ectopics, ventricular 31
Ectropion 377
Eculizumab 99
Edema 421
  idiopathic 366
  pulmonary 6, 7
Ehlers-Danlos syndrome 228
Eisenmenger syndrome 13, 14
Ekbom syndrome 355
Electrocardiogram 136, 300, 327, 328
Electrolyte 325
  imbalance 339
  loss 346
Elephantiasis 183
Elliptocytosis 90, 94
Emaciation 323
Emollient 238
Emotion, disturbance of 311
Emphysema 48, 102
Empyema 50
  nontuberculous 51
  tuberculous 51
Encephalitis 84, 257, 259, 372
  lethargica 273
Encephalomyelitis 257
  acute disseminated 280
Encephalopathy
  acute bilirubin 338
  chronic bilirubin 338
  hypertensive 9
  portosystemic 127
Endemic typhus 171
Endocardial cushion defect 342
Endocarditis 23, 178, 253
  acute 23
    bacterial 23
  bacterial 200
  infective 23
  noninfective 24

postoperative 23
signs of 11
Endocrine 43, 162, 228, 236, 289
  abnormalities 207
  diseases 84, 326
Endometrioma
  large 413
  small 413
Endometriosis 412
Endometrium 406
Endoscopic retrograde cholangiopancreatography 73
Endoscopy 68, 69, 87
Energy 310
Enoxaparin 201
Entamoeba histolytica 85, 122, 173, 335, 372
Enterobius vermicularis 184
Enterococcus faecalis 23
Enterococcus faecium 23
Enterovirus 334, 335
Entropion 377
Enzyme-linked immunosorbent assay 122
Eosinophilia, tropical pulmonary 183
Epidemic typhus 171
Epidermis 236
Epididymitis 253
Epigastric pulsation 37
Epiglottitis, acute 399
Epilepsy 286
  causes of 286
  Jacksonian 287
  temporal lobe 287
Epileptic seizure 300
Epimenorrhagia 404
Episcleritis 382
Episiotomy 423
Epistaxis 394
Epithelial casts 196
Epstein-Barr virus 117, 193, 257
Erythema
  gyratum repens 237
  multiforme 46, 241
  nodosum 55, 241
  leprosum 242
Erythrocyte sedimentation rate 91, 145, 242, 404
Erythroderma 237, 239
Erythroid hyperplasia 95
Erythromycin 47
Escherichia coli 76, 99, 121, 191, 211, 257, 423
Esomeprazole 68
Esophageal manometry 67
Esophageal spasm, diffuse 65
Esophageal varices 129
  rupture of 65
Esophagitis 65
Esophagus
  achalasia of 67
  barium swallow of 67, 68
  diseases of 65
Estrogen therapy 161
Etanercept 240
Ethambutol 264
Ethanol 301
Ethyl alcohol 301
Ethylene glycol 301
Eunuchoid body proportion, features of 344
Excessive normal saline infusion 325
External hordeolum 376
Extracellular fluid 73
Eye 222, 238, 245, 282
  changes 321, 359
  diseases of 375
  foreign body in 383
  movement desensitization and reprocessing 307
Eyelashes
  depigmentation of 378
  loss of 378
Eyelids 248
  diseases of 376

F

Face and trunk 248
Facial palsy, bilateral 263
Factitious disorder 317
Falciparum infection, severe 180
Falciparum malaria 179, 180, 191
Falx meningioma 284
Famotidine 68
Fanconi syndrome 282
Fascicular block 35
Fasting glucose, impaired 152
Fat malabsorption 87
Fatigue syndrome, chronic 314
Fatty liver disease, nonalcoholic 119
Febrile convulsion 331
  atypical 332
Febrile reaction 115
Febrile seizure 331
Felty's syndrome 243
Ferrous sulfate 65
Fetal death, intrauterine 425
Fetal macrosomia 425
Fever 44, 99, 100, 111, 164, 166, 191
  enteric 169
  hemorrhagic 108
  typhoid 169
  typhus 170
  undifferentiated 166
Fibrin degradation product 100

Fibrinogen 115
Fibrinolytic therapy 62
Fibroid
   complications of 408
   uterus 407
Fibromuscular dysplasia 214
Filariasis 183
Fine-needle aspiration cytology 55, 139, 232, 366
Fish tapeworm 93
Flaccid paraplegia 284
Flatulence 88
Flea-borne typhus 171
Fludrocortisone 146
Fluid
   intravenous 133, 348
   loss 205, 346
   restriction 201
   syndrome 366
Fluorescent treponema antibody absorption test 255
Folic acid 87, 96, 267
   deficiency 94
Food
   allergen 249
   poisoning 195
Foot
   complications 151
   diabetic 153
Forced vital capacity 40
Formic acid, metabolite 300
Fragile X syndrome 342
Friedreich's ataxia 264, 281, 283, 284
Friedreich's sign 22
Fundoscopy 421
Fungal
   infections 242
   sinusitis, allergic 395
Furosemide 201, 327
Furunculosis 388

G

Gait 271
   apraxia 271
   ataxia 321, 359
   waddling 289
Gallbladder, palpable 75
Gangrene 151
Gardnerella vaginalis 413
Gastrectomy 86
Gastric
   cancer, early 73
   erosion 65
   outlet obstruction 71, 72
   ulcer 71
      chronic 65
Gastrinoma 71, 86

Gastritis
   acute 68
   chronic 68
Gastroenteritis 84, 146
Gastroesophageal reflux disease 66
Gastrointestinal diseases 64
Gastrointestinal infection 83
Gastrointestinal loss 327
Gastrointestinal tract 74, 86, 92, 159, 226, 228, 230, 245, 302, 314, 339, 361, 408
   disease 64
   disorders 84
   loss 328
Genetics 341
   disease 228
Genitalia
   external 344
   rudimentary external 344
German measles 165
Ghon focus 58
Giant aortic aneurysm 65
Giant cell arteritis 350, 351
Giardia lamblia 85, 186, 335
Giardiasis 86, 186
Gilbert's syndrome 117
Gitelman syndrome 327
Glabellar tap 271
Glands, adrenal 143
Glasgow coma scale 190
Glaucoma 384
Globus hystericus 65
Glomerular basement membrane 354
Glomerular disease 205, 206
Glomerulonephritis 197, 201
   acute 196, 202
   focal segmental 201
   membranoproliferative 202
   mesangiocapillary 202
   postinfectious 202
   poststreptococcal 203
   rapidly progressing 199, 202
Glomerulopathy, membranous 202
Glomerulosclerosis, focal segmental 201
Glossitis 91
Glucocorticoid 146
Glucose tolerance
   impaired 152
   test 150
Glucose-6-phosphate dehydrogenase 180, 337
   deficiency 90, 94, 342
Goiter 135, 137, 138
   investigations of 139
   nodular 139
   retrosternal 65
   simple 139

toxic 139
multinodular 137, 139
nodular 138
Gonadotropin-releasing hormone 149, 364
Gonococcal infection, disseminated 252
Gonorrhea 252
Goodpasture syndrome 354
Gout 222, 227
secondary causes of 227
Gower's sign 289
Gram stain 252
Grandiose delusions 306
Granular casts 196
Granulomatosis 349, 353
Granulomatous diseases 383
Graves' disease 135-138, 250
Grey Turner's sign 74
Growth
hormone 148, 313
assay 150
retardation 87
Guillain-Barré syndrome 47, 263, 284, 285, 272
Guttate psoriasis 238
Gynecomastia 126, 343

H

Haemophilus ducreyi 254
Haemophilus influenzae 47, 234, 257, 333, 413
Hair 245
Hairless face 344
Hallucination 307, 310
gustatory 307
olfactory 307
Haloperidol 117, 274
Ham acid serum test 99
Hand, X-ray of 142
Hansen's disease 187
Hanta virus 209
Haptoglobin, low 95
Harrison's sulcus 319
Hartmann's solution 336
Hashimoto's thyroiditis 135-138, 250
Hashitoxicosis 138
Head injury 270, 315
Headache 100, 164, 261, 262
cluster 261
tension 261
unilateral 262
vascular 261
Hearing loss 390
Heart 161, 222, 230, 245
block 32
complete 5, 34
disease
congenital 3, 12
ischemic 16, 136, 198
failure 6
myxoma of 2
sound, first 1
Heat stroke 357
Heberden's node 228
Hejunal biopsy, endoscopic 88
Helicobacter pylori infection 68
diagnosis of 69
treatment of 69
HELLP syndrome 355
Hematemesis 65
Hematochezia 66
Hematological disease 243, 277
Hematology 90
Hematoma, chronic subdural 315
Hematuria 197
causes of 197
initial 197
painful 197
painless 197
terminal 197
total 197
Hemiballismus 274
Hemiblock 33
Hemiparesis 283
Hemiplegia 283
Hemochromatosis 117, 130, 222
hereditary 130, 341
primary 130
Hemoglobin
abnormality 90
concentration 90
electrophoresis 98
Hemoglobinopathy 94
Hemoglobinuria
paroxysmal
cold 97
nocturnal 95, 99
Hemolysis
evidence of 95
intravascular 100
Hemolytic anemia 46, 90, 91, 94
active 107
group of 96
hereditary 92, 95
microangiopathic 98, 100
warm autoimmune 97
Hemolytic transfusion reaction 115
Hemolytic uremic syndrome 98, 99
Hemophilia 65, 108, 110, 197
A 342
B 111, 342
pedigree of 110
Hemorrhage 408
antepartum 418

gastrointestinal 71
postpartum 419, 420
retinal 417
subarachnoid 277, 278
subconjunctival 380
Hemosiderosis, prevention of 96
Henoch–Schönlein purpura 109, 222
  treatment of 110
Hepatic iron index 131
Hepatic precoma 127
Hepatitis 47, 117
  A 117
  acute 84
    alcoholic 119
    viral 120
  B 96, 117
    virus 118, 200
  C 96, 117
    virus 118, 200
  chronic 119
  D 96, 117
  E 117
    infection 120
  viral 117, 121
Hepatobiliary system 118
Hepatocellular failure, signs of 126
Hepatolenticular degeneration 282
Hepatology 117
Hepatoma 102, 131
Hepatotropic viruses 120
Herpes simplex virus 64, 167, 253, 257, 383
  encephalitis 167, 168, 260
  types of 167
Herpes zoster virus 285
Hiatus hernia 67
Hiccough 367
High-dose dexamethasone suppression test 144
Highly active antiretroviral therapy 373
High-resolution computed tomography 148, 374
Histoplasma capsulatum 191, 257
Histoplasmosis 242
Hoarseness 397
Hodgkin's disease 111, 236, 372
Homocystinuria 278
Hookworm infestation 184
Hordeolum internum 377
Hormonal therapy 219
Hormone
  adrenocorticotropic 143
  antidiuretic 150
  assay 161
  deficiency 141
  excess 141
  follicle-stimulating 148, 364

replacement therapy 405
  benefits of 406
  complications of 406
resistance 141
therapy 405
Horner's syndrome 264
Horseshoe kidney 162
Human chorionic gonadotropin 149
Human diploid cell vaccine 169
Human immunodeficiency virus 65, 96, 200, 237, 257, 267, 315, 370, 382
  cutaneous manifestations of 372
  diagnosis of 372
  disease 371
  infection 145, 370
    prevention of 373
  natural history of 371
  transmission of 371
Human insulin 156
Human leukocyte antigen 223
Humerus, mid shaft of 269
Huntington's chorea 273
Huntington's disease 270, 315, 341
Hyaline membrane disease 425
Hydatid disease 192
Hydrocephalus 284, 293
  normal pressure 271, 294, 315
Hydrocortisone 146, 148
  intravenous 137
  suppression test 142
Hydronephrosis 162
Hydroquinone 247
Hydroxychloroquine 225
Hyperaldosteronism, primary 147, 327
Hyperbilirubinemia
  conjugated 117
  unconjugated 117
Hypercalcemia 73, 85, 146, 215
Hyperemesis gravidarum 417
Hyperfunction 143
Hyperglycemia 326
  clinical diagnosis of 155
  typical features of 155
Hyperglycemic hyperosmolar state 151, 155
Hyperkalemia 146, 208, 326, 327
Hyperkeratosis 244
Hyperlipidemia 201, 326
Hypermenorrhea 403
Hypernatremia 325
Hyperoxaluria 215
Hyperparathyroidism 85, 141, 315, 348
  primary 142
  secondary 142
  tertiary 141, 142
  treatment of 142
Hyperplasia 142
  adrenal 147

congenital adrenal 143
Hyperpyrexia 422
Hypersensitivity 64
   pneumonitis 57
   reactions 312
Hypertension 8-11, 42, 136, 144, 147, 161, 206, 208, 210, 421, 422, 425
   benign intracranial 264, 281
   complications of 8
   features of 204
   grades of 9
   idiopathic intracranial 281
   malignant 9
   pulmonary 14, 37
   refractory 9
   resistant 9
   treatment of 10
Hyperthyroidism 86, 135
Hypertriglyceridemia 73
Hypertrophy, prostatic 205
Hyperuricemia 215
Hyperuricosuria 215
Hyperventilation 129
Hypoalbuminemia 142
Hypocalcemia 142, 143
Hypocalciuria 215
Hypochondriasis 314
Hypodermis 236
Hypofunction 143
Hypoglycemia 146, 151, 157
   causes of 157
   clinical diagnosis of 155
   neonatal 425
   prevention of 157
   typical features of 155
Hypogonadism
   hale 163
   hypergonadotropic 163
   hypogonadotropic 161
   primary 163
Hypokalemia 127, 147, 214, 327, 328
Hypomagnesemia 328
Hypomania 309
Hyponatremia 146, 325
   postoperative 326
   true 325, 326
Hypoparathyroidism 142, 315
Hypopituitarism 315
   causes of 148
Hypoplasia, endometrial 160
Hypoprothrombinemia 417
Hyposmia 395
Hypotension 166, 199, 205
   orthostatic 295
Hypothyroidism 85, 90, 135, 136, 280, 315, 348
   autoimmune 343
   features of 136

   goitrous 136
   nongoitrous 136
   primary 135
   secondary 135
   spontaneous atrophic 135
   treatment of 136
Hypovolemia 85
Hypromellose 225
Hysteria 314
Hysterical conversion reaction 84

I

Ichthyosis 237
Ileal disease 93
Ileal resection 93
Ileocecal tuberculosis 82
   complications of 82
Imipramine 309
Immune thrombocytopenic purpura 65, 197, 403
Immunochromatographic test 181
Immunofluorescence assay 171
Immunoglobulin
   A nephropathy 201, 204
   M 118
Indirect fluorescent antibody test 181, 194
Indirect hemagglutination assay 181
Infections 101, 115, 135, 249, 267, 315, 406
   asymptomatic 371
   nonviral 117
   viral 117
Inflammation 135
   postinfectious 279
   postvaccinal 279
   scleral 375
Inflammatory bowel disease 77, 86, 242
Infliximab 240
Influenza 44
Injection artesunate 180
Injuries 406, 422
Insane, general paresis of 256
Insulin
   analogues 156
   therapy
      absolute indications of 156
      complications of 157
Internal malignancy, dermatological manifestations of 237
Interstitial diseases 206
Intestinal disaccharidase deficiency 86
Intestinal enteropeptidase deficiency 86
Intestinal malabsorption, features of 88
Intestinal obstruction 76, 84
Intestine 86

Intrahepatic portosystemic shunt 127
Intramuscular ceftriaxone, single dose 253
Intrauterine contraceptive device 403
Intrauterine growth
   restriction 422
   retardation 338
      complications of 339
Iridocyclitis 381
Iris inflammation 375
Iron 85, 87
   deficiency anemia 91-93
   profile 131
   therapy 93
Irritable bowel syndrome 83
Irritants 39
Ischemia 151
   myocardial 151
Isoniazid 267
Isonicotinylhydrazide 117, 259
Itching 236

J

Japanese B encephalitis 259
Jaundice 95, 117, 118, 120, 123, 417
   cholestatic 121
   hepatocellular 118
   investigations of 118
   neonatal 337
   obstructive 118, 120, 121
   painless obstructive 75
   prehepatic 118
   prolonged 337
Jod-Basedow phenomenon 138
Joints 78, 238
   magnetic resonance imaging of 232
Jugular venous pressure 1

K

Kala-azar 115, 180
Kallmann syndrome 364
Kaposi's sarcoma 64, 372
Kartagener's syndrome 395
Kayser–Fleischer ring 282
Keratitis 381
   viral 381
Keratoconjunctivitis 381
Keratomalacia 318
Kernicterus 338
Kerosene poisoning 305
Ketoacidosis 417
   diabetic 84, 151, 154
Ketone bodies 196
Kidney 78, 162
   biopsy 110, 352
   damage 207
   injury, acute 84

Kikuchi disease 365, 366
Klebsiella pneumoniae 44
Kligman's formula 247
Klinefelter syndrome 163, 343, 344
Koebner phenomenon 238, 244
Koplik's spots 164
Korsakoff's psychosis 320, 359
Krukenberg tumor 73
Kussmaul's breathing 155
Kussmaul's sign 22
Kwashiorkor 323, 324, 330
   marasmic 323

L

Lactase deficiency causing lactose intolerance 86
Lactate dehydrogenase 365
Lactic acidosis 84, 151
Lambert-Eaton myasthenic myopathic syndrome 289
Lansoprazole 68
Laryngitis
   acute 398
   chronic 399
Laryngotracheobronchitis, acute 399
Laser trabeculoplasty, selective 385
Lathyrism 284
Lead 264
Leflunomide 224
Left bundle branch block 35
Leg ulcer 243
Legionella pneumophila 44
Leishmania donovani 180
   bodies 243
Leishmaniasis 180
Lemon on matchstick appearance 144
Leprosy 187, 200, 242, 267
   classification of 187
   lepromatous 187
   types of 187
Leptospira interrogans 188
Leptospirosis 117, 188, 209
Lesion
   sites of 265
   types of 274
Leukemia 64, 104, 124, 200, 403
   acute 102, 105
      lymphoblastic 104
   chronic lymphatic 94, 106
Leukemoid reaction 107
Leukocytosis 191
Leukoencephalopathy, progressive multifocal 315
Leukoerythroblastic blood picture 102
Leukotriene antagonists 395
Lichen planus 64, 244
Lid diseases 375

Liddle's syndrome 327
Limb girdle 348
  myopathy 289, 290
Lipoprotein
  high-density 157, 406
  low-density 136, 157, 406
Liposomal amphotericin B 181, 183
Lisch nodule 292, 293
Listeria monocytogenes 257
Liver 68, 130, 282
  abscess 121
    amoebic 122, 123
    pyogenic 121, 123
  biopsy 119, 132, 133
  cirrhosis of 69, 125, 126, 326
  disease 86, 124, 236
    alcoholic 118, 119
    cholestatic 123
    chronic 119, 123, 125
    progressive 123
  failure 315
    acute 128
    fulminating 128
  function test 111, 118-123, 126, 129, 132-134, 171, 313, 355, 361
  transplantation 125, 127, 283
Louse-borne typhus 171
Low platelet count syndrome 422
Lumbar puncture 259, 266, 285, 334
Lung 68, 222
  abscess 51
  collapse of 67
  disease 329
    diffuse parenchymal 56, 226
    occupational 62
  function tests 47
  lesion 43
Lupus vulgaris 243
Luteinizing hormone 148, 207, 364
Lyme disease 263
Lymph node 68
Lymphadenopathy, generalized 255
Lymphangitis, acute 183
Lymphatic
  disease, chronic 183
  obstruction 125
Lymphogranuloma venereum 253
Lymphoma 53, 94, 111, 124, 200, 267
  intestinal 86
Lysergic acid diethylamide 317

M

Macrocytic anemia 90, 92
  causes of 91
Macrocytosis 91
Maculopapular skin rash 46
Madarosis 378

Magnesium 87
  ammonium phosphate stone 215
Magnetic resonance
  angiography 214
  cholangiopancreatography 75
  imaging 232, 259, 266, 281, 316, 349, 350
Major depression 306
Malabsorption syndrome 86
Malaise 123, 164
Malaria 115, 178
  malignant 179
Malassezia furfur, skin scraping for 251
Male erectile dysfunction 209
Malignancy 90, 107, 200
  nonmetastatic manifestation of 284
Mallory-Weiss syndrome 65, 358, 417
Malnutrition 67
Mania 309
  clinical features of 310
Mantoux test 82, 232, 243, 259, 335, 404
Marasmus 323, 330
Marfan's syndrome 38, 341
Marijuana 304
Marrow failure 99
Massive fibrosis, progressive 62
Mastitis 423
Mastoiditis, acute 390
McArdle's syndrome 289, 348
Mean corpuscular
  hemoglobin concentration 90
  volume 90
Measles 44, 164, 330
  virus 164
Mebendazole 184
Meckel's diverticulum 69
Median nerve palsy 268
Mediastinal mass 65
Mees' line 244
Megacolon, toxic 80
Megaloblastic anemia 91, 93
  causes of 93, 94
  symptoms of 93
Meglitinide 156
Meigs syndrome 124
Melanosis 244
Melasma 247
Melena 66
Menaquinone 320
Ménétrier's disease 86
Ménière's disease 295
Meningeal irritation, signs of 334
Meningioma, parasagittal 284
Meningitis 84, 253, 257, 333
  acute 372
    bacterial 257
  bacterial 333
  carcinomatous 257

complications of 258
tuberculous 259, 335
viral 258, 334
Meningococcal infection 108
Meningococcus 257, 258
Meningoencephalitis 257
Menopause 405
Menorrhagia 403
Menstrual disturbance 163, 408
Mental
change 270
retardation 343
status 190
Mesothelioma, pleural 63
Metabolic disorder 108, 383
Metastasis
features of 73, 218
secondary 315
Methanol 300
poisoning 264
Methicillin-resistant *Staphylococcus aureus* 25, 424
Methotrexate 224
Methyl xanthines 40
Metoclopramide 84
Metronidazole 122
Metrorrhagia 404
Metrostaxis 404
Microalbuminuria 153, 198
Microcytic hypochromic anemia 90
causes of 91
investigations of 92
Micturition, frequency of 198, 199, 211
Migraine 84, 261
Mineralocorticoid 146
Miscarriage 408, 410
Mite-borne 170
Mixed connective tissue disease 226, 279
Mohammedan's prayer position 74
Monoarthritis, causes of 221
Monoclonal antibody therapy 113
Mononucleosis, infectious 193
Monoplegia 283
Montelukast 42
Mood 310
disturbance of 143, 311
Moraxella catarrhalis 47
Morphea 225
Morphine 84
Motility disorders 93
Motor neuron
disease 274, 283
lower 262
Motor neuropathy 284
predominantly 268
Motor system 268, 274, 276

Mouth
mucous membrane of 255
ulcer 64
causes of 64
Multidrug-resistant tuberculosis 60
diagnosis of 60
treatment of 60
Multi-infarct dementia 294, 315
Multinodular goiter 139
complications of 139
Multiple endocrine neoplasia 75, 141
Multiple sclerosis 264-266, 284, 315
clinical courses of 266
signs of 266
symptoms of 266
types of 266
Mumps 164, 330
virus 257
Münchausen's syndrome 317
Murmur, mid-diastolic 1
Muscles
biopsy 288
deltoid 289
diseases of 288
Muscular atrophy
primary 274
progressive 274, 284
Muscular disease, classification of 289
Muscular dystrophy 289
congenital 289
hereditary 289
Musculoskeletal system 149
Myalgia 47, 164, 361
Myasthenia gravis 65, 278, 279, 289, 348
Myasthenic disease 289
Myasthenic myopathic syndrome 348
Mycobacterium 372
avium 371
bovis 58
leprae 187
tuberculosis 58, 82, 232, 257, 335
Mycoplasma 285
pneumoniae 241
Myelitis 257
acute transverse 283
transverse 279, 284
Myelodysplastic syndrome 104
Myelofibrosis 102, 107
Myeloid 107
leukemia, acute 99, 104
Myeloma, multiple 108, 114, 199, 209, 267
Myelopathy 257
Myeloproliferative disorder 102
Myocardial infarction 18, 151
acute 19
complications of 19

Myocarditis 22, 46, 174
   signs of 11
Myoclonic jerks 287
Myoclonus 274
Myoma 407
Myomectomy, indications of 408
Myopathy 289, 348
   congenital 289
   diseases of 288
   proximal 144, 348
Myophosphorylase deficiency 289
Myotonia 290
   congenita 289, 291
   dystrophica 289, 290
Myotonic dystrophy 348
Myotubular myopathy 289
Myxedema 124, 135, 136
   coma 137
   congenital 137

N

N-acetylcysteine 299
N-acetyl-P-benzoquinone imine 298
Nail-patella syndrome 200
Nails 238, 244
Narrow pulse pressure 166
Nasal
   decongestant 393
   drops, decongestant 390
   mastocytosis 395
   obstructions 393
   polyps 395
   septum, deviated 393, 395
Nausea 85, 88
Near drowning 356
Near syncope 295
Necator americanus 184
Neck, webbing of 343
Necrolytic migratory erythema 237
Negri bodies 169
Neisseria gonorrhoeae 23, 252, 379, 413
Neisseria meningitidis 191, 258, 333
Neomycin 87
Neonatal pneumonia, early onset 332
Neoplasm 395
Nephrectomy 216
Nephritic syndrome, acute 202
Nephritis, interstitial 197, 209
Nephroblastoma 217
Nephrocalcinosis 215
Nephrology 196
Nephropathy
   diabetic 153
   salt-losing 325
Nephrotic syndrome 199, 200, 326
   complications of 200
Nerve lesion 263

Nervous system 245
Neuralgia
   cranial 261
   migrainous 261
   trigeminal 265
Neurasthenia 314
Neurobrucellosis 178
Neurofibroma 292
   complications of 293
Neurofibromatosis 292, 314
Neurology 257
Neuronitis, vestibular 84
Neuropathy 289
   autonomic 86
   peripheral 94
   types of 153
Neuroprotective agents 276
Neurosyphilis 256, 315
Niacin 321
Nicotinic acid 267, 315
Night blindness 318
Night sweat 111
Nigrostriatal degeneration 270
Nikolsky's sign 240
Nipple, Paget's disease of 237
Nocturia 198
   causes of 199
Nongerm line cytoplasmic inheritance 342
Non-hepatotropic viruses 120
Non-Hodgkin's lymphoma 112, 139, 372
Nonlocalized disease 178
Nonmetastatic extrapulmonary manifestations 43
Nonsmall cell carcinoma 43, 44
Nonsteroidal anti-inflammatory drugs 65, 167, 191, 199, 229, 242, 326
Noonan syndrome 160, 162, 343
Normoblastic marrow 91
Normocytic normochromic anemia 90
   causes of 91
Norwalk virus 85
Nose 245, 392
   diseases of 386
   foreign body in 392
Nucleic acid amplification test 252
Nutritional deficiency 267
Nutritional supplementation 417
Nystagmus 266, 296
   ataxic 297
   horizontal 296
   jerky 296
   optokinetic 297
   phasic 296
   vertical 296
   vestibular 296

O

Obesity 158
  causes of 158
  complications of 158
  hypoventilation syndrome 362
Obsessive compulsive disorder 306, 309
Obstruction, bronchial 45
Obstructive sleep apnea 63
Octreotide 72
Ocular myopathy 289
Odynophagia 65
Ofloxacin 170
Oligomenorrhea 403
Oliguria 198
  causes of 198
Olivopontocerebellar degeneration 270
Omeprazole 68, 72
Ondansetron 84
Onychomycosis 246
Ophthalmia neonatorum 253, 379
Opiate 85
  poisoning 305
Opisthotonos 176
Optic
  atrophy 94, 264
  neuritis 264, 266
Oral candidiasis 225
Oral contraceptive pill 247, 404
Oral miltefosine 181
Oral rehydration solution 85, 172
Orchitis 164
Organophosphate-induced delayed polyneuropathy 302, 303
Organophosphorus
  compounds 302
  insecticides 302
Orientia tsutsugamushi 170
Orlistat 87
Oro-facio-genital syndrome 342
Oropharyngeal disease 65
Osler-Weber-Rendu disease 356
Osteitis fibrosa cystica 207
Osteoarthritis 228
Osteoarthrosis 222
Osteomalacia 207, 319, 348
Osteomyelitis, acute 234
Osteoporosis 124, 207, 228, 282
Osteosclerosis 207
Ostium primum 13
Ostium secundum 13
Otalgia 386
Otitis externa 387
  acute 388
  chronic 388
Otitis media
  acute suppurative 388, 390
  chronic suppurative 389
Otomycosis 388
Otosclerosis 391
Ovarian dysfunction 161
Ovarian fibroma 124
Ovarian tumor 408, 414
  malignant 414
Overflow incontinence 198
Oxygen 70
  therapy 369

P

Pacemaker 36
  complications of 36
  permanent 36
Packed cell volume 166
Paget's disease 237, 369
Pain 283
  abdominal 85, 88, 109
  colicky abdominal 172
  deep-seated abdominal 121
Pair therapy 193
Palmar erythema 126
Pancreatic exocrine insufficiency 93
Pancreatitis
  acute 73, 84, 124, 142
  chronic 75, 86
  hereditary 75
Panhypopituitarism 148
Panic disorder 308
Pantothenic acid 267
Papilledema 264
Papilloma 217
Paracentesis 125
Paracetamol poisoning 298
Parainfluenza 44
Paralysis
  agitans 270
  familial periodic 348, 362
  hyperkalemic periodic 289, 363
  hypokalemic periodic 289
Paraneoplastic syndrome 43, 73, 292
Paraparesis 283
Paraphimosis 205
Paraplegia 283
  noncompressive causes of 284
Paraproteinemia 326
Parathyroid gland 141
  diseases of 141
Parathyroid hormone 141
  suppression of 208
Parkinson's disease 270, 315
Parkinsonian plus 270, 271
Parotid
  enlargement 126
  glands 164
Patent ductus arteriosus 14, 342
Paucibacillary single lesion 188

Peak expiratory flow rate 40
Pefloxacin 170
Pelvic
    inflammatory disease 413
    thrombophlebitis 423
Pemphigoid 64
Pemphigus vulgaris 64, 239
Pendular nystagmus 297
Penicillamine 283
Penicillin 108
    allergy 25
Pepper pot appearance 142
Peptic esophagitis 65
Peptic ulcer
    bleeding, management of 70
    disease 69, 84
Percutaneous transluminal coronary
        angioplasty 18
Pericarditis 46
    acute 20
    chronic constrictive 21
    signs of 11
Perinuclear anti-neutrophil cytoplasmic
        antibodies 133
Peripheral blood film 87, 208, 242, 264
Peripheral nerve 281
    disease 372
Peripheral nervous system 207
Peritonitis
    spontaneous bacterial 125, 127
    tuberculous 82
Peritonsillar abscess 65, 397
Permethrin 237
Persistent active inflammation 223
Peutz-Jeghers syndrome 341
Phacoemulsification 384
Phakomatosis 293
Phalen's sign 268
Pharyngeal diverticulum 65
Pharyngeal web 65
Pharyngitis
    acute 398
    chronic 398
Pharynx 252
Phenothiazine 117, 273
Phenoxymethylpenicillin 98
Phenylketonuria 341
Phenytoin 267
Pheochromocytoma 143, 147
Phimosis 205
Phobia
    simple 308
    social 308
Phobic disorder 308
Phosphate 365
    control 208
Phylloquinone 320

Pick's disease 315
Pickwickian syndrome 362
Piperacillin 127
Pituitary gland 148
Pityriasis versicolor 245
Placenta previa 418
Plasma
    aldosterone 147
    exchange 101
    loss 205, 346
    osmolality 155
Plasmapheresis 354
Platelet 109
Pleural effusion
    right-sided 49, 122
    types of 49
Pleural fluid protein 50
Plexiform neurofibroma 293
Plummer–Vinson syndrome 65, 68
Pneumococcus 257
Pneumoconiosis 62
Pneumocystis carinii 374
Pneumocystis jirovecii 51, 374
    pneumonia 371, 374
Pneumonia 44, 258, 423
    atypical 46
    complications of 45
    delayed resolution of 45
    idiopathic interstitial 57
    late onset neonatal 332
    neonatal 332
    nosocomial 46
    recurrent 45
    treatment of 45
    types of 44
Pneumothorax 53
    primary 53
    secondary 53
Poisoning 270, 298
    common causes of 298
    severe 302
Poliomyelitis 189
    paralytic 190
    provocation 190
    types of 189
    vaccine for 190
Poliosis 378
Poliovirus 257, 259
Polyangiitis 349
    microscopic 352
Polyarteritis nodosa 124, 243, 263, 351
Polyarthralgia 109
Polyarthritis, causes of 221
Polycystic kidney disease 197, 204,
        205, 341
    infantile 204
    treatment of 205

Polycystic ovarian syndrome 162, 401
   complications of 163
   diagnostic criteria of 162
Polycythemia 102, 205
   rubra vera 102, 103
   true 102
Polydipsia, psychogenic 326
Polyhydramnios 425
Polymenorrhagia 404
Polymerase chain reaction 83, 259, 374
Polymyalgia rheumatica 222, 348, 351
Polymyositis 231, 289, 348
   primary idiopathic 231
Polyneuropathy 267
   chronic inflammatory demyelinating 267, 285
Polyposis coli, familial adenomatous 341
Polyuria 198
   causes of 199
Pontine myelinolysis, central 296, 326
Portal hypertension 130
   signs of 126
Post kala-azar dermal leishmaniasis 182
Postprandial capillary plasma glucose 157
Postvaccination 284
Potassium 87, 325
Pott disease 233, 284
Prader–Willi syndrome 160
Precordium 6
Prednisolone 109, 185
Preeclampsia 421, 425
Pregnancy 10, 41, 136, 231, 261, 266, 273, 408, 424, 425
   ectopic 404, 407
Preprandial capillary plasma glucose fasting blood glucose 157
Presbycusis 391
Presenile dementia 343
Presyncope 295
Primary angle-closure glaucoma 385
Primary open-angle glaucoma 384
Prochlorperazine 84, 270
Proctitis, active 80
Proctocolitis, extensive 80
Propylthiouracil 138
Prostate
   benign enlargement of 197, 218
   infection of 211
Prostatitis 211
Prosthetic valve endocarditis 25
Protein 196
   energy malnutrition 322, 323, 330
   malabsorption 87
Proteinuria 197, 421, 422
   nephrotic 197
   non-nephrotic 198
   orthostatic 198
Proteus mirabilis 215
Prothrombin time 100, 115, 118, 298
Proton-pump inhibitor 66
Pruritus 123, 124, 236
Psedohypoparathyroidism 142
Pseudo Meigs syndrome 408
Pseudobulbar palsy 65, 275
Pseudogout 222
Pseudohypertrophy 289
Pseudohypoparathyroidism 160
Pseudomembrane 174
Pseudomonas aeruginosa 191, 368
Pseudopolycythemia 102
Pseudoxanthoma elasticum 341
Psoralen and ultraviolet A 230
Psoriasis 11, 237, 238
   chronic plaque 237
   erythrodermic 238
   pustular 238
Psychiatric diseases 306
   classification of 306
Psychosis
   manic-depressive 306
   postpartum 306, 424
   puerperal 315
Psychotherapy 84
Pterygium 379
Ptosis 263
   bilateral 264
   unilateral 263
Puberty 161
   delayed 160
Puerperal disorders 315
Pulse 300
   intravenous methylprednisolone 101
Punch drunk syndrome 270, 280, 315
Pupil 265, 300
Purpura 107
Pus cell 196
   presence of 211
Pyelonephritis 211
   acute 209, 211, 213
   chronic 213, 215
   emphysematous 213
Pyloric stenosis 72, 84
Pyoderma gangrenosum 243
Pyogenic meningitis 333
   treatment of 258
Pyramidal signs 271
Pyrantel pamoate 184

Pyrazinamide 117
Pyrexia
   of unknown origin 121, 216
   puerperal 422
Pyridoxine 259, 321
Pyruvate kinase deficiency 90, 94
Pyuria 198

Q

Q fever 117, 171
   acute 172
   chronic 172
   endocarditis 25
Quadriparesis 283
Quadriplegia 283
Quartan malaria 200
Quinine 264

R

Rabies 168
   virus 259
Radial nerve palsy 269
Radiation colitis 86
Radiation myelopathy 284
Radiculopathy 257
Radioactive iodine uptake 140
Radioimmunoassay 150
Radiolucent stones 216
Radiotherapy 115, 150
   adjunctive 112
Raised aspartate aminotransferase 422
Raised intracranial
   pressure 84, 129, 264
   tension 129
      headache of 262
Ranitidine 68
Raynaud's phenomenon 226
Red blood cell 90, 337
   casts 196
Red cell 196
   enzyme deficiency 94
   membrane
      abnormality 94
      defect 90
Red eye 375
Red flags 375
Red urine, causes of 197
Reflux
   nephropathy 213
   vesicoureteric 213
Refractory ascites 125
Regurgitation
   aortic 5, 6
   mitral 2, 342
   pulmonary 4

Reiter's syndrome 64, 233
   triad of 233
Renal artery stenosis 214
Renal biopsy 200
Renal calculus 215
Renal cell carcinoma 102, 197, 216
Renal disease 109, 326
   end-stage 206
   intrinsic 199
   primary 199, 215
Renal failure 100, 315, 360, 422
   acute 74, 205, 325, 417
   chronic 205, 206
   septic 199
Renal function tests 111, 208
Renal loss 327, 328
Renal osteodystrophy 207
   treatment of 209
Renal pelvis, infection of 211
Renal replacement therapy, indications of 209
Renal stone 215
Renal transplantation, contraindications of 209
Renal tubular acidosis 215, 219
   clinical features of 220
Renovascular disease 206
Reproductive system 160
Respiratory diseases 39
Respiratory failure 58, 315
Respiratory rate, high 190
Restless leg syndrome 355
Resuscitation 72
Reticulocyte count 98, 338
Retinol 318
Retinopathy
   diabetic 153
   hypertensive 264
Reversible ischemic neurological deficit 276
Rh incompatibility 338
Rhabdomyolysis 360
Rheumatic chorea 273
Rheumatic fever 11, 221, 330
   diagnostic criteria of 11
Rheumatoid arthritis 2, 90, 199, 223, 243
Rheumatological disease 64
Rheumatology 221
Rhinitis 394
Rhinosinusitis, chronic 395
Riboflavin 321
Rice water stool 173
Rickets 207, 319
   familial hypophosphatemic 342
   renal 207
Rickettsia tsutsugamushi 170

Rickety rosary 319
Riedel's thyroiditis 135
Rifampicin 47, 117, 174
Right bundle branch block 34
Ringer's lactate 133, 167
  solution 336
Ringworm 246
Rinne test 392
Risus sardonicus 176
Rituximab 240
Rotavirus 85, 335
Rotor syndrome 117
Roundworm 184
Rubella 165, 383
  syndrome, congenital 165
Rupture esophageal varices, treatment of 129
Ryle's tube 76

S

Sabin-Feldman dye test 194
Salbutamol 272
Salicylate 299
Salmonella typhi 134, 169
Sarcoidosis 54, 222, 241, 257, 289, 315
Sarcoptes scabiei 237
Saturday night palsy 269
Savage's syndrome 401, 402
Scabies 237
Scalp 248
  ringworm 246
Schistosomiasis 197
Schizophrenia 306, 310, 311
Schneider's first rank symptoms 311
Scleritis 382
Sclerodactyly 226
Scleroderma 65, 225
  sine scleroderma 225
Sclerosing cholangitis, primary 117, 121, 133
Sclerosis
  amyotrophic lateral 274, 275
  diffuse cutaneous systemic 225
  primary lateral 274, 275
  systemic 86, 199, 225
  tuberous 293, 341
Sclerotherapy 129
Scrub typhus fever 170
Scurvy 108, 323
Seborrheic dermatitis 248
See-saw nystagmus 297
Seizure 100, 286, 287
  generalized 287, 288
  Jacksonian 287
  partial 287
  typical absence 287
Senile chorea 273

Sensory disturbance 266
Sensory neuropathy, predominantly 268
Sensory system 268, 276
Sepsis 190
  puerperal 423
Septal perforation 396
Septicemia 108, 211, 252
  meningococcal 146, 334
Sertoli-Leydig cell tumor 402
Serum electrolytes 147
  normal range of 325
Serum glutamic-oxaloacetic transaminase 118, 337
Serum glutamic-pyruvic transaminase 111, 337
Sex hormone-binding globulin 162
Sexual abuse 83
Sexual dysfunction 267
Sexually transmitted disease 252
Sheehan's syndrome 149, 401, 402
Shenothiazine 274
Shigellosis 172
Shock 345
  anaphylactic 347
  cardiogenic 346
  clinical features of 346
  distributive 346, 347
  hypovolemic 346
  neurogenic 348
  obstructive 346, 347
  profound 166
  septic 190, 347
Short stature 159, 343
Shy-Drager syndrome 270
Sick sinus syndrome 28
Sickle cell
  anemia 90, 97
  crises 98
  disease 94, 213
    family history of 200
Sickle chest syndrome 98
Sickle solubility test 98
Sigmoidoscopy 79
Sinoatrial block 33
Sinus
  arrhythmia 27
  tachycardia 27
Sinusitis 392
  acute 392, 393
  chronic 393
  recurrent acute 392
  subacute 393
Sister Mary Joseph's nodule 73
Sixth nerve palsy 263
Sjögren's syndrome 224-226, 279, 315, 381

Skin 43, 238, 244, 361
   appendages of 236
   disease 207, 236
   dryness of 318
   layers of 236
   lesions 109, 255, 293
   yellow discoloration of 117
Skull, X-ray of 142
Sleep 310
   apnea 63
      central 63
      syndrome 37
Small cell carcinoma 43, 44
Small pox 177
Snail tract ulcer 64
Snake bite 345
Snoring 396
Sodium 87, 325
   retention 147
   stibogluconate 182, 183
Solitary thyroid nodule 140
   treatment of 140
Somatization disorder 314
Somatoform autonomic dysfunction 314
Somatoform disorders 306, 313, 314
   general management of 314
Sore throat 164, 360
Spastic paraparesis, noncompressive causes of 284
Spastic paraplegia 233, 283
   causes of 284
   hereditary 283, 284
Speech 266, 275
Spherocytosis, hereditary 90, 94
Spinal cord 94, 266, 372
   compression 283
   disease 85
   lesion 274
   vascular disease of 284
Spiral groove 269
Spironolactone 201
Spondarthritis 222
Spondylitis, tuberculous 233
Spondyloarthropathy 222
Sponge kidney, medullary 215
Squamous cell carcinoma 43, 415
St Vitus' dance 273
Staghorn calculus 216
Standard anti-tuberculosis therapy 243
Staphylococcus albus 23
Staphylococcus aureus 23, 44, 85, 121, 191, 257, 361, 423
Staphylococcus epidermidis 211
Statins 267
Status epilepticus 288
Steatohepatitis, nonalcoholic 119

Steatorrhea 87, 88
Steele-Richardson-Olszewski syndrome 270, 280
Stem cell transplantation, allogeneic 107
Stenosis
   aortic 5, 161
   mitral 1, 65
   pulmonary 4, 343
Sterile pyuria 211, 212
Steroid 108, 247
   drops 388
   nasal sprays 393
   systemic 382
   topical 382, 395
Stevens-Johnson syndrome 46, 64, 241
Still's disease 235
Stokes-Adam attack 34
Stomach 86
Stomatitis 65
Stomatocytosis 90
Streptococcal beta-hemolyticus infection 241
Streptococcus bovis 23
Streptococcus faecalis 121
Streptococcus milleri 23, 121
Streptococcus pneumoniae 23, 44, 47, 258
Streptococcus pyogenes 361, 423
Streptococcus viridans 23
Stress 39, 83
   disorder, post-traumatic 307
   hyperglycemia 152
   incontinence 198
   reaction, acute 307
   related disorders 306
   ulcer 417
String sign 78
Stroke 273, 276
   complete 276
   ischemic 278
   partial nonprogressive 276
Strongyloides stercoralis 186
Strongyloidiasis 186
Subacute bacterial endocarditis 23, 108
   complications of 24
   symptoms of 24
Substance abuse 317
Sucrose intolerance 86
Sugar 196
Sulfasalazine 224
Sulfonamide 108, 199, 205
Sulfonylureas 156
Superior longitudinal sinus, thrombosis of 284
Superior vena cava 111
   obstruction 52

Supportive therapy 101, 114
Supraventricular tachycardia 28
Surgery 150
   history of 91
   indications of 42, 159
Sweating, disturbance of 267
Sydenham's chorea 273
Syncope 295
Syncytial virus, respiratory 39, 44
Syndrome of inappropriate antidiuretic hormone secretion 326
Synthetic vasopressin 111
Syphilis 254, 278
   acquired 255
   benign tertiary 256
   cardiovascular 256
   congenital 254
   early congenital 254
   late 256
      congenital 255
   latent 256
   meningeal 256
   meningovascular 256
   primary 255
   secondary 64, 200, 255
Syringomyelia 267, 284
Systemic disease 199, 205, 236
Systemic inflammatory
   diseases 206
   response syndrome 74, 191
Systemic lupus erythematosus 64, 90, 124, 199, 230, 239, 257, 315, 381, 396
Systemic therapy 238, 245

T

Tabes dorsalis 256, 284
Tachycardia 147, 191
   ventricular 31
Tachypnea 191
Tactile hallucination 307
Taeniasis 185
Takayasu's disease 35, 349
Tall stature 343, 344
Tazobactam 127
Telangiectasia 226
   hereditary hemorrhagic 65, 356
Temporary pacemaker, indications of 36
Temporomandibular joint disorders 386
Tension pneumothorax 54
Terbutaline 272
Testis, abnormality of 344
Tetanus 175
Tetralogy of Fallot 12, 15, 102, 342
Thalassemia 90, 94, 95
   major 107
   minor 96
Thalidomide 114
Thiamine 320
Thiazide 327
Thiocyanate 139
Third nerve palsy 263
Thomsen's disease 290
Threadworm 184
Throat 386, 396
   diseases of 386
Thrombocythemia, essential 102
Thrombocytopenia 46, 100, 231
Thrombocytopenic purpura 108
Thromboembolism 61
   pulmonary 61
Thrombophlebitis 115
   migrans 73
Thrombotic thrombocytopenic purpura 98, 100
Thyroid
   carcinoma 140
   disease 289
   function test 160
   gland 135
      diseases of 135
      tumors of 140
   medullary carcinoma of 139, 141
   nodule 140
      fine-needle aspiration cytology of 139
      single 140
   stimulating hormone 135, 313
Thyroiditis 138
   bacterial 135
   pyogenic 135
Thyrotoxic periodic paralysis 363
Thyrotoxicosis 137, 138, 348
   factitious 138
Thyroxine 148
Tics 274
Tinea
   barbae 246
   capitis 246
   corporis 246
   cruris 246
   pedis 246
   unguium 246
   versicolor 245
Tinel's sign 268
Toad's skin 318
Tocopherol 320
Togavirus 259
Tongue 275, 386
Tonic-clonic seizure, generalized 287
Tonsil 386
   tumors of 397
Tonsillitis 396

acute 65, 396
chronic 396
Tooth 386
TORCH syndrome 383
Toxic epidermal necrolysis 239
Toxic shock syndrome 361
Toxins 264
Toxoplasma 115, 194
   gondii 193, 372
Toxoplasmosis 193, 257, 383
   congenital 194
Trabeculectomy 385
Transient ischemic attack 151, 276, 316
Trauma 64, 83, 270, 284, 315
Tremor 266
   benign essential 272
   coarse 272
   types of 272
Trephine biopsy 101
Treponema pallidum 254, 265, 392
   hemagglutination 265
      assay 392
Tretinoin 247
Trichiasis 378
Trichomonas vaginalis 253
Trichophyton
   mentagrophytes 246
   rubrum 246
Tricuspid regurgitation 3, 14
Tricyclic antidepressant 300, 309
Trientine dihydrochloride 283
Triglyceride 157
Troisier's sign 73
Tropical spastic paraplegia 283, 284
Tropical sprue 86, 88
Tuberculin test 59
Tuberculoid leprosy 187
Tuberculosis 58, 107, 125, 109, 233, 386
   bone 232
   general features of 210
   intestinal 86
   joint 232
   miliary 60
   postprimary 59
   primary 58, 242
   pulmonary 59
   renal 210
   skin 243
   spine 233
   treatment of 60
Tubular acidosis, proximal 219
Tubular necrosis, acute 199, 205
Tubulointerstitial disease 199, 205
Tubulointerstitial disorder 325
Tumor 135
   adrenal 145
   gonadal 161
   lysis syndrome 365
   necrosis factor 79
   neuroendocrine 147
Turner syndrome 110, 160, 161, 343
Tylosis 237
Tympanic membrane, traumatic
   rupture of 387
Typhoid 267
   state 169

U

Ulcer 151
   aphthous 64, 65
   corneal 380
   duodenal 69
   neuropathic 243
Ulcerative colitis 64, 79, 87, 242
   types of 79
Ulnar nerve palsy 269
Ultrasonography 118, 123, 205
Unpaired anterior cerebral artery,
   thrombosis of 284
Unstable angina, treatment of 18
Upper motor neuron 267
Upper respiratory tract infection 39
Ureaplasma urealyticum 253
Ureteric calculus, bilateral 206
Ureteric stone 215
Urethra, infection of 211
Urethral syndrome 212
Urethritis 197, 211
   acute 211
   nongonococcal 253
Urge incontinence 198
Uric acid
   excess production of 227
   serum 111, 365
Urinary albumin excretion 198
Urinary bladder 408
   infection of 211
   tumors of 217
Urinary copper 282
Urinary incontinence, triad of 271
Urinary ketone body 155
Urinary tract
   infection 155, 211, 331, 423
      presentations of 211
      recurrent 212
   obstruction, chronic 213
Urinary urobilinogen, high 95
Urine
   chemical examination of 196
   incontinence of 198
   microscopic examination of 196
   routine microscopic examination
      200, 205
Urogram, intravenous 205
Urticaria 249, 250

Uterine fibroids 102
Uterus, evacuation of 409
Uveal inflammation 375
Uveitis 381

V

Vaginal agenesis 160
Vanillylmandelic acid 147
Vascular malformation 277
Vasculitis 98, 199, 231
Vaso-occlusive crisis 98
Vasovagal attack 295
Venereal disease research laboratory 265, 392
Ventricular septal defect 12, 14, 161, 342
Verapamil 85
Verbal abuse 83
Vertigo 294
  causes of 294
Vesical calculus 215
Vibrio cholerae 85, 173, 335
Vincristine 267
Vipoma 86
Viral hepatitis, chronic 126
Virchow's gland 73
Viridans streptococci 25
Viruses 85, 335
Vision, loss of 153
Visual hallucination 307
Vitamin 318
  A 87, 318
  B1 87, 267, 320, 417
    deficiency 320
  B12 87, 267, 322, 417
    deficiency 91, 93, 264
  B2 87, 321
  B3 321
  B6 321, 417
  B7 322
  C 322, 323, 417
  D 87, 319
    deficiency 141, 142
    resistant rickets 342
  deficiencies 315
  E 267, 320
  fat-soluble 318
  K 87, 320
    deficiency 417
    dependent clotting factors 320
  K1 320
  K2 320
  water-soluble 318
Vitiligo 250

Vomiting 47, 84, 85, 99, 175, 417
  causes of 84
  psychogenic 84

W

Weber syndrome 263
Weber test 392
Wegener's granulomatosis 56, 241, 349, 382
Weight loss 88
Weil's disease 188
Wenckebach phenomenon 33
Wernicke's encephalopathy 320, 359, 417
Wertheim's hysterectomy 415
Whipple's disease 86
Whipple's operation 76
White blood cell 125, 196, 326
White coat hypertension 9
White matter disease, diffuse 315
Wickham striae 244
Wilms' tumor 217
Wilson's disease 117, 127, 128, 219, 270, 273, 274, 280, 282, 315, 341
Wolff-Parkinson-White syndrome 29
Woods light examination 251
Wound
  care of 424
  infections 423
Wuchereria bancrofti 183

X

Xeroderma pigmentosum 341
Xerophthalmia 318
Xerosis 318
Xerostomia 224
X-linked dominant diseases 342
X-linked recessive disorders 341, 342

Y

Yellow fever 117
Yersinia enterocolitica 195
Young syndrome 395

Z

Zafirlukast 42
Zidovudine 348
Zinc 87, 323
  supplementation 337
Zollinger-Ellison syndrome 69, 71, 86
Zoonotic disease 177